CLINICAL CARDIOLOGY

CLINICAL CARDIOLOGY

Peter C. Gazes, M.D., F.A.C.P., F.A.C.C.

Professor of Medicine
Distinguished University Professor
of Cardiology, Medical University
of South Carolina
Charleston, South Carolina

Lea & Febiger 1990 Philadelphia • London

Lea & Febiger
600 Washington Square
Philadelphia, Pennsylvania 19106
U.S.A.
(215) 922-1330

Lea & Febiger (UK) Ltd.
145a Croydon Road
Beckenham, Kent BR3 3RB
U.K.

Library of Congress Cataloging-in-Publication Data

Gazes, Peter C., 1921–
    Clinical cardiology/Peter C. Gazes.—3rd ed.
      p. cm.
    Includes bibliographies and index.
    ISBN 0-8121-1235-0
    1. Cardiology. I. Title.
    [DNLM: 1. Heart Diseases. WG 200 G289c]
RC681.G39 1990
616.1'2—dc20
DNLM/DLC
for Library of Congress   89-12512
                                                              CIP

PRINTED IN THE UNITED STATES OF AMERICA

Print No. 4 3 2 1

Dedication

To my wife Athena and our children, Hope, Catherine, and Joanne

FOREWORD

In the preface to *Clinical Cardiology,* Dr. Gazes states that his aim is to present, in a simple and concise manner, the knowledge and technology of cardiology for use in the everyday practice of medicine. This aim is extremely well achieved in his book. Dr. Gazes is one of those rare, gifted teachers who combine genuine interest and concern for the student physician with a remarkable ability, refined over 39 years of teaching, practicing, and investigating cardiology, to select and synthesize the most important clinical information and principles and to present them in a succinct and lucid manner that makes them easy to remember. The student and eventually the student's patients benefit from this.

Over the past few decades, a remarkable array of new information, diagnostic methods, and treatment modalities for cardiac disease has become available. Changes have occurred rapidly. Many of the new diagnostic and treatment modalities have been advances of major clinical importance. Often the previous diagnostic and therapeutic approach has become outmoded. It is hard for any physician, particularly the nonspecialist who must keep up with many fields, to stay abreast of the new and clinically important developments in cardiology. This book is specifically designed to help in this task, and it fills this role excellently.

Several encyclopedic cardiology texts, which are beyond the desires or needs of many nonspecialists in cardiology, are available. Dr. Gazes' book fills a different purpose. It can be read and studied, textbook style, from cover to cover. Student physicians can be sure that they have covered all important topics because all areas of cardiology are discussed. Brevity is achieved by selectively providing detail about only the more common diseases. Less common diseases are included but discussed more briefly. If further information is desired, ample up-to-date references are provided.

The style is direct and easy to understand and remember. A simple declarative sentence summarizing the most important clinical fact or the most frequently misunderstood or misused item begins many sections of the work.

The book is organized in a manner similar to that needed by a physician when seeing a patient. It starts with the tools needed for history, examination, and diagnostic testing. Next, the pathophysiology, diagnostic tests, and treatment for the major heart diseases are presented. This is followed by treatment of heart failure, care of the cardiac patient having noncardiac surgery, and a reference list of common drugs and their dosage.

The third edition of *Clinical Cardiology* has been extensively revised to reflect newly understood pathophysiology, new diagnostic techniques, new drugs, and new procedures for treatment. For example, material is presented on Doppler echocardiography; thrombolytic therapy of myocardial infarction; coronary angioplasty; and the new drugs for heart failure, angina, and arrhythmias. The book is up to date and complete without lapsing into the detail more appropriate for encyclopedic reference texts. It remains succinct and easy to understand and remember.

Dr. Gazes brings an exceptional array of qualifications and experience as a teacher, a practicing cardiologist, and a cardiac investigator to the writing of this book. Students and physicians who read and study it will take away practical, clinically useful knowledge. Patients with heart disease will benefit.

James F. Spann, Jr., MD
Professor of Medicine
Director, Cardiology Division
Director, Gazes Cardiac Research Institute
Medical University of South Carolina

PREFACE

For many years I have lectured to physicians, medical students, and nurses with the prime aim of presenting in a simple, concise manner the new knowledge and vast technology in cardiology for use in everyday practice of medicine. This book is designed to cover these subjects. Much of the material in this book, based on my personal experience, is intended for ready reference because it is virtually impossible today for the average physician to read the voluminous literature in cardiology.

Every physician, regardless of the type of practice in which he is engaged, must deal with cardiology problems. This book is aimed at the physician, internist, surgeon, resident in medicine and family medicine, cardiology fellow, medical student, and nurse. Practicing cardiologists and cardiovascular surgeons will also find it useful. Emphasis is placed on teaching how to separate organic from functional problems without necessarily making a specific diagnosis and on recognizing common problems and emergencies and their appropriate therapy. For example, I have often wondered what an electrocardiographic report means to the physician receiving it. The chapter on electrocardiography has a section on how to interpret the electrocardiograph and explains the meaning and importance of common interpretations.

The chapter on noncardiac surgery in the cardiac patient is another example of the practical application of this book. The preoperative, operative, and postoperative management of the cardiac patient scheduled for noncardiac surgery is described. In addition, there is a section on dental and oral surgical problems in patients with cardiac disease. An outline of the usual laboratory studies ordered for a routine cardiac evaluation and other specific studies depending on the suspected problem is presented in the first chapter. This outline gives the practicing physician some idea about ordering studies for various conditions, which in itself is a learning experience.

Since the first two editions, there have been tremendous growth and advances in certain major areas of cardiology. In this third edition, old material has been extensively updated and rewritten, and new sections have been added. The expanded use of new diagnostic procedures such as echocardiography, Doppler echocardiography, color flow Doppler, and radionuclide and other imaging studies is discussed extensively in the appropriate chapters. The chapter on coronary artery disease has been expanded and revised to include more detail and updated or new sections on nitrates, β-blockers, calcium entry blockers, percutaneous transluminal coronary angioplasty (PTCA), laser angioplasty, coronary bypass surgery, and silent myocardial ischemia. The initial management of acute myocardial infarction with thrombolytic agents, adjunctive agents, and postthrombolytic management have been added. Postinfarction management has been revised to include cardiac rehabilitation, coronary risk factors and their management, antiarrhythmic agents, and antiplatelet agents. The chapter on arrhythmias has been completely rewritten and expanded to include sections on the mechanism of arrhythmia, new antiarrhythmic drugs, antitachycardiac devices, types and modes of cardiac pacing, sudden cardiac death, and management of cardiac arrest and office emergencies. The management of congestive heart failure has been extensively updated. Chapter 18 on cardiovascular emergencies has been deleted in this edition because these emergencies are included in the appropriate chapters.

Throughout the book, controversial issues are avoided as far as possible. Information of day-to-day value to the clinician is stressed. This book is not intended to be an encyclopedia of cardiology—several excellent textbooks are available that give detailed lengthy discussions on the various cardiac lesions. It does, however, cover all the cardiac problems contained in the encyclopedic texts, but they are presented in a concise and practical manner. Primarily, the complete field of adult cardiology is covered; however, congenital heart lesions in children are discussed because many of these are seen later in childhood.

The appendix contains a ready reference to preparation and doses of the various cardiovascular drugs, which are listed alphabetically by brand name with the generic and chemical names in parentheses.

The references are numerically cited and appear at the end of each chapter. Numerous schematic diagrams and figures are used to give the reader an immediate outline of the cardiac lesion without the necessity of reading the text. Pressure curves and electrocardiograms are often drawn graphically to scale for their elucidative value. Many tables give quick reference to therapy.

Although this book has one author, I wish to express my indebtedness to the members of the cardiovascular division and many other individuals without whose help this endeavor would not have been possible. Doctors Robert Leman, Michael Assey, Paul Gillette, John Heffner, Jon Levine, and Edmund Farrar have been most patient in reading portions of the manuscript and offering helpful suggestions. I also wish to thank Dr. Bruce Usher and Dr. Derek Fyfe for the preparation of the echocardiograms and Doppler figures. I acknowledge the expertise of Betty Goodwin in preparing some of the illustrations. I wish to express special gratitude to my dedicated staff assistant, Cathy Martin, who has been responsible for the typing of this manuscript and for making my task easier and more pleasant by her inestimable assistance, and also to Deb Morinelli and Linda Paddock for their most valuable help. Finally, I wish to thank R. Kenneth Bussy and the staff of Lea & Febiger for their indispensable cooperation.

Charleston, South Carolina   Peter C. Gazes

CONTENTS

Chapter 1

THE CARDIOVASCULAR EXAMINATION

The patient with suspected heart disease should have a complete medical history and physical examination even though the emphasis should be on the cardiovascular system. Diseases of the heart can be related directly or indirectly to other organs or can produce changes in other organs. Physicians should be aware of the many diagnostic (noninvasive and invasive) procedures that are performed in cardiology. However, it is tempting to order a study to arrive at a quick diagnosis rather than to get a thorough history and perform a cardiovascular examination. Many of these studies are expensive and unnecessary and in some instances may even have harmful effects. Those of us in teaching settings should be cognizant of these facts and not allow students and housestaff to get into the habit of ordering such studies prior to performing a detailed history and physical examination. It is disturbing when the students presenting a case begin with the results of studies such as the echocardiogram before giving the history and physical findings. In addition, many studies such as the ECG stress test have to be interpreted in light of the history.

HISTORY

Organic Cardiac Symptoms

Patients with heart disease may have no symptoms. If they do complain, it is because of chest pain, dyspnea, palpitations, cough, hemoptysis, abdominal swelling or discomfort, peripheral edema, or dizziness and syncope. Careful questioning may reveal that the complaints are functional or noncardiac in origin, such as those due to pulmonary disease. With experience one will learn to ask questions and evaluate answers without leading the patient. For example, patients with angina frequently deny having chest pain, yet will admit having chest discomfort. The location, duration, precipitating factors, quality, and factors that relieve pain are important in arriving at its cause. Generally, if one has discomfort anywhere above the waist (chest, arms, neck, or jaw) on exertion that is relieved by rest, angina should be considered. Some patients will answer "yes" to practically all questions pertaining to a variety of symptoms. Therefore, as far as possible, it is best to allow the patient to spontaneously mention symptoms. Sighing respirations (air hunger) must be differentiated from true dyspnea of heart disease. A simple test for evaluating dyspnea is to ask if the patient can talk without difficulty during exertion such as

1

climbing stairs. Dyspnea due to left heart failure often must be differentiated from that due to lung disease. The history is often useful. Orthopnea and paroxysmal nocturnal dyspnea, especially with little wheezing, are features that suggest left ventricular failure, whereas repeated bouts of bronchitis with chronic cough, sputum production, wheezing, and progressive dyspnea for many years suggest pulmonary disease. Nocturia may be associated with heart failure. Insomnia may be due to Cheyne-Stokes respiration secondary to decreased cardiac output.

The description of palpitation can be a clue to the type of arrhythmia. Premature beats often produce a skipping, thumping, pounding, fluttering sensation or a feeling that the heart is turning over. Polyuria can occur in association with paroxysmal tachycardias. Cough due to cardiac disease most often is noted in the recumbent position and nocturnally. It is often due to pulmonary venous hypertension secondary to left heart failure or mitral stenosis. Dyspnea often precedes the cough, whereas in patients with chronic lung disease, cough and expectoration usually precede the dyspnea. Hemoptysis demands a careful study to exclude mitral stenosis. Liver congestion can produce abdominal pain. Nausea, vomiting, dysphagia, bloating, and belching may arise from heart disease rather than gastrointestinal (GI) disease. There are many common causes of peripheral edema that should be considered prior to labeling a person as having congestive heart failure. Among them are obesity, venous stasis, varicosity and other venous diseases, psychogenic or cyclic, as well as hepatic and renal diseases. Formerly, dizziness or syncope was always related to the cerebral system. Since the advent of pacemakers, many such patients have been found to have heart disease. A clue in the history that syncope is due to an Adams-Stokes seizure is that often such patients, immediately after an attack, are mentally clear and in fact can continue their conversation as though nothing has happened. Patients with cerebral disease after syncope remain confused for variable periods. Other symptoms that can occur are fatigue, hoarseness, and fever. Fatigue is a nonspecific symptom that is usually associated with a depressed cardiac output or can be due to drugs. Hoarseness can be due to an aortic aneurysm, large pulmonary artery, or large left atrium compressing the left recurrent laryngeal nerve. Chills and fever can occur with infective endocarditis.

A meticulous history of the patient's medications is important. Often the name of a drug, unless the bottle is labeled, has to be traced by calling the pharmacy or the former physician who did the prescribing.

Functional Cardiac Symptoms

Often one must question the patient carefully to clarify whether the symptoms are functional or organic. The syndrome of neurocirculatory asthenia (soldier's heart, effort syndrome, DaCosta's syndrome, or cardiac neurosis) has been described in detail since World War I. Common symptoms of this syndrome are breathlessness, recurrent precordial pain, palpitations, fatigue, dizziness, sweating, headache, tremor, and lack of enthusiasm. The breathlessness is unrelated to effort and is frequently characterized by sighing or an inability to get enough air. The precordial pain is usually sharp or dull, stabbing, and may radiate down the left arm. It usually occurs *after* rather than during exertion, and at night, especially when the patient is lying on the left side. It may last a few minutes or hours. Palpitation, a common symptom of cardiac neurosis, is often described as a rapidly beating heart, often pounding and at times skipping. Fatigue is a pronounced symptom. The patient states that even after a good night's sleep, he awakens feeling exhausted. Light-headedness or dizziness occurs with sudden changes in head movement or change in body position. It may be associated with hyperventilation. Cool (not warm), moist sweating is a frequent complaint and is usually confined to palms of the hands, axillae, and soles of the feet. Vague, throbbing headaches are common. The patient notes tremors of his fingers, yet states that this does not interfere with his performance. He is uninterested in life and prefers to lie around doing nothing. Other patients may have cardiac anxiety, with acute emotional symptoms, that is not as long-lasting as neurocirculatory asthenia. Such patients usually give a history of some recent event that precipitated their symptoms, such as a marital problem or a cardiac death in the family.

If an adequate history has been taken, the physician will often have an impression of whether heart disease is present and, in many instances, of the type prior to the physical examination or other studies.

The cardiac symptoms, such as chest pain, dyspnea, palpitations, and others, will be considered in more detail in the chapters on specific diseases.

METHOD OF PHYSICAL EXAMINATION

Inspection and Palpation

The physical examination should be complete because a noncardiac disease may be the cause of the patient's symptoms. Inspection, palpation, and auscultation of the heart are more important today than percussion. A systematic approach will aid in avoiding mistakes. Initial inspection should include a survey of the body build, skin, neck pulsations, chest configuration and pulsations, abdomen, and extremities. I usually stand at the patient's left side to palpate the chest using my palms, fingers, and fingertips. First the patient should be examined supine, next sitting up and leaning forward, and finally while on the left side. The following areas are palpated: sternoclavicular joints, second intercostal space to the right of the sternum (aortic area), second intercostal space to the left of the sternum (pulmonic area), precordial, apical, and epigastric areas.

Auscultation

A routine should be established for auscultation. First listen with the diaphragm of the stethoscope to the aortic, pulmonic, precordial, and apical areas during regular breathing. Next this should be repeated in the sitting and standing positions, after squatting, and after performing a Valsalva maneuver. Findings also should be noted at the end of inspiration and expiration. At times auscultation after giving a vasoactive drug such as amyl nitrite may aid in clarifying a murmur. High-frequency sounds and murmurs are best heard with the diaphragm. The bell of the stethoscope also may be used in this manner, but is primarily used for low-pitched sounds at the apex, especially those heard in the left lateral position. The bell should barely touch the chest because it will simulate a diaphragm if tight against the chest. The length of the tubing of the stethoscope should be only about 12 inches.

The first heart sound has several components (i.e., related to mitral and tricuspid valve closure). Normally it may be heard as one sound or narrowly split and is best heard at the apex. The second sound is related to aortic and pulmonic valve closure and is heard best at the base of the heart, especially in the pulmonic area. Normal splitting of the second sound can occur with inspiration. A third heart sound can be heard at the apex during rapid filling of the left ventricle in normal young subjects.

Percussion

Since skills in palpation have improved, one seldom uses percussion today in the cardiac examination. The left and right borders of the heart can be outlined in some instances, such as in pericardial effusion, where palpation may not be helpful.

In addition, a complete cardiovascular examination should include close attention to the blood pressure (BP), neck veins, and arteries. Chapter 2 describes in more detail features of the physical examination.

ELECTROCARDIOGRAPHY AND VECTORCARDIOGRAPHY

Electrocardiography is an important diagnostic method but does have its limitations. The fact that the tracing is normal does not exclude heart disease; that it is abnormal does not necessarily indicate heart disease. Routinely 12 leads should be taken and repeated as indicated. Exercise stress ECG test should be performed under the direction of a physician. This is described in Chapter 4. Continuous electrocardiographic monitoring of two channels (Holter monitoring) is being used extensively for arrhythmia detection, as a guide to therapy, and also for detection of silent ischemia. Signal-averaged electrocardiography and fast-Fourier transform of the electrocardiogram, which look at frequency, amplitude, and time-duration parameters of ventricular activation as markers for risk of malignant ventricular arrhythmias, are being investigated.[1,2]

The electromotive force of cardiac activation can be represented by a vector. The sum of all the electromotive forces in the depolarizing heart at any instant may be indicated by a single instantaneous vector. If all of these instantaneous vectors could be plotted consecutively from a single reference point and their ends connected, a vector loop would be formed. Three such loops can be plotted in three planes (frontal, sagittal, and horizontal), recorded by a cathode ray oscilloscope, and photographed on Polaroid film or instantly on chart paper. These are referred to as a spatial vectorcardiogram (VCG). Since the body surface leads of the routine ECG record potential variations represented by the vectorcardiogram, these two studies interrelate. The main difference is that the ECG is a scalar representation of forces, depicting magnitude (voltage) and sense (positive or negative) but not direction. The vectorcardiogram presents all three properties. The vectorcardiogram gives little additional information (except in selected cases) and in fact is somewhat inadequate because there is no agreement on the best lead system to use for recording vectorcardiograms. Also, it gives no information in diagnosis of arrhythmia, and it is costly. The system most widely used clinically at present is the Frank system. Probably the greatest value of vectorcardiography is that it allows visualization of the approximate sequence of atrial and ventricular activation in a three-dimensional form and so gives a better understanding of electrocardiography, thus allowing the student to understand electrocardiography without memorizing various ECG patterns.

CARDIAC ROENTGENOLOGY

The four views of the chest that are routinely obtained for cardiac evaluation are the posterior-anterior (PA), right anterior oblique (RAO), left anterior oblique (LAO), and left lateral. Each of these views gives more information about a specific area of the heart, and therefore they are complementary. The PA view gives an idea of total heart size and contour, aortic and pulmonary artery abnormalities, pulmonary vein abnormalities, enlargement of the left atrium and its appendage, and enlargement of the right atrium or left ventricle. The right border of the heart in this projection starting from the diaphragm is primarily formed by the right atrium and superior vena cava, and occasionally by the ascending aorta. The left border from above downward includes the aortic knob, pulmonary artery, and left ventricle. The RAO view predominantly demonstrates the left atrium, especially as it is outlined by swallowed barium. The barium-filled esophagus is indented by the aorta, pulmonary artery, and a dilated left atrium. Enlargement of the left ventricle and left atrium will produce a diffuse esophageal indentation. The LAO view allows the aorta to be identified. The trachea and its bifurcation can be seen, and the left main-stem bronchus can be identified, especially if it is displaced upward by an enlarged left atrium. The left ventricle also can be evaluated in this view as it extends toward the dorsal spine. The lateral view identifies the right ventricle, since the anterior border behind the sternum is formed by the right ventricle and ascending aorta. The normal right ventricle is against the lower third of the sternum, whereas the upper two thirds of the retrosternal space are radiolucent. Right ventricular enlargement will occupy some of this latter space. However, the shape of the chest can alter these findings. In addition, in the lateral view the left ventricular enlargement can be noted. Normally the posterior border of the left ventricle crosses the inferior vena cava more than 2 cm above the left diaphragm. Left ventricular enlargement would cross it lower, and the point of intersection would be closer to the diaphragm.[3] Inaccuracies can occur if the film is not a true lateral view.

Figure 1–1 depicts schematically these four views. Fluoroscopy, especially with an image intensifier, allows a dynamic view of the heart. Pulsations of the heart, aorta, and pulmonary arteries can be identified and at times differentiated from noncardiac masses. Also, intracardiac or pericardial calcifications can be seen.

PHONOCARDIOGRAPHY AND OTHER GRAPHIC METHODS

Phonocardiography. The graphic recording of auscultatory events is known as phonocardiography. There is much debate about the number of components and origin of the various sounds. The first heart sound (S_1) has several components, but clinically two components are primarily recognized; namely, those associated with closure of the mitral and tricuspid valves. The main components of the second sound (S_2) are associated with aortic (A_2) and pulmonic (P_2) valve closure. In recent years, the importance of valves in the production of sounds has been considered to be less than the importance of

NORMAL HEART

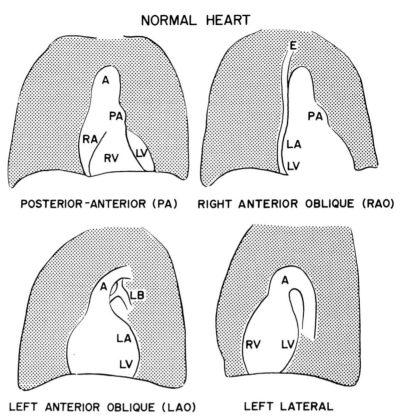

POSTERIOR-ANTERIOR (PA)   RIGHT ANTERIOR OBLIQUE (RAO)

LEFT ANTERIOR OBLIQUE (LAO)   LEFT LATERAL

Fig 1-1. Four x-ray views of the chest usually taken for evaluating the heart size and the contour of the individual chambers. A = aorta; PA = pulmonary artery; RA = right atrium; RV = right ventricle; LA = left atrium; LV = left ventricle; E = esophagus; LB = left main-stem bronchus.

ventricular events. The third heart sound (S_3) is normally heard only in young individuals, and occurs at the peak of the rapid filling phase of ventricular diastole. Atrial contraction is associated with the fourth heart sound (S_4), which is usually not heard unless there is a resistance to ventricular filling or first-degree AV block. Phonocardiography identifies normal heart sounds, splitting of the sounds, murmurs, gallops, opening snaps, ejection sounds, and clicks. Timing is aided by the simultaneous recording of the ECG, carotid pulse, and apex cardiogram, and less often by the jugular pulse. Combined phonocardiographic and echocardiographic recordings have increased our understanding of auscultatory events and have been useful diagnostically.

Carotid pulse. The upstroke of the carotid pulse is rapid. It reaches its initial peak (percussion wave) at the time ejection is at its maximum, and there follows a plateau or secondary wave (tidal) late in systole that depends on peripheral vascular tone. Following the tidal wave at the early part of the downstroke is the incisura or dicrotic notch. The first heart sound occurs just before the onset of the carotid pulse. The aortic component of the second sound occurs just prior to the dicrotic notch with the pulmonic component just after this notch.

Jugular venous pulse. Right atrial contraction produces the A wave of the jugular venous pulse which begins just before the first heart sound. The C wave follows the A wave and has no clinical significance. It is probably produced by closure of the tricuspid valve and carotid artifact. Following the C wave is the negative X wave occurring with ventricular systole and atrial relaxation. As the right atrium fills the V wave is formed with its peak just before the opening of the tricuspid valve. The second sound occurs before the peak of the V wave. The Y descent occurs as blood enters the right ventricle and follows the V wave.

Apex cardiogram. The apex cardiogram is a low-frequency recording of the precordial movements at the apex. The initial upward component A occurs with the fourth heart sound (S4). This is followed by the maximum systolic peak E occurring at the opening of the aortic valve. This is followed by a rapid descent which occurs during the initial rapid ejection phase of left ventricular systole, and during the latter half of systole the curve levels off. Point O occurs at the onset of rapid filling which is closely associated with the opening of the mitral valve. This O point is often used to time the opening snap of mitral stenosis. Figure 1–2 depicts the relationship of the phonocardiogram and the various graphic methods used for timing the cardiac events.

ECHOCARDIOGRAPHY

This is another noninvasive technique that has become a valuable clinical tool. Reflected ultrasound between two media has been applied to the study of cardiac and valvular motion. Cardiac structures return the echoes derived from the ultrasonic beam, display them on the oscilloscope, and then record them on film. The M-mode echocardiogram depicts amplitude and the rate of motion of moving objects and is usually displayed on a strip-chart recorder. It gives an "ice pick" view of the heart but it is not one-dimensional, since it has time as a second dimension. The transducer is usually positioned in the fourth intercostal space at the left sternal border. A change in the aim of the trans-

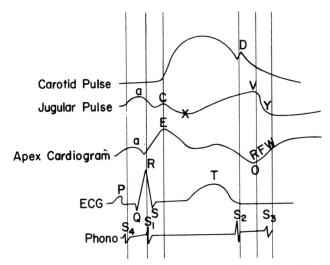

Fig 1–2. Diagram of the relationship of graphic methods used for timing of the heart sounds. S_4 occurs at the time of atrial contraction (a); S_1 just after the peak of the R wave of the ECG; S_2 at the dicrotic notch (D) of the carotid pulse and S_3 at the peak of the rapid filling wave (RFW). The O of the apex cardiogram approximates the opening of the mitral valve.

ducer will alter the path of the beam and the structures visualized. Echoes can be recorded from the pericardium, myocardium, endocardium, septum, valves, and aorta. Such abnormalities as mitral stenosis, prolapse of mitral valve leaflets, idiopathic hypertrophic subaortic stenosis, atrial septal defect, pericardial effusion, and many others can be detected. Cardiac chamber dimensions, volume, and ventricular function also can be assessed. Figure 1–3[4] depicts diagrammatically a normal echocardiogram from structures that this particular oriented ultrasonic beam traverses. By changing the direction of the ultrasonic beam as in an arc, the single view of Figure 1–3 can be augmented to give an overall view as in Figure 1–4. Figure 1–4 is a diagrammatic cross section of the heart showing the structures through which the ultrasonic beam passes and its presentation by the M-mode echocardiogram as the transducer is directed from the apex (position 1) to the base of the heart (position 4).[5] In position 1 the ultrasonic beam traverses the left ventricular cavity (LV) at the level of the posterior papillary muscle (PPM) and passes through a portion of the right ventricular cavity (RV); in position 2 it traverses the left ventricular cavity at the level of the edges of the mitral valve leaflets (AMV and PMV) or the chordae and a portion of the right ventricle; in position 3 more of the anterior mitral valve leaflet is recorded and part of the left atrial cavity (LA); and in position 4 the root of the aorta (AO), the aortic valve leaflets, and the body of the left atrium are traversed. During diastole, when the mitral valve opens, the anterior leaflet is M-shaped and the posterior leaflet is W-shaped. The two leaflets come together during systole (C-D). Echoes returned from the anterior right coronary cusp and the posterior noncoronary cusp show a systolic pattern of the aortic valve (AV) resembling a box. The tricuspid valve

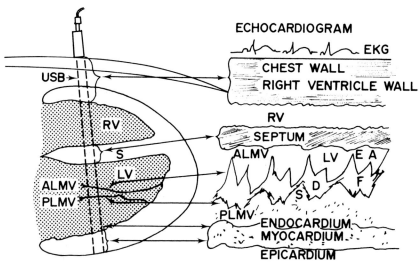

Fig 1–3. Normal echocardiogram. Path of ultrasound beam (USB) at the fourth intercostal space left sternal border shown schematically on the left. On the right is a diagram of the corresponding echocardiogram for this direction of the transducer. RV = right ventricle; S = septum; LV = left ventricle; ALMV = anterior leaflet of mitral valve; PLMV = posterior leaflet of mitral valve; S = systole; D = diastole; E = peak of rapid anterior opening of mitral valve during beginning of diastole; A = peak of anterior movement of the leaflet into the ventricle produced by atrial systole; F = position of leaflet during rapid ventricular filling. (Modified from Popp R.L. et al.: Estimation of right and left ventricular size by ultrasound. *Am. J. Cardiol.* 24:523, 1969.)

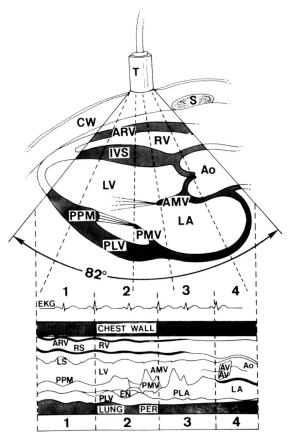

Fig 1–4. This is a diagrammatic cross section of the heart showing the structures through which the ultrasonic beam passes and its presentation by the M-mode echocardiogram (*bottom*) as the transducer is directed from the apex (*position 1*) to the base of the heart (*position 4*). It also demonstrates a two-dimensional sector scan (82 degrees) of the heart in the long axis (*top*). T = transducer; CW = chest wall; S = sternum; ARV = anterior right ventricular wall; RV = right ventricular cavity; IVS = interventricular septum; LV = left ventricle; AO = aorta; PPM = posterior papillary muscle; AMV = anterior mitral valve leaflet; PMV = posterior mitral valve leaflet; LA = left atrium; PLV = posterior left ventricular wall; RS = right septum; LS = left septum; AV = aortic valve; EN = endocardium of the left ventricle; PLA = posterior left atrial wall; PER = pericardium. (From Feigenbaum H.: Clinical applications of echocardiography. *Prog. Cardiovasc. Dis.* 14:531, 1972. Used with permission.)

resembles the mitral and the pulmonic resembles the aortic. However, usually only the diastolic position of the pulmonary leaflet and a single leaflet opening initially with systole are recorded.

M-mode echocardiography records the motion of cardiac structure parallel to the ultrasonic beam. It cannot be used for evaluating the shape of the heart structures or lateral motion. However, the latter two can be depicted by cross-sectional or two-dimensional echocardiography, which can be shown on movie film or videotape. M-mode echocardiography displays the cardiac structures in an unfamiliar format and provides only limited information regarding spatial orientation of cardiac structures. Two-dimensional echocardiography overcomes these two disadvantages and has a superficial resemblance to cardiac fluoroscopy and angiography in that the heart can be seen contracting and the valves opening and closing. However, it does not record silhouettes as fluoroscopy and angiography do; it shows tomographic or cross sections of the heart and in many more views. The usual transducer positions and views (tomograms) are shown in Table 1–1.[6] With the transducer along the left sternal border, the plane through which the ultrasonic beam sweeps is parallel to the long axis of the heart, and the heart is transected in a plane between positions 1 and 4 of 82 degrees (see Fig 1–4). The difference in this figure[7] using the two-dimensional rather than M-mode is that the beam is moving rapidly through the heart rather than remaining stationary and so shows a true anatomical slice through the heart in a plane parallel to the long axis.

Two-dimensional echocardiography is also being recorded following some form of stress as treadmill exercise or bicycle ergometry which can provoke ischemia. Beside its use for diagnosis of coronary artery disease, stress echocardiography may have prognostic importance following myocardial infarction. For those who cannot exercise, pharmacologic agents as dipyridamole or dobutamine can be used.

Esophageal echocardiography and color flow Doppler can now be obtained and are being used to monitor cardiac function during cardiac surgery. In ad-

Table 1–1. Two-dimensional Echocardiographic Examination

I. *Parasternal Approach*
  A. Long-axis plane
    1. Root of aorta—aortic valve, left atrium, left ventricular outflow tract
    2. Body of left ventricle—mitral valve
    3. Left ventricular apex
    4. Right ventricular inflow tract—tricuspid valve
  B. *Short-axis plane*
    1. Root of the aorta—aortic valve, pulmonary valve, tricuspid valve, right ventricular outflow tract, left atrium, pulmonary artery, coronary arteries
    2. Left ventricle—mitral valve
    3. Left ventricle—papillary muscles
    4. Left ventricle—apex
II. *Apical Approach*
  A. Four-chamber plane
    1. Four-chamber
    2. Four-chamber with aorta
  B. Long-axis plane
    1. Two-chamber—left ventricle, left atrium
    2. Two-chamber with aorta
III. *Subcostal Approach*
  A. Four-chamber plane—all four chambers and both septa
  B. Short-axis plane
    1. Left ventricle
    2. Right ventricle
    3. Inferior vena cava
IV. *Suprasternal Approach*
  A. Four-chamber plane
    1. Arch of aorta—descending aorta
  B. Long-axis plane
    1. Arch of aorta—pulmonary artery, left atrium

From Feigenbaum H:[6] *Echocardiography*. Philadelphia, Lea & Febiger, 1986, pg. 83. Used with permission.

dition, these studies can be done directly on the epicardium and intravascular system. Contrast echocardiography is being investigated and may be available in the future.

DOPPLER ECHOCARDIOGRAPHY

Doppler echocardiography can measure the velocity of blood flow, detect the abnormal direction of blood flow, and detect turbulent blood flow. Continuous wave Doppler uses a continuous stream of ultrasound transmitted from a piezoelectric crystal toward the heart. The back-scattered ultrasound from the blood cells and its movement produce a Doppler shift of ultrasound frequency. The receiving transmitter picks up the reflected ultrasound and estimates its direction and extent of Doppler shift. Sound reflections from all depths through which the Doppler beam has passed are simultaneously returned and analyzed. The examiner does not know where the moving signals are arising along the beam as he would know from pulsed Doppler. The transmitting and receiving transducers are mounted side by side. Simultaneous use of two-dimensional echocardiography can locate the sites of blood flow producing the Doppler shift. Continuous-wave Doppler and two-dimensional echo can estimate the severity of valvular stenosis and instantaneous pressure gradients. The pulsed Doppler system uses pulsed ultrasound and the same transducer transmits and receives the ultrasound. Sounds received only at specific times (gating) are analyzed and thus reflections can be localized and analyzed from a specific depth. Pulsed Doppler has the advantage of permitting Doppler analysis at a precise location and being obtained simultaneously with M-mode and two-dimensional echocardiograms. However, it has velocity measurement limitations. Blood moving rapidly through a stenotic area cannot be sampled rapidly enough with pulsed Doppler. This problem is referred to as aliasing. Continuous-wave Doppler can record such high velocities.

Doppler color[8] flow imaging uses multigate Doppler to produce a visible flow within the heart or great vessels. Most machines display flow toward the transducer as red and away from the transducer as blue. Turbulent, high velocity flow is displayed as a mixture of colors, often including green or turquoise. Color Doppler is especially useful in evaluating valvular regurgitation. Quantitation of valvular regurgitation by this method is now being studied. It is also being used in stenotic lesions and shunts.

The pulsed and continuous-wave methods used together can aid in the diagnosis of valvular obstruction or regurgitation and intracardiac shunts and blood flow. With the addition of color Doppler and the use of calculations, these methods may allow at best semiquantitation of some of the lesions. There are many technical details (highly operator-dependent) when there is an attempt to quantitate lesions by Doppler studies. Doppler studies record velocity and not volumetric flow, and these studies are influenced by many other factors. Until further investigation, quantitation of lesions by Doppler should be considered reasonable estimates. Application of these methods will be shown in Chapter 6 during discussion of specific valvular lesions.

RADIONUCLIDE STUDIES

Improvements in radiopharmaceutical, instrumentation, and computer technology have led to many radionuclide techniques for study of the cardiovascular system.[9-11] The radioactive tracers are given intravenously (IV). The unique properties of radionuclides enable them to be used as physiologic markers either within the cardiac bloodpool or within a specific metabolic or biochemical pathway.

Technetium 99m pyrophosphate (^{99m}Tc Pyp) is widely used for imaging an acute myocardial infarction, for this tracer will accumulate only in the infarcted area (hot spot) when calcium is deposited in the necrotic cells. Thallous chloride Tl 201 (^{201}Tl Cl or thallium 201) distributes in the myocardium in proportion to regional blood flow. Therefore, an infarcted area will show a decreased uptake (cold spot). Thallium can also be used during a stress test to detect reduced perfusion areas. In addition to planar thallium imaging, the use of single photon emission computed tomography (SPECT) has been developed.[12] SPECT imaging gives a better demonstration of the location and extension of an abnormality. It also provides better contrast for detection of perfusion abnormalities with a lack of overlap and better recognition of individual diseased vessels. Technetium 99m can be used to perform a dynamic radionuclide angiogram from which the left ventricular ejection fraction and abnormalities in regional wall motion can be noted. Dynamic radionuclide angiography is of two main types, the first-pass and the gated equilibrium techniques. In the first-pass method, ^{99m}Tc is injected rapidly IV, and its passage through the right heart, lung, and left heart is followed with a gamma camera. Once the tracer leaves the left ventricle, no more data can be obtained. In the gated equilibrium technique, ^{99m}Tc is tagged to the patient's own red blood cells or to the human serum albumin and is allowed to equilibrate in the entire bloodpool. Imaging is carried out over a period of minutes, not just during a few cardiac cycles. Count acquisition is gated to the R wave of the ECG. The total number of counts and the resolution are increased by this multiple gated acquisition bloodpool imaging (MUGA). Radionuclide angiocardiography has been used to assess ventricular performance during exercise. These techniques are discussed in detail in Chapter 4.

OTHER CARDIAC IMAGING STUDIES

Several new cardiac imaging techniques have been introduced during the past few years: digital subtraction angiography, positron emission tomography (PET), magnetic resonance (MR) and computed x-ray tomography (Cine CT). These are still under investigation with increasing evidence of their clinical importance being reported daily in the diagnosis and assessment of cardiac disease. When a fluoroscopic image is converted to a digital format by an analog to the digital converter, a digital angiogram is obtained. Initial angiography by this method has been obtained following intravenous contrast media. For cardiac use, this has no advantage, but when used intracoronary or in the ventricle, it has enhanced contrast angiograms.

Recent PET scanners have spatial resolutions to allow adequate imaging of myocardial tracer uptake.[13] PET is being used to measure regional blood flow to the myocardium and study regional myocardial metabolism. Blood flow tracers (^{13}N-ammonia and Rubidium 82) are being investigated for clinical use. Recent studies using these tracers during exercise or after infusion of dipyridamole show high sensitivity and specificity for detecting coronary artery disease. Metabolic imaging (markers of fatty acid metabolism) should be sensitive for identifying ischemic myocardium. Since receptors, neurotransmitters, and cardiac drugs can be labeled, the direct effect of these on cardiac tissue in the future may be clarified by PET.

Magnetic resonance imaging (MRI) is a spatial two- or three-dimensional map of nuclei resonating at a characteristic frequency when placed in a magnetic field and subjected to intermittent applied radio frequency signals. Its prime clinical use is to demonstrate pathologic anatomy, which has been useful for the evaluation of patients with coronary artery disease, pericardial disease, cardiomyopathies, congenital heart disease, thoracic aortic disease, and neoplastic disease. There is justification for further pursuing MRI in cardiovascular diseases because it has excellent resolution, is sensitive to blood flow, lacks ionizing radiation, is three-dimensional, and has morphologic imaging capabilities.[14]

CT scanners of the heart require scanners specifically designed to evaluate central cardiovascular anatomy and function. CT scan has been used to evaluate regional wall motion, myocardial perfusion, myocardial infarction, patency of bypass grafts, pericardial disease, masses in the pericardium and paracardiac areas, congenital heart disease, and diseases of the thoracic aorta.

HEART CATHETERIZATION AND SELECTIVE ANGIOCARDIOGRAPHY

Right and left heart catheterization are extensively utilized today for diagnosis and assessment of the degree of congenital and acquired heart lesions. Pressures in the chambers and vessels can be measured by passing a catheter from the venous or arterial side, and shunts can be determined by measuring oxygen saturation (oximetry) and by indicator dilution curves. Selective angiocardiography can be performed by injecting radiopaque agents directly into the heart chambers or vessels. Cineangiocardiography has become very popular, and now coronary arteriography is being performed in most centers. The normal values for pressure and oxygen saturations in the various vessels and chambers of the heart are seen in Figure 1–5.

Diagnosis, degree of the abnormality, and cardiac function can be established by the pressure measurements. For example, in pulmonary stenosis the systolic pressure in the right ventricle is elevated compared with that in the pulmonary artery, producing a gradient across the pulmonic valve. With right heart failure and in constrictive pericarditis the right ventricular end-diastolic pressure is elevated. The pulmonary artery pressure is elevated with increased pulmonary vascular resistance, increased pulmonary blood flow, or an elevated pulmonary venous pressure. The pulmonary artery wedge (capillary) pressure closely reflects the left atrial pressure and is elevated in mitral valve disease (especially stenosis) and in left ventricular failure. The left ventricular systolic pressure corresponds with the systemic pressure unless aortic stenosis is present, in which case it is elevated above the systemic pressure. The left ventricular end-diastolic pressure is elevated in the presence of left ventricular failure or a stiff left ventricle (loss of compliance).

If a higher oxygen saturation in the blood is noted in a right-sided chamber or vessel than was present proximal to it, a left-to-right shunt is present such as at the atrial, ventricular, or pulmonic levels. Systemic arterial unsaturation in the absence of lung disease or congestion usually indicates a right-to-left shunt. Small shunts (less than 25% of systemic blood flow) may not be detected

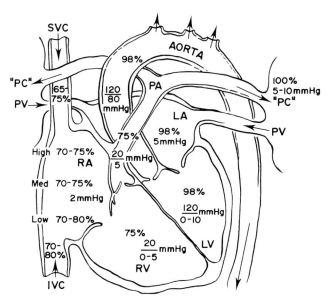

Fig 1–5. The normal values for pressures and oxygen saturation in the various vessels and chambers of the heart. SVC = superior vena cava; IVC = inferior vena cava; RA = right atrium; RV = right ventricle; PA = pulmonary artery; PC = pulmonary capillary; PV = pulmonary vein; LA = left atrium; LV = left ventricle.

by the oxygen saturation. Dye dilution curves also may detect shunts and can be used for estimation of valvular regurgitation and cardiac output. This latter procedure involves measuring the concentration of a dye (such as indocyanine green) at one site in the circulation after it has been injected in another site. Normal appearance time and recirculation of the dye will be noted if there is a left-to-right shunt and early appearance time if there is a right-to-left shunt if the dye is injected IV and sampled from a peripheral artery.

Shunts (even small) can be localized by varying the sites of injection of dye and sampling sites in the cardiac chambers and vessels during heart catheterization. Shunts also can be detected by the use of a hydrogen electrode and by selective angiocardiography. Cardiac output can be determined by the Fick method or the indicator dilution method. Thermodilution (cold saline is the indicator) has become a popular method for measuring cardiac output.

The indications for cardiac catheterization and angiographic studies are to establish a specific diagnosis, exclude heart disease, evaluate the severity of the lesion, and evaluate for cardiac surgery and the surgical results.

SWAN-GANZ CATHETERIZATION

Use of a balloon-flotation catheter[15] for hemodynamic monitoring at the bedside is helpful in the evaluation and management of several acute and chronic conditions (Table 1–2). The catheter can be inserted into the antecubital, subclavian, or internal jugular vein, and its position is monitored by observing the pressure waveforms displayed on an oscilloscope. The inflated balloon allows passage through the cardiac chambers into the pulmonary capillary wedge position. After a pulmonary capillary wedge pressure is obtained, the balloon is deflated and a pulmonary artery pressure reappears. The pul-

Table 1–2. Situations in Which the Swan-Ganz Catheter May Be Helpful

1. When there is need to know the fluid status (left ventricular filling pressure)
   a. Acute myocardial infarction with hemodynamic instability
   b. Acute, and sometimes chronic, renal failure
   c. Third space fluid loss
   d. Septic shock
   e. Acute volume depletion, particularly in the patient with underlying cardiac disease
   f. Adult respiratory distress syndrome
   g. Diffuse pulmonary disease
2. When there is a need to obtain diagnostic information
   a. New cardiac (holosystolic) murmur (acute mitral regurgitation vs. ventricular septal defect)
   b. Obtaining mixed venous Po_2 in a patient with "combined systems" disease (e.g., anemia + low cardiac output, COPD)
   c. Right ventricular myocardial infarction
   d. Equalization of pressure in cardiac tamponade
3. When IV vasodilator therapy is required
   a. Acute, severe mitral or aortic insufficiency, pending surgery
   b. Hypertensive crisis (particularly in patients with coronary disease)
   c. Spontaneous idiopathic lactic acidosis, treated with sodium nitroprusside
4. At times on initiation of oral vasodilator therapy as treatment for congestive heart failure in a poorly compensated patient

From Assey M.E.:[16] The use of Swan-Ganz pulmonary artery catheters in community hospitals. *J. SC Med. Assoc.* 75:410, 1979. Used with permission.

monary capillary wedge pressure reflects the filling pressure of the left ventricle, which is one of the determinants of left ventricular stroke volume. This pressure, the left ventricular end-diastolic pressure, and the pulmonary artery end-diastolic pressure are for clinical purposes equal except when conditions such as pulmonary hypertension or mitral stenosis are present. The central venous pressure (CVP) is a measurement of the right ventricular filling pressure and does not give information pertaining to the left ventricle. With the Swan-Ganz catheter, the right atrial, right ventricular, pulmonary artery, and pulmonary capillary wedge pressures can be obtained (Fig 1–6).[16] The cardiac output can also be obtained with a thermistor (triple-lumen catheter) that allows measurement of blood flow through the heart by the thermodilution technique. Systemic and pulmonary vascular resistances can also be calculated. In addition, the Swan-Ganz catheter can have a separate ventricular pacing probe through a dedicated right ventricular lumen. Thus hemodynamic monitoring and temporary ventricular pacing can be done on demand.

ORDERS FOR EVALUATING THE CARDIAC PATIENT

Weed's[17] problem-oriented record system has given us a method to assess the quality of education and patient care. The data base includes the history, physical examination, and routine laboratory studies. From these data a problem list is created with assigned numbers. For each problem a plan is outlined and orders are written. The plan and orders maintain the same number as the respective problem. Likewise, the same assigned numbers are keys for subsequent progress and discharge notes.

The following is an outline of usual laboratory studies (data base) we order

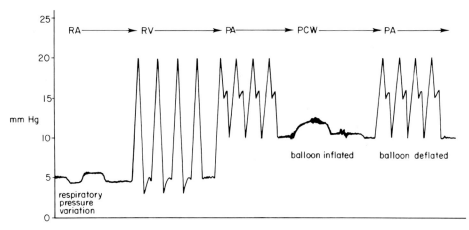

Fig 1–6. Characteristic pressure waveforms as the Swan-Ganz catheter is advanced from the right atrium to the pulmonary artery. RA = right atrium; RV = right ventricle; PA = pulmonary artery; PCW = pulmonary capillary wedge. (From Assey M.E.: The use of Swan-Ganz pulmonary artery catheters in community hospitals. *J. SC Med. Assoc.* 75:410, 1979. Used with permission.)

for a routine cardiac evaluation (first 7) and other specific studies depending on the suspected problem and whether the patient can tolerate the procedure:

Routine

1. Complete blood cell count, hematocrit
2. Urinalysis
3. BUN, creatinine
4. Electrolytes (Na, K, Cl, CO_2)
5. Fasting and 2-hr Pc blood sugar
6. ECG
7. PA, lateral, x-ray views of chest, or, as case dictates, right and left oblique or portable AP view.

   The following are additional studies ordered depending on the suspected problem:

Coronary Artery Disease

8. Stress ECG, thallium 201, and radionuclide angiocardiography
9. Vectorcardiogram and cardiac fluoroscopy in certain cases
10. Uric acid
11. Glucose tolerance
12. Cholesterol, triglycerides, lipid electrophoresis
13. Prothrombin time, Lee-White clotting time, activated partial thrombo-plastin time (APTT)
14. Cardiac enzymes (SGOT, lactic dehydrogenase [LDH] and isoenzymes, creatine phosphokinase [CPK] and isoenzymes)
15. ^{99m}Tc Pyp uptake, thallium 201 perfusion, radionuclide angiocardi-ography
16. Echocardiography and Doppler (as case dictates)
17. Coronary arteriography and left ventriculogram when indicated.

Hypertension and Hypertensive Heart Disease

The following tests are requested depending on the history, physical examination, and the routine (first 7) laboratory studies.

8. Urine culture
9. 24-hr urine for volume, protein, creatinine, urea, uric acid, and electrolytes
10. Creatinine, endogenous creatinine clearance
11. Serum calcium and phosphorus
12. Triiodothyroxine (T_3), thyroxine (T_4)
13. Serum protein electrophoresis, bilirubin, alkaline phosphatase, SGOT, SGPT
14. Cholesterol, triglycerides, lipid electrophoresis
15. Minute sequence hypertensive pyelogram
16. Radioisotope renogram and renal scans
17. Serum and 24-hr urine catecholamines, vanillylmandelic acid, or metanephrines (pheochromocytoma)
18. Plasma renin activity and bilateral renal vein renin (renovascular hypertension)
19. Serum and/or urine aldosterone (primary aldosteronism)
20. Dexamethasone suppression test (Cushing's syndrome)
21. Aortography (aorta and renal arteries)

Rheumatic Fever and Rheumatic Heart Disease

8. Sedimentation rate
9. C-reactive protein (CRP)
10. Antistreptolysin-O (ASO) titer, anti-deoxyribonuclease B (anti-DNase B), antihyaluronidase, antistreptozyme test (ASTZ)
11. Throat culture
12. Serum LDH
13. Phonocardiogram in certain cases
14. Echocardiogram and Doppler (including color flow)
15. Radionuclide angiocardiographic studies at rest and with exercise in certain cases
16. Cardiac fluoroscopy in certain cases
17. Cardiac catheterization and angiocardiography when indicated

Congenital Heart Disease

8. Cardiac fluoroscopy in certain cases
9. Phonocardiogram in certain cases
10. Echocardiogram and Doppler (including color flow)
11. Vectorcardiogram in certain cases
12. Chromosome blood analysis in certain cases (Turner's and Down's syndromes)
13. First-pass radionuclide angiocardiography (intracardiac shunts)
14. Cardiac catheterization and angiocardiography when indicated

Pulmonary Heart Disease

8. Pulmonary function studies

   9. Lung scan
10. Arterial gas studies (pH, P_{CO_2}, O_2 saturation)
11. Echocardiogram
12. First-pass radionuclide angiocardiography
13. Lung biopsy when indicated
14. Pulmonary arteriogram when indicated

Cardiovascular Syphilis

   8. Serum VDRL, fluorescent treponemal antibodies (FTA-ABS), *Treponema pallidum* immobilization test (TPI)
   9. Echocardiogram and Doppler
10. Radionuclide studies
11. Cardiac catheterization and angiocardiography when indicated

Pericardial Disease

   8. Viral studies (Coxsackie B, influenza, echo), acute and convalescent
   9. Purified protein derivative (PPD) and fungal skin tests
10. Fungal serology
11. Serum protein electrophoresis
12. Lupus erythematosus (LE) cell test
13. Rheumatoid (RA) factor
14. Serum antinuclear antibody (ANA) (lupus)
15. Blood cultures
16. Cold agglutinins (mycoplasma)
17. Heterophils (infectious mononucleosis)
18. Serum T_3, T_4, TSH (hypothyroidism)
19. ASO titer, anti-DNase B, antistreptozyme (rheumatic fever)
20. Serum complement levels
21. Echocardiogram
22. Cardiac fluoroscopy in certain cases
23. Pericardial scan in certain cases
24. Pericardial tap when indicated
25. Pericardial biopsy when indicated
26. Pericardial fluid for smear (cells, bacteria, fungi, parasites), culture (routine, tuberculosis, fungi), guinea pig inoculation (tuberculosis), cell count, protein, LE cell, enzymes, cytology, complement levels
27. Cardiac catheterization and angiocardiography when indicated

Bacterial Endocarditis

   8. Blood cultures (aerobic, anaerobic)
   9. Special cultures for fungi
10. Sedimentation rate
11. Serologic test for teichoic acid (*Staphylococcus aureus* infection)
12. Gallium scan (myocardial abscess)
13. Echocardiography (vegetations) and Doppler
14. Tube dilution sensitivity test
15. Tube dilution test for serum bactericidal level
16. Radionuclide studies
17. Cardiac catheterization and angiocardiography when indicated

Myocardial Disease (Myocarditis and Cardiomyopathy)

8. Cardiac fluoroscopy in certain cases
9. Echocardiogram
10. Sedimentation rate
11. CRP
12. ASO titer
13. Protein electrophoresis
14. Serum calcium and phosphate
15. Serum enzymes (SGOT, LDH, CPK, SGPT)
16. LE cell (lupus)
17. Serum ANA (lupus)
18. Rheumatoid factor (rheumatoid arthritis)
19. Serum complement levels
20. X-ray appropriate joints and spine (rheumatoid arthritis), x-ray of hands (Marfan's syndrome)
21. Skin test PPD, fungal, and fungal serology
22. Viral studies (Coxsackie B, echo, influenza, mumps), acute and convalescent
23. Blood cultures
24. Serum and urine for heavy metals (lead, mercury, phosphorus)
25. Barium swallow (scleroderma)
26. Liver studies, plasma iron level and iron-binding capacity (hemochromatosis), and liver biopsy if indicated
27. Urinary mucopolysaccharides (Hurler's syndrome)
28. 5-Hydroxyindole acetic acid (5HIAA) (carcinoid)
29. Biopsy of node (sarcoidosis), skin and muscle (dermatomyositis, polyarteritis nodosa), gum and rectum (amyloidosis)
30. Endomyocardial biopsy when indicated
31. Radionuclide studies
32. Cardiac catheterization and angiocardiography when indicated

Thyroid and the Heart

8. Serum T_3, T_4, TSH
9. Radioactive iodine uptake
10. Cholesterol
11. Echocardiogram

Digitalis Toxicity

8. Digoxin blood level
9. Digitoxin blood level
10. Serum magnesium level

These are many of the studies that are performed in evaluating cardiac problems. Naturally, some of them cannot be performed in all community hospitals. However, this outline gives the practicing physician some ideas about ordering studies, which in itself is a learning experience.

The New York Heart Association nomenclature and criteria[18] for diagnosis of diseases of the heart and great vessels is an excellent classification, especially for the medical student and others in training. In 1973 it was revised.

Table 1–3. Cardiac Status and Prognosis

Cardiac Status	Prognosis
1. Uncompromised	1. Good
2. Slightly compromised	2. Good with therapy
3. Moderately compromised	3. Fair with therapy
4. Severely compromised	4. Guarded despite therapy

From *Nomenclature and Criteria for Diagnosis of Diseases of the Heart and Great Vessels.* The Criteria Committee of the New York Heart Association; ed. 7. Boston, Little, Brown & Co., 1973.

The three major diagnostic categories—etiologic diagnosis, anatomical diagnosis, and physiologic diagnosis—are still emphasized. However, the fourth category, the functional and therapeutic classification, has been deleted and replaced by a new classification of the patient's overall cardiac status and prognosis. This is an important improvement, since the previous editions classified the patient's cardiac status on the basis of symptoms alone, without regard to the other diagnostic categories. The grading of cardiac status and prognosis is presented in Table 1–3. Specific recommendations should be mentioned after this classification.

An example of the use of these diagnostic categories could be as follows:

Etiologic—Congenital anomaly

Anatomic—Atrial septal defect (ostium secondum), enlarged heart (right ventricle), dilatation of the pulmonary artery

Physiologic—Normal sinus rhythm, left-to-right shunt

Cardiac status and prognosis—2.2

Specific recommendations—Significant left-to-right shunt demonstrated at the atrial level by cardiac catheterization; surgery recommended

REFERENCES

1. Kanovsky M.S., Falcone R.A., Dresden C.A., et al.: Identification of patients with ventricular tachycardia after myocardial infarction: signal-averaged electrocardiogram, Holter monitoring, and cardiac catheterization. *Circulation* 70:264, 1984.
2. Cain M.E., Ambos H.D., Wilkowski F.X., et al.: Fast-Fourier transform analysis of signal-averaged electrocardiograms for identification of patients prone to sustained ventricular tachycardia. *Circulation* 69:711, 1984.
3. Hoffman R.B., Rigler L.G.: Evaluation of left ventricular enlargement in the lateral projection of the chest. *Radiology* 85:93, 1965.
4. Popp R.L., Wolfe S.B., Hirata T., et al.: Estimation of right and left ventricular size by ultrasound. *Am. J. Cardiol.* 24:523, 1969.
5. Feigenbaum H.: Clinical applications of echocardiography. *Prog. Cardiovasc. Dis.* 14:531, 1972.
6. Feigenbaum H.: *Echocardiography.* Philadelphia, Lea & Febiger, 1986, pg. 83.
7. Feigenbaum H.: Echocardiography, in Braunwald E. (ed.): *Heart Disease.* Philadelphia, W.B. Saunders Co., 1980.
8. Feigenbaum H.: Doppler Color Flow Imaging, in Braunwald E. (ed.): *Heart Disease Update,* Philadelphia, W.B. Saunders Co., 1988.
9. Wisenberg G., Schelbert H.R.: Radionuclide techniques in the diagnosis of cardiovascular disease. *Curr. Probl. Cardiol.* 4:6, 1979.
10. Berger H.J., Zaret B.L.: Nuclear cardiology (pt. 1). *N. Engl. J. Med.* 305:799, 1981.
11. Berger H.J., Zaret B.L.: Nuclear cardiology (pt. 2). *N. Engl. J. Med.* 305:855, 1981.
12. Iskandrian A.S., Heo J., Askenase A., et al.: Thallium imaging with single photon emission computed tomography. *Am. Heart J.* 114:852, 1987.
13. Jacobson H.G. (ed.): Application of positron emission tomography in the heart. Council on Scientific Affairs. *JAMA* 259:2438, 1988.
14. Jacobson H.G. (ed.): Magnetic resonance imaging of the cardiovascular system. *JAMA* 295:253, 1988.

15. Swan H.J.C., Ganz W., Forrester J.S., et al.: Catheterization of the heart in man with use of balloon-tipped catheter. *N. Engl. J. Med.* 283:447, 1970.
16. Assey M.C.: The use of Swan-Ganz pulmonary artery catheters in community hospitals. *J. SC Med. Assoc.* 75:410, 1979.
17. Weed L.L.: *Medical Records, Medical Education, and Patient Care.* Cleveland, The Press of Case Western Reserve University, 1971.
18. Criteria Committee of the New York Heart Association: *Nomenclature and Criteria for Diagnosis of Diseases of the Heart and Great Vessels,* ed. 7. Boston, Little, Brown & Co., 1973.

Chapter 2

DIAGNOSTIC CLUES IN CARDIOVASCULAR DISEASE

Careful physical examination has again become important in detecting clues to cardiovascular diagnosis. This is not to decry the value of instrumentation and highly specialized procedures such as echocardiography, Doppler, radionuclide studies, and heart catheterization. These mechanical devices have aided tremendously in correlating bedside findings with specific disease states. This chapter describes some of the diagnostic signs easily detected at the bedside.

SKIN

The color and texture of the skin may give the first clues to cardiovascular disease. Cyanosis of the skin and mucous membranes may suggest congenital heart disease in the child and pulmonary disease in the adult. If the hands are warm and the nail beds are cyanotic, the cyanosis is central, since peripheral cyanosis is usually seen in cool areas. Clubbing of the fingers and toes is often associated with central cyanosis. Obliteration of the angle or groove (nail fold) between the base of the nail and the proximal skin is the earliest sign of clubbing. Chronic pallor is often due to anemia, which can precipitate heart failure in a patient with subclinical heart disease or produce intractable heart failure in a patient with known heart disease. Acute pallor in a person with chest pain may be a sign of angina or myocardial infarction. Fine, silky, warm skin may indicate hyperthyroidism and dry, coarse skin, myxedema. Tight, smooth, glossy skin on the fingers may be noted with scleroderma. These findings occasionally unveil the etiology of unexplained cardiomegaly.

Erythema marginatum of acute rheumatic fever is confined primarily to the trunk; sometimes it occurs on the extremities, but never on the face. These crescentic lesions are evanescent but may recur long after the acute phase of rheumatic fever has subsided. Rheumatic subcutaneous nodules develop on the extensor surface of the elbows or on any bony prominence such as the spine, skull, or dorsum of hand or foot. They vary from the size of a pinhead to about 2 cm in diameter. The skin moves freely over these nontender nodules.

Xanthomas are often noted in persons with an abnormal lipid disorder and associated coronary disease. They are of several types. Xanthelasmas have predilection for the eyelids; xanthoma tendenosum, the tendons, especially the Achilles tendon; xanthomas tuberosum, the bony tubercles, especially the elbows; and eruptive xanthomas, the trunk, buttocks, arms, and legs. The smooth tendenosum variety may cause the tendon to be thickened rather than lumpy and, except in the obese, should be suspected in a smooth Achilles tendon with a diameter greater than the person's index finger. The color of the tuberosum and eruptive types varies from flesh color to yellow, orange, or pink. Persons with xanthelasma, xanthoma tendenosum, and tuberosum often have Fredrickson's[1] type II hypercholesterolemia lipid disorder, whereas those with the eruptive type have Frederickson's type I, IV and V hyperlipoproteinemia disorders. Xanthomas in the creases of the palms and fingers and the tuberoeruptive type on the extensor surfaces of the extremities are seen in patients with Fredrickson's type III abnormality.

Petechiae often support a diagnosis of bacterial endocarditis, especially in association with fever and a heart murmur. One should palpate for thrills and auscultate for continuous murmurs over all scars to exclude an arteriovenous fistula that can produce high-output heart failure.

HEAD

Subluxation of the lens with tremulous iris (iridodonesis) is a characteristic of Marfan's syndrome. Arcus senilis, gray ring around the iris (usually type II lipid abnormality), and cataracts in the middle-aged male may be associated with coronary disease. However, arcus senilis in blacks, in whom it often occurs, usually does not reflect a lipid disturbance or vascular disease. If a patient has a small pupil that fails to react to light but constricts on accommodation (Argyll-Robertson pupil), one must consider syphilis as the cause of the associated aortic insufficiency regardless of the patient's social status.

A hoarse voice may indicate congenital heart disease or mitral valve disease. These conditions can dilate a pulmonary artery, causing pressure on the left recurrent laryngeal nerve and producing hoarseness. This may also be a sign of an aortic arch aneurysm. Such patients are often first seen by the otolaryngologist.

The head may give other clues to the etiology of undiagnosed heart disease. Macroglossia is found with myxedema and amyloidosis, in which there may be cardiac involvement. Increasing hat size and shrinking body stature may indicate Paget's disease. The head's appearance can be the clue to congenital heart defects. Widely set eyes (hypertelorism) can be associated with pulmonary stenosis. Hypertelorism, low ears, wide mouth, upturned nose, and pointed chin can be the facies (elfin type) of supravalvular aortic stenosis.

NECK

Webbing of the neck suggests Turner's syndrome with coarctation of the aorta or Noonan's syndrome with pulmonary valvular stenosis. Aortic valvular stenosis occurs less frequently in both of these syndromes. The neck should be examined carefully for thyroid enlargement and nodules.

Arterial and venous pulsations are visible in the neck and afford several valuable clues. The external jugular veins have valves, and pulsations from the right atrium are not transmitted beyond these valves. The deep internal jugular veins without valves show pulsations that can be seen when the patient is recumbent, but are barely visible above the clavicles or not seen at a 45-degree angle from the horizontal. These venous pulsations can only be seen transmitted to the neck, for the internal jugular veins cannot be seen and are not palpable. Venous pulsations are wavelike and more diffuse than arterial pulsations and are influenced by alterations in posture, respiration, or abdominal pressure. Moderate pressure on the neck with a pencil below the level of pulsations obliterates jugular but not carotid pulsations. The main visible components of the venous pulsations are A waves (atrial contraction) and V waves (atrial filling), but most often only the A wave is clearly seen, unless it is absent because of atrial fibrillation or over-shadowed by the prominent C-V waves of tricuspid insufficiency. The systolic expansion of the internal jugulars from tricuspid insufficiency may cause the patient's head to move from side to side ("no-no" sign).[2] After the A wave there is an X descent associated early with atrial diastole and then with ventricular systole. When the tricuspid valve opens and there is a rapid fall in right atrial pressure, a Y descent is noted in the venous wave. These X and Y descents are more noticeable in abnormal states.

The 45-degree position is used to examine most patients with cardiac disease. If the jugular venous pressure is low, 30 degrees is best and if high 60 degrees or above may be best to see jugular vein pulsations. With the patient at a 45-degree angle from the horizontal, it is best to look for the silhouette of the right neck's internal jugular pulsations by standing on the left side and shining a light tangentially to the neck. One should look for the top level of jugular pulsations. The top level of pulsation is like a fulcrum of movement showing less pulsation at the very top level. Many reference levels have been used as zero to interpret the height of the internal jugular pulsations, most often the sternal angle of Louis (junction of the manubrium and gladiolus where the second rib articulates). At the 45-degree position the upper limit of normal from the sternal angle to the top level of pulsation is usually 3 cm. However, occasionally it may be up to 4.5 cm[3] (Fig 2-1). Attempts have been made to add this level, with the distance from the sternal angle to the middle right atrium, to give an estimate of the venous pressure. However, since the distance between the sternal angle and the right atrium is so variable, it is not considered a reliable measurement. The pulsations ascend over 3 cm with congestive failure and may reach the ear lobes. The pulsations become less visible if the internal jugular veins are tensely distended from the very high venous pressure of congestive heart failure or pericardial constriction. Early congestive heart failure should be suspected when sustained pressure applied over the right upper abdomen produces an increase of greater than 3 cm in the height of neck vein distension (positive hepatojugular reflux) at the 45-degree position. Ducas et al. showed that, after 10 seconds of abdominal pressure, the venous pressure did not change over the next 60 seconds.[4] Pressure on the liver is not essential for this test. However, use of the term hepatojugular reflux is retained because it has been used for many years. Compression over any part of the abdomen can be used. The venous pressure rises with abdominal compression in the presence of congestive heart failure because of the increased venous tone and blood volume in this condition. In addition, right upper quadrant compression could interfere with left ventricular filling.[5]

Any obstruction from the pulmonary arterioles to the tricuspid valve can produce prominent A waves. These are seen in conditions in which outflow from the right atrium is impeded, such as pulmonary hypertension, pulmonary stenosis, or tricuspid stenosis.

When the atria and ventricles are dissociated, large A waves are visible

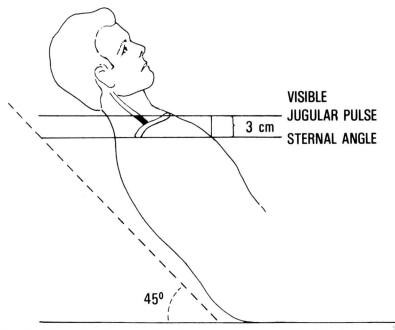

VISIBLE
JUGULAR PULSE
3 cm
STERNAL ANGLE

45°

Fig 2–1. Bedside method for measuring the venous pressure. Patient is placed at 45 degrees horizontally. Horizontal lines are shown through the top of the visible jugular venous pulse and sternal angle. The upper normal distance from the sternal angle to the horizontal line which represents the top of the visible jugular venous pulse is 3 cm.

during intervals when the P waves follow the QRS complexes. These cannon A waves are produced by atrial systole when the tricuspid valve is closed, forcing blood up the superior vena cava to the jugular veins. They can be seen intermittently as sudden, prominent venous pulsations in any type of atrioventricular (AV) dissociation as in complete AV heart block and in some cases of ventricular tachycardia or regularly with nodal (junctional) rhythm.

The X descent becomes prominent with pericardial tamponade because of more complete ventricular emptying in an attempt to maintain cardiac output. The Y descent can be deep and noticeable in constrictive pericarditis and in tricuspid regurgitation and is related to the rapid fall in ventricular pressure. Slow rate of Y descent occurs with tricuspid stenosis.

The V wave can become prominent with tricuspid regurgitation (eventually the C and V waves will merge), congestive heart failure, or rapid atrial filling (such as that due to exercise, hyperthyroidism, or atrial septal defect).

Obstruction of the superior vena cava or the innominate veins may produce unilateral or bilateral venous distention without pulsation. An atherosclerotic aorta can compress the innominate vein against the sternum and distend the neck vein on the left side.

Arterial pulsations are brisk and palpable. Carotid arterial pulsations are usually equal but may be diminished in carotid artery insufficiency. This condition is often associated with transient monocular blindness and contralateral hemiplegia. A systolic or continuous bruit may be audible over the narrow carotid artery segment. However, benign bruits are often heard over the neck arteries in children and young adults, usually loudest in the supraclavicular fossae.

Bounding, vigorous, rapidly rising carotid arterial pulsations suggest aortic valvular insufficiency, patent ductus arteriosus, arteriovenous fistula, or other high-output syndromes. Slowly rising pulsations suggest aortic stenosis (valvular, or discrete subvalvular). Combined aortic stenosis and insufficiency, idiopathic hypertrophic subaortic stenosis, and, pure severe aortic insufficiency may give a double-peaked carotid pulsation (pulsus bisferiens). The two peaks occur during systole with the percussion and tidal waves separated by a distinct midsystolic dip. In aortic regurgitation the major factors are the large stroke volume (percussion) and reflected waves from the periphery (tidal). In idiopathic hypertrophic subaortic stenosis the first peak is a rapid ejection of blood into the aorta (percussion). This is followed by a decrease in the pulse due to the obstruction, then a second peak due to the slower ejection from the ventricle and reflected waves from the periphery (tidal). The wave after the dicrotic notch (see Fig 1–2) can become prominent and palpable; it is called a dicrotic wave and may give the appearance of a bisferious pulse. It is usually associated with a low cardiac output and an elastic aorta and is most often noted in severe congestive failure, cardiac tamponade, and conditions with a low stroke volume. Supravalvular aortic stenosis often produces a more prominent pulsation of the right carotid artery than of the left. Kinking of the right common carotid artery may appear as a prominent pulsation in the supraclavicular area, simulating an aneurysm of this artery or of the innominate. When the chest is short, the innominate pulsation on the right can simulate an aneurysm.

CHEST

Inspection and Palpation Clues

On examining the chest, one should always palpate the right and left sides for dextrocardia. Dextrocardia with situs inversus is often innocuous, but isolated dextrocardia may be associated with serious congenital heart disease.

Chest deformities such as pectus excavatum and the straight back syndrome may produce insignificant cardiac findings that simulate organic heart lesions. An emphysematous-appearing chest or anterior bowing in the area of the manubrium sterni in a child suggests pulmonary hypertension such as that occurring with ventricular septal defect. This is especially important in the presence of a balanced shunt and no murmur.

Prominence over the precordium or parasternal area often indicates right ventricular enlargement. This bulge, when high in the area of the second and third intercostal spaces, suggests an atrial septal defect. Lower prominence, in the area of the fourth or fifth spaces, suggests a ventricular septal defect.

The sternoclavicular, aortic, pulmonary, parasternal or anterior precordium, apical, and ectopic areas also should be examined. Abnormalities of the aortic arch can produce pulsations of the sternoclavicular joints. Such pulsations in a patient with chest pain suggest a dissecting aneurysm. A right aortic arch can produce pulsations of the right sternoclavicular joint. Tetralogy of Fallot is the most common congenital lesion associated with right aortic arch. Occasionally, pulsations are noted in the right sternoclavicular joint in the older patient with a tortuous innominate artery.

Abnormal pulsations in the aortic area usually indicate an abnormality of the ascending aorta. Valvular aortic stenosis often produces a systolic thrill in this area. In the pulmonic area, abnormal pulsations usually indicate an abnormality of the pulmonary artery (due to increased pressure or flow or both in the pulmonary artery). Pulmonary stenosis often produces a thrill in this area.

A slight retraction is normally palpable in the lower left parasternal or anterior precordial area, except in young people with thin chests, in whom a short outward tap can be felt. Conditions with right ventricular hypertrophy or dilatation can cause abnormal pulsations in the left parasternal area. Pulsations due to volume loads associated with left-to-right shunts, such as those at the atrial or ventricular level, give a vigorous, brisk pulsation with a short outward and longer inward movement compared with the slower, sustained outward lift of resistant loads that are seen in pulmonary hypertension or pulmonary stenosis. In these conditions with right ventricular enlargement and a parasternal lift there is associated middle or lateral chest retraction. In biventricular enlargement, such as with a ventricular septal defect, in addition to a parasternal lift there may be another rise in systole at the apex with an area of retraction between them. Moderate or severe mitral insufficiency produces a most forceful, brisk left parasternal thrust (left atrial lift), predominantly in late systole and related to the regurgitant jet into the left atrium, pushing the right ventricle against the chest wall.[6] Ventricular septal defects often produce thrills in the parasternal area.

The size and character of the apical impulse are more important than its location. The location depends upon many factors, such as the shape of the chest and position of the diaphragm. It is usually smaller than 2 cm or a half-dollar in diameter and occupies less than two intercostal spaces in the same phase of respirations in the normal person in the supine position.[7] In many normal persons, it may be palpable only in the left lateral decubitus position. Eilen et al.[8] noted that, in patients without left ventricular hypertrophy, an apical impulse greater than 3 cm in the left lateral decubitus position was sensitive (92%) and specific (91%) for left ventricular enlargement. An apical impulse with greater distance than 10 cm or lateral to the midclavicular line was sensitive but not specific for left ventricular enlargement. The early systolic outward motion of the apical area is produced by isovolumetric contraction of the left ventricle and is palpable during the first heart sound or just before the carotid upstroke. This outward motion lasts only for the first third of systole.

Rather diffuse, active apical impulses are seen with the volume loads of aortic or mitral insufficiency, which produce left ventricular dilatation. Resistant loads with resultant hypertrophy, such as those seen with aortic stenosis, produce a forceful and sustained apical lift throughout systole. This is often palpable but difficult to see. Palpation sometimes can be superior to the chest x-ray or the ECG in detecting concentric left ventricular hypertrophy. Double or bifid apical impulses can occur when an outward movement during systole due to left ventricular dilatation or hypertrophy is combined with a diastolic component due to an S_3 or S_4 gallop. Hypertrophic subaortic stenosis and left bundle-branch block can produce a bifid apical impulse during systole.

Cardiac pulsations noted in ectopic areas, i.e., between the pulmonary artery and apex, are often due to ischemic heart disease. These ectopic impulses can occur transiently with angina or over a long period with myocardial infarction, and they may remain as a feature of a ventricular aneurysm.

Auscultatory Clues

There is still much debate concerning the number of components and mechanisms of the first sound. Muscular, valvular, and vascular events contribute to the first sound.[9] Some investigators have shown that there is a delay of the first sound after the mitral valve closure and that it occurs with the halting of the valve at its maximum displacement into the left ventricle. The abrupt accelerations and especially decelerations of blood associated with the checking action of valves and the degree of systemic and pulmonary vascular resistances and capacity probably contribute to all normal and abnormal sounds. Clinically, we assume that valve closures are responsible for the major components of heart sounds. The first sound lasts approximately 0.1–0.12 seconds and is best heard at the apex. The second sound is associated with closure of the semilunar valves. However, just as for the first sound, there are proponents for valvular, muscular, or vascular events producing their origin.[10,11] The second sound splits normally with inspiration. The inspiratory increase in stroke volume of the right ventricle causes delay in pulmonic valve closure (P_2). The low pulmonary vascular impedance and large capacity probably also contribute to the delay. Other factors may be involved in this splitting, such as early closure of the aortic valve (A_2) due to bloodpooling in the lung with inspiration which causes a decrease in venous return to the left heart, resulting in a shortened left ventricular systole. Deceleration of blood also may be a factor because of the low systemic vascular capacity and increased peripheral impedance. In adults, the second sound is heard loudest in the primary aortic area and is of shorter duration than the first sound. A physiologic third heart (S_3) sound in early diastole is often heard in persons under the age of 20.

The following features of a cardiac murmur should be recorded: timing, intensity, site of maximum intensity, duration, radiation, quality, and response to maneuvers and to vasoactive drugs. The intensity of murmurs can be graded[12] from 1 to 6. One has to form his own interpretation of grading through experience. Generally, if a murmur is difficult to hear initially, it is grade 1; if easily heard and faint, grade 2; if a thrill is present with a murmur, grade 4 or greater; if it can be heard without the stethoscope against the chest, grade 6. Systolic ejection murmurs start just after the first sound and end before the second sound, whereas regurgitant murmurs usually extend from the first into the second sound.

It should be remembered that murmurs produced by a valve may not necessarily be heard over the specific anatomical area of the valve but may be referred to another section of the chest. For example, it is not unusual to hear the murmur of aortic valvular stenosis best at the apex. For this reason, I like to teach students to recognize the character and quality of a murmur rather than to be overly concerned with timing and location. The murmurs most commonly confused are those of aortic stenosis and insufficiency and mitral stenosis and insufficiency. The systolic murmur of aortic stenosis is harsh, ejection-type (crescendo-decrescendo, diamond-shaped), and often sounds like the bark of a bulldog. Such a murmur is rarely produced by the mitral valve; therefore, even if it is best heard at the apex, it should be considered due to aortic stenosis.

The diastolic murmur of aortic insufficiency is high-pitched, sounding like a pistol shot or blowing into a jug. Often this murmur is heard best along the left sternal border or at times even at the apex rather than in the primary aortic area. Actually, it makes no difference where you hear this murmur because most often it is due to aortic valvular insufficiency. The only other murmur that resembles this is pulmonic insufficiency, which is rare and usually associated with pulmonary hypertension. Mitral insufficiency is best heard at the apex and is a regurgitant high-pitched systolic murmur usually of equal intensity throughout systole. There are exceptions to this, which will be discussed in Chapter 6. Mitral stenosis is a rumbling, low-pitched diastolic murmur best heard at the apex and usually in the left lateral recumbent position. Whereas the other murmurs are best heard with the diaphragm of the stethoscope, mitral stenosis is best heard with the bell.

For many years emphasis was placed on the heart murmurs. Today the heart sounds and extra sounds that occur are equally emphasized. Splitting of the heart sounds, ejection sounds, clicks, and gallops often give the clue to a diagnosis. Any abnormal situation that causes a delay in pulmonic valve closure can produce wide splitting of the second sound in inspiration and expiration such as right bundle-branch block, atrial septal defect, and pulmonic valvular stenosis. Rarely, early closure of the aortic valve (shortened left ventricular ejection) such as with mitral insufficiency can produce splitting. Paradoxical or reversed splitting of the second sound only with expiration can occur with lesions which cause a delay of aortic valve closure, such as left bundle-branch block, severe aortic stenosis, and myocardial dysfunction of any cause.

There are two main types of ejection sounds, aortic and pulmonic. These are associated with milder degrees of aortic stenosis or pulmonic stenosis and vibrations in a dilated root of the aorta or pulmonary artery. Sudden deceleration of blood is a factor in their production. The aortic ejection sound is often heard best at the apex and the pulmonic ejection sound in the pulmonic area. These give the impression of splitting of the first sound, with the ejection sound being the loud component just after the first sound. In pulmonary valvular stenosis the ejection sound behaves differently on inspiration from the usual right-sided events. Usually with right-sided lesions the intensity of the murmur or sound increases on inspiration with the increased blood flow to the right side. However, in pulmonary valvular stenosis the ejection sound decreases or disappears during inspiration. This is probably due to the elevation of the right ventricular diastolic pressure during inspiration, which exceeds the low pulmonary arterial pressure causing the pulmonary valve to move to its open position prior to ventricular systole so that right ventricular contraction cannot produce an ejection sound.[13]

Clicks usually occur in midsystole or late systole. For years these were considered to be extracardiac in origin, e.g., due to pericardial or pleural adhesions, but studies have shown that abnormalities of the mitral valve leaflets or chordae tendineae and dysfunction of the papillary muscle can produce these sounds with or without a late systolic murmur of mitral insufficiency. Most often the clicks are associated with prolapse of one or both mitral leaflets into the left atrium during late systole.

An S_3 (ventricular gallop) has always been considered a serious finding of myocardial dysfunction. The S_4 gallop (atrial gallop) only recently has been given attention. It also indicates some myocardial dysfunction with impaired filling due to an elevated ventricular end-diastolic pressure or decreased compliance. However, it is not as significant as an S_3 and may be heard in older people who have no other manifestations of cardiac disease.[14] It also may occur with a long P-R interval. Both of these sounds are low-pitched and sound like the cadence of a horse; they should not be confused with the higher-pitched split sounds and the ejection sounds. The significance of an S_3 sound depends on the setting. It can be physiologic in the young, or it may be associated with severe mitral insufficiency (referred to as a third heart filling sound). In the presence of severe myocardial dysfunction it is referred to as a gallop. In all cases the third heart sound has the same phonocardiographic characteristics and probably the same mechanism. It probably results from vibrations in early diastole originating within the left ventricular wall as its active rapid expansile motion is suddenly halted. Other mechanisms considered responsible for its genesis are a valvular mechanism and the impact of the left ventricle against the chest wall.

Second sound splitting must be differentiated from an S_3 gallop, an opening snap of mitral stenosis, and a pericardial knock. Splitting of the second sound is best heard at the left second and third intercostal spaces near the sternum and may vary with respirations. The interval between splitting of the second sound is shorter than that between the second sound and an S_3 gallop. The S_3 gallop is low-pitched and often palpable. An opening snap is high-pitched and often heard best at the fourth left intercostal space near the sternum or at the apex. In addition, the latter is usually associated with other findings of mitral stenosis. Likewise, a pericardial knock is associated with other evidence of constrictive pericarditis. It most often occurs after the time of the opening snap and before the time of the usual third heart sound.

Splitting of the first sound must be differentiated from an S_4 gallop and systolic ejection sound. Splitting components are usually close and heard best in the tricuspid area (lower left sternal border). A left ventricular S_4 gallop is low-pitched, widely separated from the first sound, and heard best at the apex and during expiration. An ejection sound is very high-pitched. The aortic ejection sounds do not vary with respiration, whereas the pulmonic ejection sounds due to pulmonary valvular stenoses decrease in intensity with inspiration.

ABDOMEN

There are several causes of pulsations in the upper abdominal area. With tricuspid stenosis or insufficiency, the liver pulsates in an AP plane. A large right ventricle, such as that noted with chronic lung disease and cor pulmonale, may cause downward pulsation under the xiphoid. However, the shape of the fixed anterior chest hides this enlargement. An aortic aneurysm gives forward and lateral pulsations.

The liver should not be considered enlarged unless the distance between its dull upper edge and lower palpable edge is more than 11 cm. With a low diaphragm, the liver may be descended into the right pelvis, yet be of normal size. A palpable spleen can be associated with bacterial endocarditis or even heart failure, especially if the failure is associated with secondary tricuspid insufficiency.

There are many causes of abdominal murmurs, such as normal flow types, renal stenosis, atherosclerosis of abdominal aorta and its branches, and hepatic AV shunts. Over 50% of patients under age 25 have normal flow abdominal systolic murmurs of any length. Occasionally patients may have a venous hum above and to the right of the umbilicus over the inferior vena cava.

EXTREMITIES

The hands often give diagnostic clues to underlying cardiovascular disease.[15] Polydactylia and variation in shape and size of the fingers or their joints may be associated with congenital heart lesions. The thumb may be like a finger in patients with atrial septal defects who have the Holt-Oram syndrome. When the fist is closed over the thumb and it extends beyond the ulnar side of the hand and the fingers are long and spider-like, one should consider Marfan's syndrome. Warm feet, especially in a female, often suggest hyperthyroidism even though no other overt signs are present. A patient with big shoulders and arms and small legs may have coarctation of the aorta.

All peripheral pulses should be equal. Rarely, the radial artery takes an aberrant deep course and is not readily palpable, but a nonpalpable radial pulse also can indicate thrombosis or embolism. Five to eight percent of normal persons do not have dorsalis pedis pulsations. Absent or weak femoral pulsations with good radial pulses suggest coarctation of the aorta unless there is peripheral vascular disease.

Pressure over or proximal to a suspected arteriovenous fistula can raise the diastolic pressure, stimulate the vagus (Marey's reflex), and cause bradycardia (Branham's sign). The scalenus anticus syndrome may be present if the radial pulse can be obliterated or diminished by elevating the chin and rotating the neck to the affected side during deep inspiration (Adson maneuver).

Blood pressure (BP) should be checked routinely in both arms and legs. The standard 12-cm cuff can indicate an erroneously high BP in arms with a large diameter and too low a pressure in thin arms. The same cuff often indicates a pressure in the legs 30 mm Hg or more higher than in the arms. A cuff of about 16 cm is preferable for the legs. The width of the compression cuff should be about 20% greater than the diameter of the extremity.[16] The systolic and diastolic pressures, if taken simultaneously, can vary between the arms by 10 mm Hg or more in 5% of subjects. It is best to record the diastolic pressure at the point when Korotkoff's sounds disappear, although in certain cases (e.g., aortic insufficiency) it is best to record both when the sounds are muffled and when they disappear. At times, if the arm is large and especially if it is shaped like a cone, it is best to place the cuff on the forearm and auscultate at the radial artery. High BP in a sweaty, thin patient whose heart rate increases in the standing position may indicate pheochromocytoma.

Pulsus alternans indicates left ventricular failure and is best detected by using the BP cuff. After detecting the top systolic pressure, allow the cuff pressure to drop a few millimeters of mercury at a time and note whether every other impulse disappears or becomes weak. This can occur for a few millimeters or through the entire BP reading. Pulsus alternans can occur secondary to tachycardias even in normal persons. A PVB can start a short run of pulsus alternans in patients with heart failure. It may appear only during exercise or it can be exaggerated or produced by decreasing the venous return to the heart by standing. It is associated with alternation of stroke volume together with alternation of either left ventricular contractility or end-diastolic volume.

Likewise, always check for pulsus paradoxus with the BP cuff. After detecting the top systolic pressure, note whether the sounds disappear during inspiration as the cuff pressure is reduced a few millimeters at a time. Significant pulsus paradoxus is present if this occurs for at least 10 mm Hg, and it is diagnostic of pericardial effusion and occurs less frequently in patients with chronic constrictive pericarditis. However, this phenomenon can occur in myocardial disease and in airway obstruction, such as emphysema or bronchial asthma. The neck veins can aid in differentiating pericardial disease from airway obstruction when pulsus paradoxus is present. On inspiration, these veins fill in pericardial disease and collapse in airway obstruction. During cardiac tamponade, inspiration causes a fall in the elevated intrapericardial pressure, which results in an increase in venous return and an increase in right ventricular volume and bulging of the septum toward the left ventricle and a further decrease in left ventricular volume.[17,18] Other mechanisms have been postulated. In patients with asthma or chronic obstructive lung disease, the exaggerated fluctuation in intrathoracic pressure can produce variations in venous return and in the pulmonary blood volume, and there may be transmission of the more negative intrathoracic pressure during inspiration to the aorta and great vessels.

A wide pulse pressure can occur with a variety of conditions, namely, aortic insufficiency, arteriovenous fistula, patent ductus arteriosus, anemia, complete heart block, hyperthyroidism, or beriberi, and is especially common in older persons with great vessel sclerosis. A narrow pulse pressure occurs with aortic stenosis (usually a late finding), constrictive pericarditis, shock, and heart failure.

Ulcers on the legs are often a diagnostic clue. Characteristically, the brownish venous ulcers are present on the inner aspect of the ankles just above the malleoli. Hypertensive ulcers (due to degenerative changes in the arterioles) often are found on the lateral or posterolateral aspect of the lower third of the leg, and ulcers associated with arteriovenous fistula usually occur at the distal parts of the foot, i.e., between the toes.

Subcutaneous edema does not occur with heart failure until at least 10 lb of fluid has accumulated. Peripheral edema is most unusual in a patient with heart failure unless he has cardiomegaly, neck vein distention, and hepatomegaly. The most common cause of peripheral edema is not heart failure. There are many common noncardiac causes, such as obesity, venous stasis, varicosities, venous disease, and menopausal, psychogenic, hepatic, and renal abnormalities. Psychogenic edema is very common, especially in young females with edema of the hands and feet occurring during tension states. Studies in such cases have shown an abnormal water tolerance. These patients often become dependent on diuretics and cannot be convinced that the edema will subside with lessening of their problems.

REFERENCES

1. Fredrickson D.S., Lees R.S.: A system for phenotyping hyperlipoproteinemia. *Circulation* 31:321, 1965.
2. De Leon A.C.: Diagnostic fine-tuning based on pulsation, waves, and sounds. *Consultant,* p. 111, March, 1984.
3. Constant J: *Bedside Cardiology,* ed. 2. Boston, Little, Brown & Co., 1976.
4. Ducas J., Magder S., McGregor M.: Validity of the hepatojugular reflux as a clinical test for congestive heart failure. *Am. J. Cardiol.* 52:1299, 1983.

5. Hamosh P., Cohn J.N.: Mechanism of the hepatojugular reflux test. *Am. J. Cardiol.* 25:100, 1970.
6. Armstrong T.G., Meeran M.K., Gotsman M.S.: The left atrial lift. *Am. Heart J.* 82:764, 1971.
7. Conn R.D., Cole J.S.: The cardiac apex impulse: Clinical and angiographic correlations. *Ann. Intern. Med.* 75:185, 1971.
8. Eilen S.D., Crawford M.H., O'Rourke R.A.: Accuracy of precordial palpation for detecting increased left ventricular volume. *Ann. Intern. Med.* 99:628, 1983.
9. Luisada A.A., MacCannon D.M., Kumar J., et al.: Changing views on the mechanism of the first and second sounds. *Am. Heart J.* 88:503, 1974.
10. Sabbah H.N., Stein P.D.: Relation of the second sound to diastolic vibration of the closed aortic valve. *Am. J. Physiol: Heart Circ. Physiol.* 3:H 696, 1978.
11. Smith D., Craige E.: Influence of the aortic component of the second sound on left ventricular maximal negative dP/dt on the dog. *Am. J. Cardiol.* 55:205, 1985.
12. Freeman A.R., Levine S.A.: The clinical significance of the systolic murmur: A study of 1,000 consecutive "noncardiac" cases. *Ann. Intern. Med.* 6:1371, 1933.
13. Hultgren H.N., Reeve R., Cohn K., et al.: The ejection click of valvular pulmonic stenosis. *Circulation* 40:631, 1969.
14. Spodick D.H., Quarry-Pigott V.M.: Fourth heart sound as a normal finding in older persons. *N. Engl. J. Med.* 288:140, 1973.
15. Silverman M.E., Hurst J.W.: The hand and the heart. *Am. J. Cardiol.* 22:718, 1968.
16. Burch G.E., DePasguale N.P.: *Primer of Clinical Measurement of Blood Pressure.* St. Louis, C.V. Mosby Co., 1962.
17. Shabetai R., Fowler N.O., Fenton J.C., et al.: Pulsus paradoxus. *J. Clin. Invest.* 44:1882, 1965.
18. Settle H.P., Adolph R.J., Fowler N.O., et al.: Echocardiographic study of cardiac tamponade. *Circulation* 56:951, 1977.

Chapter 3

CLINICAL ELECTROCARDIOGRAPHY

The ECG is recorded on a background of horizontal and vertical lines. The horizontal lines measure duration and are separated at 0.04-second intervals. The vertical lines measure amplitude and are divided in 1-mm squares. Every fifth horizontal and vertical line is thickened (Fig 3–1). The ECG is properly standardized when 1 mm amplitude represents 0.1 mV. Tracings are usually recorded with standardization of 10-mm deflection (1 mV).

BASIC PRINCIPLES

The spread of the impulse through the atria produces the P wave of the ECG, which is normally upright in leads I and II and in the left precordial leads. Its amplitude should not exceed 2.5 mm, and its duration is normally about 0.08 second. The interval from the beginning of the P wave and the beginning of the QRS complex is the P-R interval. The P-R interval represents conduction time from the SA node through the atria, AV node, and the His bundle and its branches. It normally has a range from 0.12 to 0.20 second.

The QRS complex represents activation (depolarization) of the ventricles. To understand its genesis, it is important to realize that our instrumentation is engineered so that when an impulse goes toward an electrode, an upright complex is produced, and when an impulse goes away from the electrode, a downward complex is produced. In ventricular depolarization a component above the baseline is called an R wave. A downward component below the baseline and preceding the R wave is called a Q wave. If the downward component occurs below the baseline after the R wave, it is designated an S wave (Figs 3–1 and 3–2). Ventricular depolarization will be approached first as it is recorded by the precordial leads. The position of the exploring electrode on the chest for these recordings is as follows: V_1, right of the sternum at the fourth intercostal space; V_2, left of the sternum at the fourth intercostal space; V_4, left midclavicular line at the fifth intercostal space; V_3, on a line between V_2 and V_4; V_5, left anterior axillary line at the fifth intercostal space; V_6, left midaxillary line at the fifth intercostal space.

In applying the above facts to the genesis of the precordial patterns, one will note (Fig 3–3) that initially depolarization occurs from left to right through the septum prior to activation of the remaining myocardium. Therefore, an electrode in the V_1 position will record a small R wave, and one in the V_5 or V_6 position a small Q wave. Next, in view of the sequence of depolarization from

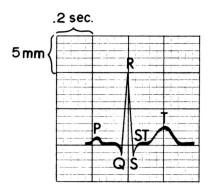

Fig 3–1.   Time and amplitude measurements with a typical ECG of a cardiac cycle.

the right ventricle to the larger left ventricle mass, there will be recorded an increment in R wave amplitude and a decrease in S wave size from the V_2 through the V_5 or V_6 positions. In other words, the impulse reaches the thin right ventricular surface early, and, therefore, the deep S wave recorded from the right ventricular electrode represents the impulse going away from it, activating the left ventricle. Simultaneously, an electrode over the left ventricle records a high R wave as the left ventricle is depolarized. The precordial lead that records a QRS complex with equal amplitude of the R and S waves represents the transitional zone. Clockwise rotation of the heart on its longitudinal axis is present if the transitional zone is in V_5 or V_6 and counterclockwise rotation if it is in V_1 or V_2. These rotations are noted looking up from below the diaphragm. From this view, if the heart rotates on its longitudinal axis toward the right, counterclockwise rotation is present, and if to the left, clockwise rotation is present. The normal transitional zone is usually in V_3 or V_4.

From the sequence of activation of the ventricles, the six limb leads also can be derived. The impulse is usually traveling away from the right arm lead (aV_R); therefore, a downward QS complex is recorded in that lead. The configuration of the complexes of the left arm lead (aV_L) and the left leg lead (aV_F) depends on whether the heart is in an electric horizontal, vertical position or some intermediate position. In the horizontal position aV_L will demonstrate a tall R wave, and in the vertical position this will be noted in aV_F. Lead I displays potential differences between aV_L and aV_R; lead II, between aV_F and

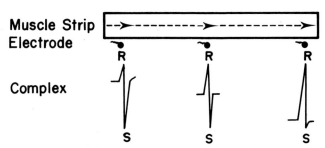

Fig 3–2.   A stimulated muscle strip showing an R wave as the impulse travels toward the electrode and an S wave as the impulse goes away from an electrode. An electrode in the middle of the strip will record R and S waves of equal amplitude.

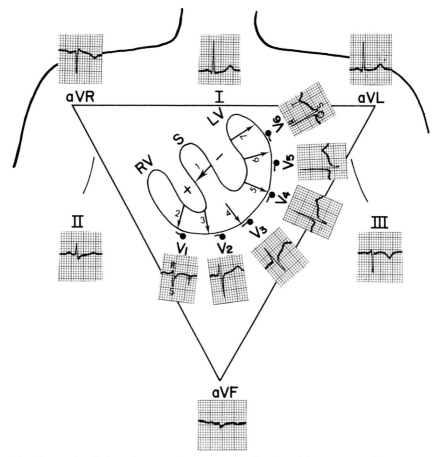

Fig 3–3. Vectors 1 to 7 show the normal sequence of activation of the septum and ventricles. The 12 routine ECG leads are shown with a normal recorded ECG. RV = right ventricle; S = septum; LV = left ventricle.

aV_R; and lead III, between aV_F and aV_L. In view of these relationships, leads I and aV_L will often record almost similar complexes and lead III will record almost similar complexes to aV_F. Lead II is equal to the sum of the potentials of leads I and III (Einthoven's equation). This can be used to check the accuracy of the electrode placement on the extremities. Figure 3–3 depicts a normal ECG with the heart in the horizontal position and the transitional zone in V_3.

The duration of the normal QRS is usually between 0.06 to 0.10 second, with an average of 0.08 second. The limb lead total QRS amplitude normally is usually over 5 mm, and in the precordial leads more than 10 mm. The upper limit of the R wave voltage is 30 mm in the adult. A normal Q wave width is 0.03 second or less, with a variable depth.

The ST segment is between the end of the QRS and the beginning of the T wave and usually in a normal person is at the baseline (isoelectric). The T wave represents the recovery phase (repolarization) and is shown in Figure 3–1. The T wave normally is upright in leads I and II and in V_3 through V_6. It is inverted in aV_R and variable in leads III, aV_L, and aV_F, and in V_1 and V_2. These T wave configurations are those seen in normal adults. The normal amplitude of the T wave in the limb leads varies from 1 to 5 mm, and in the precordial leads from 1 to 10 mm. The Q-T interval is measured from the beginning of the QRS complex to the end of the T wave. This interval varies according to the heart rate, sex, and age. The Q-T interval for various heart rates can be calculated by the following formula:

$$Q - T_c = \frac{Q - T \text{ (measured in sec)}}{\sqrt{R - R \text{ interval in sec}}}$$

It is considered abnormal if the Q-T interval is more than 0.42 sec. Ashman and Hull[1] have a table with measurements calculated to give the upper limits of normal of the Q-T interval. It may be very difficult to measure if the T wave is followed by a U wave. The Q-T interval is usually less than half the preceding R-R interval if there is normal sinus rhythm.

Each of the 12 routine ECG leads records potential variations of the whole heart and not just the electric potential of one localized area. However, the area facing an electrode does have considerable influence on the recording. The precordial leads (V_1 through V_6) record potential variations of the anterior surface of the heart, and leads II, III, and aV_F record those from the diaphragmatic or inferior surfaces. Leads I and aV_L record potential variations from the anterolateral surface of the heart. This information aids in localizing abnormalities such as, e.g., the area involved in acute myocardial infarctions.

The QRS axis depicts the heart's electric position in the frontal plane. The mean QRS vector can be drawn as an arrow to represent the mean QRS axis. The mean frontal plane QRS axis is normally between -30 and $+120$ degrees as plotted on the hexaxial reference system (Fig 3–4). Pathologic left axis is between -30 and -90 degrees, and pathologic right axis is between $+120$ and $+180$ degrees. The gray zone is between -90 and -180 degrees, which can indicate either extreme right or extreme left axis. The mean T wave axis normally is in the same direction as the QRS axis. If the angle between the QRS and T axes is greater than 50 degrees, then the tracing is abnormal.[2] The axes can be determined from the limb leads. On quick inspection one can locate the axis by the fact that the QRS complex or the T wave with the highest amplitude will have its mean vector parallel to the lead in which it is recorded. In addition, the QRS complex or T wave that is equiphasic or has the smallest deflection will have its mean vector perpendicular to the lead in which it is recorded. For example, the axes for the ECG of Figure 3–3 are calculated in

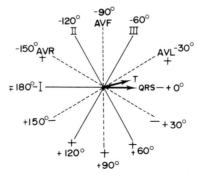

Fig 3–4. Hexaxial reference system used to determine the mean QRS and T axes in the frontal plane. The QRS and T axes shown were calculated from the normal ECG of Figure 3–3.

Figure 3–4. In Figure 3–3 the R wave is highest in lead I; therefore, the mean QRS vector should be near parallel to this lead and perpendicular to lead aV_F, where the R and S waves are almost equal and the total QRS deflection is small. The mean QRS axis is 0 degrees. The T wave amplitude is highest in leads I and aV_L; therefore, the mean T wave vector should be near parallel to these leads and is placed an equal distance between them. The mean T wave axis is −15 degrees. From the precordial lead transitional zone, one can determine whether these axes are pointing forward or backward. The angle between the mean QRS and T vectors is within normal range, 15 degrees.

MYOCARDIAL INFARCTION

To understand the current of injury, it is best to review normal depolarization and repolarization (Fig 3–5) in more detail than in Figure 3–2. When the muscle strip is at rest, the positive charges are on the outer surface of the cell membrane and the negative charges on the inside. This is the polarized state. With stimulation of the muscle cell, an electric current flows across the membrane, and the positive charges move inward and the negative charges to the outside surface. When the entire muscle is activated (depolarized), an R wave is recorded because positive charges are facing the epicardial electrode, and an electrode on the endocardial side records a Q wave. The activated muscle remains in the activated state at the baseline for a short time (ST segment),

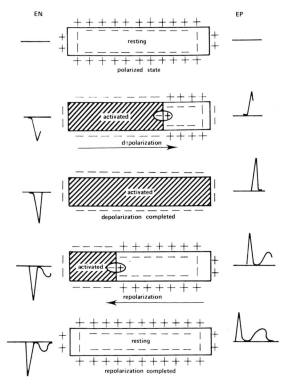

Fig 3–5. The potentials recorded by an endocardial (EN) and epicardial (EP) lead during depolarization and repolarization of a normal cardiac muscle fiber. See Text. (Modified from *Diagnostic Electrocardiography and Vectorcardiography*, ed. 2, by H.H. Friedman. Copyright © 1977 by McGraw-Hill, Inc. Used with the permission of McGraw-Hill Book Company.)

then repolarization occurs. Repolarization in cardiac muscle starts where depolarization ends (opposite direction of depolarization). The positive and negative charges are restored to their resting states. As repolarization occurs away from the epicardial electrode, an upright T wave is recorded, and an electrode facing its path on the endocardial surface records a negative T wave. When the epicardial portion of the muscle is injured (Fig 3–6), it is partially depolarized, the negative charges are on the outer surface, and the baseline is shifted downward (injury deflection) as recorded in the electrode facing that area. When this muscle is stimulated at the other end and activation begins, the positive charges on the endocardial surface will begin to move inward, the negative charges outward, and the epicardial lead starts to record an R wave, which begins from the injury deflection. With further activation the R wave goes toward the true baseline. Once depolarization arrives at the injured area and the whole segment is activated, the R wave returns to the true baseline. The activated muscle remains at this true baseline for a short time (ST segment), and then repolarization occurs with the T wave recorded in the epicardial lead ending at the injury deflection. The end result is a monophasic curve in which the ST segment elevation and the T wave are merged. This is referred to as a diastolic current of injury.[3] Therefore, this current of injury is actually TQ segment depression. However, this is not how it turns out in the ECG recording, for the current of injury is neutralized by a compensatory current

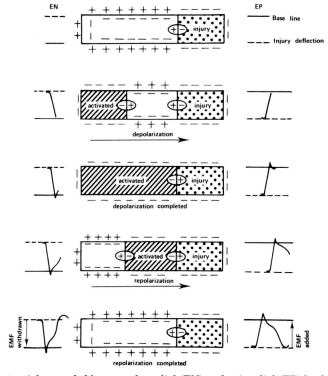

Fig 3–6. The potentials recorded by an endocardial (EN) and epicardial (EP) lead during depolarization and repolarization of a cardiac muscle fiber with subepicardial injury. See Text. EMF = electromotive force. (Modified from Barker J.M.: *The Unipolar Electrocardiogram.* New York, Appleton-Century-Crofts, Inc., 1952. Used by permission.)

(EMF) from the ECG (by the capacitor-coupled amplifier), the baseline is brought back automatically to the isoelectric, and thus the ST segment appears as elevation above the true baseline and not below (TQ). Another theory[4] (systolic current of injury) indicates that during activation, injured partially depolarized cells do not have further excitation or show early repolarization producing a true ST segment shift above the baseline. A combination of both mechanisms (systolic and diastolic current of injury) is thought to produce the ST segment elevation.[5] However, a more recent study suggests that the diastolic current plays the major role.[6] As expected, an electrode at the endocardial surface will show ST depression.

The following three facts can be helpful clinically in understanding the ECG changes in myocardial infarction and other causes of injury and myocardial damage: (1) An electrode facing necrotic muscle will record a Q wave, since the impulse is traveling away from the dead area through the contralateral healthy muscle. (2) An electrode subtending a current of injury will record ST elevation. (3) An electrode facing healthy muscle with a current of injury on the opposite side will record an R wave and ST segment depression. Figure 3–7 diagrammatically depicts these findings. Therefore, in an acute anterior wall myocardial infarction the precordial leads V_1 through V_6 (depending on the extent of the infarct) facing dead tissue and an acute current of injury will record Q waves and ST elevation. These changes when present in the V_1, V_2, and V_3 positions indicate an anteroseptal myocardial infarction; in V_3 and V_4, midanterior; and in V_4, V_5, and V_6, positions anterolateral. An anterolateral infarction also may show changes in leads I and aV_L. The healthy area on the opposite side of the anterior infarction will record R waves such as in leads II, III, and aV_F. However, since these electrodes have good muscle between them and the current of injury on the opposite side, their recordings will show ST

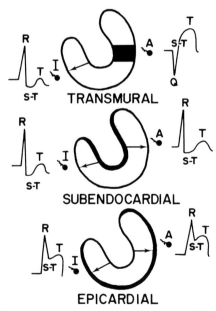

Fig 3–7. Diagrammatic illustration of changes in acute myocardial infarction (transmural and subendocardial) and in epicardial injury.

depression. This reciprocal ST depression occurs in the very early stage of an infarction and is usually transient, whereas the ST elevation over the injured area persists longer. The significance of precordial ST depression during an acute inferior infarction and of the inferior ST depression during an acute anterior infarction has created much debate. One study suggested that the ST depression in the precordial leads (V_1 to V_4) in the presence of an inferior infarction can indicate ischemia due to significant left anterior descending disease.[7] However, other studies indicate that the ST segment depression is related to the severity of the ischemia of the infarct-related artery and not to disease in the noninfarct-related arteries.[8,9] Figure 3–8 depicts the findings in an acute anterior infarction. A diaphragmatic or inferior wall infarction will show Q waves with ST elevation in leads II, III, and aV_F and R waves and ST segment depression in the precordial leads (Fig 3–9). Right ventricular infarction can be detected in the ECG when there is ST segment elevation in the right precordial lead V_4R. In one study, the sensitivity was 82.7%, specificity 76.9%, positive predictive value 70%, and negative predictive value 87.7% in 58 patients documented by autopsy, radionuclide studies or a combination of these with echocardiography or hemodynamic monitoring.[10] Since right ventricular infarction is most often associated with an inferior infarction, V_4R should be recorded routinely in such cases. Strictly posterior myocardial infarction occurs up near the base of the heart (not the same as an inferior). The only lead that may show this damage is V_1, in which the R wave may become tall, slurred, and often wide. An esophageal lead may show a Q wave. In such cases a vectorcardiogram may be helpful. Subendocardial infarctions will re-

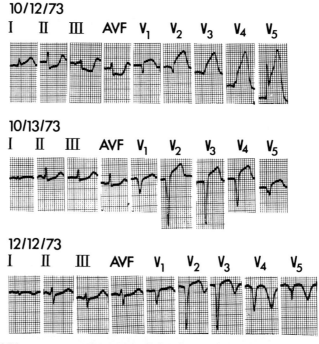

Fig 3–8. 10/12/73—acute anterior myocardial infarction. 10/13/73—less ST elevation. 12/12/73—evolutionary changes, ST segments isoelectric and T waves inverted (coved) in leads V_2 to V_5.

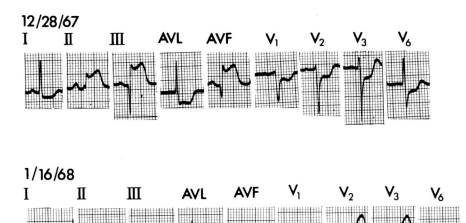

Fig 3–9. 12/28/67—acute inferior (diaphragmatic) infarction. 1/16/68—evolutionary changes, ST segments isoelectric and T waves inverted (coved) in leads II, III, and aVF.

cord R waves, but they may be of decreased amplitude. In such cases the electrodes are opposite healthy muscle, but there is a current of injury on the opposite side; therefore, these will record ST segment depression (see Fig 3–7). When there is only epicardial injury, depending on the extent, the electrodes in all leads except aV_R and at times V_1 will be facing a current of injury and will record ST segment elevation (see Fig 3–7). Usually when there is diffuse ST elevation, pericarditis is considered rather than an epicardial injury of an infarction. The latter is most often localized. When an infarction follows its normal evolutionary course, the ST segments will return to the baseline, and the T waves will become inverted or coved. These findings are usually noted within one week. The Q waves most often remain; however, the T waves may eventually become upright. If the ST segment elevation persists for months, then a ventricular aneurysm should be considered. Often tracings of myocardial infarction are seen where there are abnormal Q waves followed by late R waves. These tracings also may show widened QRS complexes. The late R waves indicate activation of healthy muscle which is depolarized late and is facing the electrode.

It is often difficult to make a diagnosis of infarction of the free left ventricular wall in the presence of a left bundle-branch block, since septal activation is reversed. The abnormal right-to-left septal activation will show R waves in the precordial leads instead of the expected Q waves, as are seen when electrodes face necrotic tissue (Fig 3–10).

There are at least 100 noncardiac situations reported that are associated with ECG patterns that may simulate changes seen with acute myocardial infarction secondary to coronary disease. The majority of these have emphasized ST segment and T wave changes.[11] However, there are many causes other than myocardial infarction that also will produce Q waves in addition to ST and T changes. Several of these are shown in Figures 3–11 and 3–12. The

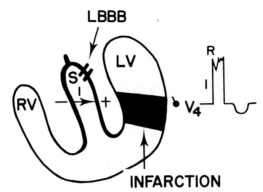

Fig 3–10. Left bundle-branch block and transmural myocardial infarction of the free left ventricular wall. The abnormal right to left septal activation produces an R wave in V_4 and obscures the expected Q wave.

following causes (proved at autopsy) produced the changes seen in Figure 3–11:

A. Acute diffuse myocarditis in a 76-year-old man
B. Viral myocarditis in an 11-month-old girl
C. A 2 cm gastric ulcer in the supradiaphragmatic area eroding into the inferior myocardial surface, penetrating the posterior descending branch of the right coronary artery with active bleeding from this artery in a 63-year-old woman
D. Bacterial endocarditis with a septic embolism to the right coronary artery in a 9-year-old girl
E. Periarteritis nodosa with rupture of the myocardium in a 61-year-old woman
F. Cerebellar pontine angle tumor (neurilemmoma of the acoustic nerve) in a 56-year-old woman
G. Angioendothelial sarcoma (of Kaposi) of right AV origin, with formation of a right coronary artery to right atrial fistula and with occlusion of the midportion of the right coronary artery by this tumor in a 52-year-old woman

The ECGs in cases A, C, D, and G simulate an inferior myocardial infarction and that of B an anterior infarction. Cases E and F simulate an apical infarction (anterior and inferior). Autopsies in these cases showed no evidence of significant coronary atherosclerosis. Figure 3–12 shows two cases of the Wolff-Parkinson-White syndrome (see Chapter 15) that simulated inferior infarctions.

VENTRICULAR HYPERTROPHY

Unfortunately, there are no specific criteria for ventricular hypertrophy. This is particularly true for left ventricular hypertrophy. Many criteria give false-positive or false-negative results when correlated with autopsy reports. If there is right ventricular hypertrophy, the R wave amplitude should be increased to the right in the V_1 and V_2 positions; and if there is left ventricular hypertrophy, the R wave amplitude should be increased to the left in the V_4

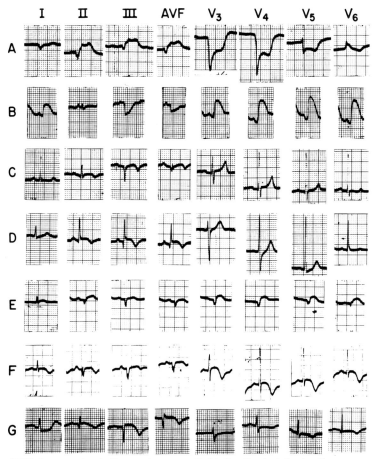

Fig 3–11. ECG changes simulating acute myocardial infarction but due to other causes (see text).

through V_6 positions. Associated with these R wave increments, there should be ST-T changes (opposite in direction to the mean QRS vector) due to the strain or ischemic changes secondary to the hypertrophy. The voltage criteria of Sokolow and Lyons for left ventricular hypertrophy include $R_1 + S_{III}$ equal or greater than 25 mm; R in AVL greater than 12 mm; R in AVF greater than 20 mm; S in V_1 equal or greater than 24 mm; R in V_5 or V_6 greater than 26 mm; and S in $V_1 + R$ in V_5 or V_6 greater than 35 mm.[12] Increased QRS voltage criteria alone for the diagnosis of left ventricular hypertrophy are nonspecific, since the voltages can vary with the shape and diameter of the chest and body build in general. Diagnosis is more specific if there are associated ST-T changes (opposite in direction to the mean QRS vector) especially in the absence of cardiac drugs. I prefer the Romhilt and Estes[13] point system for diagnosis of left ventricular hypertrophy, which is as follows:

1. 3 points if the largest S wave in V_1 or V_2 or if the largest R wave in V_5 or V_6 is 30 mm or more, or if the largest R or S wave in the limb leads is 20 mm or more
2. 3 points for ST-T changes
   1 point for ST-T changes with digitalis

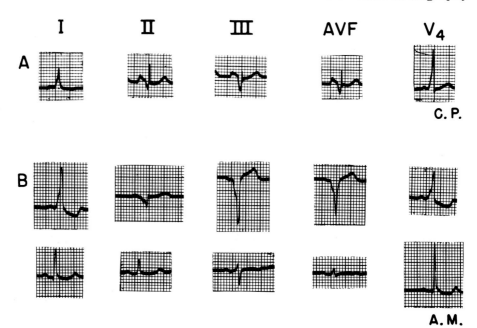

Fig 3–12. **A,** Wolff-Parkinson-White syndrome simulating an inferior infarction. **B,** Wolff-Parkinson-White syndrome simulating an inferior infarction. With normal conduction (bottom tracing) these findings have cleared.

3. 2 points for axis deviation of −30 degrees or more to the left
4. 1 point if the QRS interval is 0.09 second or more or if the intrinsicoid deflection in V_5 or V_6 is 0.05 second or more (this is the time interval measured from the beginning of the QRS to a perpendicular line drawn from the peak of the R wave to the baseline)
5. 3 points if left atrial enlargement is present in the absence of mitral disease (terminal negativity of the P wave in V_1 of 1 mm or more in depth and 0.04 second or more in duration).

Four points indicate probable left ventricular hypertrophy, and five or more definite left ventricular hypertrophy. Echocardiographic and anatomic studies show a sensitivity of about 50% for the Romhilt-Estes point system and about 25% for the Sokolow-Lyons voltage criteria.[12,13] Both have a specificity of about 95%.[14] An example of left ventricular hypertrophy is seen in the diagrammatic drawing of Figure 3–13.

In right ventricular hypertrophy, the R wave is increased in height in the right precordial leads with an R:S ratio of greater than 1.0. The QRS configuration in V_1 at times can give a clue to the diagnosis. A qR complex indicates that the right ventricular pressure exceeds that in the left as seen with pulmonary hypertension or severe pulmonic stenosis, especially if the R remains tall in V_2 and V_3; R or rR suggests that the pressure in the right and left ventricle is equal as noted with tetralogy of Fallot (R in V_2 usually is smaller); and rsR^1 suggests that right ventricular pressure is lower than left as noted with an atrial septal defect. Deep S waves in V_5 and V_6 (R:S ratio equal or less than 1.0) are usually associated with these findings. The limb leads usually will record right axis of +110 degrees or more. A diagrammatic drawing of

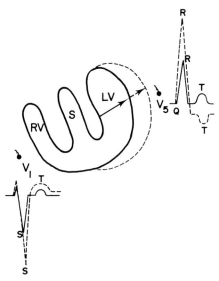

Fig 3–13. Left ventricular hypertrophy shown diagrammatically. Dotted lines show the ECG changes of increased R wave amplitude in V_5 with ST-T changes and deep S waves in V_1. Solid lines superimposed show a normal tracing. RV = right ventricle; S = septum; LV = left ventricle.

right ventricular hypertrophy is seen in Figure 3–14. In the presence of right bundle-branch block, it is difficult to make a diagnosis of right ventricular hypertrophy. However, left ventricular hypertrophy can be detected in the presence of right bundle-branch block. Left bundle-branch block obscures the hypertrophy patterns of both ventricles.

ATRIAL ENLARGEMENT

Atrial enlargement may produce ECG changes because of dilatation, hypertrophy, or disease of the atrial wall. In right atrial enlargement, the P waves are tall and pointed in leads II, III, aV_F, and occasionally in V_1. The P wave

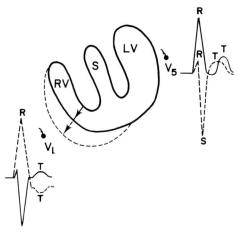

Fig 3–14. Right ventricular hypertrophy shown diagrammatically. Dotted lines show the ECG changes of increased R wave amplitude in V_1 with ST-T changes and deep S waves in V_5. Solid lines superimposed show a normal tracing. RV = right ventricle; S = septum; LV = left ventricle.

amplitude is usually 2.5 mm or more. However, there may be pseudo–right atrial enlargement due to rotations of the heart and chest deformities. In left atrial enlargement the P waves are wider than 0.12 second (usually in leads I, II, and aV_L), or its terminal component below the baseline (representing left atrial activation) is prominently negative in the V_1 position. In the V_1 position, this terminal component should be 1 mm or more in depth and 0.04 second or more in width prior to considering left atrial enlargement. Figure 3–15 shows drawings of right and left atrial enlargement.

BUNDLE-BRANCH BLOCK

Depolarization of the septum and ventricles produces a QRS average width of 0.08 second. Hypertrophies of the ventricles and myocardial damage can produce some prolongation of the QRS complexes. When the QRS complexes measure 0.1 second or more, bundle-branch block should be considered. Bundle-branch block patterns can be described in simple terms. If the right bundle is blocked (Fig 3–16), the septum will still be depolarized normally to give an initial R wave in V_1 and a Q wave in V_5 (vector 1). Next, activation of the left ventricle (vector 2) will produce an S wave in V_1 and an R wave in V_5, and then conduction to the right ventricle will occur late (vector 3) because the impulse is now outside of conducting tissue and traveling through muscle. This late activation of the right ventricle will give a slurred terminal R' in the V_1 position and a terminal slurred S wave in the V_5 position. On the other hand, if left bundle-branch block is present, there will be a delay of forces activating the left ventricle and slurring of the terminal R' in the left ventricle leads, namely, V_4, V_5, or V_6 (Fig 3–17). Since the septal activation is from right to left, there are usually Q waves in the right precordial leads. However, at times right ventricular apical activation may give small R waves in these leads. Often a full left bundle-branch block can be preceded by an incomplete left bundle which shows an absence of the initial septal vector and a QRS width between 0.10 and 0.12 sec. This can simulate an old anteroseptal infarction. Left bundle-branch block most often has ST-T changes in opposite directions from that of the QRS. At times the ST segment may be isoelectric and the T wave concordant with the QRS vector (so-called primary T-wave changes). This was once considered an indication of a myocardial abnormality independent of the left bundle-branch block, but the correlation has been poor. Left bundle branch block is often associated with a normal QRS axis. At times there

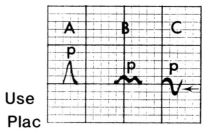

Use
Plac

Fig 3–15. Atrial enlargement shown diagrammatically. **A,** right atrial enlargement. Pointed P waves of 3 mm (leads II, III, and aV_F). **B,** left atrial enlargement. P width of 0.12 sec and notched (usually leads I, II, and aV_L). **C,** left atrial enlargement. Terminal component (*arrow*) of the P wave below the baseline representing left atrial activation with a depth of 1 mm and a duration of 0.04 sec (V_1).

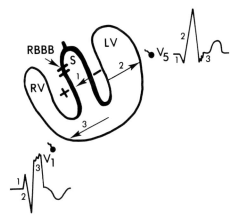

Fig 3–16. Right bundle-branch block (RBBB) shown diagrammatically. Vectors (1 to 3) show sequence of activation. RV = right ventricle; S = septum; LV = left ventricle.

may be associated left or right axes which have no clear explanation. Many of the patients have cardiomyopathy. The combination of left bundle-branch block and left axis is often associated with myocardial dysfunction, more advanced disease of the conducting system, and earlier mortality.[15] At times the limb leads resemble left bundle-branch block and the precordial leads right bundle-branch block. In the past this often was referred to as "masquerading" bundle-branch block. Such tracings probably indicate a right bundle-branch block with a left anterior fascicular block. Bundle-branch blocks can be rate-related. Most often they occur with a rapid rate (critical rate), but rarely they can occur with a slow rate ("bradycardia-dependent"). The slow type is referred to as phase 4 action potential phenomenon, but this has no clear cut explanation. The hemiblock syndromes are described in Chapter 15.

THE ST SEGMENT AND THE T WAVE

There are many causes of ST or T wave changes, as presented later in this chapter. The interpreter should be aware of the clinical findings. However, if this information is not available, the configuration of the ST segment and T

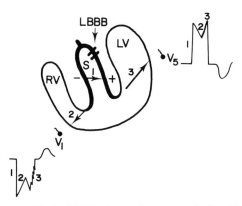

Fig 3–17. Left bundle-branch block (LBBB) shown diagrammatically. Vectors (1 to 3) show sequence of activation. RV = right ventricle; S = septum; LV = left ventricle.

wave may suggest a cause. Figures 3–18 and 3–19 describe some of these features. The ST elevation of early repolarization is concave upward, up to 5 mm in many leads, especially the right precordial leads. It is often a normal finding in blacks. The ST segment of epicardial injury is frequently convex downward. This is seen in the early phase of an acute myocardial infarction, and in such cases is often localized. It is most often diffuse in acute pericarditis. Subendocardial injury produces a flat, sagging, horizontal type of ST segment depression, which can occur transiently with angina or as the initial finding of a subendocardial infarction. The ST segment depression characteristic of digitalis has a cup-shaped, scooped-out appearance or may resemble "Dick Tracy's" chin. A long QT interval with sagging ST depression and T wave inversion is seen with hypokalemia, quinidine, cerebral lesions, tricyclic antidepressants, congenital heart disease, ischemic heart disease, and phenothiazines, and in some cases of mitral valve prolapse. In such cases the base of the T wave is widened. This accounts for most of the Q-T interval prolongation. Strain patterns are usually associated with hypertrophy of the ventricles. Subendocardial ischemia will produce tall, upright T waves but not as peaked as those seen with hyperkalemia. In addition, the base of the T wave is narrow with hyperkalemia and the Q-T interval is shortened. Hypercalcemia produces a short Q-T interval, with the proximal limb of the T wave ascending abruptly. Digitalis also shortens the Q-T interval. Hypocalcemia is characterized by a prolonged Q-T interval with an upright or inverted T wave. The prolongation of the Q-T interval is due to the ST segment, since the T base is narrow. Subepicardial ischemia produces a pointed or coved inverted T wave.

Other ECG findings will be discussed with cardiac problems as these come up in subsequent chapters. The ECG features of arrhythmias are described in Chapter 15.

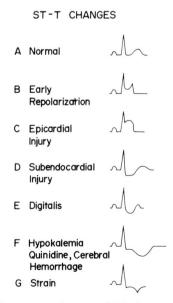

ST-T CHANGES

A Normal

B Early Repolarization

C Epicardial Injury

D Subendocardial Injury

E Digitalis

F Hypokalemia Quinidine, Cerebral Hemorrhage

G Strain

Fig 3–18. Diagrammatic configurations of various ST-T changes.

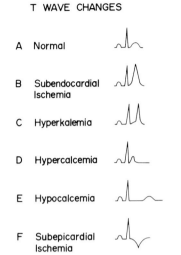

T WAVE CHANGES

A   Normal

B   Subendocardial Ischemia

C   Hyperkalemia

D   Hypercalcemia

E   Hypocalcemia

F   Subepicardial Ischemia

Fig 3-19. Diagrammatic configurations of various T wave changes.

HOW TO UNDERSTAND ELECTROCARDIOGRAPHIC INTERPRETATIONS

The two greatest hazards of an ECG report are the interpreter's overreading of a tracing and the physician's failure to understand the interpretation. I have often wondered what an ECG report means to the physician receiving it. Not only do reports vary among interpreters depending on their training and locale, the information provided about the patient, and so on; but the same individual on different occasions may give different interpretations of the same tracing.

Some interpreters use confusing terminology. Obviously this puzzles the physician, who cannot understand the report unless he communicates with the interpreter and gives the proper information. Unfortunately, physicians lean heavily on the ECG report, which, if misleading, can create problems in diagnosis and therapy, with psychological, social, and economic consequences. This section will explain the meaning and importance of common interpretations.

Axis deviation. This term is used to designate the heart's electric activity in the frontal plane. The mean QRS axis should be expressed in degrees and is normally between -30 and $+120$ degrees. The axis can be normal in the presence of definite evidence of heart disease. Left-axis deviation recently has assumed more importance. Left-axis deviation[16] is present when the mean electric axis is between $+30$ and -90 degrees. A deviation to the left of -30 degrees or more is usually abnormal. This abnormality is most often due to block or delay in the left anterosuperior fascicle of the left bundle (left anterior hemiblock) and can be caused by many conditions. A list of the more common organic causes follows:

1. Nonspecific fibrosis or sclerodegenerative changes of the conducting system[17,18]
2. Acute and chronic coronary artery disease
3. Left ventricular hypertrophy and left bundle-branch block

4. Congenital heart disease (ostium primum atrial septal defects, ventricular septal defects, tricuspid atresia)
5. Myocardial disease (cardiomyopathy, myocarditis)
6. Hyperkalemia
7. Wolff-Parkinson-White syndrome
8. Surgically induced

A shift of axis of −30 degrees or more is rarely due to abnormal anatomical position of the heart as can occur with chest deformities or with a very high diaphragm. Although not clearly understood, left axis of this degree can be seen with pulmonary emphysema (so-called pseudo−left axis).

Right-axis deviation[16] is present when the axis is between +90 and −90 degrees. In adults, right-axis deviation of +110 degrees or more to the right is abnormal. The following are the most common causes:

1. Right ventricular hypertrophy (congenital heart lesions, cor pulmonale, mitral stenosis)
2. Chronic lung disease with or without cor pulmonale
3. Acute myocardial infarction
4. Pulmonary embolism (especially if the right axis is transient)
5. Block or delay in the posteroinferior branch of the left bundle (left posterior hemiblock)
6. Dextrocardia
7. Factitious, due to reversal of the right and left arm leads
8. Wolff-Parkinson-White syndrome

Chest deformities such as pectus excavatum may produce an axis of greater than +110 degrees.

Left bundle-branch block. This is usually reported as complete or incomplete depending on the QRS width. If the QRS is between 0.10 and 0.12 seconds in width, the term incomplete is used, and if it is over 0.12 seconds, the term complete is used. Actually, it would be best not to use the term complete, since over the years the QRS width in a patient with complete bundle-branch block may increase from 0.12 second. The plain term left bundle-branch block can cover all degrees of block. Left bundle-branch block is usually attributed to the following:

1. Coronary artery disease
2. Hypertensive cardiovascular disease
3. Cardiomyopathy
4. Rheumatic heart disease
5. Nonspecific fibrosis
6. Aortic valvular disease
7. Trauma
8. Myocarditis

Rarely, apparently healthy persons have isolated left bundle-branch block without demonstrable cardiovascular disease.[19] The cause of left bundle-branch block in these apparently healthy persons is not clear, and the disorder is rarely congenital. Perhaps it is a degenerative fibrotic process involving the aortic sinuses; pars membranacea septi interventricularis cordis; summit of the ventricular septum, central fibrous body, and mitral annulus (sclerosis of the left side of the cardiac skeleton); or myocarditis in a small critical area at the origin of the left bundle before its bifurcation. Often a diagnosis of coronary artery disease is made, but coronary arteriograms for many of these patients are normal.

The etiologic factors are usually the same in both transient and fixed forms of complete or incomplete left bundle-branch block. Complete AV block can develop in some of these patients, since it is commonly caused by bilateral bundle-branch block.

The prognosis for patients with left bundle-branch block without demonstrable associated heart disease is better than for those with heart disease. In the latter, the prognosis depends on the associated type of disease, not on the conduction defect.[20]

Right bundle-branch block. This is associated with such disorders as:

1. Coronary artery disease
2. Hypertensive cardiovascular disease
3. Rheumatic heart disease
4. Congenital heart disease
5. Myocarditis
6. Pulmonary embolism (transient)
7. Cor pulmonale
8. Nonspecific fibrosis
9. Cardiomyopathy
10. Trauma

Right bundle-branch block may occur either as an isolated congenital anomaly or asymptomatically without other abnormalities. These two latter types are seen more often in patients with right bundle-branch block than in those with left bundle-branch block, and the prognosis is better in the former. Incomplete right bundle-branch pattern may be due to a heritable focal hypertrophy of the right ventricle rather than to delayed conduction within the right bundle branch.[21]

Hemiblock. This is a term that Rosenbaum et al.[17] used to explain intermittent conduction block in the anterior superior (left anterior hemiblock) and posterior inferior (left posterior hemiblock) divisions (fascicles) of the left bundle branch. Hemiblock is of great importance when associated with right bundle-branch block, because this combination may be the forerunner of bilateral bundle-branch block, which leads to advanced and third-degree AV conduction disturbances (trifascicular blocks). Hemiblocks and bundle-branch blocks derive from the same causes.

Left ventricular hypertrophy. This is a frequent ECG interpretation and does not always correlate with the evidence found clinically, roentgenographically, echocardiographically, or at autopsy. Its identification by ECG is not simple, because many criteria may be used.[13,22] Highly sensitive criteria lead to overdiagnosis, especially in young patients. Other criteria sacrifice sensitivity for increased specificity.

Left ventricular hypertrophy usually indicates changes secondary to the following:

1. Hypertension
2. Aortic valvular disease
3. Mitral insufficiency
4. Cardiomyopathies
5. Congenital heart disease

Cabrera and Monroy[23] used the term systolic overload to describe hypertrophy secondary to a resistant load, such as in aortic stenosis, and the term diastolic overload to describe hypertrophy secondary to volume overload, such as in aortic insufficiency. They used these terms in an attempt to correlate ECG alterations with hemodynamic and anatomical changes. Systolic overloading of the left ventricle shows the typical left ventricular hypertrophy pattern, whereas diastolic overloading shows increased R wave amplitude in V_5 and V_6, with very prominent upright T waves in these leads.

Left atrial hypertrophy or enlargement. This is often associated with left ventricular hypertrophy. As an isolated ECG finding, left atrial hypertrophy may be the clue to mitral stenosis or insufficiency (P mitrale). Left atrial enlargement can result from left ventricular dysfunction that is associated with an increase in left ventricular end-diastolic pressure, which increases the resistance to left atrial emptying.

Left ventricular strain. This is a term that has been used extensively but has not been generally accepted because of its mechanical rather than electric implication. ST-T changes often are present without voltage increase, and this alone does not fulfill most criteria for left ventricular hypertrophy. These findings should be designated as nonspecific ST-T changes, since other findings must be known to clarify their significance.

Right ventricular hypertrophy. This is usually associated with the following:

1. Congenital heart disease (pulmonary stenosis, tetralogy of Fallot, pulmonary hypertension)
2. Mitral stenosis (especially if associated with left atrial hypertrophy)
3. Cor pulmonale

Right ventricular hypertrophy is usually interpreted most accurately when it is due to congenital heart disease, less accurately when it is due to mitral stenosis or cor pulmonale, and least accurately when it is secondary to left heart failure. Systolic overload refers to a resistance to the ejection of blood during systole, such as in pulmonary stenosis or pulmonary hypertension, whereas diastolic overload refers to an increased volume of blood during diastole, such as in atrial septal defect.[23] Systolic overloading of the right ventricle shows the typical right ventricular hypertrophy pattern, whereas diastolic overloading shows the pattern of complete or incomplete right bundle-branch block due to hypertrophy of the basal area of the right ventricle.[24]

S_1, S_2, S_3 **syndrome.** This is often reported and can be seen in the following:

1. Normal variant
2. Right ventricular enlargement in congenital or acquired heart disease

3. Emphysema with or without cor pulmonale
4. Myocardial infarction

Right atrial hypertrophy or enlargement. This is commonly associated with right ventricular hypertrophy, such as in congenital heart disease or in cor pulmonale. Often as an isolated finding right atrial hypertrophy is referred to as P pulmonale. Pseudo P pulmonale can occur in some patients with pure left heart disease with no specific reason.[25] The P waves may be tall and notched in tricuspid valvular disease.

Biventricular hypertrophy. This is most often diagnosed by electrocardiography when the cause is a congenital heart lesion, such as ventricular septal defect, and less often when the cause is acquired heart disease.

Nonspecific T waves. These are frequent interpretations used by many and may or may not be important. The interpreter, lacking clinical and laboratory data, usually will describe T wave changes as nonspecific. This term is vague and annoying to some, but I would rather use it than diagnose ischemic changes due to coronary artery disease from the findings shown in the tracing alone.

Levine[11] has listed 67 causes for T wave changes. The T waves can be affected by the following factors that affect cellular metabolism:

1. Primary or secondary cardiac disease
2. Physiologic stimuli (e.g., anxiety, hyperventilation, posture, cold, eating, exercise)
3. Pharmacologic agents (quinidine, procainamide, digitalis, diuretics, tranquilizers, antidepressants)
4. Reversible noncardiac disease (electrolyte disturbances, anemia, uremia, acute abdominal lesions, hypothyroidism, shock, cerebrovascular lesions)

Many of these causes often can be excluded, and the changes can be considered normal variants, as in the juvenile pattern (persistent T wave inversion in the right precordial leads), or due to physiologic stimuli. Changes resulting from the latter can be clarified by a repeated ECG after standing, hyperventilating, fasting, ingesting glucose or potassium, or receiving atropine or propranolol.

Inverted T waves often are erroneously interpreted as due to coronary heart disease, a diagnosis that can produce a catastrophic effect on a patient's life, with psychologic, social, and economic consequences. Although the terms myocardial ischemia and coronary insufficiency are often used in an ECG report, they should be accepted only when they have been evaluated in conjunction with findings other than those of T wave changes alone. The appearance of the T waves may suggest to the interpreter a specific cause, but the interpretation should be made only after consideration of all other data.

Nonspecific ST changes. ST changes with or without T wave changes also are often reported as nonspecific. These changes can be associated with the same conditions noted for the nonspecific T waves.

Positive exercise stress test. The diagnostic accuracy of the exercise ECG test in detecting coronary artery disease has recently been questioned, especially since it may produce many false-positives in the female.[26] In addition, positive tests can occur in other forms of heart disease, such as the cardiomyopathies. False-positive test results can occur with digitalis therapy, autonomic changes, and the Wolff-Parkinson-White syndrome, and interpretation is difficult in the presence of left ventricular hypertrophy and left bundle-branch block.

Exercise responses often are reported as positive, suspicious, or negative. Angina pectoris is a clinical diagnosis, and the ECG changes should be used as an adjunct to the clinical findings, particularly in patients with atypical symptoms. A suspicious test result is even more confusing and should be evaluated in conjunction with other findings. A negative test result does not exclude coronary artery disease. The greatest difference of opinion among interpreters is on evaluating results of exercise stress tests. It may be best if the interpreter described only the exercise and postexercise changes, rather than giving a specific diagnosis.

Much has been written about the sensitivity (percent of patients with documented coronary artery disease having an abnormal stress test), specificity (percent of negative results in subjects without disease), and predictive accuracy (percent of positive results that are true positives). Bayes's theorem, as was emphasized by Rifkin and Hood,[27] states that a test cannot be adequately interpreted without reference to the disease (pretest) in the population, even though the reliability of diagnostic tests is based on the sensitivity and specificity.

Junctional S-T depression. This is frequently a normal finding, often seen with sinus tachycardia after an exercise stress test or similar activity.

Early repolarization. This is a normal variant that is often reported in the black subject.[28] It can simulate the injury potential of acute pericarditis or myocardial infarction. The clinical picture, enzyme values, and serial ECG findings should establish the correct diagnosis.

Acute pericarditis. This is usually reported in the following conditions:

1. Infections (bacterial, viral, fungal)
2. Rheumatic
3. Collagen-type diseases (rheumatoid arthritis, lupus)
4. With myocardial infarction, dissecting aneurysm, or postinfarction syndrome
5. Malignancies
6. Uremia
7. Trauma
8. Drug use (procainamide, hydralazine)

Seldom do the acute ECG changes of pericarditis occur with tuberculous pericarditis. Tuberculous pericarditis occurs insidiously, and most often is seen in the evolving stage.

Low voltage. This is seen with the following:

1. Pericardial effusion
2. Constrictive pericarditis
3. Anasarca
4. Ascites
5. Pneumopericardium
6. Pleural effusion

   7. Emphysema
   8. Myocardial disease
   9. Myxedema
  10. Obesity
  11. Diffuse ischemic disease
  12. Drug use—Adriamycin (doxorubicin)

Myocardial infarction. This is an ECG interpretation which often is of considerable clinical diagnostic assistance. However, it must be realized that many other lesions can give ECG changes which simulate those of an infarction (see Figs 3–11 and 3–12), such as brain lesions, myocarditis, tumors of the heart, Wolff-Parkinson-White syndrome, pulmonary embolism, hypokalemia, muscular dystrophy, and hypertrophic cardiomyopathy. These and many other conditions can simulate infarction; therefore, knowledge of the patient is of the utmost importance.

The interpreter may indicate the site of the infarction as subepicardial, transmural, intramural, or subendocardial. Further localization is designated as anteroseptal, midanterior, anterolateral, high lateral, diaphragmatic or inferior, inferolateral, apical, strictly posterior, or posterobasal. At times such localization of an infarction is useful. For instance, in an inferior infarction we anticipate AV heart block, since the right coronary artery supplying the inferior surface of the heart also supplies the main branch of the AV node in 90% of patients. The SA node is supplied by the right coronary artery or the left circumflex in approximately equal numbers. This branch arises near the origin of these vessels; therefore, when it is involved, the occlusion is proximal, producing a rather large lesion. These patients are prone to atrial arrhythmias, namely, atrial fibrillation or flutter.

An interpretation of left bundle-branch block does not rule out an infarction, because this condition often obscures the ECG features of infarction.

If the initial tracing is normal, serial ECGs should be taken, because changes may take days to appear. Evolutionary changes can occur over hours, days, weeks, months, or even years. These evolutionary stages are designated as acute, subacute, evolving, healing, or old. They can be obscured by many factors, especially cardiac drugs, old myocardial infarctions, and repeated episodes of coronary insufficiency. The tracings do not provide much information about functional recovery and should not be the determinants for the speed and degree of mobilization of the patient or the duration of hospital stay. It is hazardous to predict the outcome of a patient on the basis of the ECGs. It is misleading to designate an infarction as massive or small by an ECG. A patient with a clinically severe infarction may have a tracing that is atypical, borderline, or even normal. Emphasis should be placed on the clinical setting and not on the ECG alone. Often a patient with chest pain is delayed at home in order to obtain a tracing. This practice should be discouraged, since cardiac arrest often occurs during the first 2 hours of the onset of an infarction.

After an infarction, the tracing can return to normal. In one study, 21 of 480 consecutive patients were found to have normal resting ECGs associated with complete or nearly complete occlusion of one or more major coronary vessels.[29] Others have noted disappearance of the ECG features of necrosis in 12% of 775 patients with healed infarction.[30] The explanation may be viable muscle surrounding the scarred area, or the infarction may have occurred in an area not contributing to the genesis of the ECG. At times a routine tracing has the features of an old infarction, yet the patient cannot recall attacks (silent infarct).

Ventricular aneurysm. This may be suspected by the interpreter when the ECGs show persistent changes of acute myocardial infarction. However, other factors can be responsible for persistent ST elevation in an infarction, such as cardiac drugs or superimposed bouts of coronary insufficiency. Rarely, tumors of the heart can produce such changes.

Ischemia. This is a frequently used term with many connotations. As indicated previously, there are many causes for T wave changes besides coronary artery disease. This interpretation therefore should take into account clinical findings and other laboratory findings.

Electrolyte imbalance. This can be due to hypokalemia, hyperkalemia, hypocalcemia, hypercalcemia, or hypomagnesemia. The ECG may give the first clue to its presence.

Digitalis effect. This usually refers to the ST changes, does not signify toxicity, and does not correlate with degree of digitalization or with clinical results.

Dextrocardia. This is most often detected by electrocardiography. The electrocardiographer must not confuse this with reversal of the right and left arm leads. It is frequently a normal variation when associated with situs inversus. When it exists as an isolated finding, it is usually associated with a serious congenital heart lesion.

Electric alternans. This is less common than pulsus alternans, but usually has the same significance, being associated with left ventricular failure. It also can be seen with pericardial effusion, hypertension, digitalis intoxication, and various other conditions.

Preexcitation syndromes (Wolff-Parkinson-White, Lown-Ganong-Levine, Mahaim). All three of these syndromes have accessory pathways that bypass the AV node.[31] The Wolff-Parkinson-White syndrome (WPW) is the most common; its accessory pathway is from the atria to the ventricles (Types A and B). Patients may have recurrent attacks of arrhythmias, especially supraventricular. Often there is no evidence of other cardiac disease, but at times it can be associated with a congenital heart lesion such as Ebstein's anomaly. In the Lown-Ganong-Levine syndrome the bypass tract from the atria enters the lower AV node. Tachycardias can also occur in such patients. Mahaim tracts that connect the lower AV node or bundle of His to the ventricular myocardium are rare. It is not known how often tachycardias can occur with this type.

COMMON ARRHYTHMIA INTERPRETATIONS

Sinus tachycardia. This often occurs in a normal heart and represents a response to disease (infection, anemia, hyperthyroidism) or to a physiologic or pharmacologic stimulus.

Sinus bradycardia. This is frequently noted in or with the following:

1. Normal persons (especially athletes)
2. Pharmacologic agents (digitalis, morphine, β blockers)

3. Inferior infarction
4. Disease of SA node or atrium
5. Obstructive jaundice
6. Myxedema
7. Increased intracranial pressure

Sinus arrhythmia. This is caused by variations in the rate of discharge of the sinus node. It is associated with vagal tone and respirations. In the phasic variety, related to respirations, the heart rate increases with inspiration and slows with expiration. It is often a normal finding in children and young adults. In the elderly it is frequently associated with carotid sinus hypersensitivity.

Premature beats. These are common findings noted in routine ECGs. Depending on their site of origin, they are referred to as atrial, junctional, or ventricular (right or left ventricular origin can be determined). The term junctional is now used instead of nodal, since no pacemaker cells have been noted in the AV node proper. Studies have shown that cells producing automaticity are noted in the lower part of the AV node or at its junction with the common bundle and in the bundle.[32] The prevalence of both supraventricular (atrial and junctional) and ventricular ectopic beats increases with age. In the absence of other evidence of heart disease, they have been considered innocent. They may be precipitated by exercise, anxiety, caffeine beverages, alcohol, tobacco, fatigue, infection, or stimulating drugs. An epidemiologic study suggested that PVBs may not always be innocuous, but may be associated with an increased risk of coronary artery disease and sudden death in persons over 30 years of age.[33] Frequent PVBs, occurring in runs, multifocally, and early near the preceding normal conducted beat, may be associated with heart disease and may lead to more serious arrhythmias. Yet, such complex findings can occur in individuals with no evidence of cardiac disease and who can have a good long-term prognosis.[34] Premature ventricular beats originating from the left ventricle may be more serious than those whose site of origin is from the right ventricle.

Parasystole is a term used when PVBs of a similar contour appear with a varying interval in relation to the preceding normal conducted beat. The parasystolic focus is considered to be continuously active and protected. It has its own rate and does not appear when it finds the ventricles refractory because of stimulation by the sinus focus. At times it will arrive simultaneously with the sinus impulse to activate the ventricles and thus produce a fusion beat.

Premature atrial beats may occur early and be blocked or may find the ventricles partially refractory and so be aberrantly conducted.

Wandering or shifting SA pacemaker. This refers to the shifting of the pacemaker from the sinus node downward within the atrium to the junctional tissue, at times with intervening atrial fusion beats. This is seen most often in children and in elderly persons with fluctuating vagal tone. It is frequently a normal finding in the young, but can indicate heart disease in the elderly.

Escape beats. These represent passive rather than active impulse formation and usually follow a long pause, as in various arrhythmias (e.g., SA block, sinus arrest, marked sinus bradycardia or arrhythmia, heart block, and premature beats). These are usually junctional (nodal) or ventricular junctional escape beats and are often seen in normal individuals.

AV junctional rhythm. This can result from suppression of the sinus node activity by vagal stimulation, digitalis, propranolol, SA block, and many other conditions. Once this was called nodal rhythm. The usual rate is between 45 and 60 beats per minute.

Paroxysmal supraventricular tachycardia. Paroxysmal atrial tachycardia (PAT) has been used to denote a sudden, rapid (150–230 beats per minute) supraventricular rhythm. However, recent studies[35] have shown that most of these are AV nodal re-entrant tachycardias rather than ectopic atrial tachycardias. For re-entry to occur, at least two pathways must be available for impulse conduction and a unidirectional block in one pathway. The upper portion of the AV node appears to have longitudinal dissociation into pathways to account for most of these tachycardias. An ectopic or automatic focus accounts for the minority of cases of paroxysmal supraventricular tachycardia. The accessory pathways and the normal AV node pathway account for the supraventricular re-entrant tachycardias associated with the Wolff-Parkinson-White syndrome.

Nonparoxysmal AV junctional tachycardia. This is due to enhanced automaticity in the AV junction. The rate is usually 70 to 130 beats per minute, and it does not occur in patients without demonstrable heart disease. It is most commonly due to acute myocardial infarction, myocarditis, acute rheumatic fever, open heart surgery, and digitalis toxicity. Often this is associated with atrioventricular dissociation.

Atrial flutter. This is most often associated with organic heart disease and is seldom seen in normal individuals. It occurs in response to a rapid series of impulses from an ectopic atrial focus or intra-atrial re-entry. It is most common in ischemic heart disease, rheumatic heart disease, and myocardial diseases.

Atrial fibrillation. This is one of the most prevalent of the chronic rhythm disorders and can be due to any type of heart disease. It is especially common in the following conditions:

1. Rheumatic mitral disease
2. Hypertension
3. Coronary artery disease
4. Thyrotoxicosis
5. An isolated finding (lone or idiopathic)
6. Cardiomyopathy
7. Pericarditis
8. Cor pulmonale
9. Apparently normal persons (precipitated by excessive alcohol intake, infection, smoking, anxiety, or fatigue)

Even in persons without evidence of heart disease, it is not innocuous, because atrial thrombi can develop. About 30% of persons with long-standing atrial fibrillation will have emboli, especially those who have repeated episodes of this arrhythmia. It also can impair cardiac function, especially if there is an underlying heart lesion. Fibrillatory waves described as coarse are seen with rheumatic mitral disease and thyrotoxicosis, and waves described as fine are seen with coronary and hypertensive heart disease.

Multifocal atrial tachycardia. This irregular rhythm is due to frequent PABs from several foci and often occur in runs. It is most commonly seen in chronic obstructive pulmonary disease.

Ventricular tachycardia. This is usually serious; it occurs in persons with heart disease and rarely in normal persons. It originates from an ectopic focus in a ventricle or is due to re-entry. Coronary artery disease is the most common associated disease. Numerous factors, such as digitalis, sympathomimetic drugs, cyclopropane, exercise, and excitement, may precipitate attacks. It can be diagnosed with certainty with the ECG in only 50% of instances, because it is often impossible to distinguish from supraventricular tachycardia complicated by bundle-branch block or aberration.

Monomorphic ventricular tachycardia. This is a repetitive type of ventricular tachycardia occurring often in the young without evidence of significant heart disease. Usually there are three or more premature ventricular beats with identical configuration which are interrupted by normal sinus beats.

Accelerated idioventricular rhythm. This ectopic ventricular rhythm has a rate of usually 60 to 100 beats per minute and is common with acute myocardial infarction (usually inferior). This rhythm has also been noted in subjects with no evidence of cardiac disease.

Polymorphic ventricular tachycardia. This unusual ventricular arrhythmia has a rate of usually between 200 and 240 beats per minute. The peaks of the QRS complexes appear to twist around the isoelectric line. The arrhythmia usually occurs in the setting of prolongation of the Q-T interval and then it is called torsades de pointes. In fact, drugs that prolong the Q-T interval, such as quinidine, procainamide, and disopyramide, can precipitate or aggravate attacks. It appears to be an arrhythmia transitional between the usual ventricular tachycardia and ventricular fibrillation.[36]

Sinoatrial block. This is usually due to heart disease or to a toxic reaction to drugs, the most frequently implicated of which is digitalis. Coronary artery disease and myocarditis are common causes. It can be noted in healthy subjects with increased vagal tone or with a hypersensitive carotid sinus. The impulse forms in the SA node normally, but its conduction to the atria is blocked. With SA pauses, the SA node fails to discharge one or more impulses. The sick sinus node syndrome has been described to include SA block, sinus pauses, or any form of sinus node depression. It may be associated with tachybrady arrhythmias (bursts of atrial tachyarrhythmia alternating with periods of sinus node depression or slow junctional rhythm). This syndrome can be due to coronary artery disease, inflammatory diseases, cardiomyopathy, and many other conditions.

Atrioventricular block. This is usually designated by degree. First-degree block is found at times in apparently normal persons. Second-degree block is referred to as Mobitz type I (Wenckebach's phenomenon) or Mobitz type II. Both are often associated with heart disease, but type II in most instances is more serious and type I can occur in normal persons, especially athletes. Until recently the Wenckebach block always was thought to occur in the AV nodal region, but Narula and Samet[37] have shown that it also may occur in the

His-Purkinje system. In such cases, prognosis should be the same as for type II. Third-degree block can be in the AV node, bundle of His, or in both bundles (trifascicular block).

The most common causes of AV block are:

1. Fibrosis involving both bundles
2. Coronary heart disease
3. Cardiac drugs (digitalis, antiarrhythmic drugs)
4. Myocarditis (e.g., diphtheria)
5. Acute rheumatic carditis
6. Calcific aortic stenosis
7. Congenital
8. Trauma
9. Tumors
10. Surgical intervention
11. Sarcoidosis (especially in persons below age 40)

Rarely, rheumatoid disease or thyroid disease also may produce AV heart block. Acute heart block most often is due to myocardial infarction. Inferior infarction involves the AV node, and anterior infarction usually involves the septum and both bundles.

Atrioventricular dissociation. This is a term that has produced considerable confusion, since it can refer to any arrhythmia in which the atria and ventricles are beating independently. Occasionally beats can be conducted from the atria to the ventricles (interference or capture beats). Ventricular tachycardia, third-degree AV block, and nonparoxysmal AV junctional (nodal) tachycardia are examples of AV dissociation. However, many electrocardiographers use this term only in describing nonparoxysmal junctional tachycardia with AV dissociation, wherein impulses are blocked retrograde to the atria, but some can be conducted from the independently beating SA node to the ventricles. This latter arrhythmia has been called "interference dissociation" and "AV dissociation with interference." Preferably, it should be called "AV dissociation with nonparoxysmal AV junctional tachycardia." Usually it is secondary to use of a cardiac drug (especially digitalis), infection, acute rheumatic fever, myocarditis, open heart surgery, or acute myocardial infarction.

Concealed conduction. This occurs when an impulse penetrates the conducting tissue but fails to completely traverse it and can be inferred from its influence on subsequent events. A simple example is the prolonged P-R interval seen after a ventricular extrasystole (usually interpolated type) because the extrasystole penetrated retrograde the AV node and thus affected the next normal antegrade conduction. Many complex arrhythmias can be explained by this mechanism.

Digitalis intoxication. This is often recognized by ECG evidence of arrhythmias. PVBs (often as coupling), AV dissociation with nonparoxysmal junctional tachycardia, AV block, atrial tachycardia with AV block, ventricular tachycardia, and bidirectional tachycardia can be due to digitalis and are often the first indications of toxicity. Atrial flutter or fibrillation is rarely due to digitalis intoxication.

REFERENCES

1. Ashman R., Hull E.: *Essentials of Electrocardiography*. New York, Macmillan Publishing Co., 1945.
2. Grant R.P.: *Clinical Electrocardiography: The Spatial Vector Approach*. New York, McGraw-Hill Book Co., 1957.
3. Nahum L.H., Hamilton W.F., Heff H.E.: Injury current in the electrocardiogram. *Am. J. Physiol.* 139:202, 1943.
4. Eyster J.A.E., Meek W.J.: Cardiac injury potentials. *Am. J. Physiol.* 138:166, 1942.
5. Samson W.E., Scher A.: Mechanism of S-T segment alteration during acute myocardial injury. *Circ. Res.* 8:780, 1960.
6. Vincent G.M., Abildskov J.A., Burgess M.J.: Mechanisms of ischemic ST-segment displacement. Evaluation by direct current recordings. *Circulation* 56:559, 1977.
7. Salcedo J.R., Baird M.G., Chambers R.D., et al.: Significance of reciprocal ST segment depression in anterior precordial leads in acute inferior myocardial infarction: Concomitant left anterior descending coronary artery disease? *Am. J. Cardiol.* 48:1003, 1981.
8. Little W.C., Rogers E.W., Sodums M.T.: Mechanism of anterior ST segment depression during acute inferior myocardial infarction. *Ann. Intern. Med.* 100:226, 1984.
9. Lew A.S.: Ups and downs of reciprocal ST changes in acute MI. *Cardiology,* Jan. 1988, p. 59.
10. Klein H.O., Tordjman T., Ninio R., et al.: The early recognition of right ventricular infarction: Diagnostic accuracy of the electrocardiographic V_4R lead. *Circulation* 67:558, 1983.
11. Levine H.D.: Non-specificity of the electrocardiogram associated with coronary artery disease. *Am. J. Med.* 15:344, 1953.
12. Sokolow M., Lyon T.P.: The ventricular complex in left ventricular hypertrophy as obtained by unipolar and limb leads. *Am. Heart J.* 37:161, 1949.
13. Romhilt D.W., Estes E.H. Jr.: A point-score system for the ECG diagnosis of left ventricular hypertrophy. *Am. Heart J.* 75:752, 1968.
14. Reichek N., Devereux R.B.: Left ventricular hypertrophy; relationship of anatomic, echocardiographic, and electrocardiographic findings. *Circulation* 63:1391, 1981.
15. Dhingra R.C. et al.: Significance of left axis deviation in patients with chronic left bundle branch block. *Am. J. Cardiol.* 42:551, 1978.
16. New York Heart Association: *Nomenclature and Criteria for Diagnosis of Diseases of the Heart and Great Vessels,* ed. 7. Boston, Little, Brown & Co., 1973.
17. Rosenbaum M.B., Elizari M.V., Larrari J.O., et al.: Intraventricular trifascicular blocks. *Am. Heart J.* 78:450, 1969.
18. Lev M.: Pathology of bundle branch block. *Heart Bull.* 16:107, 1967.
19. Beach T.B., Gracey J.G., Peter R.H., et al.: Benign left bundle branch block. *Ann. Intern. Med.* 70:273, 1969.
20. Rotman M., Triebwasser J.H.: A clinical and follow-up study of right and left bundle branch block. *Circulation* 51:477, 1975.
21. Moore E.N., Boineau J.P., Patterson D.F.: Incomplete right bundle branch block: An electrocardiographic enigma and possible misnomer. *Circulation* 44:678, 1971.
22. Baxley W.A., Dodge H.T., Sandler H.A.: A quantitative angiocardiographic study of left ventricular hypertrophy. *Circulation* 37:509, 1968.
23. Cabrera E.C., Monroy J.R.: Systolic and diastolic overloading of the heart: II. Electrocardiographic data. *Am. Heart J.* 43:669, 1952.
24. Walker W.J., Mattingly T.W., Pollock B.E., et al.: Electrocardiographic and hemodynamic correlation in atrial septal defect. *Am. Heart J.* 52:547, 1956.
25. Chou T., Helm R.A.: The pseudo P pulmonale. *Circulation* 32:96, 1965.
26. Weiner D.A., Ryan T.S., McCabe C.H., et al.: Exercise stress testing: Correlations among history of angina, S-T segment response and prevalence of coronary artery disease in the coronary artery surgery study (Cass). *N. Engl. J. Med.* 301:230, 1979.
27. Rifkin R.D., Hood W.B. Jr.: Bayesian analysis of electrocardiographic exercise stress testing. *N. Engl. J. Med.* 297:681, 1977.
28. Goldman M.J.: RS-T segment elevation in mid and left precordial leads as normal variant. *Am. Heart J.* 46:817, 1953.
29. Martinez-Rios M.A., DaCosta B., Cecena-Seldner F.A., et al.: Normal electrocardiogram in the presence of severe coronary artery disease. *Am. J. Cardiol.* 25:320, 1970.
30. Kalbfleish M.M., Shadakharappa K.S., Conrad S.L.: Disappearance of the Q deflection following myocardial infarction. *Am. Heart J.* 76:196, 1968.
31. Gallagher J.J., Pritchett E.L., Sealy W.C., et al.: The preexcitation syndrome. *Prog. Cardiovasc. Dis.* 20:285, 1978.
32. Hoffman B.F., Cranefield P.F.: The physiological basis of cardiac arrhythmias. *Am. J. Med.* 37:670, 1964.

33. Chiang B.N., Perlman L.V., Ostrander L.P. Jr., et al.: Relationship of premature systoles to the coronary heart disease and sudden death in the Tecumseh epidemiologic study. *Ann. Intern. Med.* 70:1159, 1969.
34. Kennedy H.L., Whitlock J.A., Sprague M.K., et al.: Long-term follow-up of asymptomatic healthy subjects with frequent and complex ventricular ectopy. *N. Engl. J. Med.* 312:193, 1985.
35. Peters R.W., Scheinman M.M.: Emergency treatment of supraventricular tachycardia. *Med. Clin. North Am.* 63:73, 1979.
36. Smith W.M., Gallagher J.J.: "Les Torsades de Pointes": An unusual ventricular arrhythmia. *Ann. Intern. Med.* 93:578, 1980.
37. Narula O.S., Samet P.: Wenckebach and Mobitz type II A-V block due to block within the His bundle and bundle branches. *Circulation* 41:947, 1970.

Chapter 4

CORONARY HEART DISEASE

Coronary or ischemic heart disease results from partial or complete occlusion of one or more coronary arteries producing impairment of the blood supply to the heart. It is the leading cause of death in the United States. Almost 1.5 million attacks of myocardial infarction occur annually, and more than 700,000 coronary heart disease deaths occur per year (nearly 200,000 under age 65). Angina pectoris and myocardial infarction are the main clinical syndromes that result from coronary heart disease.

ANGINA PECTORIS

Angina pectoris is related to a disproportion between myocardial oxygen requirement and oxygen supply. Since the advent of invasive and noninvasive procedures, many causes of angina have been clarified and new causes identified (Table 4–1). Coronary atherosclerosis is the most common underlying disease. Yet some patients with severe coronary disease may not experience angina during their lives, and others with normal coronary arteries have it. There are several causes of angina with normal coronary arteriograms, and these should be sought because specific therapy is available for some of them.

Coronary Atherosclerosis

The pathogenesis of atherosclerosis is currently thought to begin with endothelial injury. Platelets are activated in this area and release ADP and thromboxane A_2 (vasoconstrictor), which causes the platelets to aggregate. This can lead to thrombosis and platelet-derived growth factor (PDGF) with proliferation of smooth muscle cells. Monocytes also migrate into the injury site, become macrophages, and produce growth factor. These reactions produce intimal hyperplasia which is the earliest phase of the atherosclerotic lesion. Cholesterol is taken up in the cells of the early lesion to form foam cells which, with the connective tissue and thrombus, form the atheroma, which can narrow the coronary vessel. The atherosclerotic anginal syndrome can be classified as shown in Table 4–2. Stable angina (chronic effort angina) can be defined as predictable and recurrent, with no change in pattern or severity for 12 weeks or longer. The syndrome of coronary artery disease that falls between stable angina and myocardial infarction has been given a variety of names, such as preinfarction angina, acute coronary insufficiency, coronary failure, intermediate syndrome, accelerated angina, and many others. The term unstable angina is now used by the majority for this entity. Many criteria for unstable angina have been presented. I prefer the four types listed in Table

65

Table 4–1. Classification of Causes of the Anginal Syndrome

Coronary atherosclerosis
Syndrome X
Coronary artery spasm
Mitral valve prolapse
Myocardial bridges
Hypertrophic cardiomyopathy
Aortic valve disease
Hypertension (systemic or pulmonary)
Unusual causes (congenital anomalies, polyarteritis, arteritis of lupus, rheumatoid, and that associated with many other conditions)

4–2. Crescendo angina refers to angina that is increasing in frequency, intensity, and duration, and often occurs at rest. This type may be of initial onset or may occur suddenly in a patient with known stable angina. A second type of unstable angina results in episodes of prolonged pain, 15 minutes or longer, occurring at rest without evidence of significant myocardial infarction as demonstrated by serum enzyme rises or ECG changes. Precipitating factors, such as anemia or arrhythmias, should be excluded. I prefer the term intermediate syndrome for this type. Often with these two types of unstable attacks, ST depression or T wave changes occur. Patients may have a combination of types 1 and 2. A third type of unstable angina can be noted in some cases of variant angina (ST segment elevation during pain and at times ventricular arrhythmia or heart block). Such patients often have prior effort-induced angina or myocardial infarction and on study have a high-grade proximal stenotic atherosclerotic lesion with superimposed spasm. Spasm rarely occurs alone with no evidence of a coronary lesion. Although the right coronary artery is usually involved in the cases with spasm alone, it is at times clinically difficult to distinguish those with presumed spasm alone from those with significant fixed obstructive lesions without performing coronary arteriography. Any of the three types of unstable angina can be considered in a high-risk subgroup (type 4) if patients have prolonged episodes of angina at rest, usually continuing in the hospital and responding poorly to nitrates, have transitory ST-T changes during episodes of chest pain, and usually have a history of stable angina or a previous infarction or both.[1]

The pathophysiology of angina has become much clearer with the use of continuous electrocardiographic monitoring, coronary arteriography, and newly developed, high resolution flexible fiberoptic angioscopes. Sherman et al.[2] visualized intracoronary lesions in patients during coronary artery bypass surgery who had stable and unstable angina. Patients with unstable angina

Table 4–2. Classification of Coronary Atherosclerotic Anginal Syndromes

Stable angina
Unstable angina
  Type 1: Crescendo
  Type 2: Prolonged pain (intermediate syndrome)
  Type 3: Variant angina (Prinzmetal's)
  Type 4: High-risk subgroup

had complex plaques with ulceration, intraplaque hemorrhage, and thrombus and the atheroma with stable angina had a smooth surface without hemorrhage or ulceration. In addition, in all types of angina, dynamic stenosis can occur.[3] Dynamic stenosis may be due to "physiologic" increase in coronary tone with constriction or spasm of a segment of coronary artery. Physiologic increase in smooth muscle tone is most likely important in determining the variability of exercise tolerance and episodes of rest ischemia in patients with chronic stable angina. In addition, all types of angina can have silent ischemia, as has been demonstrated by Holter monitoring and other methods.[4]

Angina with Normal Coronary Arteriograms

Syndrome X. The term syndrome X has been coined for those patients who have angina with angiographically normal coronary arteries and no other reason as spasm of the epicardial coronary vessels (even after ergonovine) or ventricular hypertrophy to account for the angina.[5] The prevalence of this syndrome is not known but has been estimated to be between 10 and 20% of patients who are studied for symptoms suggestive of myocardial ischemia and have normal coronary arteries. It occurs more frequently in women.

Pathologic changes and/or spasm in the small coronary vessels could explain the clinical features of syndrome X, since the small coronary arteries supply blood to the myocardium, sinoatrial and atrioventricular nodes, and the conducting system. Symptoms of angina, conduction disturbance, and arrhythmias could result. This syndrome should be considered if the electrocardiographic or radionuclide stress test is abnormal; left bundle branch block is present at rest or with stress; atrial pacing produces a decrease in great cardiac vein flow and increased lactate production, reduced vasodilatory reserve, echocardiographic and Doppler findings of abnormal diastolic function, and no impairment of ventricular function (echo) when dipyridamole produces ST segment depression and chest pain;[6] or endomyocardial biopsy shows changes (Table 4–3). Abnormal vasodilatory reserve of the coronary microcirculation appears to be a significant factor.[7] However, the mechanism responsible for this is not clear and may be related to dynamic factors. Yet intrinsic abnormalities of the smooth muscle cells, abnormal neural or humoral factors, or structural changes should be considered. Therapy for this syndrome is not clear, but the prognosis usually appears to be good. However, one study concluded that those with left bundle branch block had progressive deterioration of left ventricular function and possibly had early or latent congestive cardiomyopathy.

Coronary Artery Spasm. This can exist alone or be superimposed on an

Table 4–3. Diagnostic Clues for Syndrome X

1. Typical angina
2. Resting ECG—Left bundle branch block (LBBB)
3. Positive ECG stress test (ST depression or LBBB)
4. Abnormal radionuclide stress test
5. Reduced compliance of left ventricle (Echo and Doppler)
6. Dipyridamole—Echo test
7. Lactate production with atrial pacing
8. Normal epicardial coronary arteries

atherosclerotic lesion. Therefore, it is probably better to use the term variant angina than Prinzmetal's,[8] which refers to patients with lesions and superimposed spasm. Such patients have angina at rest with ST elevation. Usually the spasm alone or a lesion plus spasm can be localized by the ECG changes. Spasm alone is seen more often in the right coronary artery, with the ST elevation localized in the inferior leads. It may be precipitated during coronary arteriography by the use of the ergonovine provocative test if normal coronary arteries are noted. Variant angina also reacts to the cold pressor test with typical spasm and pain. The spasm is usually localized near the origin of the vessel, but may occur in the distal segment. During an episode of pain, ST elevation may be detected. Catheter-induced spasm can be differentiated because it does not produce pain or ST changes. Holter monitoring may detect ST elevation at times even without pain. Thallium radioisotopic imaging during an attack has demonstrated poor perfusion, with subsequent normal perfusion when the syndrome resolves. Ventricular arrhythmias and subsequent heart block can be recorded during an attack of pain and ST segment elevation. Exercise may produce ST elevation or even ST depression. The pathophysiology of coronary artery spasm is not clear. Coronary spasm has been considered to be due to stimulation of the CNS, hyperactivity of the autonomic nervous system, and a variety of metabolic and humoral influences. All of these factors play a part in calcium influx in various ways. Calcium ions influence coronary artery smooth muscle contraction and are required for the activation of myofibrillar adenosine triphosphatase (ATPase). Hydrogen ions compete with calcium ions at the myofibrillar ATPase. Vasoconstriction occurs if calcium ion concentration increases or hydrogen ion concentration decreases. Coronary spasm can be produced by infusion of TRIS-buffer and hyperventilation, which decreases hydrogen ion.[9] Calcium antagonists have become very important agents for relief of coronary spasm. In addition, prostaglandins have also been implicated in spasm. Thromboxane A_2 is synthesized by platelets and stimulates platelet aggregation and vasoconstriction. Prostacyclin, which is synthesized in vessel walls, seems to counteract the vasoconstriction caused by thromboxane A_2. Chest pain is not a constant feature of attacks. However, when present, it always follows hemodynamic responses and ST changes. The left ventricular systolic pressure falls and the end-diastolic pressure rises with practically no rise in heart rate.[10] These changes precede the ST elevation. Whereas angina at rest with ST elevation is referred to as Prinzmetal's angina, it has been demonstrated that spasm can occur in all syndromes of coronary disease, as with exertional angina, unstable angina of all types, and even myocardial infarction.

Mitral Valve Prolapse. This systolic click murmur syndrome has been noted commonly since the advent of echocardiography (see Chap. 6). Patients may be detected clinically by finding on auscultation an isolated click or multiple clicks. The midsystolic click often is followed by a late systolic apical murmur. These findings can be altered by hemodynamic or pharmacologic interventions. The diagnosis in most instances can be confirmed by echocardiography. However, sometimes clinical findings may be noted with no echocardiographic changes or vice versa. Patients with this syndrome have an unusual amount of chest pain, but most often it is of the nonanginal type; a few patients do have typical angina. Electrocardiographic changes at rest (ST-T changes in the inferolateral leads) are seen in up to one third of patients and almost 25% have a positive ECG stress test. Arrhythmias may occur at rest or with exertion. The cause of angina in this syndrome is not known. Coronary arteries are most often normal on arteriography. In a few cases coronary artery spasm has been demonstrated. Increased tension on the papillary muscle has also been considered as a cause of myocardial ischemia.[11] Thallium imaging has shown perfusion defects in a limited number of patients at rest and also with stress.

Myocardial Bridges. Muscular overbridging of coronary arteries may critically constrict the vessel during systole and produce myocardial ischemia and angina. The prevalence of this in autopsy series has been as high as 27%, yet most clinical studies detected it in only 0.5 to 1.6% of coronary arteriograms. A retrospective review of 465 consecutive coronary arteriograms noted bridging in 7.5%, yet the prevalence of the initial catheterization report was only 1.7%.[12] The increased frequency in this report suggests that if one is specifically looking for bridging, it will not be overlooked. Bridging most often occurs at the junction of the proximal and middle thirds of the left anterior descending coronary artery, but it can involve all of the major epicardial vessels. Frequently a marked dip is noted in the course of the left anterior descending artery at the point of bridging. This probably represents the downward turn of the mural segment of the coronary artery. It may occur as an isolated entity in patients with normal coronary arteries or it may be noted in patients with coronary artery disease. In most cases, it is of no hemodynamic significance. However, rapid heart rates and more severe systolic bridge narrowing can produce myocardial ischemia. Sudden death in otherwise healthy individuals with myocardial bridging has been reported. Permanent relief of symptoms can be achieved by surgical excision of the myocardial bridges.[13]

Hypertrophic Cardiomyopathy. Many patients with hypertrophic cardiomyopathy have angina with angiographic normal coronary arteries. The mechanism for myocardial ischemia in such cases can result from several factors (e.g., LV mass, systolic and diastolic properties).[14] The increased myocardial mass can cause an imbalance between oxygen supply and demand. In the obstructive type, elevated left ventricular systolic pressure can be associated with increased myocardial oxygen consumption and evidence of myocardial ischemia. In addition, patients with hypertrophic cardiomyopathy have diastolic dysfunction. The left ventricle is stiff, producing impaired diastolic relaxation and filling with associated elevation of the left ventricular end diastolic pressure, which can produce subendocardial ischemia. Another factor that could contribute to myocardial ischemia is obstruction of the small intramyocardial arterioles with resulting inadequate coronary flow reserve. A recent study showed thallium perfusion abnormalities in 41 of 72 patients (57%).[15] Fixed or only partially reversible defects were noted in 17 patients and completely reversible perfusion defects were noted in 24 patients. The coronary arteriograms were normal in those that had this procedure. Echocardiography has increased our diagnostic acumen for the hypertrophic syndrome.

Aortic Valve Disease. Aortic valvular stenosis or insufficiency can be associated with angina. About 50% of patients with calcific aortic stenosis also have coronary artery disease. However, angina can occur in the presence of normal coronary arteries in view of increased oxygen demand of the hypertrophied muscle with increased systolic wall stress and reduction of oxygen supply due to excessive compression of the coronary vessels. Angina is less frequent in aortic insufficiency. In addition to the increased oxygen demand with aortic insufficiency, the low diastolic pressure reduces the oxygen supply to the myocardium. Nocturnal angina can occur with aortic insufficiency when the diastolic pressure drops and the heart rate slows. Patients with severe aortic stenosis should not be stressed, since major arrhythmias and syncope can occur. Patients with aortic insufficiency at times may tolerate stress on the treadmill better than can be prediced from their clinical findings. The peripheral vasodilatation with exertion reduces the afterload and lessens the amount of the aortic insufficiency.

Systemic Hypertension. Hypertension alone can produce angina, although most often such patients have coexistent coronary artery disease.[16] Myocardial oxygen demand can be increased because of the tension developed by the myocardial tissue. In hypertension this tension is increased because of cardiomegaly (increase in left ventricular size) and the increase in systolic pressure. In addition, hypertension with left ventricular hypertrophy may produce angina, even though the coronary arteriogram is normal, because of small vessel arteriole obstruction and reduced coronary blood flow (abnormal vasodilator reserve) as has been noted with dipyridamole. Other factors that may increase myocardial oxygen consumption are an increase in heart rate and circulating norepinephrine that can occur with hypertension. The incidence of myocardial infarction in patients having left ventricular hypertrophy with normal epicardial coronary arteries is not known.

Pulmonary Hypertension. The right ventricular myocardial tension is increased not only by the increase in systolic pressure but also by the enlarged right ventricle. This tension is a major factor for myocardial oxygen demand. Low cardiac output and hypoxemia are also factors. In addition, since right ventricular coronary flow occurs with systole (right ventricle exerts less compressive forces than left ventricle) and diastole, the increased right ventricular pressure may impede systolic flow to the right ventricle. Dyspnea, dizziness, or syncope can also occur with exertion.

Unusual Causes of Angina. There are rare and unusual causes of impaired coronary flow as noted with anomalous origin of the coronary arteries, coronary AV fistula or aneurysm, arteritis often secondary to collagen diseases, luetic coronary ostial arteritis, and others.

The discussion in this chapter will primarily relate to the coronary atherosclerotic type of angina.

THE DIAGNOSIS OF ANGINA PECTORIS

Coronary artery disease is ubiquitous and can occur with or without pain. Patients who die suddenly or have pulmonary edema, chronic heart failure, abnormal ECGs, cardiac arrhythmias, abnormal x rays, or abnormal coronary arteriograms may have significant coronary disease but no painful episodes. Most patients without premonitory symptoms who have been resuscitated from sudden death due to ventricular fibrillation have been shown by coronary arteriography to have severe coronary disease. Pulmonary edema may be the first manifestation of coronary disease. Perhaps in such cases the discomfort is obscured by the acute dyspnea. It is most unusual for a patient with coronary disease to present with chronic heart failure without having had some coronary events. Electrocardiographic changes have been noted in asymptomatic individuals who subsequently, on coronary arteriography, have coronary disease. This can also be noted in individuals with cardiac arrhythmias. Generally, if there is x-ray evidence of cardiomegaly due to coronary disease, a patient has had coronary symptoms. Today many individuals are having ECG stress tests. If the test is strongly positive at a low level of exercise, coronary arteriograms are performed, and coronary disease has often been found. However, it should be emphasized that patients with coronary disease usually have some symptoms. In spite of all the sophisticated studies of today, the history is still an essential feature in the clinical diagnosis of angina pectoris regardless of the cause. Electrocardiography and radionuclide studies at rest and with exercise and coronary arteriography can be normal in the presence of typical angina. A carefully taken history will usually elicit the diagnosis.

History

Heberden in 1772[17] established the concept that the history is the essential feature in the clinical diagnosis of angina pectoris due to coronary disease. This is essentially unchanged, but the development of exercise stress electrocardiography, radionuclide tests, and coronary arteriography have given us objective studies. Recent progress in therapy makes early and correct diagnosis essential. Coronary arteriography is considered the gold standard, yet it must be recognized that this study may be normal in the presence of typical angina. Coronary arteriography has taught us that the history is more classic than it was once thought to be.

The anginal distress may be described according to the location, quality, intensity, duration, and precipitating factors. It may vary considerably from person to person, but can remain constant in the individual patient. It is then appropriately referred to as "his discomfort."

Ischemia activates the cardiac afferent sympathetic nerves, which carry impulses to the cervical and upper thoracic sympathetic ganglia and then to the spinal cord via the dorsal roots of the first five thoracic segments. The anginal distress is referred to somatic nerves and is classically located in the retrosternal area (T_1 to T_6) with radiation to the inner aspect of the left arm (T_1), hypothenar eminence (C_8), and fourth and fifth fingers (C_7 and C_8). It may be referred to the neck and corresponding areas of the right arm, to both arms, and to the lower jaw. It may also be noted only in the interscapular area or across the shoulders, or may radiate to these areas. Thus, the areas of reference can extend from C_2 to T_{10} (Fig 4–1). However, the distress of angina may occur in only a segment of this distribution; it may be only in the chest, only in the jaw, only in the neck or throat, only in the left arm, or even only in the right arm. In fact, discomfort only in these areas other than the chest, occurring usually with exertion, should not be considered atypical because it is more diagnostic of angina than chest pain, which has so many causes. The psychoneurotic patient with a complaint that brings to mind angina is usually specific and pinpoint his discomfort on the chest with one finger, whereas the patient with angina is rather vague and uses his entire hand to designate the area.

The difficulty experienced by the patient with angina is often described as a

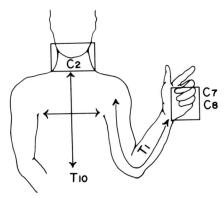

Fig 4–1. The area of reference of cardiac pain.

distress or discomfort, not as a pain. Frequently the patients become annoyed and object to the word "pain." Characteristically, angina distress is described as a burning sensation, tight squeezing sensation, or heavy feeling. It may be described as constricting, expanding, boring, a dull aching, or pressing. It may be a mild oppression, slight smothering, gassy fullness, a sense of weakness, or faintness with mild nausea. The elderly and some diabetics with angina may complain of dyspnea, weakness, faintness, or mild nausea on exertion without chest discomfort. These types of symptoms are often referred to as anginal equivalents. It is known that ischemic pain can spare many diabetic patients. Faerman et al.[18] found abnormal morphologic changes of cardiac sympathetic and parasympathetic nerves in heart specimens from diabetic patients who died with painless myocardial infarctions. Such findings were not noted in specimens from a control group of diabetic patients who died from painful infarctions.

Sometimes the feeling is interpreted as dyspnea when in fact it is a band-like feeling across the chest which restricts breathing, or a localized oppressive dyspnea in the substernal area. However, dyspnea may be the only symptom of myocardial ischemia. There may be severe aching, burning, numbness or tingling in arms, hands, and fingers. There may be an aching, tingling, or bursting sensation in the throat, neck, or lower jaw. Others may complain of indigestion that is relieved by eructation. Seldom is it so sharp that the patient refers to it as "pain." It may begin as sharpness in the substernal area, but almost immediately it spreads out as a heavy or tight feeling.

The angina sensation usually develops gradually. It begins mildly and progressively mounts in intensity over a period of approximately 30 seconds to 5 minutes. It is rarely excruciating or intolerable. The period seems longer to the patient. The distress subsides rapidly with rest (within 3 to 5 minutes), particularly if nitroglycerin is given. Variant forms tend to be more severe and of longer duration. The discomfort of angina is usually brought on by increased cardiac work (increase in heart rate, BP, ventricular volume, or contractility), such as that associated with exertion (walking uphill, walking after a meal or in cold weather), or with emotional tension. Myocardial ischemia occurs when the myocardial oxygen consumption (MVo_2) exceeds the capacity of the diseased coronary vessels to deliver oxygen. The attacks do not occur regularly each day unless they are related to exercise or emotion. The variability of ischemic threshold is related to the change in vasomotor tone of the coronary vessels, especially at the site of the stenoses. Minor exertion in the morning on arising can precipitate an attack, yet the patient may not have further attacks with even more severe exertion during the rest of the day. The attacks often demonstrate a circadian increase occurring between 6:00 A.M. and 12:00 P.M.[19] Rarely, patients can walk through their angina. Nitroglycerin used prophylactically prevents the anginal distress and at times eliminates abnormal precordial cardiac pulsations that occur during the anginal attack. Angina usually responds in less than 3 minutes to sublingual nitroglycerin. This is not diagnostic of angina, since esophageal and sphincter of Oddi spasm can respond as dramatically to nitroglycerin.

As mentioned previously, patients with unstable angina may have their discomfort at rest and at times as prolonged attacks without necrosis, as seen with the intermediate syndrome and variant angina.

It is important to recognize that patients have multiple types of chest pain and that they are more concerned about the sharp, noncardiac type and may not mention the heavy, constricting anginal type. Often, while relating the history, they will wander from one type to the other.

Physical Examination

The physical examination is often not helpful in patients with angina. Even if the patient has cardiomegaly or other evidence of heart disease, this does not imply that his chest pain is angina. Our index of suspicion should be high if an individual has hypertension, diabetes, hypercholesterolemia, hypertriglyceridemia, xanthomata, or gout. An S_3 gallop, paradoxical splitting of S_2, abnormal chest pulsation, or mid or late apical systolic murmur (papillary muscle dysfunction due to ischemia) occurring during pain may be a clue to the diagnosis of angina. An S_4 sound may be constantly present or appear only during attacks. A diagonal earlobe crease and/or canal hair was reported to be a marker for coronary artery disease.[20,21] However, this was not confirmed by other studies, especially since the prevalence of earlobe crease and coronary artery disease increases with age.[22]

Levine[23] demonstrated that anginal pain could be relieved by carotid sinus massage. Levine considered this response to be diagnostic in many instances. The right carotid sinus is massaged with the patient seated or recumbent. If this does not bring relief, the left carotid sinus is massaged. Auscultation of the heart is carried out during the maneuver, and massage is stopped if the heart slows significantly. Massage should not be done on both sides at once or for more than 3 to 5 seconds at a time. The test is positive for angina pectoris if distress is relieved within seconds, usually accompanied by slowing of the heart. When relief without slowing of the heart occurs, the carotid massage may be interrupting sympathetic reflex arcs or sensory pathways. A negative response does not rule out angina.

Stress Electrocardiogram

A randomly taken ECG is often normal in patients with angina, yet physicians still rely heavily on this and make the mistake of reassuring the patient. A properly performed stress test is more useful for the detection and evaluation of underlying coronary artery disease.

Food, coffee, and smoking should be omitted for at least 2 hours before the stress test. It also is preferable that drugs be withheld for at least several days before testing, proportional to the duration of their pharmacologic effects. The Master's test was an important impetus that led to frequent use today of exercise stress testing. We now give a near maximal or maximal exercise test graded by heart rate as performed by Sheffield and co-workers.[24] Instead of heart rate, oxygen consumption as measured or estimated during an exercise test may be used to regulate intensity, as can metabolic equivalents (METS). One MET is the energy requirement at complete rest and is equivalent to 3.5 to 4.0 ml O_2/kg of body weight/minute. We attempt to achieve at least 90% of the maximal heart rate for the patient's age (Table 4–4). It really does not make any difference what type or means of exercise is used to reach the desired rate. A bicycle ergometer or a treadmill can be used. There are many protocols available for performing a stress test. We follow the multistage exercise test protocol of Bruce et al.[25] using the treadmill (Table 4–5). Routinely, prior to exercise, an ECG should be taken with the patient in the lying and upright positions. In addition, a tracing should be taken during and after the patient hyperventilates for up to 60 seconds. Three or more leads can be monitored during exercise. Monitoring several leads rather than one increases the sensitivity of exercise testing, but the specificity of taking multiple leads remains to be demonstrated. Inferior leads will probably have more false-positives than the precordial leads. Immediately after exercise, a complete tracing is taken in the lying position. The tracing is repeated after exercise at 1 minute, 3 minutes, 5 minutes, 8 minutes, or until the tracing returns to the control. Often we see tracings taken only immediately after exercise. These are inadequate tests, since abnormalities may not appear until later. The BP is recorded with each stage of exercise. If any significant symptoms (angina, undue fatigue or dyspnea, or light-headedness), major arrhythmias, ataxic gait, cyanosis, excessive BP rise or fall, or more than 3 mm horizontal or downsloping ST depression appear before the patient reaches the expected target heart rate, the test is stopped and postexercise tracings are taken. In many instances patients who previously have given only vague histories will report a classic description of angina while exercising. For this reason, as well as to prevent any undue attack of prolonged coronary insufficiency or even occlusion, the physician should be present during the test. A defibrillator should be available.

Often an attempt to reproduce the patient's symptoms by exposing him to the factor that precipitated his anginal distress may be rewarding, and an

Table 4–4. **Target Heart Rate for Graded Exercise Test Based on Age and Activity***

Ages (yr)	20	25	30	35	40	45	50	55	60	65	70
Untrained											
M.H.R.†	197	195	193	191	189	187	184	182	180	178	176
90% M.H.R.	177	175	173	172	170	168	166	164	162	160	158
Trained											
M.H.R.	190	188	186	184	182	180	177	175	173	171	169
90% M.H.R.	171	169	167	166	164	162	159	158	156	154	152

*Data from Sheffield T., et al.:[24] Submaximal exercise testing. *J. S.C. Med. Assoc.* 65:18, 1969.
†M.H.R. = maximum heart rate.

Table 4–5. Multistage Exercise Capacity Test*

Stage	Duration (min)	Speed (mph)	Grade (%)	METS (unit)	VO₂ (ml/kg/min)
First	3	1.7	10	5	18
Second	3	2.5	12	6–7	25
Third	3	3.4	14	8–10	34
Fourth	3	4.2	16	10–12	46
Fifth	3	5.0	18		58
Sixth	3	5.5	20		70
Seventh	3	6.0	22		

*From Doan A.E., Peterson D.R., Blackmon J.R., Bruce R.A.:[25] Myocardial ischemia after maximal exercise in healthy men. *Am. Heart J.* 69:11–21, 1965.

ECG taken at that time may be significant. Abnormalities have been seen in such instances, even though an exercise test has been negative.

Interpretation of the Stress Electrocardiogram

The greatest difference of opinion among interpreters concerns evaluating results of exercise stress tests. All interpreters of stress ECGs are guilty of giving a different opinion of a given stress test on another occasion. Exercise responses are often reported as positive (abnormal), suspicious (borderline), or negative (normal). It may be more appropriate to describe the changes during and after exercise than to use these latter terms. The ECG changes should be used as an adjunct to the clinical findings. A positive test does not definitely indicate coronary artery disease, and a negative test result does not exclude it.

The P-Q or P-R interval should be used as a baseline for ST displacement with at least three consecutive complexes on a straight baseline drawn through the point of onset of each QRS complex. The ST segment displacement can be expressed in millimeters or millivolts. We consider a stress test abnormal if the ST segment is depressed 1 mm (0.1 mV) or more horizontally or downward sloping, with or without T wave inversion[26] (Fig 4–2). Numerous studies suggest that manifestations of coronary heart disease are proportional to the degree of ST segment displacement.[27,28] If depressed, downsloping ST changes occur in the first three minutes of exercise with a rate under 70% of the predicted maximal heart rate and persist for six minutes or more, the more likely it is that coronary disease is present and often very severe. These and

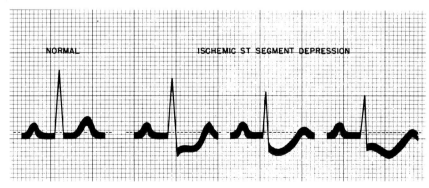

Fig 4–2. Ischemic right angle ST segment depression. Note that the degree of ST depression is measured from the top of the continuation of the P-R interval. (From Gazes P.C., et al.: The diagnosis of angina pectoris. *Am. Heart J.* 67:830, 1964.)

other markers have been used to estimate the extent of coronary artery disease. Since heart rate is directly related to myocardial workload during exercise, heart rate adjustment of ST segment depression may be a more accurate method to detect the presence and extent of coronary artery disease than the extent of ST segment alone. However, this relationship in patients with coronary artery disease is not linear throughout the test; therefore, the delta ST/HR index (dividing maximum ST depression during exercise by the corresponding heart rate change from upright preexercise control) can only approximate the heart rate normalized magnitude of ST depression that occurs with ischemia. The ST/HR slope calculation can best give this; this is time-consuming to perform manually, but software will become available to do it from computer-measured ST segments.[29] It also has been proposed that the ST segment depression be adjusted for R-wave amplitude. This appears to be helpful only for great ST depression and not for ST depression that approximates 1 mm which is the usual criterion of abnormality.[30] Transient ST segment elevation of 1 mm or more above the base line during or after exercise is considered as a manifestation of myocardial ischemia. Patients with old Q wave infarctions may have ST elevation with exercise which could be due to segmental wall motion abnormalities in the infarcted area rather than myocardial ischemia. It is probably due to transmural ischemia, if it occurs without underlying Q waves. Inverted U waves (Fig 4–3) also indicate a positive stress test. The mechanism of this rare occurrence is not known. In one study[31] an exercise-induced U wave inversion was considered as a marker of stenosis of the left anterior descending coronary artery. In 36 patients in whom this was observed, 33 had proximal left anterior descending or left main coronary involvement. It is often obscured by the rapid heart rate and is, therefore, noted more often after exercise when the rate slows. Bonoris et al.[32] considered the R wave amplitude in treadmill stress testing as a good predictor of coronary artery disease. According to those authors, R wave changes are related to left ventricular volume (Brody effect). In normal individuals, tachycardia and catecholamine release with exercise produce a decrease in left ventricular volume and a decrease in R wave amplitude. The ischemic heart with exercise shows no change or an increase in R wave amplitude. An increase in R wave amplitude during stress testing suggested impaired left ventricular function with elevated systolic and diastolic volumes and pressures. In this study, R wave amplitude changes proved to be more sensitive and more specific than ST changes in detecting coronary artery disease which was confirmed by coronary arteriography.

However, Battler et al.,[33] using radionuclide studies, showed that R wave amplitude changes during exercise testing have little diagnostic value and are not related to exercise-induced changes in volume or left ventricular function. Morales-Ballejo et al.[34] reported that an increase in Q-wave amplitude in CM5 with exercise is a normal response and if it occurred in the presence of ST depression, this would identify the ST depression as false-positive. In the presence of significant coronary disease, most had no Q-wave or no increase in Q-wave amplitude. A more recent study[35] concluded that the Q-wave analysis is no more sensitive for detecting coronary artery disease than the ST segment response, but if a decreased Q-wave occurred, it most often predicted multivessel coronary artery disease with left anterior descending disease. However,

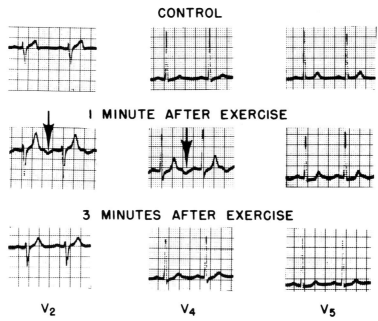

Fig 4–3. Note inverted U wave (*arrows*) 1 minute after exercise, which cleared by 3 minutes after exercise.

until further studies are done, most do not use R and Q wave amplitude changes in the diagnoses of coronary diseases.

Several abnormalities observed during or after exercise imply an increased risk related to coronary artery disease, but available data are insufficient to establish their significance. They are bundle-branch block, inverted T waves becoming upright or increasing in amplitude, arrhythmias, and T wave inversion. With maximal exercise, occasional unifocal premature ventricular complexes occur in up to 42% of a clinically normal population. Even complex ventricular arrhythmias are common in healthy subjects.[36] Their reproducibility in serial testing is not much greater than by chance alone. Patients with coronary artery disease may have multifocal or runs of premature ventricular complexes, and more than ten per minute occurring with heart rates below 70% of the predicted maximal heart rates. However, ventricular arrhythmias alone with exercise cannot be used as a criterion for the diagnosis of coronary heart disease, but do have significance in the presence of other abnormalities.[37] It also should be recognized that ventricular arrhythmias can disappear with increasing exercise even if the individual has ischemic heart disease. Junction J point (end of QRS complex) displacement by itself seems not to imply increased risk. However, upsloping ST segment with 2-mm ST depression measured 0.08 second from the J point is considered borderline and even positive by many when the pretest risk is high[38,39] (Fig 4–4). Atrial repolarization (T of P depression) where the P-R interval has a downward course, which often occurs with rapid heart rates, as the only change has no coronary artery disease implication. Autonomic changes (vasoregulatory abnormality) and changes occurring in the presence of left ventricular hypertrophy, left bundle-branch block, Wolff-Parkinson-White syndrome (Fig 4–5),[40] chest de-

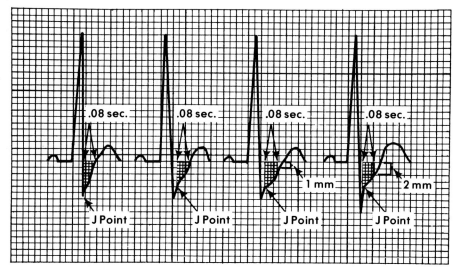

Fig 4–4. Upsloping ST depression measured 0.08 second from the J point (end of QRS). First two complexes show no depression. The third complex has 1-mm ST depression, and the fourth has 2-mm ST depression below the baseline (P-R interval). (Gazes P.C.: Angina pectoris— classification and diagnosis. *Primary Cardiology* 5:60, 1979. Used with permission.)

formities, or therapy with cardiac drugs (namely, digitalis) and diuretics impose difficulties in interpretation and often give false-positive changes. Autonomic ST-T changes can usually be detected because they occur primarily in the standing position or with hyperventilation and can be blocked by giving a β-blocker.

A majority of exercise studies could not correlate an increase in ST depression in the presence of left bundle-branch block with coronary artery disease.[41]

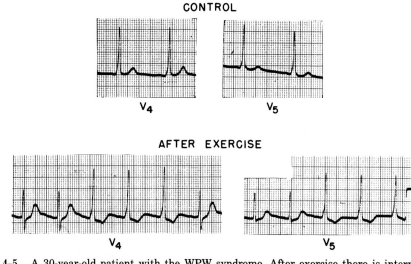

Fig 4–5. A 30-year-old patient with the WPW syndrome. After exercise there is intermittent normal and WPW conduction. During the WPW conduction, ST depression with inverted T waves can be seen that did not occur in the normal conducted beats. (From Gazes P.C.: False-positive exercise test in the presence of the Wolff-Parkinson-White syndrome. *Am. Heart J.* 78:13, 1969).

However, there is a good correlation in the presence of right bundle-branch block when the ST depression occurs in leads V_4 to V_6.[42] ST segment depression limited to leads V_1 to V_3 with right bundle-branch block represents a false-positive exercise test.

Many so-called false-positive tests may be due to mitral valve prolapse, idiopathic hypertrophic subaortic stenosis, and syndrome X. Therefore, these are not actually false positive results, but simply are due to diseases other than coronary artery disease.

The diagnostic accuracy of the exercise ECG test in detecting coronary artery disease has been questioned, especially since it may produce many false-positives in women.[43] Much has been written about the sensitivity (percentage of patients with documented coronary artery disease having abnormal stress tests), specificity (percentage of negative results in subjects without coronary artery disease), and positive predictive accuracy (percentage of positive results that are true positive). Positive predictive value depends not only on the sensitivity and specificity of the test, but also on the proportion of subjects who have the disease in the population being tested. Bayes's theorem states that a test cannot be adequately interpreted without reference to the prevalence of the disease (pretest) in the population, even though the reliability of a diagnostic test is also based on the sensitivity and specificity. This was emphasized by Rifkin and Hood[44] in the interpretation of the stress test. One can use curves showing the probability of disease as a function of the pretest. The pretest in Figure 4–6 is based on clinical judgment and on studies as reported by Friesinger et al.[45] Figure 4–6 shows that if a patient has 1.0- to 1.49-mm downsloping ST depression and falls in the clinical pretest category 1 (typical anginal pectoris of effort), the probability of his having coronary artery disease is at least 90%. There are many other conditions besides coronary disease that can produce ST segment depression, such as left ventricular pressure overload, increase in left ventricular end diastolic pressure, abnormal activation sequence, drugs, and autonomic changes. Therefore, the sensitivity and specificity of a stress test depend on the population studied, the electrocardiographic criteria, other factors that affect the ST segment, and the amount of exercise performed. The amount of exercise and the heart rate can be altered by drugs such as β-blockers. Even if the diagnostic value of the stress test is questioned, the test still has great value in explaining unusual exercise-related symptoms, detecting arrhythmias, determining patient exercise capacity, and in following therapeutic interventions.

Blood Pressure Responses to Stress

Recording of BP during ECG stress testing is important, even though at times it can be difficult to measure. Automated methods to date have not been entirely satisfactory. The double product (systolic BP multiplied by the heart rate) is a good index of myocardial oxygen consumption. Normally, with exercise the systolic BP should rise. It should fall just as the exercise is completed and again momentarily rise when the patient lies down. The BP usually rises about 10 mm Hg per stage of exercise. There is no set level of rise when the exercise should be stopped. Our group has arbitrarily chosen a systolic level of 235 mm Hg. In addition, we do not subject to stress someone with a resting

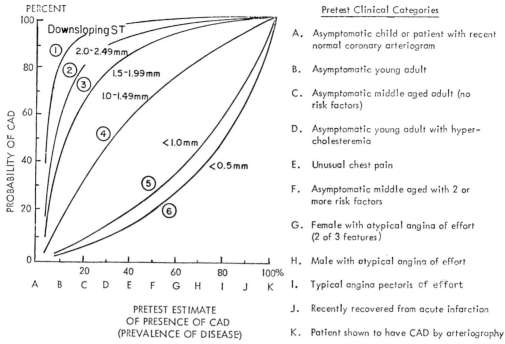

Fig 4–6. Curves based on ST segment changes noted during exercise. Pretest risk is on the X-axis (abscissa) and probability of disease on the Y-axis (ordinate). (Modified and reprinted by permission from Rifkin R.D., Hood W.B., Jr.: Bayesian analysis of electrocardiographic exercise stress testing. *N. Engl. J. Med.* 297:681, 1977. Pretest clinical categories adapted by permission from Humphries J.O., based on the studies of Friesinger G.C., et al.: Prognostic significance of coronary arteriography. *Trans. Assoc. Am. Phys.* 83:78, 1970.)

level of 180/110 mm Hg or greater. A fall in systolic pressure early during exercise, with or without ST changes, may be indicative of left main or triple-vessel disease.[46] In addition, an increase in diastolic BP of more than 15 mm Hg is an abnormal response and may be indicator of coronary artery disease, even in the absence of ST segment changes.[47] Normally, the diastolic BP response to exercise is no change or a decrease.

Radionuclide Studies in Angina

Exercise radionuclide techniques, such as planar thallium scintigraphy and radionuclide angiography in conjunction with exercise electrocardiography, have significantly enhanced the sensitivity, specificity, and predictive accuracy for coronary artery disease detection compared with exercise electrocardiography alone. Thallium imaging depends on coronary flow and looks at reduced perfusion with stress, and radionuclide angiography looks at the effects of stress on global and regional ventricular systolic function. The maximum level of exercise (just as for the ECG stress test) should be reached before thallium is injected, and exercise should be continued for another 30 to 60 seconds. Imaging is performed within 5 to 10 minutes of the injection. An abnormal myocardial region is visualized as an area of relatively decreased tracer uptake (cold spot). However, this can represent a viable but transiently ischemic zone or a chronic scar, such as from an old infarct. Imaging should be repeated several hours (usually 4 hours) after injection. At times repeat imaging may be necessary 24 hours after injection, especially if there is some redistribution at 4 hours. Redistribution will reflect cell viability, and the cold spot should clear if there was just ischemia, whereas it would remain if an old scar was present. Thallium redistribution defect with exercise, especially if associated with abnormal lung uptake (increase in left ventricular diastolic pressure), is often indicative of coronary artery disease. Thallium stress imaging is used clinically in the situations noted in Table 4–6.

Dynamic imaging of the heart has become possible with the application of computer technology to nuclear medicine. Dynamic radionuclide angiography is of two types. In the first-pass technique, ^{99m}Tc is injected IV as a rapid bolus, its passage through the heart is followed with the gamma camera, and data are obtained until the tracer has been ejected from the left ventricle. The counts are limited to a few cardiac cycles. The total number of counts and resolution can be increased by multiple-gated acquisition bloodpool imaging (MUGA). It is performed by the use of ^{99m}Tc bound to the patient's own red blood cells. Imaging is begun 10 to 15 minutes after the tracer has equilibrated with blood. Information from many segments of each cardiac cycle is stored in the computer memory, and composite images can be displayed in a flicker-free movie format. Exercise is usually performed using a bicycle ergometer in either the supine or the erect position, and data of ventricular function are obtained during and after exercise. Radionuclide angiography stress imaging is used clinically in situations noted in Table 4–7. The stress MUGA is considered abnormal if the left ventricular ejection fraction fails to increase by more than 5% or declines during stress or regional wall motion abnormalities are noted. MUGA studies are also being performed after handgrip and cold pressor tests in patients who cannot exercise supine.

In a review study of 2,048 patients collected from 22 studies reported in the literature, the sensitivity of thallium stress test was 83% and the specificity 90%, and the sensitivity for the ECG stress (1.0 mm or greater ST depression) was 58% and specificity 82%.[48] Exercise radionuclide regional wall motion abnormality had a sensitivity of 76% and a specificity of 95% and failure to increase the left ventricular ejection fraction by 5% or more with exercise showed a sensitivity of 88% and specificity of 76%. Combining new regional

Table 4–6. Clinical Use of Thallium Stress Test

Diagnosis of coronary artery disease
  a. Atypical chest pain
  b. False positive ECG stress test
  c. Chest pain and negative ECG stress test
Stress test in patients with resting ECG abnormalities, such as left bundle-branch block, left ventricular hypertrophy, drug effect (Digoxin)
Evaluate physiologic significance of lesions detected by coronary arteriography
Evaluation of patency of coronary bypass grafts
Evaluation of adequacy of PTCA
To differentiate viable myocardium from scar
Guide to effectiveness of medical treatment

Table 4–7.   Clinical Use of MUGA Stress Test

Diagnosis of coronary artery disease
Determine severity of coronary artery disease
Assess response to medical, PTCA, or surgical therapy
Assess ventricular function

wall abnormality and failure to increase ejection fraction gave a sensitivity of 86% and specificity of 91%. It can generally be stated that if these radionuclide tests are normal, the chance of significant coronary artery disease is approximately 10%. This level of probability could be sufficient for some physicians to manage such patients. Improvement in radionuclide tests in the future may improve sensitivity and specificity. A newer method of thallium imaging has emerged with the use of single photon emission computed tomography (SPECT),[49] (Fig 4–7). This has advantages over planar images, namely, better contrast of images, lack of superimposition of normal and abnormal areas, sensitivity of about 94% and specificity of 91% and a three-dimensional view of the site and extent of perfusion abnormalities. It is also better for identifying individual diseased vessels. Instead of exercise, intravenous infusion of dipy-

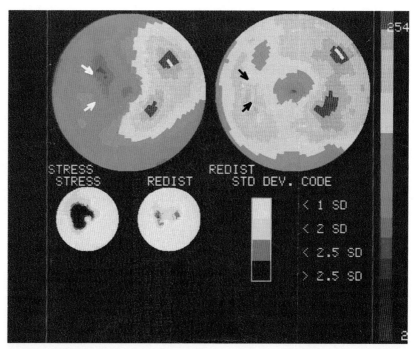

Fig 4–7.   Stress thallium (SPECT). Images of left ventricle (on left, white arrow) reveal markedly decreased perfusion of the septal and anterior wall extending to the apex, which at 4 hours after redistribution fills in extensively (on right, black arrows). These findings are consistent with stress-induced ischemia in the distribution of the left anterior descending coronary, which, on arteriography, had a proximal high-grade obstruction. (Courtesy Dr. Grady H. Hendrix.)

ridamole has been used for myocardial perfusion imaging with thallium. This is considered for patients who have orthopedic or other problems and cannot perform physical exercise. Dobutamine has also been used in such patients.

Exercise two-dimensional echocardiography in some centers has shown promise in detecting segmental wall motion abnormalities induced by the development of ischemia. Sensitivity and specificity have been reported up to 90%. This has not been used extensively because of technical difficulties.

Coronary Arteriography

We reserve coronary arteriography (Table 4–8) for patients with chest pain in whom we cannot establish a definite diagnosis by other means, those with coronary disease who may benefit from percutaneous transluminal angioplasty (PTCA) or revascularization surgery, and patients scheduled to undergo surgery for aortic or mitral valve disease, especially if they have a history of angina. In fact, today it is appropriate to perform coronary arteriography on most patients who have had any coronary event such as a myocardial infarction or any degree of angina. The diagnosis of angina can most often be made by the history and associated electrical or radionuclide stress tests, but except for a few subsets (such as the early positive ECG stress test), the degree of anatomic involvement cannot be suspected; i.e., patients with infrequent angina may have left main coronary disease. Asymptomatic men with strongly positive ECG stress tests at low work-loads should be studied. Since women often have false-positive tests, if they are symptomatic and have an early positive stress test, I perform a thallium stress test and, if this is positive, proceed with coronary arteriography. Asymptomatic patients resuscitated after sudden cardiac arrest often have significant coronary disease and should have coronary arteriography. In addition, it is often used to evaluate patients after PTCA or revascularization surgery. The mortality associated with coronary arteriography should be below 0.1% and associated acute myocardial infarction 0.2% or less.

The studies of Proudfit et al.[50] have shown a 95% correlation between stenotic lesions and typical angina of effort without rest pain. The correlation fell to 79% in patients with rest pain only and to 65% in those with atypical angina. It appears from several studies that up to 10% of patients with angina and a positive ECG exercise test have normal coronary arteriograms. The reason for this is not clear. Some of these patients have a cardiomyopathy or small arteriole disease.

Table 4–8. Indications for Coronary Arteriography

Undiagnosed chest pain
Patients considered for coronary artery bypass surgery or PTCA
Strongly abnormal ECG stress test
Some patients successfully resuscitated
Some patients prior to valvular and other types of open heart surgery
Determine graft patency
Determine adequacy of PTCA

Differential Diagnosis

Chest pain is a common symptom and produces anxiety among patients, their families, and even physicians. Angina pectoris must be differentiated from the discomfort of anxiety neurosis, muscular skeletal disease or deformities, organic and functional disturbances of the GI tract with pain referred to the chest, and Tietze's syndrome (costochondritis). The main differential fact is that these conditions produce more prolonged pain than angina, and the attacks are not associated with exertion.

Anxiety, often associated with hyperventilation, produces stabbing precordial pain which the patient can pinpoint with one finger, whereas the anginal pain is vague, and the patient uses his entire hand to designate the area of discomfort. The pain often occurs after and not during the exertion. In addition, these patients have dizziness, at times syncope, palpitations, paresthesias of the extremities, and ST-T changes at rest and with exercise. Voluntary hyperventilation can reproduce their symptoms. One must be careful in interpreting the symptoms, since patients with angina frequently have associated anxiety symptoms.

Muscular skeletal lesions, such as cervical disks, osteoarthritis, spondylitis, neuritis, myalgia, fibrositis, and subdeltoid bursitis produce pain that is usually not related to exertion and can be reproduced by pressure, twisting, or bending. Lower cervical or thoracic nerve root compression can mimic angina. The pain is generally sharp and piercing, but can be boring, constricting, dull, or deep in the chest and down the arms. Usually these radicular syndromes can be reproduced by movement of the body, coughing, and sneezing. Various maneuvers such as bending, hyperextension of upper spine, stretching the arms, pressure on top of the head, and palpation can produce the pain symptoms and also associated paresthesias. Symptoms may be noted after prolonged recumbency, and jogging or running can produce root pain. Thoracic outlet syndromes can be identified by maneuvers such as the Adson maneuver (obliteration of the radial pulse when the scalenus anticus muscle is put on tension by extending the neck with the head turned to the affected side while the patient takes a deep breath) for detecting the scalenus anticus syndrome. Painful chest syndromes can be detected by chest pressure. Tietze's syndrome causes a painful, tender, swollen costochondral or sternoclavicular junction and can be relieved by local injections of lidocaine or steroids.

Digestive tract disorders often cause chest pain, especially those of the esophagus, for the autonomic nerve supply of the heart and esophagus are similar, so symptoms may be similar. Stomach, duodenum, biliary tract problems, and, less commonly, pancreatic, hepatic, or colonic conditions can produce chest pain. These disorders usually are readily differentiated from cardiac pain. Often digestive tract disorders coexist with cardiac diseases.

Pain of esophageal origin is often of the heartburn, esophageal spasm, or swallowing type. Heartburn may mimic angina, for it can be described as substernal burning, fullness, pressure, or a burning from the xyphoid to the suprasternal notch. It can radiate to the back but seldom to the neck and arms.[51] Gastroesophageal reflux may be demonstrated by such tests as barium swallow (videoesophagography) and esophageal manometry. At times esophagoscopy, biopsy, Bernstein test, and pH probe are necessary to demonstrate esophagitis. Diffuse esophageal spasm can produce chest, arm, jaw, and back pain. It may be spontaneous or occur after swallowing (namely, cold liquids). It is usually caused by a motor disorder, may be relieved by nitroglycerin and may be produced by ergonovine. However, this discomfort is not brought on by exertion. Yet it must be differentiated from rest angina such as Prinzmetal's angina, which is associated with ST segment elevation during pain. Diagnosis can be made of diffuse esophageal spasm by barium swallow, esophageal manometry, and radionuclide transient studies,[52] especially if such studies are done during an attack. Ergonovine can provoke attacks in both situations, but with esophageal spasm, no ST-T changes occur. Sliding hiatal hernias are common and are seldom symptomatic. If associated with esophageal reflux, symptoms can occur to simulate angina on recumbency, after a large meal, and with bending, but are relieved by antacids and are not produced by exertion. Often patients with angina have a small sliding hiatal hernia, and it is tempting, especially if the patient is a close friend or relative, to consider that the hernia is producing the symptoms.

Functional GI tract disorders can also cause chest pain and are more difficult to identify than structural disorders. The splenic flexure syndrome produces left upper quadrant pain, which may radiate to the left chest and shoulder. The pain is exacerbated by meals, especially those high in fat content, and patients may have diarrhea, constipation, or both, and mucus in the stools. Often symptoms clear after passage of flatus. Usually the diagnosis is made by typical symptoms and exclusion of other disease with a normal upper intestinal study and barium enema.

Premature beats before or after exercise are often associated with short, stabbing chest sensations. Patients with angina may have unnecessary dental extractions because of pain in the jaw and teeth.

Chest pain is a common symptom and should be approached by the clinician in a systematic way. The history and physical examination findings may be sufficient to make the diagnosis. These findings may lead one to order x rays and other tests for skeletal or GI tract problems. Exercise stress testing (electrocardiography and radionuclide) are valuable not only for diagnostic purposes, but also for determining the patient's functional capacity. However, in the final analysis, when in doubt, coronary arteriography is currently the only way to establish the diagnosis, and the physician should not be content with statistical probabilities.

MEDICAL TREATMENT OF ANGINA PECTORIS

The major determinants of myocardial oxygen demand are contractility, heart rate, and wall tension. An increase in these parameters increases myocardial oxygen demand. Wall tension is increased by an increase in intraventricular pressure or volume. Coronary blood flow can be altered by coronary atherosclerosis, coronary spasm (epicardial and intramyocardial coronary vessels) and the pressure gradient during diastole (the difference between aortic diastolic pressure and the left ventricular end diastolic pressure). In addition, collateral vessels and myocardial arteriolar autoregulation can increase coro-

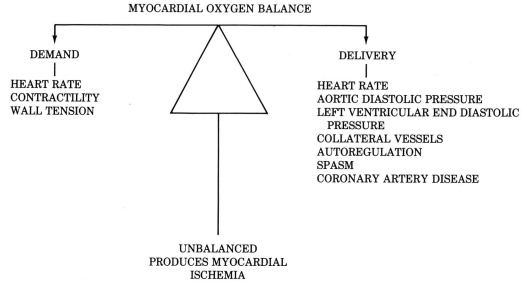

MYOCARDIAL OXYGEN BALANCE

DEMAND

HEART RATE
CONTRACTILITY
WALL TENSION

DELIVERY

HEART RATE
AORTIC DIASTOLIC PRESSURE
LEFT VENTRICULAR END DIASTOLIC
  PRESSURE
COLLATERAL VESSELS
AUTOREGULATION
SPASM
CORONARY ARTERY DISEASE

UNBALANCED
PRODUCES MYOCARDIAL
ISCHEMIA

Fig 4–8.   Balance between demand and delivery.

nary flow. Oxygen delivery by the coronary arteries must increase to meet any demand; otherwise, myocardial ischemia will occur, producing angina pectoris. Figure 4–8 shows the necessary balance between demand and delivery. The treatment is aimed at reducing the myocardial oxygen requirements or increasing the supply. For treatment purposes, angina can primarily be divided into two types, stable and unstable. The treatment program for both types is summarized in Table 4–9.

STABLE ANGINA

Angina is considered stable when it has been present for several months without change in duration or frequency, is usually precipitated by a known amount of exercise and anxiety, and is relieved by rest and nitroglycerin.

Activity

Patients with stable angina should be advised to avoid activities that are known to precipitate angina, such as walking in the cold or after a large meal, or to take nitroglycerin before such activities. Having sexual intercourse, driving a car, and flying commercially are among the many activities that must be discussed with each patient because of the variability of the precipitating factors. It is not unusual for a patient to perform a rather strenuous act without an attack, yet have pain from some minor activity. Only the patient can identify his angina.

It is important to avoid invalidism by not imposing unnecessary restrictions. It is equally important for the physician to interview members of the patient's family because they often are responsible for the patient's invalidism. I have frequently heard a well-meaning wife say to her husband, "Darling, be careful. Lifting that chair may cause you to have another attack and die." As a result

Table 4–9. Treatment of Angina Pectoris

Stable Angina	Unstable Angina
Avoidance of precipitating factors	Hospitalize
Control risk factors	IV nitroglycerin
Nitrates	Same drugs as for stable angina
Beta-blockers	Aspirin
Calcium-blockers	Heparin
Treatment of associated disorders	Intra-aortic balloon
Surgery	Surgery
Percutaneous transluminal coronary angioplasty (PTCA)	Percutaneous transluminal coronary angioplasty (PTCA)

of the anxiety caused by this remark, the husband may have angina, whereas lifting the chair would not have resulted in an attack.

A patient often thinks he is totally disabled if he cannot pursue his usual occupation. He must be convinced that he can do some type of work. At times this presents a problem, because he may be disabled for his usual job, yet be unable to obtain other jobs because he lacks training. It is important that he receive counseling and be directed to the proper agency for vocational rehabilitation. Work classification units are available to evaluate the working capacity of patients with heart disease. If the physician is not interested in employment for these patients, how can the patients be motivated? I fear that we physicians are responsible for industry's shunning the cardiac patient.

Later in this chapter, control of risk factors such as exercise, smoking, diet, and others will be discussed for all clinical syndromes of coronary disease.

Drugs

Nitrates. The nitrates have been used for years in treating angina; however, their mechanism of action has only recently been clarified. Nitrates relax vascular smooth muscle and so dilate both systemic arteries and veins, the predominant effect being on the venous circulation. The decreased venous return to the heart reduces the preload and ventricular dimensions, and this reduces wall tension and afterload. As a result, the myocardial oxygen requirements are reduced. These drugs also increase regional myocardial blood flow, usually with a redistribution of blood flow to ischemic zones, by directly dilating the coronary arteries and by increasing collateral blood flow. Since coronary lesions are eccentric, nitrates can dilate the compliant portion of the vessel at the site of the coronary narrowing. At the cellular level, nitrates with sulfhydryl groups induce an increase in cyclic guanosine monophosphate (cGMP) production, which accelerates calcium release from vascular smooth muscle cells and thereby reduces calcium stores.[53]

Nitroglycerin remains the drug of choice for acute attacks, and it usually relieves the pain within 2 to 4 minutes. The psychoneurotic patient often does not obtain relief until after 15 minutes or longer, which indicates that the pain probably was not angina. However, nitroglycerin is not specific for angina; it can relieve spasm in some GI disorders such as cardiospasm, pylorospasm, or colic due to gallstones. Also, failure to respond to nitroglycerin does not exclude angina, especially the unstable variety. In some instances, lack of response is the result of loss of potency of the nitroglycerin tablets. The supply should be replenished if the tablets do not produce burning of the tongue or some fullness in the head. Some formulations of nitroglycerin, such as Nitrostat, have been recommended as providing improved stability and more uniform tablet potency.

The patient and his family should be instructed carefully in the proper use of nitroglycerin. The drug can be inactivated by heat and moisture as well as by air, light, and time, and thus should not be carried close to the body; that is, an outside pocket is preferable to an inside pocket. A 2-week supply of tablets should be kept in a stoppered, dark glass bottle or vial or a special insulated container, since nitroglycerin is volatile. The use of metal pillboxes should be discouraged.

The cotton packing should be removed from the bottle and discarded to expedite removal of a tablet in an emergency. It is not unusual to see a dead patient with an open bottle of nitroglycerin tablets lying nearby, the cotton only partially removed. The main supply of the drug should be refrigerated. Before the personal supply is replenished, the bottle from the refrigerator should be warmed to room temperature to prevent condensation of water on cold tablets. The unused portion of the main supply of tablets should be replaced by a fresh supply every 6 months.

To avoid headaches, the patient should be instructed to begin his course of nitroglycerin therapy with the smallest effective dose. Patients who have had a headache caused by the drug frequently are reluctant to take the medication. Thus it is wise for the physician to observe the patient's reaction on taking his first nitroglycerin tablet. In the event that nitroglycerin cannot be tolerated, the sublingual isosorbide dinitrate (Isordil and Sorbitrate) or transmucosal tablets (Susadrin) under the lip or buccal pouch may be substituted.

The initial sublingual dose of nitroglycerin should be 0.16 mg (1/400 grains) or 0.32 mg (1/200 grains). An increase in dosage may be necessary until a feeling of warmth or a pounding headache is produced. This at least will establish that the drug has not lost its potency. The patient should be advised that nitroglycerin may be taken repeatedly without becoming ineffective or habit-forming, and that tolerance is uncommon. At times the dosage may have to be increased. I usually advise the patient to take 1 tablet every 5 minutes for a total of 3 tablets and to seek medical aid if the pain persists, because a coronary occlusion may be developing. A sublingual nitroglycerin spray that gives a metered aerosolized dose of 0.4 mg can be more usable, especially for the elderly.

Postural hypotension can occur with excessive use of nitroglycerin, especially in the elderly. However, the drug is short-acting and does not accumulate in the body; thus, the series of 3 tablets may be repeated after 15 minutes if angina recurs. I advise patients with angina to use nitroglycerin if they are uncertain about whether they are having an attack, because the drug is relatively harmless. Nitroglycerin also may be used prophylactically in anticipation of angina that is known to occur with certain activities, such as sexual intercourse. Patients should be instructed to record the number of tablets used daily, so that any change in the anginal pattern can be noted. Occasionally, angina worsens with the use of nitroglycerin, which suggests that the cause may be severe aortic stenosis or idiopathic hypertrophic subaortic stenosis.

Many long-acting organic nitrates such as isosorbide dinitrate or nitroglycerin ointment are available for the prevention of anginal attacks. At present, isosorbide dinitrate is widely used. Initially it was thought to work only sublingually, which necessitated giving tablets of 2.5 to 10 mg every 2 to 3 hours. The smaller oral doses used previously probably were ineffective because not enough was given to saturate the liver and allow a sufficient amount to get into the circulation. It may take up to 20 to 40 mg or more three times per day orally to produce a hemodynamic effect.[54] Oral isosorbide-5-mononitrate (a metabolite of isosorbide dinitrate) may be more suitable for long-term therapy because it lacks first-pass hepatic metabolism. Nitrol ointment may be applied to the skin in 1 to 2 inches three times per day. Recently several transdermal methods (Transderm-Nitro, Nitro-Dur, and Nitro-Disc) have made the delivery of nitroglycerin easier and much less messy by using a strip resembling an adhesive bandage.

Long-term therapy with such patches has produced conflicting results. The majority have shown improvement of exercise tolerance for only 4 to 6 hours and considerable attenuation of therapeutic effect by 24 hours.[55] In addition, the effective dose of nitroglycerin has not been resolved. Recently the FDA issued a preliminary report on a multicenter dosage cooperative study of the three types of patches involving 450 patients.[55a] Exercise treadmill tests were performed each week at the time a new dosage was given; the first one just before receiving a new dose; the second one four hours after application; the last one 24 hours after application. This study concluded that the transdermal patches increased the time patients could exercise on the treadmill before experiencing angina up to 4 hours for several doses, but no differences were found compared to placebo at 24 hours. Tolerance developed rapidly and could not be overcome by increments of dose from 15 mg up to 105 mg/24 hours. However, there was a trend in reduction of anginal attacks in patients with frequent baseline attacks suggesting a possible dissociation between nitroglycerin effects on exercise tolerance and on angina frequency. Another study showed that intermittent therapy with larger doses of 15 to 20 mg of transdermal nitroglycerin was more beneficial than the commonly prescribed dosages of 5 to 10 mg.[55b] Present patches contain about 5 to 15 mg of nitroglycerin. It is best to start with 5 to 10 mg and increase to 15 mg depending on the patient's response to therapy until further studies are done.

Nitrate tolerance can develop with all forms of chronic nitrate administration. The mechanism of tolerance is thought to be due to a deficiency of reduced sulfhydryl groups and decreased production of nitrosothiols and cyclic GMP. It appears that preparations and dosages that produce constant plasma and tissue concentrations exhibit rapid tolerance, whereas those that produce nitrate-free intervals exhibit only partial tolerance. Therefore, at present, I recommend that oral nitrates be given three times per day with the last dose at the time of the evening meal and that the patches be removed after 16 hours.[56,57] However, the optimal timing for the nitrate-free period can vary depending on the timing of the ischemic events. Most ischemic events, both symptomatic and asymptomatic, occur early in the day. If a patient experiences angina frequently at night, it may be necessary to change the nitrate timing or adjust the β-blocker or calcium blocker to cover this night time interval.

β-Blockers. For many years, the nitrates have been the main drugs used for angina. With the advent of β-blockers, the management of angina has improved tremendously. β-blockers are probably the most significant drugs introduced in clinical medicine in this century. Numerous double-blind control studies (especially with propranolol) have well substantiated the value of β-blockers in the management of angina. Relatively few patients with angina cannot be helped by the use of these drugs. Direct sympathetic nerve stimulation mediates most of the β_1 response and norepinephrine is the usual neurotransmitter. Epinephrine accounts for most of the β_2 effects. The β-blockers' antianginal effect is almost entirely due to β_1 blockade. Thus they can reduce myocardial oxygen needs by decreasing myocardial contractility, slowing the heart rate, and lowering systolic blood pressure.[58] The left ventricular volume (preload) may increase with such drugs and so increase the myocardial oxygen requirements. β_2 receptor blockade may allow peripheral vasoconstriction (increase afterload), since it leaves the alpha-adrenergic effect to predominate. Theoretically, coronary vasoconstriction can occur with β-blockers because they allow unopposed coronary vasoconstrictor impulses to prevail. However, this is rarely noted clinically and then occurs primarily in the nonischemic areas and so may direct blood to the ischemic zone. Comparing these hemodynamic actions with those of nitrates and calcium blockers, it appears that the β-blockers act complementarily with nitrates and calcium blockers (Table 4–10). Usually β_2 blockade produces side effects such as bronchospasm, vasoconstriction, and suppression of glycogenolysis. In addition, recent studies have shown that excessive catecholamines (namely, β_2 stimulation) can enhance inward movement of potassium from the extracellular compartment into the intracellular compartment and thus can produce hypokalemia.[59] This potassium shift cannot be blocked by blocking β_1 receptors. However, β_2 blockade such as occurs with nonselective β-blockers can blunt the shift and thereby decrease the potential for hypokalemia.[60] Increased sympathetic drive in the presence of hypokalemia may lead to cardiac arrhythmias, particularly in patients with coronary artery disease. Other possible mechanisms of β-blockers in angina are their inhibition of oxygen-wasting effect of free fatty acid metabolism (reduces myocardial oxygen demands) and their reduction of platelet aggregation.

The β-blockers (Table 4–11) can be divided into the lipophilic types (propranolol, timolol, pindolol, and metoprolol) and the hydrophilic types (nadolol, acebutolol, and atenolol).[61] The lipophilic types are absorbed well and cross the brain barrier. They are metabolized by the liver and have a plasma half-life of about 6 hours. Timolol is largely metabolized by the liver and is less lipid-soluble than propranolol or metoprolol. The hydrophilic types are not absorbed

Table 4–10. Complementary Action of β-Blockers

	Nitrates	β-Blockers	Calcium Blockers
Heart rate	— or ↑	↓	—, ↑, or ↓
Contractility	—	↓	— or ↓
Blood pressure	— or ↓	↓	↓
Preload	↓	↑	— or ↓
Afterload	— or ↓	— or ↑	↓
Coronary vasodilation	↑	— or ↓	↑

↑ = Increased.
↓ = Decreased.
— = No effect.

Table 4–11. Beta Blockers

Lipophilic	B_1 Blockade	B_2 Blockade	PVR	ISA	MS	Daily Mg Dosage
Propranolol	+	+	—	—	+	40–320
Metoprolol	+	*lesser	—	—	+	100–400
Timolol	+	+	—	—	—	20–40
Pindolol	+	+	↓	+	+	5–40
Hydrophilic						
Nadolol	+	+	—	—	—	40–80
Atenolol	+	*lesser	—	—	—	50–100
Acebutolol	+	*lesser	↓	+	+	200–800

ISA = Intrinsic sympathetic activity.
PVR = Peripheral vascular resistance.
MS = Membrane stabilizing activity.
↓ = Decreased.
— = No effect.
* = Dose-related.

well, do not cross the brain barrier, are excreted by the kidney, and have a half-life of up to 24 hours. Metoprolol, acebutolol, and atenolol are cardioselective (lesser blockade of Beta$_2$ receptors); however, in higher doses this selectivity is lost. The average dose of propranolol is usually 160 mg daily, with a maximum of about 320 mg daily. It is best to begin with 10 mg four times per day and increase the amount depending on the response. At times daily, Inderal-LA capsules of 80 to 160 mg may be best, especially if the patient has a compliance problem. The β-blockers should not be given in the presence of congestive heart failure, greater than first-degree AV block, or in patients with chronic lung disease with asthmatic bronchitis. Metoprolol (Lopressor), atenolol, and acebutolol have been used with some success in lower doses in patients with chronic lung disease. One should be careful in giving these drugs to diabetic patients, for they can mask and prolong hypoglycemia. Urticaria has been rarely noted. Peripheral vascular disease may be aggravated. Sudden withdrawal of such drugs can produce an exaggerated cardiac β-adrenergic responsiveness, with a marked exacerbation of angina, precipitation of arrhythmias, or even acute myocardial infaction.[62] The hydrophilic types may produce less fatigue and fewer cerebral symptoms, since they do not cross the brain barrier. Nadolol (Corgard) therapy is usually begun at a dosage of 40 mg daily and increased as necessary. If one changes from propranolol to nadolol, it is best to begin with a dosage that is half the amount of propranolol that the patient was taking. Because nadolol is excreted predominantly in the urine, its half-life increases in renal failure, and therefore the dosage interval should be increased. At times such patients may require a dose only every other day. Atenolol (Tenormin) is usually begun at a dosage of 50 mg daily. β-blockers with intrinsic sympathetic activity (pindolol and acebutolol) exhibit low-grade β stimulation when sympathetic activity is low. When sympathetic activity is high, as with stress or exertion, they act like the usual β-blockers. They are useful in patients with angina and a slow resting heart rate or in those who get severe sinus bradycardia with the conventional β-blockers. Membrane-stabilizing activity (quinidine-like effect) is noted with propranolol, metoprolol, acebutolol and pindolol, but only in doses much larger than those used clinically. Table 4–11 compares the effects and dosages of the various β-blockers.

A β-blocker can be expected to cause sinus bradycardia, which indicates that the drug has been absorbed and is producing a pharmacologic effect. Physicians unfamiliar with such a drug will discontinue prescribing it because of the slowed heart rate. This reaction alarms the patient, who becomes reluctant to take the drug again and thinks he will become weak because of the slow heart rate. We usually begin with a low dose of β-blocker and increase it depending on anginal relief, reactions, and heart rate. Generally the resting heart rate is not allowed to fall below 55 beats per minute. With adequate β-blockades, the heart rate will increase less than 20 beats per minute after about 10 sit-ups on the examining table.

Long-term administration of β-blockers may produce lipid changes.[63] It appears at present that the nonselective types are the most unfavorable (they increase triglycerides, decrease HDL, and have variable effects on total cholesterol), the cardioselective types have fewer lipid adverse effects, and those with intrinsic sympathetic activity are the most favorable (they may decrease cholesterol, increase HDL, or may be neutral). However, further long-term studies are needed to confirm such findings.

Calcium-entry Blockers. Recently it has been shown that spasm can occur with all types of coronary syndromes (stable and unstable angina). This may be due to physiologic increase in coronary tone with constriction or segmental spasm of a coronary vessel. Physiologic increase in smooth muscle tone is probably important in determining variability of exercise tolerance and episodes of rest ischemia in patients with chronic stable angina. Approximately 42% of patients with rest angina have spasm, and if ST elevation is associated with the chest pain, 93% have spasm. Usually the spasm is superimposed on an atherosclerotic lesion. However, at coronary arteriography 5% may have normal vessels and 11% may have less than 50% narrowed vessels. Calcium-entry blockers have been shown to be effective in the management of angina because calcium plays an important part in spasm. Whereas nitrates and calcium blockers relieve spasm of epicardial coronary arteries, calcium-blockers also relieve spasm of the intramyocardial arterioles. Nitrates and calcium blockers (less so) reduce left ventricular end-diastolic pressure and lessen diastolic compression of the subendocardial capillaries and improve diastolic filling. In addition, calcium blockers dilate peripheral arteries and reduce the afterload. Some also decrease the heart rate, reduce conduction velocity through the AV node, and decrease myocardial contractility (Table 4–12). Those available at present for angina are nifedipine (Procardia), verapamil (Calan and Isoptin), and diltiazem (Cardizem). They vary considerably to the extent that they produce the above actions. Verapamil has a greater negative inotropic effect and should not be given if left ventricular function is greatly decreased. Nifedipine has a more potent peripheral vasodilator effect, which reduces afterload and lessens its negative inotropic effect. However, this effect can produce reflex tachycardia. Verapamil and diltiazem block the slow channel calcium response in the AV node. Nifedipine does not have this effect. The usual dosage for nifedipine is 10 to 30 mg q 6 to 8 h, for verapamil 80 to 120 mg q 6 to 8 h and for diltiazem 30 to 60 mg q 6 to 8 h. Such drugs can produce postural hypotension, dizziness, nausea, headaches, and peripheral edema (not due to heart failure). Constipation can occur with verapamil. If left ventricular dysfunction is present, it is best not to prescribe other negative inotropic agents as beta-blockers and disopyramide (Norpace) with verapamil. Verapamil can in-

Table 4–12. Clinical Effects of Calcium Blockers

Dosage	Diltiazem 30–60 mg tid	Nifedipine 10–30 mg tid	Verapamil 80–120 mg tid
Coronary vasodilation	+ +	+ + +	+ +
Peripheral arteriolar vasodilation	+	+ + +	+ +
Myocardial contractility	—	↓ ↑	↓
Heart rate	↓	↑	↓ ↑
AV nodal conduction	↓ ↓	—	↓ ↓ ↓

↓ = Decreased.
↑ = Increased.
— = No effect.
+,+ +,+ + + = Increasing degree of effect.

crease the serum digoxin level. There have been conflicting reports that ni-fedipine can do this. Table 4–13 shows the calcium blockers of choice for angina when it is associated with other problems or conditions. In addition, occasionally combinations of calcium blockers may be effective because they have different ways and sites of inhibiting calcium entry. Recently, nicardipine (Cardene), which has actions similar to those of nifedipine, has been released for angina and hypertension. Other calcium blockers will soon be available for hypertension, such as isradipine (Dynacirc) and nitrendipine (Baypress).

Many studies have been done comparing the various agents (nitrates, β-blockers, calcium blockers) but the results have been variable. The efficacy of one drug over the other depended on the relative dose and the population being studied. Calcium-entry blockers have been found to be as effective as a β-blocking drug or a long-acting nitrate in reducing the frequency of angina and improving exercise tolerance. In some studies, combined therapy with two or more drugs has been shown to be more effective than monotherapy. In my experience, often patients end up requiring triple therapy (nitrate, calcium-blocker, and β-blocker). The mechanisms of action of these drugs are very similar but do differ sufficiently to suggest that combination therapy may be useful. However, on such triple therapy, patients should be observed closely for orthostatic hypotension. In addition, patients with reduced left ventricular function and conduction system disease must be observed closely, for such patients have been excluded from the reported studies.[64]

Ambulatory ECG monitoring has shown that patients with angina have a circadian variation of transient myocardial ischemia.[65] Frequency of symp-

Table 4–13. Angina and Other Conditions

	Nifedipine	Verapamil	Diltiazem
SA or AV node disease	√	—	—
BBB	√	√	√
SVT	—	√	√
LV dysfunction	√	—	√
Pulmonary disease, PVD, diabetes	√	√	√

√ = Can be used.
— = Should not be used.
BBB = Bundle branch block.
SVT = Supraventricular tachycardia.
LV = Left ventricular.
PVD = Peripheral vascular disease.

tomatic and asymptomatic (silent ischemia) episodes of ST segment displacement are maximum in the morning between 6 a.m. and 12 noon. Myocardial infarction, sudden death and stroke are also more likely to occur during these hours.[66,67] Factors that may be responsible for this are the following that occur in the morning: increased coronary tone, hypercoagulable state, increase in platelet aggregability, decrease in fibrinolytic activity, and increase in systemic blood pressure. In view of this, antianginal medication should be timed to provide protection during these morning hours.

Associated Aggravating Conditions

Hypertension, diabetes, and hyperuricemia should be treated aggressively. Anemia, thyrotoxicosis, heart failure, and arrhythmias must be recognized and appropriately treated.

UNSTABLE ANGINA

Patients with unstable angina (criteria listed in Table 4–2) should be treated as outlined in Table 4–9. They should be hospitalized and monitored in a cardiac care unit. In some cases, control of precipitating factors, such as arrhythmias, emotion, hypotension from any cause, hypertension, anemia, insulin reaction, thyrotoxicosis and pulmonary emboli, will stabilize the situation. Intravenous nitroglycerin should be started at a rate of 5 μg/min and increased as necessary as long as hypotension does not occur (mean arterial pressure should not be reduced by more than 10%). This reduces the need of other forms of nitrates. In addition, the patient should receive a β-blocker and calcium blocker as recommended for stable angina. Once the patient is stable, coronary arteriography should be performed. However, if in spite of therapy angina continues (Table 4–2, type 4:high risk subgroup), coronary arteriography should be done immediately.[1] If hemodynamic instability is present, before coronary arteriography, an intraaortic balloon for counter pulsation should be inserted. The Veterans Administration Study and the Canadian Study showed that aspirin reduced mortality and fatal or nonfatal acute myocardial infarction by 51% in patients with unstable angina.[68,69] The Veterans Study gave 324 mg daily and the Canadian study, 325 mg four times daily. A recent study tested the usefulness of 325 mg aspirin twice daily, heparin 1,000 units per hour by I.V. infusion, and a combination of the two in the early management of 479 patients with unstable angina in a double-blind, randomized, placebo-controlled trial.[70] Aspirin or heparin was associated with a reduced incidence of myocardial infarction (trend favoring heparin) and heparin reduced the incidence of refractory angina. At present we recommend that heparin be administered to all patients, unless there is a contraindication, until patients have coronary arteriography. Because many of our patients come to surgery, we wait until after this procedure to start 325 mg aspirin per day since the effect of aspirin cannot be reversed immediately and bleeding can occur. However, if the patient is a candidate for PTCA, aspirin is given prior to the procedure even though there is a risk that the patient may need emergency bypass surgery. The role of thrombolysis in unstable angina is still being tested. In patients with unstable angina, intraluminal thrombus frequently persists, despite heparin treatment. A study by Gold et al. gave a 12-hour infusion of rt-PA with heparin which lysed the thrombus and stabilized the patient but was associated with an unacceptably high incidence of bleeding.[71]

Some patients with Prinzmetal's variant angina can be classified (Table 4–2) as having unstable angina. This entity has been described earlier in this chapter. Usually in such cases spasm is superimposed on an atherosclerotic lesion, producing rest angina and ST elevation. Coronary arteriography in patients with Prinzmetal's angina has revealed in several studies that 5% have normal vessels, 11% have mildly (less than 50%) narrowed vessels, 43% single-vessel disease, 21% double-vessel disease, and 20% have triple-vessel disease.[72,73] Patients with Prinzmetal's angina with attacks can have major ventricular arrhythmias and Stokes-Adams attacks, especially with spasm of the right coronary artery. Spasm in patients with normal coronary arteriograms is more common in the right coronary artery and less in the left anterior descending and circumflex vessels, and rarely occurs in the left main coronary artery. In fact, only catheter-induced spasm has been reported in the normal left main coronary artery,[74] and there have been no reports of spontaneous occurrence. As mentioned early in this chapter, calcium plays an important part in spasm. Calcium blockers and nitrates have been effective in the management of such cases. Studies have shown that such drugs can block ergonovine-provoked spasm.[75] β-blockers have produced variable responses in Prinzmetal's angina and at times may even aggravate the situation by unmasking the alpha-adrenergic response. Aspirin is of no value and in high dosage may block biosynthesis of the vasodilator prostacyclin (PGI_2) and increase the anginal attacks.

PERCUTANEOUS TRANSLUMINAL CORONARY ANGIOPLASTY

Percutaneous transluminal coronary angioplasty (PTCA) has been used successfully to dilate stenotic coronary arteries as well as saphenous vein grafts. This procedure has been used since 1964 to dilate peripheral arterial obstructions[76] and recently has been expanded by combining it with laser. Gruntzig et al. modified this procedure for peripheral vessel dilation and in 1978 dilated coronary artery lesions.[77] The basic equipment consists of a guiding catheter which is inserted into the femoral or brachial artery and advanced and positioned in the orifice of the coronary artery requiring dilation; through this a dilating catheter aided by a flexible guide wire is placed in the stenotic arterial branch (Figs 4–9 and 4–10). The dilating catheter has a double lumen to allow for pressure measurements, contrast injection, and inflation of the balloon. Inflation and deflation of the balloon are controlled by a calibrated pressure pump.[78] Intimal splitting, desaturation of liquid plaque elements, plaque compression, and increased outer arterial diameter occur to improve vessel caliber and increase coronary blood flow. Originally, patients for the procedure were carefully selected, and had to have single-vessel disease, discrete, concentric, noncalcified proximal coronary obstruction, and good left ventricular function and were candidates for coronary bypass surgery. Advances in catheter and guide wire technology and operator experience have extended the procedure for selected patients with multiple-vessel disease, vein-graft and internal mammary-graft stenosis (anastomotic site has best result), and for patients who have had a myocardial infarction with or without thrombolytic therapy. Calcification is no longer a contraindication. The avail-

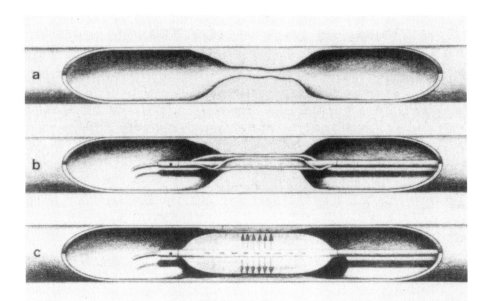

Fig 4–9.   Percutaneous transluminal coronary angioplasty. Stenosis in a coronary artery (*a*). The double-lumen balloon catheter is introduced by the use of a guiding catheter into the stenotic area. A side hole is connected to the main lumen of the dilating catheter for pressure recordings and contrast-material injection (*b*). The balloon is inflated across the stenosis (*c*). (Reprinted by permission from Grüntzig A.R., et al.: Nonoperative dilatation of coronary-artery stenosis: Percutaneous transluminal coronary angioplasty. *N. Engl. J. Med.* 301:61, 1979.)

ability of longer balloons and angled balloons has expanded their use. Generally, a surgeon should be available for emergency coronary bypass if it becomes necessary. However, this is not necessary in some individuals in whom angioplasty may be of value, but surgery is contraindicated as in patients with severe pulmonary disease. Objective evidence of myocardial ischemia should be obtained. In general, the indications for coronary angioplasty are the same as those for bypass surgery if the coronary anatomy is suitable, until the results from controlled clinical trials are known. Angioplasty is successful in up to 90% of patients with single-vessel disease. Complications that can occur are coronary artery dissection, prolonged angina, arrhythmias, coronary spasm, hypotension and ventricular fibrillation. New procedural modalities are reducing the major complication rates. Less than 5% of cases require emergency surgery. The success rate is almost as high with multiple vessel angioplasty, but the long-term results are not as favorable. After PTCA, patients should have exercise thallium-201 myocardial perfusion scintography. One study[98a] showed by sequential studies that there may be delayed improvement after PTCA (up to 2 to 9 months). Thus an abnormal thallium stress test a few days after PTCA does not necessarily reflect residual coronary artery stenosis or recurrence of coronary artery disease. Early abnormal scans could represent stunned or hibernating myocardial perfusion state or transient effect of local trauma at the site of angioplasty. Restenosis occurs in approximately 20% of cases with chronic stable angina (most are candidates for repeat angioplasty), usually within 6 months of PTCA. Restenosis may be higher in unstable angina and in the setting of an acute myocardial infarction (where thrombus is

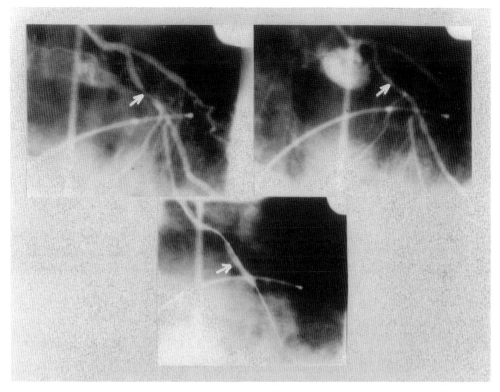

Fig 4–10. Right oblique view. Left upper figure depicts 95% proximal lesion in the circumflex coronary artery (arrow). Lower figure shows balloon (3 mm) inflated in the stenotic area, and upper right figure after percutaneous transluminal coronary angioplasty reveals the vessel completely open. (Courtesy of Dr. Michael E. Assey.)

likely). Aspirin, dipyridamole, fish oil and anticoagulants are being used to decrease this rate of stenosis.[79] One study comparing dipyridamole and aspirin to placebo showed no reductions in the 6-month rate of restenosis in both groups after successful angioplasty, but the antiplatelet group reduced the incidence of transmural infarction during or soon after PCTA.[80] Intracoronary stents are also being evaluated to prevent restenosis.[81] The NHLBI registry reported an in-hospital mortality rate of 1% and nonfatal myocardial infarction rate of 4.3% for patients having PTCA in 1985 to 1986.[82] Long-term results with angioplasty up to 6 years show an actuarial event-free survival (freedom from death, myocardial infarction, and bypass surgery) of 79% at 6 years.[83] Long-term follow-up and comparisons with bypass surgery need further investigation. At present, two large trials are in progress to establish safety and efficacy in multivessel disease.

LASER ANGIOPLASTY

A significant number of patients cannot be treated by angioplasty or bypass surgery, and many have reocclusions after these procedures and need further therapy. Laser recanalization, which can ablate the obstructive lesion into water vapor, carbon dioxide, and other combustion products appears to offer another method of therapy.[84] Its beam can be passed through small optical fibers, leaving a smooth surface which may reduce restenosis characteristic of balloon angioplasty. Currently, several continuing-wave lasers have been used such as CO_2, Argon-Ion and Neodymium Yttrium Aluminum garnet (ND:YAG). Excimer is a pulsed laser which produces less thermal injury and can ablate calcified lesions. Laser wavelengths vary from deep infrared to ultraviolet (excimer laser). Lasers are now used routinely for peripheral arterial obstruction. Clinical trials are investigating the use of lasers in coronary artery obstructions by the percutaneous method and in the operating room during bypass surgery. Preliminary studies have shown some promising results in both peripheral and coronary arteries. Lasers with bare optical fibers have been used and with encapsulated heated metal caps (hot-tips). The latter method allows the passage of a guide wire and subsequently balloon angioplasty. More recently, a sapphire lens at the tip of the optical fiber has been used to create a larger channel and so balloon angioplasty may not be required. Arterial perforation has been one of the major limitations of the use of lasers. A steerable "monorail" guide wire system may reduce this complication. The "smart" laser is a new system that employs fluorescence spectroscopy to identify atherosclerotic plaques during laser angioplasty. Many studies are now under way exploring alternate sources of heat (including electrical and thermal) and more flexible catheter systems for coronary arteries.

SURGICAL TREATMENT OF CORONARY ARTERY DISEASE

Saphenous vein and internal mammary artery bypass grafts from the aorta distal to the segmental coronary obstruction (Fig 4–11) has become the most widely used revascularization technique at present. Fortunately, about 70% of lesions are in the proximal segment of the coronary arteries. As mentioned

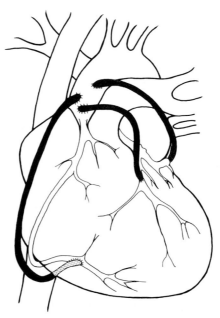

Fig 4–11. Drawing of saphenous vein grafts to the right, left anterior descending and circumflex coronary arteries.

earlier, because symptomatology and stress tests may not define the coronary anatomy involved, it is best to perform coronary arteriography in most patients who have had any coronary event. Several studies have shown that patients with significant left main coronary artery lesions or triple-vessel disease with impaired left ventricular function have a statistically significant greater survival for at least 7 years with surgery as compared to medical therapy.[85,86] The European Coronary Surgery Study,[87,88] a prospective randomized trial of medical and surgical treatment, showed that the groups that benefited most from surgery were those with left main (5-year survival, 62% for medical and 93% for surgery) and three-vessel disease (85% for medical and 95% for surgery). This study also showed that patients with two-vessel disease in whom one of the involved vessels is in the proximal portion of the left anterior descending coronary artery also had a longer survival with surgery. Surgery should be recommended depending on symptoms, ventricular function, coronary anatomy, age, and general health of the patient. Even though there are many criteria for surgery at present, I feel that it should be offered to patients with angina not responding well to medical therapy, those who react to drugs or do not feel comfortable with the life style produced by the angina, and those with significant left main coronary artery stenosis or three-vessel coronary artery disease, especially if there is left ventricular dysfunction. Patients with single- and two-vessel disease have to be individualized. The European Study has shown that those with two-vessel disease have longer survival with surgery if the left anterior descending coronary artery is one of the involved vessels. Those with multivessel disease who have discrete lesions and are candidates for surgery can be considered first for angioplasty. Kumpuris et al.[89] have shown that stenosis of the left anterior descending coronary artery is a heterogeneous disease. The extent of jeopardized myocardium depends on the site of stenosis. Patients with proximal lesions (prior to the first septal branch) and a myocardial infarction had greater decrease in ejection fraction and more abnormal segmental wall dysfunction than those who had obstruction with infarction in the middle (after the first septal branch and before the first diagonal branch) or distal (2 cm distal to origin of the first diagonal branch) segments of the left anterior descending coronary artery. However, ejection fraction and segmental wall dysfunction were similar, with proximal and distal stenosis of the right coronary artery and inferior infarction. I recommend angioplasty or surgery for a patient with a proximal left anterior descending lesion especially when the left anterior descending is a long vessel going around the apex, for obstruction of such a vessel might cause serious damage to the left ventricle, which can lead to a ventricular aneurysm, cardiogenic shock, or serious electric conduction defects. Angioplasty or surgery is offered for single-vessel right coronary lesion, circumflex or middle or distal left anterior descending if there is objective evidence of diffuse ischemia with a large area compromised that can produce serious ventricular damage, or the patient is symptomatic in spite of medical therapy. Often after coronary arteriography "compelling anatomy" may influence one's decision. This term is subjective and difficult to define.

Benefits from bypass surgery progressively decrease with time because atherosclerosis progresses in the grafted and ungrafted arteries and in the grafts. The Veterans Administration Cooperative Study[86] showed that after 7 years the surgical survival benefits declined for patients with three-vessel disease and decreased left ventricular function. In addition, patients who had surgery for any coronary involvement had an increase in symptoms and a decrease in exercise tolerance to levels similar to those of medically treated patients at 10 years. Fibrous thickening of intimal, media, and adventitia, endothelial damage, medial hypertrophy, intimal lipid deposition, and aneurysmal dilation can occur in the grafts.[90] Elevation of blood lipids appears to be a major factor for the development of intimal fibromuscular proliferation or atheroma.[91] Early occlusion rate per distal anastomosis of vein grafts has been reported to be about 8 to 18% in the first month after surgery.[92] In the same period, the occlusion rate per patient, with one or more distal anastomoses occluded, ranges from 21 to 38%. By the end of the first year, the overall occlusion rate per distal anastomosis is about 16 to 26%. During that time, about 41 to 47% of patients will have one or more distal anastomoses occluded. A study by Lytle et al.[93] showed that the patency of internal mammary artery (IMA) grafts within 5 years of operation is 97% and for vein grafts 82%, and for over 5 years, 96% for IMA versus 55% for vein grafts. In another study,[94] the 10-year actuarial survival rate for those receiving IMA grafts compared to vein grafts was 93.4% versus 88% for those with one-vessel disease; 90% versus 79.5% for those with two-vessel disease; and 82.6% versus 71% for those with three-vessel disease. Whenever feasible, the internal mammary artery should be used instead of a vein graft. Aspirin and dipyridamole can decrease the incidence of vein graft occlusion.[92,95] Those with elevated lipids should have dietary counseling and lipid-lowering agents if necessary. The National Heart, Lung, and Blood Institute is now sponsoring a multicenter study in postcoronary bypass graft patients on the impact of various interventions (diet regimen, cholesterol-lowering drugs, and antithrombotic therapy) on saphenous vein graft patency.

Often patients coming to coronary artery bypass surgery have asymptomatic carotid artery bruits. A recent study[96] concluded that the presence of carotid bruits increased the risk of stroke after bypass surgery, but the absolute magnitude of this risk is small (2.9%) and is comparable to the reported risk of stroke from carotid endarterectomy. Several studies have confirmed that patients with asymptomatic cervical bruits and significant occlusive carotid disease have a higher incidence of stroke than those without significant obstruction.[97,98] However, whether surgical intervention will reduce this stroke risk in such patients has not yet been established. At present, for the patient with neurologic symptoms, staged carotid reconstruction several days before elective coronary bypass surgery appears to be the safest method. Combined procedures may be necessary for those with active neurologic symptoms and unstable coronary artery disease.[99]

SILENT MYOCARDIAL ISCHEMIA

Silent myocardial ischemia can be defined as objective evidence of ischemia without pain or other recognized complaints. Cohn[100] has classified silent myocardial ischemia into three types as follows: (1) patients with coronary artery disease who are asymptomatic and presumably healthy individuals; (2) patients who have had a myocardial infarction and demonstrate silent ischemia; (3) patients with angina who have silent ischemia. Type 1 patients are usually detected by a positive stress test (ECG or radionuclide) and subsequent coronary arteriography. Erikssen[101] screened 2014 men (ages 40 to 59) and found that 50 (2.5%) had silent myocardial ischemia on exercise testing and significant coronary artery disease on coronary arteriography. Type 2 cases are also usually detected by a positive stress test. The stress test study of Theroux of 210 consecutive postmyocardial infarction patients showed that 17% had ST depression without experiencing angina, and these along with those who had angina are at a high risk for further cardiac events and death.[102] In one study ischemic ST changes on Holter monitoring (majority silent) occurred in nearly one third of high-risk postinfarction patients and are significantly associated with 1-year mortality.[103] Type 3 patients can show a positive stress test or ST changes during Holter monitoring not associated with angina. Four to 5 million people in the United States have silent myocardial ischemia, and of these 1 to 2 million are asymptomatic (type 1), about 50,000 are patients asymptomatic postinfarction (type 2), and 3 million have angina (type 3).[100] Fifty percent of patients with coronary artery disease initially have an acute myocardial infarction or sudden death. Deanfield et al.[104] studied patients with stable angina using 4 days of ambulatory Holter monitoring and showed that of 1934 episodes of ST segment depression, only 24% were associated with angina. In addition, with these silent episodes the heart rate did not increase in 77%, indicating a decrease in myocardial oxygen supply rather than an increased demand. This suggests that spasm may be a factor, although the mechanism is not clear. Some individuals may have a defective anginal warning system and differences in pain threshold. Currently it appears that beta-endorphins do not play an essential role in the pathophysiology of silent myocardial ischemia.[105] Symptomatic episodes are usually more severe and longer as determined by the magnitude of ST changes. Ischemia of sufficient degrees to produce ECG changes may not be sufficient to produce angina. Approximately 25% of acute myocardial infarctions are silent. Two major problems at present confronting the practicing physician are the following: (1) Who should be screened for silent ischemia? (2) How should it be managed? At present, I would suggest that patients with known coronary artery disease and those with significant risk factors should have an ECG or radionuclide stress test. Ischemia noted by Holter monitoring is most always detected in stress ECG testing. There are many ongoing studies of the natural history and prognosis of silent myocardial ischemia that may answer the treatment question. Gottlieb[106] had Holter monitors on 70 patients with unstable angina on triple therapy (nitrates, β-blockers, calcium blockers) and found that 37 of these patients had silent ischemia. In 1 month 6 sustained acute myocardial infarction, whereas only 1 of 33 without silent ischemia had an infarction. Assey et al.[107] of our institution evaluated 55 patients with known coronary artery disease and positive thallium stress tests and found that at 30 months follow-up 6 of 28 patients with no angina during the stress test had myocardial infarctions and 3 died, and only 1 infarction occurred in the 27 patients who had angina during the test with no deaths. Such studies in the future will clarify the need of therapy for the silent episodes. At present we should make an attempt to eliminate with therapy (as in symptomatic angina) these silent episodes, especially concentrating therapy when such episodes are more likely to occur. Several studies have shown a circadian pattern of myocardial ischemia with frequency of episodes (silent and painful) increasing in the early morning to noon and then becoming less. During these hours it also has been shown that acute myocardial infarction and sudden death occur most often. Recently, mental stress was shown to precipitate silent myocardial ischemia in patients with coronary artery disease.[108] Such stress should be controlled.

ACUTE MYOCARDIAL INFARCTION

Coronary occlusion with resulting infarction is usually due to coronary atherosclerosis. Rarely, there are other causes, such as localized coronary artery spasm, platelet thrombi, embolism, or collagen diseases. Atheroma, thrombosis, or hemorrhage is present in most cases of coronary occlusion due to atherosclerosis. The role of thrombosis appears to be related to the time of study (coronary arteriography or autopsy) after the onset of chest pain. DeWood et al.[109] used coronary arteriography to study the degree of coronary obstruction in 322 patients admitted within 24 hours of an acute infarction. Total coronary occlusion was noted in 87% who were evaluated within 4 hours of the onset of symptoms and decreased to 65% when patients were studied 12 to 24 hours after the onset of symptoms. The authors suggested that coronary spasm or thrombus formation with subsequent recanalization or both may be important in the evolution of infarction. It appears that there may be a dynamic interaction between coronary spasm, platelet aggregation, thrombosis, and the atherosclerotic plaque that leads to coronary occlusion in the early phase of an acute infarction. Coronary occlusion can occur without infarction if adequate collaterals are present. Acute myocardial infarction, coronary occlusion, and coronary thrombosis often are used as synonyms. This is not the case. Acute coronary occlusion can occur other than by thrombosis and without infarction developing. In addition, acute infarction can occur without evidence of an acute arterial occlusion.

Each year in the United States, approximately 1,500,000 persons suffer an acute myocardial infarction. About 540,000 die, and 350,000 of the deaths occur outside the hospital.[110] One study showed that 180,000 die within 1 hour of the onset of acute symptoms, and 300,000 die within 2 hours.[111] Ventricular fibrillation is probably the mechanism of death in the majority of cases.[112] Many of these deaths can be prevented, or the patient can be resuscitated. Therefore, early recognition of acute myocardial infarction is most important for the expeditious entry of these patients into the medical care system, in either a mobile or a stationary facility. In addition, measures to limit infarction size will probably be most effective if applied early after the onset of infarction.

DIAGNOSIS OF ACUTE MYOCARDIAL INFARCTION

Symptoms

Prodromal Symptoms. Unfortunately, by the time the patient calls the physician, he has usually been experiencing symptoms for several hours. The first 2 hours are the most potentially lethal.[113] The earlier the patient can seek therapy the better, especially in view of the newer modalities of treatment. Patients should be educated about chest pain, especially those with known coronary artery disease. Delay is most often due to the patient (self-treatment and communication with other lay persons) and is also related to patient-physician contact. Office visits and inappropriate triage by nurses and receptionists are also important factors in physician delay.[114] In one study, a third of the patients who had an acute myocardial infarction made their own diagnosis prior to admission; another third interpreted the chest pain as indigestion; and the remaining patients were unable to explain the nature of their chest pain.[115] Prodromal symptoms may be present several weeks prior to the attack. In fact, in a study of 100 patients[116] admitted to a coronary care unit with acute myocardial infarction, prodromata occurred in 65%. Prodromal symptoms in that report usually were present 24 hours or longer (longest, 2 months) before the occurrence of the definitive attack of acute myocardial infarction. Chest pain was the most common symptom, and it usually was recurrent and progressive. Pain in 18% was associated with other symptoms such as dyspnea, diaphoresis, and light-headedness. In 9% pain was absent, and symptoms included burning in the chest, dyspnea, vertigo, weakness, and fatigue. Patients with previous coronary artery disease may note a sudden change or return of anginal symptoms.

The Acute Attack. The majority of patients with acute myocardial infarction have chest pain that is similar in location and quality to that of angina. The distress is classically located in the retrosternal area with radiation to the inner aspect of the left arm, hypothenar eminence, and fourth and fifth fingers. It may be referred to the neck and corresponding areas of the right arm, to both arms, and to the lower jaw. However, just as for angina, the distress may occur in only a segment of this distribution—it may be only in the chest, only in the interscapular area, only in the jaw, only in the neck, only in the left or right arm, and at times in only a part of the arms. It is usually described as a tight, squeezing, burning, indigestive, heavy, expanding, or boring sensation. Seldom is it sharp. It may begin as a sharpness and then develop into a heavy, squeezing feeling. The pain of acute myocardial infarction differs from angina in that it lasts 30 minutes to several hours; also, it frequently occurs at rest. Many patients have nausea and vomiting due to activation of vagal reflexes or to activation of cardiac receptors, namely in the left ventricle, which initiate impulses that travel in the vagus to the vasomotor centers and inhibit sympathetic discharge (Bezold-Jarisch reflex), especially in patients with inferior infarction.

Various epidemiologic and autopsy studies have shown that 20 to 60% of all myocardial infarctions are unrecognized. A 5-year prospective study in Israel reported an incidence of 39.8% unrecognized infarcts.[117] Half of these subjects had no recollection of any symptoms or illnesses since their last examination, and their infarctions were classified as silent. Another 42.3% had atypical symptoms that neither the subject nor the physician associated with a heart attack. Among the remaining 7.7%, the physicians thought that their symptoms might be related to infarcts, but the ECGs were not initially interpreted as such. However, the next survey examination of these subjects showed tracings interpreted as infarcts. American studies[118] report 30% of all infarcts as unrecognized, half of which are classified as silent. While it is impossible to make an accurate prediction of the incidence of unrecognized infarcts, studies suggest that for every clinical infarct detected there is probably at least one that is unrecognized in the same population group. However, in my experience many of these patients on further questioning will remember a vague episode of substernal discomfort that they had passed over as indigestion or some other condition. In other cases, pain is obscured by anesthesia, a cerebrovascular accident, shock, or initially by an Adams-Stokes attack. The pain may be overlooked if acute pulmonary edema develops rapidly. The presenting symptoms may be nausea, vomiting, excessive sweating, and weakness (especially in the elderly). The unrecognized infarction appears to be more frequent in patients with diabetes.

PHYSICAL EXAMINATION

The patient with acute myocardial infarction may have evidence of some of the risk factors. Funduscopic examination may reveal hypertensive, diabetic, or lipemic changes. Xanthomas may be noted as xanthelasmas around the eyelids; tendenosa in the tendons; tuberosa around the bony tubercules; or eruptive type about the trunk, buttocks, arms, or legs. Patients may have no significant complications, or the first conspicuous finding may be a complication.

Uncomplicated Case. Usually the patient appears sweaty and ashen. Hypotension may be present, and sometimes hypertension during pain or apprehension even though the patient was not previously hypertensive. An abnormal cardiac apical pulsation or an ectopic precordial impulse may be detected even in the absence of cardiomegaly. The ectopic pulsations are usually palpable or visible in the third or fourth intercostal spaces, superior and medial to the apical impulse, and often disappear in a few weeks unless a ventricular aneurysm develops. An atrial (S_4) gallop is present in the majority of patients with acute infarction. The first sound may become faint. Rarely, there is paradoxical splitting of the second sound, unless left bundle-branch block is present. The heart rate can be within normal range, or a sinus tachycardia or bradycardia (usually with an inferior infarct) may be present. During the first few days PVBs are noted in the majority of patients. Fever (seldom more than 101°F but sometimes as high as 103°F) usually develops after 24 hours, and a pericardial friction rub may appear after this period. The fever and pericardial rub can persist for several days. When pericarditis follows a myocardial infarction, the chest pain may be wrongly attributed to spread of the infarct, especially if no friction rub is audible.

Complicated Cases. Disturbances in the rhythm and conduction of the heart can be noted by physical examination. Final differentiation depends on the ECG. Major arrhythmias include persistent PVBs in excess of six beats per minute, as coupling, in pairs, or multifocal; paroxysmal supraventricular tachycardia; junctional, or ventricular tachycardia; and atrial flutter or fibrillation. Conduction disturbances can appear as AV block or the development of right (with or without hemiblocks) or left bundle-branch block. Left ventricular failure may present with persistent sinus tachycardia, pulmonary congestion, a ventricular (S_3) gallop, or as frank pulmonary edema. Later, right ventricular failure can develop with an elevated jugular venous pulse, hepatomegaly, and peripheral edema. Cardiogenic shock should be differentiated from hypotension. Often the BP may fall below 90 mm Hg, yet the patient is warm and has adequate urinary output. The patient in shock is usually cold and clammy, and the urine output is less than 0.5 ml per minute. An apical systolic murmur due to papillary muscle dysfunction may become audible. This murmur is usually late systolic, but can be holosystolic or midsystolic. A loud, prolonged apical systolic murmur may indicate papillary muscle rupture. Rupture of the ventricular septum produces a loud, rasping systolic murmur, often associated with a thrill, along the left sternal border. If the septal rupture is near the apex, its murmur may be difficult to distinguish from that of papillary muscle rupture.

Even though the left ventricle is usually damaged in acute myocardial infarction, it is now recognized that with acute inferior and posterior infarcts the right ventricle can be involved. This should be suspected in patients with such infarcts when there is an elevated systemic venous pressure (nearly equal to or greater than the pulmonary wedge pressure) without clinical or x-ray evidence of significant pulmonary congestion. Occasionally, prominent systolic C-V waves can be seen in the jugular venous pulses as a result of tricuspid insufficiency because of infarction of the right ventricular papillary muscle. Hypotension, cardiogenic shock, and bradyarrhythmias can occur. Pericarditis, Kussmaul's sign, and right ventricular S_3 or S_4 sounds have been noted in the majority of cases.[119] The combination of jugular venous distention, clear lungs, and hypotension can suggest acute pulmonary embolism; the presence of a pericardial rub with pulsus paradoxus can suggest acute cardiac tamponade. Abnormal right ventricular wall motion and dilatation of the right ventricle can be noted by echocardiography, gated bloodpool imaging, and the diagnosis can be confirmed by right heart catheterization at the bedside, using a Swan-Ganz flow-directed balloon-tipped catheter.

These and other complications, such as thromboembolism, postmyocardial infarction syndrome, and cardiac rupture, will be discussed later, along with management of acute myocardial infarction.

Laboratory Tests

Since the appearance of serum enzymes, the leukocytosis and the elevated sedimentation rate that occur with myocardial infarction have been ignored. Moderate leukocytosis is usually present after the first day and persists for a week. The sedimentation rate rises by the second day and remains elevated for several weeks. Serum glutamic oxalacetic transaminase (SGOT), lactic dehydrogenase (LDH) and isoenzymes, α-hydroxybutyrate dehydrogenase (HBD), and creatine kinase (CK or CPK) and isoenzymes are enzymes that are released from irreversibly injured myocardial cells into the circulation and can be measured. The SGOT was the first enzyme used clinically, but it is not used often today because it is nonspecific. The SGOT rises in 12 hours, peaks at 24 to 48 hours, and returns to control by 3 to 4 days. The enzymes LDH and HBD begin to rise in 12 hours but peak later than the SGOT, at 48 to 72 hours, and do not return to control for 7 to 10 days. These are helpful if the patient does not seek aid until 48 hours after the episode of pain. The enzyme CK rises in 4 to 6 hours, peaks by 24 hours, and returns to normal in 72 hours (Fig 4–12). The SGOT, LDH, and HBD are often elevated because of noncardiac disorders, such as liver disease or liver congestion. The CK is not found in the liver but is prominent in skeletal muscle. The serum level can be elevated by any muscle trauma, even that due to intramuscular injections. It should be mentioned that the serum CK can rise after heart catheterization, particularly selective

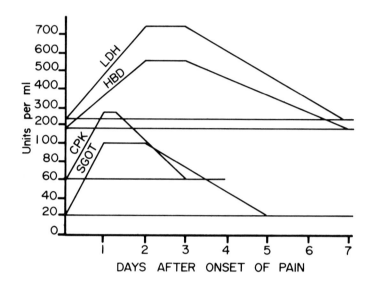

Fig 4–12. Changes in serum enzymes following an acute myocardial infarction. Horizontal lines indicate the top normal levels.

coronary arteriography. However, the other enzymes and isoenzymes do not exceed the accepted clinical range. This often presents a problem when a patient experiences pain after heart catheterization, and the diagnosis of infarction has to be excluded. It must be recognized that infarction can be present without elevation of the enzymes if there is a small area of necrosis. The setting of chest pain and an enzyme elevation to peak and then decline is suggestive of infarction. Serum enzymes not only aid in diagnosis, but also give a rough idea of the size of the infarction, which is related to their increase. Coodley[120] found a direct relationship between amplitude of enzyme rise and early mortality and morbidity. There was a mortality of 56% in patients with levels six times normal. If the level was four to five times normal there was an increased incidence of arrhythmias, heart failure, and cardiogenic shock.

Isoenzymes as MB fraction of CK and the flipped ratio of LDH_1 to LDH_2 (LDH_1 level higher than LDH_2) are more specific for myocardial infarction than total levels of CK and LDH. The MM, BB, and MB isoenzymes of CK have been identified. The skeletal muscle contains predominantly MM, the brain and kidney BB, and the cardiac muscle MM and MB. The CK-MB is the most sensitive and specific for myocardial necrosis. Measurement of CK by radio-immunoassay has improved sensitivity, specificity, and accuracy. At times, small amounts of CK-MB in the patient with infarction who has no significant rise in total CK can be detected. In such cases, however, the total CK and CK-MB show a classic rise and fall as seen with large infarcts, even though the total CK does not exceed the upper limits of normal. Usually in such a case the total CK activity for that individual may be at the low end of normal, and even if it rises threefold it still may not go above the upper limit of normal. One study[121] showed that among patients believed to have normal CK but elevated CK-MB levels, a real elevation of CK may be missed if too few samples are obtained or may be misinterpreted if the entire rise and fall are within the normal range, especially if the baseline value is low. Therefore, timing of samples in relationship to the clinical event and looking at the entire characteristic of the curve are most important rather than having an arbitrary cut-off level as normal. It takes about 6 hours for CK-MB to become elevated and it peaks within 12 to 24 hours. Generally, for optimum detection of an acute myocardial infarction, it is best that blood be drawn for CK-MB on admission and a minimum of two samples taken at 12 and 24 hours after onset of symptoms. The CK-MB peaks earlier (10 to 12 hours) in non-Q wave infarctions.[122] Samples with negative values obtained before 12 hours or after 24 hours cannot be used to exclude the diagnosis of infarction.[123] Improper timing accounts for most false-negatives. False-positives can occur with electric cardioversion, but are usually noted with high energy levels of shock; peak blood levels occur very early, at 4 to 6 hours, and disappear in 24 hours. Cardiac surgery can also cause a rise in CK-MB and cannot be used alone in the diagnosis of perioperative infarction. The creatine kinase MB isoenzyme in the evaluation of myocardial infarction has been extensively reviewed by Navin and Hager.[124]

Serum lactic dehydrogenase has five isoenzymes. The heart contains LDH_1, which usually rises within 12 to 24 hours after the onset of symptoms of an infarction and exceeds the level of LDH_2. An $LDH_1 > LDH_2$ ratio is not specific for acute myocardial infarction, since injury to other tissues, such as renal injury or hemolysis of RBCs, will also cause this to occur. The absence of this ratio does not exclude the presence of an infarction. It is now recognized that it is most cost-effective to routinely have only serial levels of total CK and CK-MB rather than routinely ordering all the various enzymes.

Electrocardiographic Findings

The ECG findings of myocardial infarction are discussed in more detail in Chapter 3. Myocardial infarction may be present with a typical clinical history, yet there may be no physical abnormalities or ECG changes. Unfortunately, during the early hours after the onset of myocardial infarction when the patient is more susceptible to primary ventricular fibrillation, the ECG may be normal. If serial tracings are obtained, 90% of patients with infarction will show abnormal changes. It may take several days for changes to develop, especially in the nontransmural types. After an infarction, the tracing can return to normal. The site of the infarct may be indicated as transmural (Q waves), intramural (T wave inversion), subendocardial or nontransmural (ST depression), or subepicardial (ST elevation). The significance of reciprocal ST depression in an anterior or inferior infarction is still debated. However, most

agree that myocardial infarctions with ST segment depression in remote myocardial areas represent more extensive myocardial necrosis, and if such
changes persist beyond the immediate peri-infarction period, more cardiac
events are likely to occur because of multivessel coronary artery disease.[125]
Right ventricular infarction is most often noted with an inferior infarction.
Therefore, findings of an inferior infarction will usually be present and often
in the right chest leads, especially in RV_4, the ST segments will be elevated.
Such changes often lessen the anterior lead reciprocal ST segment depression
noted with inferior infarctions.

Surface mapping of RS-T segment (from 35 to 72 points on the chest) occasionally may be of value in diagnosis of acute myocardial infarction when the
standard ECG is normal.[126] Recording over a wider area may reveal a site of
infarction which is inaccessible to the standard tracing. Such mapping is being
used for determining infarct size and detecting infarct extension.

Vectorcardiographic Findings

Vectorcardiography plays a secondary and minor role in the diagnosis of
acute myocardial infarction in general practice. It may be superior to the
routine ECG in demonstrating a true posterior, high posterior, or posterobasal
infarct.

X ray of the Chest

The x-ray examination of the chest often discloses no abnormality following
acute myocardial infarction. Complications may produce findings such as pulmonary congestion, cardiomegaly, pulmonary infarction, and a ventricular
aneurysm. The x ray may show pulmonary congestion due to left ventricular
dysfunction at times when there is no clinical evidence of heart failure. In fact,
the heart size may be normal.

Echocardiography

The echocardiogram can aid in differentiating ischemic heart disease from
other abnormalities by demonstrating contractility disturbances. Two-
dimensional echocardiography provides a method superior to M-mode for determining the extent and type of ventricular contraction abnormalities. Localized akinetic, hypokinetic, and dyskinetic segments have been primarily
associated with coronary artery disease. Diffuse hypokinetic left ventricles
usually occur with cardiomyopathies of other etiologies. Two-dimensional
echocardiography is especially useful in detecting the complications of acute
myocardial infarction such as ventricular aneurysm and pseudoaneurysms,
pericardial effusion, ventricular septal rupture, papillary muscle rupture, mural thrombi, and right ventricular infarction. Doppler can detect and assess the
degree of mitral or tricuspid regurgitation and the site of ventricular septal
rupture and the shunt across the defect.

Radionuclide Studies

Technetium-99m pyrophosphate is widely used for imaging an acute myocardial infarction, for this tracer will accumulate only in the infarcted area
(hot spot) when calcium is deposited in the necrotic cells (Fig 4–13). Such
scans are positive in over 90% of patients with transmural infarction,[127] but

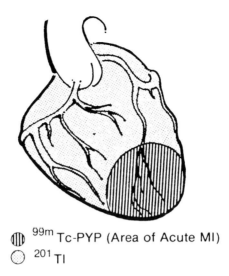

⬭ ^{99m} Tc-PYP (Area of Acute MI)

◯ ^{201} TI

Fig 4–13. Myocardial imaging of acute myocardial infarction (MI). Thallium 201 (^{201}TI) is taken up in the normal myocardium, leaving a defect in the area of the infarct, whereas technetium 99m pyrophosphate (^{99m}Tc-PYP) is taken up in the infarcted area. (Reproduced with permission from *Cardiovascular Imaging and Image Processing: Theory and Practice.* Bellingham, Wash., Society of Photo-Optical Instrumentation Engineers, 1975, pp. 245–260.)

nontransmural infarcts are less reliably detected. The scans become positive in about 24 hours after the onset of pain and remain so for 5 to 7 days, then gradually become negative. The technetium scan can aid in the diagnosis of perioperative infarction following coronary artery bypass surgery unless the patient has undergone resection of an aneurysm. Technetium scans are most useful diagnostically in equivocal cases of acute chest pain, especially in the presence of left bundle-branch block or an old myocardial infarction where the ECG often is of limited value and other laboratory evidence is nondiagnostic. Scans also are of value in detecting right ventricular infarction and estimating infarct size. Unfortunately, abnormal scans can occur with unstable angina[128] and ventricular aneurysm, and after repeated high-energy cardioversion.[129]

Thallium 201 distributes in the myocardium in proportion to regional myocardial blood blow. Therefore, an infarcted area will show a decreased uptake (cold spot; see Fig 4–13). It will be positive earlier than the technetium scan, usually within the first 24 hours; however, it does not differentiate acute involvement from an old scar. Defect resolution on delayed imaging suggests coronary spasm, since old or new infarcts would not change. Today, this imaging is most often made with single photon emission computed tomography (SPECT) that can detect small infarcts.[49]

Radionuclide angiography (either as single-pass or multigated image acquisition study [MUGA]) ejection fractions correlate well with the clinical status of the patient. In addition, by this method wall-motion abnormalities or left ventricular aneurysms can be detected.

Cardiac Catheterization and Angiocardiography

Such studies may become necessary in anticipation of angioplasty or surgery in the presence of an acute myocardial infarction if the patient has continuing episodes of pain, septal rupture, or papillary muscle rupture. It is also done after thrombolytic therapy.

Other Studies

Preliminary studies show that urine[130] and serum myoglobin[131] levels appear sooner after myocardial infarction than the serum enzymes. The latter report demonstrated that peak levels in the serum of patients with acute myocardial infarction usually occurred within 3 to 20 hours after onset of symptoms. In addition to appearing earlier than CK, the myoglobin levels peaked earlier and returned to normal more rapidly, and also occurred in multiple bursts. Elevated levels can also be seen in patients with renal failure or skeletal muscle disorders. These data require further confirmation and comparison with isoenzymes prior to becoming routine in the clinical setting of screening patients with chest pain on admission to the hospital.

DIFFERENTIAL DIAGNOSIS

Chest pain usually means cardiac pain to most patients, although the causes are diverse and numerous. The differential diagnosis of acute myocardial infarction should include other cardiovascular causes and noncardiovascular problems. The evaluation of acute chest pain is a frequent problem in daily clinical practice and demands a quick diagnosis. Initially it is important to exclude those causes with a high risk of sudden death, such as myocardial infarction, dissection of the aorta, and pulmonary embolism. The history should be taken in detail and include questioning about the character, duration, severity, location, and radiation of the pain; precipitating events; change in severity of the pain with respiration and position; response to medications; and other symptoms associated with the pain. The history in conjunction with the physical examination and the necessary supportive laboratory tests provide the most useful diagnostic clues.

Acute Pericarditis. At times this may be difficult to differentiate from infarction. This is especially true if the infarction is in the subepicardial area. If the pain is worse with deep breathing, coughing, or change in position or if it has a sharp component, pericarditis is most likely. Early fever and a pericardial friction rub prior to the first 12 hours is more diagnostic of pericarditis. This is especially important when there is only transient ST elevation or minor T wave changes. Yet pericarditis may be present without a friction rub. Minimal serum enzyme rises are noted with pericarditis, but the MB fraction of CK is usually normal unless there is associated epicardial inflammation.

Pulmonary Embolism. Dyspnea is the predominant symptom due to pulmonary embolism. The chest pain is more often pleuritic, but a large embolism with hypotension can mimic an infarction. The ECG, serum enzymes, chest x rays, blood gases, pulmonary scan, or evidence of peripheral thrombophlebitis aid in the differential. Definitive diagnosis may require pulmonary arteriography.

Dissecting Aortic Aneurysm. The pain with dissection is more tearing and maximum at onset and often radiates down to the abdomen, back, flank, and legs. Persistent hypertension, development of aortic insufficiency, loss or decrease of peripheral pulses, or a pulsating sternoclavicular joint also suggest a dissecting aneurysm. The ECG is nonspecific and rarely reveals a transmural infarction unless the dissection is into the coronary arteries. Ultrasound, CT scanning, MRI, and aortography may be necessary to confirm the diagnosis.

Spontaneous Pneumothorax and Mediastinal Emphysema. The pain with spontaneous pneumothorax is sudden and knife-like and is accompanied by severe dyspnea. A crunching sound may be heard with mediastinal emphysema. These lesions can be confirmed by x-ray examination.

Gastrointestinal Lesions. Acute esophagospasm, hiatal hernia, cholelithiasis, and peptic ulcer may initially be confused with infarction, but after x-ray studies the lesions are clarified.

Anxiety State. Patients with anxiety state and hyperventilation frequently have chest pain. For many years these patients were easily separated, but now, unfortunately, with all the information available to the public, they may subconsciously mimic the chest pain of infarction. In addition, ST-T changes can occur with this unstable autonomic state. These patients are repeatedly admitted to the hospital, and this is the main clue that their attacks are noncardiac, since it would be most unusual for a patient to have so many attacks without more significant objective findings eventually appearing. In such cases coronary arteriography is useful.

TREATMENT OF ACUTE MYOCARDIAL INFARCTION

Despite a growing public awareness of coronary risk factors and recent encouraging evidence that the incidence of death due to coronary artery disease is on the decline, the treatment of acute myocardial infarction remains a major challenge for the primary care physician. Treatment is best considered in four parts: prehospital and general management care, treatment of cardiac arrhythmias, management of other complications, and posthospital care and rehabilitation.

PREHOSPITAL AND GENERAL MANAGEMENT

Since approximately 50 to 60% of the deaths after acute infarction occur outside the hospital, the importance of recognition by the patient of warning symptoms and treatment by paraprofessional and lay personnel cannot be overemphasized. As physicians, we must enthusiastically support and participate in this educational pursuit. Much has been written about prehospital care.[132] Patients with chest pain should immediately be transferred to a hospital facility equipped with cardiac monitoring. Ideally, this should be done by an emergency medical system (EMS) or helicopter service equipped with cardiac drugs and defibrillatory capability. Often the patient can save time by going directly to a hospital emergency room. Approximately 50% of patients have early evidence of parasympathetic overactivity with bradycardia, and some of these have hypotension. One third will show sympathetic overactivity with tachycardia and at times transient hypertension.[133] Mobile coronary care units have been effective and have reduced the prehospital mortality significantly by the rapid recognition and treatment of potentially lethal arrhythmias and the immediate initiation of cardiopulmonary resuscitation when cardiac arrest occurs. In addition, by getting the patient to the hospital quickly, infarct size can be limited by early thrombolytic therapy, nitrates, calcium blockers, β-blockers, and early management of complications.

Many factors contribute to delay in early hospitalization of these patients.

The patient may not seek medical aid immediately. The family doctor may not be aware of the high risk of sudden and preventable death in an apparently mild attack or may consider it to be an anginal attack. When the patient gets to the hospital, there may be a delay in transfer from the emergency room or admitting office to the coronary care unit.

As soon as these patients reach a hospital, they should be treated in coronary care units or cardiac intensive care units. Treatment in such units has been credited with saving up to one third of the hospitalized patients who formerly would have died from acute myocardial infarction.

The requirements of a coronary care unit vary today depending on the availability of staff. Beside the basic equipment, some units are sophisticated and have arrhythmia detection computers. All hospitals, regardless of size, should have these units. Many small hospitals cannot afford to set beds aside for this service or to provide trained staff. However, in a small hospital a two-bed unit can be set up next to the main general nursing station where both patient and monitor can be easily observed. In such a small hospital having few patients with coronary attacks, the unit might be called a cardiac intensive care unit rather than a standard coronary care unit and might provide monitoring of patients who have not sustained an acute myocardial infarction but have life-threatening arrhythmias or other cardiac complications. General-duty nurses can be trained to recognize life-threatening arrhythmias and to begin resuscitation procedures when cardiac arrest occurs. In this setting, a policy of giving priority to patients with coronary attacks and transferring other patients from the unit would be mandatory.

The nursing personnel should be highly trained and in constant attendance. They should have at least a 2-month training course consisting of lectures, demonstrations, and job training in the unit under the supervision of an approved nursing staff. Recognition and emergency treatment of arrhythmias should be emphasized. The nurses gain experience in defibrillation by performing elective cardioversions under the supervision of a physician.

The nurses' responsibilities vary depending on the type of hospital and the availability of housestaff or other physicians. Especially in hospitals without a housestaff, in addition to using the defibrillator, nurses may be permitted to give IV lidocaine, atropine, and other medications on their own initiative in situations defined in a unit protocol. Authorization for these procedures should be approved by the medical and nursing staff and the hospital board; in some states this may require legislative action. Licensed practical nurses and nurses' aids also can be trained to recognize arrhythmias, but should not be allowed to initiate therapy. Staff physicians should have special training if responsible for the unit. Many training courses and teaching aids are available to provide continuing refresher courses necessary for physicians and nurses in charge of a coronary care unit.

A team of physicians should be responsible for establishing and maintaining the unit policy. Successful operation of these units depends on the cooperation of all physicians who admit patients to them. These physicians must abide by the policies of the unit. It is our policy to admit to the unit all patients with suspected or known acute myocardial infarction, regardless of the severity of the attack. After 3 to 4 days patients are transferred elsewhere in the hospital if their condition is stable. In some units patients are monitored for longer periods, or monitoring is continued telemetrically after patients leave the unit. Some hospitals have intermediate coronary care units, since ventricular tachycardia and fibrillation can occur in the late myocardial infarction period, accounting for 10 to 30% of total hospital deaths.

Coronary patients have many psychologic stresses and go through many emotional phases. The physician and nurse therefore should discuss with them their condition, care, and future. Surprisingly, patients may become attached to the coronary care unit and feel so secure there that they do not want to be transferred. Most patients, when they are admitted to the coronary care unit, realize that they have had a heart attack and are anxious. For many, this is their first illness, and they are frightened by all the equipment and personnel activity. The physician should explain the coronary care unit procedures to the patient, reassure him that he is not dying, and emphasize that the unit allows early detection and better treatment of complications. For example, I am amazed that many patients think they are in a terminal state when oxygen is given. After the initial anxiety state and as the patient improves, he may wonder if he really had a heart attack and begin to demonstrate denial. In a few days he realizes that his attack is real, and then dependency sets in. After this stage the patient may develop one of several behavioral patterns such as severe depression, tension, or independency. Our aim should be to anticipate the patient's problems and guide him through the various mental phases to recovery. In addition, the patient's family should be given a clear understanding of the disease. Often we overlook the fact that the patient is upset because of his family's anxiety. For example, the wife may feel guilty about having precipitated the attack, if it occurred during sexual intercourse. It is important to discuss with her the details of the onset of the attack and emphasize that most attacks occur at rest; in fact, the patient may be awakened from sleep. Also, wives and other members of the family should be cautioned not to ask questions about the prognosis in the patient's presence. Often they have asked at the bedside, "Doctor, will he live?" Naturally, this is startling to the patient.

INITIAL MANAGEMENT

During the past few years, the treatment for acute myocardial infarction has changed considerably. Prompt intervention may limit damage in evolving myocardial infarctions. Figure 4–14 shows an approach to the initial management of patients with acute myocardial infarction.

Opiates and Oxygen

On arrival at the unit, an IV infusion should be started. When first seen, the patient with acute myocardial infarctions should immediately receive oxygen, opiates, and nitroglycerin for relief of pain. Pain is related to ongoing ischemia and in turn can cause coronary spasm and stimulate excretion of catecholamines, which can produce an increase in heart rate, cardiac output, heart work, and arrhythmias. However, opiates may decrease alveolar ventilation with increased right-to-left shunting and decreased Pa_{O_2}. Focal atelectasis and ventilation-perfusion abnormalities can occur because of the decrease in frequency and depth of respirations. Many different opiates can be used.

The right coronary artery usually supplies the inferior and true posterior areas of the heart and in 90% of cases the AV node. If it is occluded, these

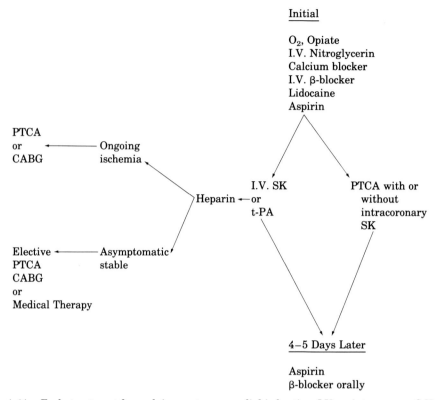

Fig 4–14. Early treatment for evolving acute myocardial infarction. I.V. = intravenous, S.K. = streptokinase, t-PA = tissue plasminogen activator, PTCA = percutaneous transluminal coronary angioplasty, CABG = coronary artery bypass surgery.

patients are prone to bradyarrhythmias, especially AV heart block. Therefore, morphine, a vagomimetic agent, may in patients with inferior or posterior infarctions aggravate or even precipitate sinus bradycardia, slow idioventricular rhythms, and AV heart block. However, it still remains the drug of choice, particularly if pulmonary edema is present, but should be used cautiously. Four to 10 mg of morphine can be given I.V. and repeated at variable intervals until the pain is relieved. Meperidine (Demerol), although not as effective as morphine, can be used in a dosage schedule of 50 to 100 mg every 3 to 4 hours. I prefer to give Demerol if an inferior or posterior infarction is present, especially if there is an associated bradyarrhythmia. Pentazocin (Talwin) is not recommended, for it may elevate the left ventricular filling pressure and increase ventricular afterload by increasing systemic vascular resistance, and as a result may augment myocardial oxygen requirement and thus exacerbate ventricular ischemia.[134] It also has a direct negative inotropic effect. If hypotension is not present and the patient is anxious, diazepam (Valium) 2 to 5 mg orally three to four times a day is helpful. Flurazepam (Dalmane) 15 to 30 mg may be used as a hypnotic.

Arterial hypoxemia most often results from ventilation-perfusion abnormalities.[135] Analgesic-induced hypoventilation and atelectasis may exacerbate the problem. Moreover, Madias et al.[136] showed that oxygen reduces the degree of ST segment evidence of myocardial ischemia. We routinely use oxygen, although this creates anxiety in an occasional patient who considers it a sign of dire illness, it rarely causes CO_2 retention in patients with obstructive pulmonary disease. If arterial oxygenation is depressed one hundred percent oxygen can safely be given to patients with myocardial infarction by nasal prongs or mask. Patients in pulmonary edema or cardiogenic shock may require endotracheal intubation.

Nitroglycerin and Calcium Blockers

Intravenous nitroglycerin (which reduces oxygen demand and wall stress by decreasing preload and afterload, reduces or eliminates coronary spasm, and recruits collaterals) can be started at a rate of 5 μg per minute and increased up to 200 μg or more, if necessary, for pain relief. There is also some evidence that it can reduce mortality and infarct size.[137] For continued pain, nifedipine (which reduces oxygen demand by decreasing blood pressure and contractility) 10 mg is swallowed after the capsule has been bitten through or punctured, since it is not absorbed well sublingually through the buccal mucosa.[138] Naturally, such drugs should be given cautiously to avoid hypotension. Administration of calcium blockers early during myocardial infarction has not been shown to limit infarct size. However, a recent multicenter trial showed that diltiazem reduced the reinfarction rate of non-Q-wave infarction by 51.2% during the first 14 days.[139] Another multicenter diltiazem study reported on 2466 patients with previous myocardial infarction who were randomized to receive diltiazem or placebo and followed for 12 to 52 months (mean, 25 months). In 1909 patients without left ventricular dysfunction (pulmonary congestion and ejection fraction 40% or less), diltiazem was associated with a reduced number of cardiac events (mortality from cardiac causes or nonfatal reinfarction) and an increase in cardiac events in 490 patients with left ventricular dysfunction.[140] No major trial to date has evaluated a combination of a calcium blocker and thrombolytic therapy in patients with infarction.

β-Blockers

β-blockers (which reduce oxygen demand by reducing heart rate and blood pressure) have been studied extensively in acute myocardial infarction.[137,141] There are several collaborative studies regarding their use early and late during the course of infarction. Several recent studies have indicated the importance of beginning β-blocker treatment early after the onset of infarction. Trials with timolol (International Collaborative Study),[142] metoprolol (Miami Trial),[143] and atenolol (ISIS-1 Trial)[144] suggest that these are of benefit in myocardial infarction when given early. Propranolol (Milis Study) did not reduce infarct size.[145] It appears that the rate of cell necrosis can probably be delayed by a β-blocker for several hours, but at 24 hours the drugs have no apparent beneficial effect on the infarct size.[146] This suggests that an early combination of thrombolytic therapy with a β-blocker may be beneficial. In fact, the early report of the TIMI II B trial at the American Heart Association meeting in November 1988 indicated that 15 mg of metoprolol (immediate group 696 patients) given I.V. over 6 minutes followed by 50 mg orally b.i.d. for 1 day and then 100 mg b.i.d. reduced recurrent ischemia and reinfarction incidence significantly during the first week as compared to results in patients with thrombolytic therapy who did not receive a β-blocker until 6 days (deferred group 694 patients) after the onset of symptoms. Fatal or non-fatal reinfarction occurred in 18 patients (2.6%) and recurrent ischemia in 107 patients (15.4%) in the immediate group and 31 (4.5%) and 147 (21.2%) respectively in the deferred group. The ejection fraction in both groups was the same. Therefore, it appears that a β-blocker should be given early with thrombolytic therapy unless there is a contraindication. Certainly patients with hypertension, sinus tachycardia, or continuous pain should receive it. One study showed that patients previously receiving a β-blocker who sustained an acute infarction may have their β-blocker abruptly discontinued if clinically indicated with no withdrawal phenomena occurring.[147] Data are available to support the importance of β-blockers given 4 to 5 days after the onset of the infarction on a long-term basis. This will be discussed later.

Lidocaine

The risk of ventricular fibrillation is 15 times higher in the first 4 hours after infarction than it is from the fourth to the twelfth hours. Hence, many studies have been performed to evaluate the value of lidocaine to prevent ventricular fibrillation. A review of 11 randomized trials by McMahon and Yusuf et al.[148] showed that the incidence of ventricular fibrillation and fatal asystole among the untreated patients to be 1.4% and 0.2% among the treated patients. Lidocaine reduced the risk of ventricular fibrillation by 36%. However, the risk of fatal asystole doubled, leaving a small reduction in mortality associated with prevention of ventricular fibrillation by lidocaine. A recent study showed that primary ventricular fibrillation occurring in a coronary care unit is a negative predictor of short-term survival in patients with acute myocardial infarction.[149] In view of this study and other studies that have shown that lidocaine prevents primary ventricular fibrillation, even though the value of prophylactic use of lidocaine in acute myocardial infarction has not been resolved, I prefer to give it routinely unless there is a contraindication. Lidocaine has an elimination half-life of 2 to 4 hours. Therefore, if a patient were given only the usual maintenance infusion of 2 to 4 mg/min, therapeutic range would not be reached for 6 hours or more. To reach the therapeutic range more rapidly, a loading dose should be administered.[150,151] This loading dose is usually about 200 to 250 mg according to body weight and should be given in divided amounts every 5 minutes over a period of about 20 minutes. Once the loading dose is started, the patient should be placed on the maintenance infusion. Toxic manifestations as central nervous system (CNS) symptoms, hypotension, bradyarrhythmia are more apt to occur in the elderly or patients with heart failure, hypotension, or liver disease. The loading and maintenance dosage should be reduced to at least half in such situations. Usually in the absence of ventricular arrhythmia, infusion is terminated in about 48 to 72 hours. It is not necessary to reduce the rate of lidocaine slowly; because of its elimination half-life, it can be stopped abruptly and yet have a sufficient plasma concentration for several hours.

Thrombolytic Therapy

It is now well established that acute myocardial infarction is almost always due to thrombolytic occlusion of a coronary artery at the site of an ulcerated atheromatous plaque. DeWood et al.,[152] during bypass surgery, removed a thrombus in 52 of 59 patients (88%) who had total coronary obstruction. Necrosis after coronary occlusion occurs over several hours and therefore can be arrested by reperfusion with thrombolytic agents, and thus some ischemic but still viable myocardium can be salvaged. The following criteria are usually required for a patient to be eligible for treatment: (1) Chest pain characteristic of myocardial ischemia lasting for 30 minutes or more; (2) ST segment elevation of 0.1 mV or more in two or more contiguous leads that persists despite sublingual nitroglycerin with or without Q-wave development; and (3) passage of less than 6 hours from the clinical onset of myocardial infarction. Patients with chest pain that can mimic infarction, such as those with dissecting aneurysm, pericarditis, and early repolarization, should be excluded. Streptokinase (SK) and urokinase are first-generation thrombolytic agents; t-PA and single chain urokinase plasminogen activator (scu-PA or pro-urokinase) are second-generation drugs; mutants of t-PA and scu-PA are third-generation drugs; and hybrids of t-PA and scu-PA are fourth-generation drugs.[153] At present, streptokinase, urokinase, and t-PA are available and the others are being studied. In addition, the effects of combinations of these are being evaluated. The aim is to have a thrombolytic agent that is clot-specific, has a long half-life and fewer side reactions, and can be given as one bolus I.V. or intramuscularly. In clinical practice today, intravenous thrombolytic therapy has become almost routine unless there is a contraindication such as poorly controlled severe hypertension, recent or remote cerebrovascular accident, CNS surgery within 6 months, bleeding diathesis or active internal bleeding, and post-traumatic cardiopulmonary resuscitation. In the following conditions, the risk of therapy should be weighted against the anticipated benefits: age over 75, recent major surgery, history of G.I. bleeding, left heart thrombus, cerebrovascular disease, and history of hypertension. Streptokinase is currently the most widely used agent. Data confirm that the earlier the therapy is started, the greater the frequency of early reperfusion.[154] Therapy should be started at least within the first 2 to 3 hours after the onset of symptoms. However, in some cases with subtotal coronary occlusion, in the presence of collaterals to the ischemic zone or when there is ongoing ischemia ("stuttering" infarction), necrosis may progress more slowly and thrombolytic therapy may still be effective beyond 3 hours from the onset. Nitroglycerin can recruit collaterals and may lengthen the window of opportunity for thrombolytic therapy. The ISIS-2 study showed that even if streptokinase was given up to 24 hours after the onset of symptoms, it reduced mortality. The usual routine is to give 1.5 million units of streptokinase I.V. over 1 hour. Streptokinase should not be given at a rate over 500 U/kg/min because hypotension can occur.[155] In some cases, corticosteroids and antihistamines may be given to prevent adverse reactions to streptokinase. Three to 5 hours after streptokinase, if the partial thromboplastin time (PTT) decreases to 50 sec, heparin should be given (1000 units per hour usual dosage) to maintain PTT at about twice the control. The heparin is continued until cardiac catheterization is performed and afterwards (with sheath in) until a decision is made about definitive therapy. Heparin resistance can be induced by intravenous nitroglycerin.[156] Therefore, patients receiving both of these agents should be monitored closely with PTT levels and the heparin dosage should be decreased when the I.V. nitroglycerin is stopped to avoid hemorrhage. Tissue plasminogen activator (t-PA) has now been extensively studied. Streptokinase induces clot lysis by forming a complex with plasminogen that converts both circulating and fibrin-bound plasminogen to plasmin. Urokinase in contrast to streptokinase activates plasminogen directly. Tissue plasminogen activator has a high affinity for fibrin, and therefore plasmin is formed preferentially at the site of the thrombus. In phase I of the Thrombolysis in Myocardial Infarction Trial (Timi),[157] predominately two-chain t-PA had an efficacy of 62% compared with streptokinase that had an efficacy of 31%. There was significantly less depletion of fibrinogen or increase of fibrinogen degradation products with t-PA compared to streptokinase. The hemorrhagic events were almost identical in the two groups. There were no episodes of intracranial hemorrhage. In this study, 80 mg of two-chain t-PA was given intravenously or, alternately, 1.5 million units of streptokinase. Single chain t-PA at a comparable dose produces a less reperfusion rate than two-chain t-PA. The reperfusion rate with 100 mg single-chain t-PA rose to 71% and with 150 mg of single-chain t-PA to 76%.[158] However, the 150 mg dosage group had an incidence of 1.6% (16 of 1,014 patients) intracranial hemorrhages which dropped to 0.6% (8 of 1,452 patients) incidence in the group receiving 100 mg.[159] Systemic fibrinogenolysis was much less with 100 mg of single chain t-PA than with 80 mg of two-chain t-PA. Tissue plasminogen activator cannot distinguish between a coronary thrombus and a protective hemostatic plug, even though it is relatively clot-specific.[160] The incidence of stroke (no distinction between hemorrhagic or thrombolytic infarction was made) with streptokinase in the Gruppo Italiano per lo Studio Della Streptochinasi Nell'Infarto Miocardico (GISSI) trial was 0.2% (10 of 5,860 patients).[161] In the Second International Study for Infarct Survival (ISIS-2) Trial, the incidence with intracranial hemorrhage was 0.1% (9 of 8,377 patients).[162] From these studies it appeared that streptokinase produced lower rates of intracranial hemorrhage. However, the Anglo-Scandinavian Study of Early Thrombolysis (ASSET)[163] randomized 5011 patients with suspected myocardial infarction to receive either t-PA or placebo (all received heparin) and showed that hemorrhagic strokes developed in only 0.3% of patients and the rate in controls was about 0.1%. The most effective dose with less complications for t-PA is 10 mg as an I.V. push and another 50 mg of t-PA during the first hour, followed in the next 2 hours by 20 mg each hour for a total of 100 mg. Heparin is started during the first hour of t-PA. When administering t-PA intravenously within 3 hours of the onset of symptoms, it is 84% effective in achieving reperfusion after coronary thrombosis and streptokinase is 69% effective. After 6 hours, the t-PA efficacy diminishes to 67% and that for streptokinase to 33%.[164] Both decrease mortality by 25%. The GISSI study was the first to show a decrease in hospital mortality (47% reduction) when intravenous streptokinase was given within 1 hour of the onset of the infarction.[161,165] Several studies have shown improvement in ventricular function at 7 to 14 days when these agents were given early after onset of the coronary occlusion.[166–169] It appears logical at present that either can be used in the first 3 hours after the onset of infarction, but beyond this time, t-PA would be preferable until further studies are done comparing these two agents. Urokinase has not been used as extensively as streptokinase and t-PA. One study concluded that urokinase (3 million units) and t-PA (70 mg) given intravenously over 90 minutes had similar efficacy and safety in the treatment of acute myocardial infarction.[170] However, reocclusion during the first 24 hours may be less frequent with urokinase. The use of thrombolytic agents for inferior infarction has been controversial because generally it is associated with less enzyme rises and better ventricular function and less congestive heart failure or death as compared to an anterior infarction. Several randomized studies did not demonstrate a significant survival benefit in patients with inferior infarctions when given streptokinase or t-PA. However, all of those studies had limitations because of low patency rate and small sample size. Some patients are right coronary dominant and are at great risk of having a large infarct with significant loss of muscle function if this vessel is occluded.[171] It is difficult initially to detect which patients fall into this category. However, Bates[172] reviewed the data on inferior infarction and concluded that thrombolytic therapy should be given to all patients with inferior infarction if seen within 3 hours of the onset of symptoms since improvement in left ventricular function has been demonstrated in such cases. He also stated that patients seen within 6 hours of onset of symptoms should be given thrombolytic therapy only if there is precordial ST depression since such patients have a similar prognosis to that for patients with anterior infarction. I feel it is reasonable to give all patients (especially the relatively young) with inferior infarction thrombolytic therapy unless there is a contraindication. Whereas streptokinase, t-PA, and urokinase are now available, other products are being investigated, namely, prourokinase (scu-PA) and anisoylated plasminogen streptokinase activator complex (APSAC). APSAC can be given as an intravenous bolus safely. It has a half-life of about 120 minutes compared to 20 minutes for streptokinase. Small studies have shown early recanalization in 50 to 60% of patients.[173] A recent multicenter trial[174] compared intravenous APSAC given to 123 patients to intracoronary streptokinase given to 117 patients within 6 hours of onset of symptoms. In patients treated 4 hours or less after onset of symptoms, APSAC was successful in 60% and intracoronary streptokinase in 60%. After 4 hours, the success rate with APSAC dropped to 33% and intracoronary streptokinase remained at 61%.

Further studies are needed comparing APSAC or urokinase with intravenous streptokinase or with t-PA.

Adjunctive Agents with Thrombolytic Therapy

Adjunctive agents with thrombolytic therapy such as aspirin, heparin, nitrates, β-blockers, calcium blockers, antioxidant agents, and combinations of thrombolytic agents are still being evaluated. The Second International Study of Infarct Survival (ISIS-2)[175] randomized 17,187 patients within 24 hours (median 5 hours) after the onset of suspected acute myocardial infarction into the following groups: (1) One hour of intravenous infusion of 1.5 million units of streptokinase. (2) One month of 160 mg daily of enteric-coated aspirin. (3) Both active ingredients. (4) Neither. Streptokinase alone and aspirin alone produced a significant reduction in 5-week vascular mortality as compared to placebo. The combination of streptokinase and aspirin was significantly better than either agent alone. The combination as compared to those allocated neither had significantly fewer reinfarctions (1.8% versus 2.9%), stroke (0.6% versus 1.1%), and deaths (8.0% versus 13.2%). These differences for streptokinase and aspirin remain highly significant after the median of 15 months follow-up. Unless there is a contraindication, I would give 325 mg aspirin early after the onset of an infarction along with a thrombolytic agent.

Heparin has been given following thrombolytic therapy to prevent reocclusion. The thrombolysis and angioplasty study in myocardial infarction (TAMI-III) randomized 131 patients receiving t-PA to t-PA alone or t-PA and 10,000 units of heparin and there was no significant difference in hemorrhagic complications or arterial patency between the two groups.[176] Likewise, the TIMI trial and the Italian GISSI trial showed no direct benefit of heparin. However, these studies did not approach this question specifically and their findings were retrospective. Other small studies showed that heparin prevents reocclusion. These studies to date have been conflicting. Ongoing randomized prospective trials may answer this problem.

Hackett et al.[177] performed arteriography in patients with acute myocardial infarction and showed intermittent coronary occlusion during intracoronary infusion of streptokinase, which could be prevented by giving intracoronary isorbide dinitrate. It appears that coronary tone is heightened during acute myocardial infarction and thrombolytic therapy. Therefore, nitrates may be of benefit.

Several studies have shown that β-blockers can be given safely in acute myocardial infarction. As mentioned earlier, the TIMI II B trial has confirmed that it can be given safely with thrombolytic therapy with benefit.

No major trials have combined thrombolytic therapy with calcium-channel blockers. However, as mentioned previously, diltiazem has reduced the reinfarction rate in patients with non-Q-wave myocardial infarctions.

When cells become ischemic, oxygen-derived free radicals are produced and cause reperfusion injury and myocardial dysfunction (myocardial stunning). Superoxide dismutase, allopurinol, and desferoxamine are agents that may inhibit the formation and enhance catabolism of these free radicals in experimental animals and are currently being studied in combination with thrombolytic agents in humans.[178,179]

Combinations of thrombolytic agents (t-PA and urokinase-TAMI pilot study) produced no improvement in patency rate but did decrease the reocclusion rate.[180] Smaller doses of each may decrease fibrinogen depletion and decrease hemorrhagic complications.

Post-Thrombolytic Management

The benefits of thrombolysis may be temporary in many cases. After clinical successful thrombolysis, reocclusion of the infarct-related vessel (about 20%), reinfarction (8 to 12% in first week), recurrent angina, and no return of ventricular function can occur. Pooled data from several studies showed that nonfatal reinfarction occurred in 4.5% of patients, early reocclusion in 19%, and recurrent angina in approximately 16%, which may be due to persistent high-grade lesions after thrombolysis.[181] Reocclusion was more likely if the residual stenosis was 90% or greater. Because of these facts, some patients with a patent infarct-related vessel after thrombolysis may require more definitive therapy. At the bedside, signs of coronary reperfusion are clearing of the chest pain, resolution of ST-T changes and the occurrence of ventricular arrhythmias, especially accelerated idioventricular rhythm (AIVR). A recent study showed that none of these clinical criteria individually is predictive of infarct artery recanalization.[182] However, if all three are present, specificity and predictive value increases to 100%. Most often, only one or two of the parameters will be present and the sensitivity and predictive value of these fall. Therefore, after thrombolysis, angiography should be considered and coronary angioplasty (PTCA) or bypass surgery should be considered, depending on the findings. Timing of these procedures recently has been extensively studied. Several studies have shown that angioplasty need not be performed immediately following thrombolysis and waiting 2 to 7 days does not cause reocclusion or loss of ventricular function. The TAMI trial[183] randomized 197 patients with arterial patency after t-PA therapy who were candidates for PTCA into an immediate PTCA group and a group for PTCA several days later (elective group). Recurrent ischemia required PTCA before 7 days in 16% of the elective group. Patency and reocclusion rate and ventricular function were not different between the groups. In the elective group, 14% had a reduction in stenosis at the seventh day following angiography and did not require revascularization. Mortality was higher in the immediate group. The European Cooperative Study, the TIMI-II A trial, and TAMI study also indicate that immediate PTCA does not provide an advantage and may be harmful (more ischemic events, bleeding, and emergency bypass surgery).[184–186] In addition, recently the TIMI-II B trial was reported at the American Heart Association meeting, November 1988.[187,187a] This trial had a conservative group (1626 patients) that received t-PA but did not have coronary arteriography unless patients had recurrent angina or documented ischemia by exercise. This group was compared to those (1636 patients) who had t-PA, heart catheterization in 18 to 48 hours, and angioplasty if there was appropriate anatomy. At 42 days, the reinfarction rate and death rate were similar in both groups. At hospital discharge or 6 weeks after randomization, there were no significant differences between the two groups in the ejection fraction at rest or during exercise. Sixteen percent of the conservative group crossed over to catheterization and angioplasty and 10.5% to coronary-artery bypass grafting within 42 days. At 1 year, the survival was 93% in both groups. After thrombolytic therapy, the residual plaque may be denuded or may rupture and angioplasty may increase the risk of reocclusion and the risk of progression to immediate bypass surgery. Serial coronary arteriograms in one study indicated that many infarct-related coronary arteries after intracoronary urokinase are associated with a complex underlying structure, probably composed of some portions of ruptured atheromatous plaque with or without an adherent thrombus.[188] During emergency coronary angioplasty in such cases, the guide wire may easily go into the plaque cavity and produce complications. Therefore, it appears from these studies that there is no need for immediate PTCA or surgery unless patients have continuous evidence of ischemia. Although immediate angioplasty may not be necessary, consideration should be given for early angiography because this is the most reliable method of identifying patients who failed thrombolytic therapy. It identifies coronary anatomy and may identify low and high risk patients. Surgery, instead of angioplasty, should be considered in high-risk patients having left main disease or severe triple vessel disease with left ventricular dysfunction.

In summary (see Fig 4–14), in view of the various trials, I recommend thrombolytic therapy for all patients with an acute myocardial infarction who are seen within 4 hours of the onset of symptoms or after this if there is evidence of ongoing ischemia unless there is a contraindication. The GISSI study[165] showed that if streptokinase is given within the first hour, mortality is reduced by 50%; if given between the first and third hour, it is reduced by only 10%. This emphasizes the importance of the community hospitals who first see such patients and can initiate early therapy. Tissue plasminogen activator (t-PA) appears to be the best choice, but until further data are available, streptokinase is a good alternative, especially if it is given early. The final word will not be in until large-scale studies, comparing the two agents head-to-head, are completed. In addition, the patient should chew a 325 mg tablet of aspirin immediately prior to thrombolytic therapy unless there is a contraindication. Heparin should also be started with t-PA or after streptokinase. Oxygen, opiates, nitroglycerin, lidocaine, β-blocker, and calcium blocker should be given as recommended earlier. If the patient has recurrent ischemia after thrombolytic therapy, immediate coronary arteriography, if available, should be done and, if not available, the patient should be transferred to a tertiary care center. Such patients should be considered, depending on the anatomy, for immediate angioplasty or bypass surgery. However, if the patient is stable after thrombolytic therapy, coronary arteriography can be delayed for 24 to 48 hours and then, depending on these findings and noninvasive studies, the patient can be considered for more definitive therapy. However, as mentioned in the TIMI II B trial,[187] this latter group can be watched and have heart catheterization only if they become symptomatic or show ischemia on exercise test.

It should be realized that only 20 to 30% of patients with acute myocardial infarction meet the present-day criteria for thrombolytic therapy. The in-hospital mortality from acute myocardial infarction originally was 30%, dropped to 15% with coronary care units, and today, with present therapy, has declined to less than 5%. However, it should be recognized that the reduction to less than 5% in mortality is in the special trial group patients and does not necessarily refer to the general population. This field is undergoing evolution, and physicians should keep abreast of ongoing studies and adapt to new changes. Often a decision has to be made depending on each patient's problem.

Since thrombolytic therapy is more effective the earlier it is given, intracoronary streptokinase has become less attractive. Good results have also been achieved by using PTCA immediately prior to thrombolytic therapy and, if it is ineffective, intracoronary streptokinase can be given followed by PTCA. However, I.V. streptokinase or t-PA logistically saves time compared to direct angioplasty unless the patient has the coronary occlusion while in the hospital and coronary arteriography is immediately available.

If β-blockers or aspirin were not started initially, then 4 to 5 days after the onset of the infarction, they should be given unless there is a contraindication. As mentioned previously, several studies have confirmed the beneficial effect of β-blockers when given several days after the onset of the infarction. When several randomized double blind and placebo-controlled trials were pooled, it appears that aspirin is of long-term benefit.[189] Much debate continues about the dosage of aspirin because higher doses may block prostacyclin, which is a vasodilator. However, it appears reasonable to give one aspirin per day (325 mg) if there is no contraindication such as recent active duodenal ulcer or bleeding disorder. Further discussion of these two agents will be taken up later along with postinfarction management.

Figure 4–15 shows an approach to the management of acute myocardial infarction that can be followed if no thrombolytic agent is used or is used and is unsuccessful in opening the vessel. The initial use of oxygen, opiate, nitroglycerin, calcium blockers, β-blockers, lidocaine, and aspirin are the same as for the evolving infarct just described. However, if the patient has an anterior infarction with an akinetic or dyskinetic area, full angicoagulation should be given and the aspirin stopped.[190,191] Approximately one-third of patients with acute anterior infarction (46% of those with an akinetic or dyskinetic segment) develop mural thrombus, usually between the 5th to 21st day after the acute attack.[192] This is unusual in an inferior infarction. Two-D echocardiography can detect the wall changes and mural thrombi. However, at the bedside, if a patient has an anterior infarction by ECG and a diffuse apical impulse or an ectopic impulse outside of PMI, he most likely will have an akinetic or dyskinetic area. In such patients, emboli usually occur at 1 to 3 months from the initial onset of the infarction. Therefore, these patients should receive heparin 5000 to 10,000 units by I.V. bolus and then 1000 units per hour, maintaining PTT 1.5 to 2 times normal. After 3 to 5 days, warfarin should be added and the heparin stopped after the prothrombin is maintained between 18 to 20 seconds. Warfarin should be continued for at least 3 to 4 months.[193] At that time, if echo shows no thrombus or a flat one attached to the wall, the anticoagulant can be discontinued. However, if a protruding thrombus is present,[194] or thrombus was present and resolved and abnormal wall motion is still present, the anticoagulant should be continued and the patient rechecked by echo periodically. If warfarin is given to such patients, then at 4 to 5 days, a β-blocker can be administered, but not aspirin. A recent study concluded that 12,500 units of heparin given subcutaneously every 12 hours for 10 days to patients with acute anterior transmural myocardial infarction is more effective in preventing left ventricular mural thrombosis than 5,000 units of heparin every 12 hours.[194a] Mural thrombosis was observed by 2-D echocardiography on the 10th day after infarction in 10 of 95 patients (11%) in the high-dose group and in 28 of 88 (32%) in the low-dose group.

Results with "rescue" angioplasty in patients with unsuccessful throm-

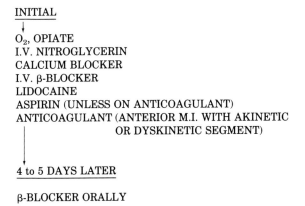

INITIAL
↓
O$_2$, OPIATE
I.V. NITROGLYCERIN
CALCIUM BLOCKER
I.V. β-BLOCKER
LIDOCAINE
ASPIRIN (UNLESS ON ANTICOAGULANT)
ANTICOAGULANT (ANTERIOR M.I. WITH AKINETIC
    OR DYSKINETIC SEGMENT)

4 to 5 DAYS LATER

β-BLOCKER ORALLY

Fig 4–15. Treatment for completed acute M.I. (no thrombolytic agent or agent unsuccessful). M.I. = Myocardial infarction, I.V. = intravenous.

bolytic therapy have been conflicting and associated with a high frequency of complications and needs further study. Most studies have excluded patients for thrombolytic therapy with pump failure (severe pulmonary edema and/or cardiogenic shock). Such patients may have a "stunned" myocardium that may benefit from reperfusion and so reverse pump failure. The European Cooperative Study group is planning a thrombolytic trial in this group. The role of thrombolytic therapy in patients with infarction and ST depression and no ST elevation also needs study. These and many other unanswered questions with regard to thrombolytic therapy need further evaluation in this rapid and expanding field.

There have been many other methods and approaches in the initial management of acute myocardial infarction to limit infarct size. Review of the literature does not provide conclusive evidence that infarct size is reduced by treatment by some of these such as polarized solution (glucose-insulin-potassium) and steroids.

Bed Rest and Activity

In 1952 Levine and Lown[195] demonstrated that a patient could be moved into an armchair during the initial stages of an acute myocardial infarction without deleterious effects. This was the first step toward shortening bed rest and the length of hospital stay.

Prolonged bed rest can decrease tolerance of the upright posture and produces a fall in BP. In addition, it results in diminished physical work capacity, elevated pulse rate response to submaximal work, and a reduced cardiovascular functional capacity as measured by maximal oxygen uptake. The circulating blood volume also is reduced. All of these changes can adversely affect the cardiac responses and may result in cardiovascular deconditioning. In the presence of coronary atherosclerosis, such changes as orthostatic hypotension decrease blood flow and can result in further ischemic damage or extension of myocardial damage. A study[196] showed that uncomplicated cases can be discharged 1 week after acute myocardial infarction. These patients at the 6-month follow-up had a low incidence of late serious complications, no more than in the control group.

Initial mobilization should be gradual and under supervision. Table 4–14 outlines phase I (inpatient) of our cardiac rehabilitation program. Phases II and III (outpatient rehabilitation program) will be discussed later. An increasing number of patients are being enrolled in such programs, which have great promise in the physical and emotional rehabilitation of the patient. Generally, I allow the patient with an uncomplicated acute myocardial infarction to sit in a bedside chair by the third day. A bedside commode is allowed immediately. However, the patient usually will not require this for 2 days or longer because of the light diet and narcotics. The patient is allowed to sit up on his own and is not lifted onto the armchair or commode. By the end of the first week, complete self-care is allowed (feeding, washing, brushing teeth, combing hair, or shaving), as well as walking slowly in the room, hall, and to the bathroom. If no complications occur, activity is gradually increased so that the patient is ambulating (with monitoring of heart rate and blood pressure) as much as desired within the hospital room and hall prior to discharge at 10 to 14 days. Studies have shown that there are no special benefits to be gained by pro-

Table 4–14. Phase I: Inpatient Cardiac Rehabilitation Program*

Acute Phase—Approximately day 1–2	MET Level
LEVEL I	
1. Bed rest; BSC with assistance if not contraindicated.	1;3
2. Bed bath by nurse or attendant.	1
3. May help feed self with HOB elevated.	1
4. a. passive ROM all extremities 5× BID	1
b. active ankle movement 5× qh w.a.	1
c. deep breathing 2× qh w.a.	1
LEVEL II	
1. Dangle legs with feet supported over edge of bed 15′ BID	1
2. Wash hands, face, perineal area.	2
3. Brush teeth gently, slowly.	
4. a. active/assistive ROM all extremities 5× BID	1
b. continue ankle movement and deep breathing	1
SUBACUTE PHASE—approximately day 3–5	
LEVEL III	
1. Bedside chair 15–60 minutes TID	1
2. Partial bath (exclude back, legs)	2
3. Shave self, apply makeup, comb hair (at bedside)	2
4. Chair and bed ROM exercises 5–10× TID	2
5. Bathroom privileges with assistance	2
LEVEL IV	
1. Bedside chair 1 hour QID	1
2. Complete bath at bedside (or sitting at sink)	2
3. Continue chair and bed exercises QID	2
4. Begin standing ROM exercise (1–4) TID	2
5. Begin ambulation in hall 5–7 minutes TID	2
AMBULATORY PHASE—approximately day 6–14 +	
LEVEL V	
1. Bedside chair ad lib	1
2. Stand at sink to bathe and shave	2
3. Additional standing ROM exercises (5–8) BID	2
4. Ambulate in room ad lib	2
5. Ambulate in hall 7–10 minutes TID	2
LEVEL VI	
1. Shower or tub bath	3
2. Continue standing ROM exercises TID	2
3. Ambulate in hall 10–12 minutes TID	2
4. Walk down one flight of stairs (take elevator up) with supervision	3.5
LEVEL VII	
1. Ambulate in hall 12–15 minutes TID (unsupervised)	2
2. Continue standing ROM exercises TID	2
3. Walk up and down 1 flight stairs (10 steps) w/supervision	4–5
4. Keep record of own pulse response to exercise	

*MET = Metabolic equivalent; BSC = bedside commode; HOB = head of bed; ROM = range of motion; BID = twice per day; qh = every hour; w.a. = while awake; TID = three times a day; QID = four times per day; ad lib = at pleasure.

longed hospitalization beyond 2 weeks. In addition, expenses are reduced, and patients convalesce better at home in their customary surroundings.

These activities are modified if persistent chest pain, shock, severe heart failure, or major arrhythmias occur. Usually activities are begun after complications have been successfully treated.

Diet

The patient usually should be allowed to feed himself from the start. Clear liquids on day 1, full liquids on day 2, and mild sodium restriction are our general rule. We do not restrict fluids, unless there is evidence of hyponatremia or uncontrolled congestive heart failure. After this, the diet depends on lipid analysis, body weight, carbohydrate metabolism, and other factors. Lipid analysis and resulting long-term dietary therapy are best evaluated at 3 months, although one study[197] suggested a good correlation between lipid levels taken on day 1 after an infarct with levels obtained 3 months later. An often-overlooked task is lipid analysis of the children and siblings of the patient. Twenty percent of patients under 60 who survive a myocardial infarction have a genetic hyperlipoproteinemia. Familial combined hyperlipidemia is the most common type. One study showed that hot and cold liquids did not produce deleterious effects.[198]

Bowel Function

Opiates, bed rest, anxiety, and change of diet predispose the patient to constipation. To prevent later straining, a combination of 30 ml of milk of magnesia and 100 mg of dioctyl sodium sulfosuccinate (Colace) is given twice a day and is effective. Severe cathartics and enemas should be avoided. Bedpans are not used, but a bedside commode is allowed. Our patients have bathroom privileges by 3 to 5 days if there are no complications.

Bladder Function

Urinary retention is especially common in elderly patients given opiates and is even more likely to occur if atropine is used for bradyarrhythmias. An indwelling catheter is used for a few days if urinary retention develops.

Anticoagulants

The use of anticoagulants in patients with acute myocardial infarction has been extensively studied with variable results. These studies were performed prior to the development of the methods now used to reduce infarct size. Earlier in this chapter, the use of heparin after thrombolytic therapy and the use of full anticoagulation in those who have anterior infarction and develop an akinetic or dyskinetic area was discussed. In addition, full anticoagulation should be considered for those who have severe heart failure, thrombophlebitis (present or past), pulmonary or systemic emboli, or cardiogenic shock. In the absence of such conditions, low-dose heparin (5000 units subcutaneously every 8 to 12 hours) is recommended during the hospitalization.

DYSRHYTHMIA

Arrhythmias were present in 94 of our first 100 patients with acute myocardial infarction monitored in 1965, and they accounted for at least 40% of the deaths.[199] If frequent premature ectopic beats are excluded, the number of patients with arrhythmia is 84 (present at the time of admission in 29). Others have reported a similar incidence.[200]

A breakdown of the arrhythmias according to type of infarction (Table 4–15) showed, as expected, a greater incidence of AV heart block and sinus bradycardia with inferior infarctions than with other types. Subdividing the anterior infarctions (36) into anteroseptal, midanterior, and anterolateral categories pointed out only one important factor: in this group anteroseptal infarctions (17) accounted for all six instances of cardiac asystole. Quite likely, in these six cases bilateral bundle-branch block was followed by complete heart block and asystole.

Since these first 100 patients were monitored, aggressive treatment has brought a considerable reduction in the incidence of major arrhythmias (ventricular tachycardia, ventricular fibrillation, atrial flutter and fibrillation, heart block, and cardiac arrest).

As yet there is no full agreement about the use of antiarrhythmic drugs prophylactically in cases presenting with a regular sinus rhythm. One study[201] showed that procainamide afforded highly significant protection against all types of active ventricular arrhythmias, markedly reduced the need for acute therapy of arrhythmia, and prevented deaths from active arrhythmias, but the total number of deaths was the same as in the placebo group. In this study patients with shock, heart block, or severe heart failure were excluded. Almost similar results were noted in a prophylactic study with quinidine.[202] Prophy-

Table 4–15. Arrhythmias in 100 Monitored Patients With Acute Myocardial Infarction*

Type of Arrhythmia	Number (Percentage) of Patients	Type of Infarction				
		Anterior (36)	Inferior (38)	Subendocardial (16)	Apical (4)	Unknown (6)
PVBs	76	29	28	13		6
Ventricular ectopic rhythms	32	15	12	5		
Ventricular fibrillation	9	4	3	1		1
PABs	42	14	15	9	2	2
Atrial tachycardia (ectopic)	5		1	3		1
Atrial flutter and fibrillation	14	4	7	2		1
Supraventricular tachycardia	9	2	4	3		
Sinus tachycardia	41	12	17	8	3	1
Sinus bradycardia	22	4	16	1	1	
First-degree AV block	18	1	14	1	1	1
Second-degree AV block	14	1	11	2		
Third-degree AV block	16	1	12	2		1
Asystole	10	6	1	2		1
AV dissociation with junctional rhythm	3	1	1	1		
Right bundle-branch block	8	4	2	1		1
Left bundle-branch block	8	2		2		4

*Modified from Gazes P.C.[199]: Treatment of acute myocardial infarction: 1. General management. *Postgrad. Med.* 47:143, 1970.

laxis with disopyramide phosphate (Norpace) was associated with a decrease in ventricular arrhythmias, incidence of reinfarction, and mortality in a small group of unmonitored patients in an open ward.[203] Later in this chapter, the results of several multicenter clinical trials with β-blockers (timolol, propranolol, metoprolol) in acute myocardial infarction will be further discussed. Several studies[204-206] with prophylactic lidocaine showed a reduction in the frequency of ventricular tachyarrhythmias. In fact, Lie et al.[206] reported nine instances of ventricular fibrillation in a placebo group compared with none in the lidocaine group. In these studies the risk of ventricular fibrillation was not always presaged by warning arrhythmias. Although not conclusive, such studies[207] and others mentioned earlier in this chapter argue strongly for the use of lidocaine prophylactically.

TACHYARRHYTHMIAS AND PREMATURE BEATS

Sinus Tachycardia

Sinus tachycardia is most often noted in patients with anterior infarction. It may be harmful because it increases myocardial oxygen consumption and reduces time for coronary perfusion. Anxiety, persistent pain, hypovolemia, pericarditis, fever, and certain drugs can produce sinus tachycardia. When it is due to pump failure (hypotension or heart failure) and is persistent, the prognosis is poor. Enhanced sympathetic activity associated with activation of myocardial receptors is probably contributory to the sinus tachycardia. Unless there is overt heart failure, digitalis seldom reduces the rate. Small doses of a β-blocking agent frequently slow the rate, allow for better coronary perfusion, and prevent the associated catecholamine release and ventricular arrhythmias. Naturally, β-blockers should not be given if there is severe hypotension or heart failure.

Atrial and Junctional Arrhythmias

Atrial or nodal (junctional) premature beats may be associated with the development of heart failure or may be forerunners of supraventricular tachycardias. Atrial fibrillation or flutter is often preceeded by PABs. It has been estimated that approximately one fourth of patients with acute infarctions have atrial tachyarrhythmias. PABs preceded atrial fibrillation or flutter in 10 of 14 cases in our initial series.[199] Patients are prone to have these supraventricular tachyarrhythmias if there is left atrial distention, pericarditis, or if the sinus node artery is occluded. The artery to the sinus node arises from the right coronary artery in approximately 55% of cases and from the proximal left circumflex coronary artery in 45% of instances.

If the PABs occur more frequently than six per minute and there is no heart failure or hypotension, then they can be suppressed by giving 0.3 g of quinidine orally every 6 hours. If they occur in the presence of heart failure, digitalis should be given.

Atrial fibrillation occurs more often than atrial flutter and paroxysmal supraventricular tachycardia (re-entrant or ectopic) in acute myocardial infarction. These arrhythmias occur more frequently in the early phase of infarction, usually anterior, and are associated with an increase in mortality.[208] The prognosis in such cases is often poor, not so much because of the arrhythmia, but because the infarct is large as shown by hemodynamic and clinical findings. Atrial infarction and left atrial dilatation secondary to left ventricular failure are factors contributing to the occurrence of such arrhythmias.

The supraventricular tachyarrhythmias shorten diastole, compromise cardiac output, and may lead to extension of the infarction.[209] They tend to recur and classically are best treated with digitalis if the patient is hemodynamically stable. We prefer to use digoxin, giving 0.5 mg initially and then 0.25 mg every 2 to 4 hours until the ventricular rate is less than 100 beats per minute, regular sinus rhythm appears, or a total of 1.5 mg has been given. In the presence of acute myocardial infarction, the heart is more sensitive to digitalis, and extreme caution is necessary to avoid toxicity. The first dose is usually given slowly I.V.; the route of administration thereafter depends on the status of the patient. We use direct-current (dc) countershock initially if severe heart failure, cardiogenic shock, or persistent chest pain is present. Otherwise, it is reserved for patients who maintain a ventricular rate of greater than 140 beats per minute in spite of digitalis or for those whose condition is beginning to deteriorate because of heart failure or hypotension (Fig 4–16). If there is no heart failure or hypotension and if the ventricular rate is over 140 beats per minute, some advocate the use of 1 to 2 mg of propranolol I.V. in divided doses, 3 minutes apart, which may produce a regular sinus rhythm or slow the ventricular rate. Five-mg verapamil I.V. can be used for atrioventricular nodal re-entrant supraventricular tachycardia. Others prefer to use dc countershock initially for controlling the supraventricular tachyarrhythmias, especially for atrial flutter, which often is resistant to digitalis and is sensitive to low-energy shock, such as 25 watt-seconds. Rapid atrial stimulation by a transvenous intra-atrial electrode has been used successfully in atrial flutter. It has advantages over dc cardioversion in that it can be used in the presence of digitalis

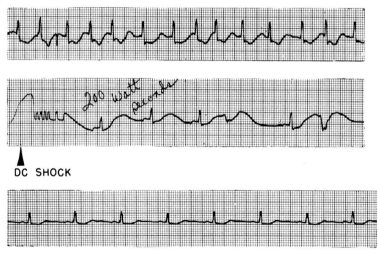

DC SHOCK

Fig 4–16. Acute myocardial infarction with atrial fibrillation. After 1.5 mg of digoxin was given, the ventricular rate was still rapid, and hypotension developed. Direct-current shock was administered. Note the ventricular coupling occurring immediately after the shock (*middle strip*) followed by regular sinus rhythm (*bottom strip*). (From Gazes P.C.: Treatment of acute myocardial infarction. *Postgrad. Med.* 47:143, 1970.)

with less chance of producing other arrhythmias and can be repeated as necessary for recurrent atrial flutter.

Recurrent atrial arrhythmias can be prevented by giving maintenance digoxin daily or 0.3 g of quinidine every 6 hours, or a combination of these. Small doses of propranolol may also be required to prevent or control the ventricular response if atrial arrhythmia recurs.

Ventricular Arrhythmias

Premature Ventricular Beats. Premature ventricular beats are common in patients with acute myocardial infarction and occurred in 76% of the first 100 patients treated in our coronary care unit.[199] Premonitory ventricular ectopic beats were seen in 20 of 22 patients with ventricular tachycardia.[210] In the past we did not institute therapy promptly unless the PVBs were more frequent than six per minute, were multifocal or in pairs, or occurred at the peak of the T wave (vulnerable phase) of the preceding beat. Studies[211,212] have shown that R on T is not a critical determinant of primary ventricular fibrillation. In addition, Roberts et al.[213] reported that repetitive ventricular arrhythmias in patients with acute myocardial infarction are often precipitated by late rather than early premature ventricular complexes. Furthermore, warning arrhythmias were found by Lie et al.[214] in only 60% of patients in whom ventricular fibrillation developed. Despite the variable results, these data suggest that lidocaine prophylactically should be given to all patients with an infarction. No clear definition is available at present regarding the nature and type of ventricular beat that should be prevented or suppressed. However, it appears to us that therapy should be initiated at the first indication of any type of PVB irrespective of its time in the cardiac cycle because these may herald ventricular tachycardia and fibrillation.

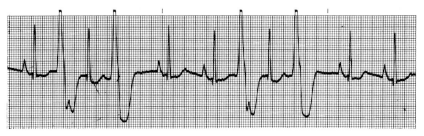

BEFORE LIDOCAINE

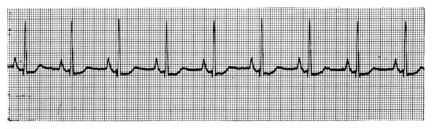

AFTER 50MG I.V.

Fig 4–17. Clearing of ventricular ectopic beats after administering IV lidocaine in a patient with acute myocardial infarction.

Lidocaine hydrochloride (Xylocaine) is the drug of choice (Fig 4–17). The method of administering it was discussed earlier in this chaper.

If the lidocaine is ineffective, 1 to 2 mg/kg of procainamide hydrochloride (Pronestyl) or 0.5 mg of propranolol hydrochloride (Inderal) can be given I.V. If necessary, the medication can be repeated in a few minutes. Maintenance procainamide (20 to 80 μg/kg/min) may be necessary. At times patients with sinus tachycardia and PVBs may respond better to β-blockers than to lidocaine.

After several hours of maintenance infusion of lidocaine, the rate of administration may have to be reduced because the extravascular pool may become saturated, and the blood level will rise. The constant infusion can be stopped abruptly after 48 hours if no ventricular arrhythmias are present. It need not be tapered because 100 minutes after lidocaine infusion is stopped, the plasma concentration has declined by one half, and by 400 minutes it has completely disappeared. This type of decline in plasma level occurs because the drug leaves the peripheral compartment and reenters the central compartment.[215,216] If PVBs recur after lidocaine is stopped, oral antiarrhythmic drugs such as procainamide, quinidine, disopyramide (Norpace), propranolol, tocainide or mexiletine can be given as described in Chapter 15. Three hundred seventy-five to 500 mg of procainamide is given orally every 4 to 6 hours, or 300 mg of quinidine sulfate every 6 hours, at least throughout hospitalization. If these agents are ineffective in preventing recurrence of PVBs, 100 to 200 mg of disopyramide phosphate or 10 mg of propranolol given orally every 6 hours can be tried. The propranolol dosage can be increased, provided that side effects do not occur. The usual dosage for tocainide is 400 to 600 mg q 8 to 12 hours, and for mexiletine 150 to 300 mg q 6 to 8 hours. Occasionally a combination of these drugs is necessary. Common early side effects are fever from procainamide, and diarrhea, nausea, and vomiting from quinidine sulfate. Disopyramide, because of its anticholinergic effect, can produce urinary retention. Since it is excreted by the kidneys, it should be given cautiously and in smaller doses in the presence of kidney disease. It also can aggravate heart failure. Its action is essentially the same as that of quinidine, but it does have fewer GI side effects. Propranolol must be used with caution if incipient failure is present or if the patient is diabetic. It is contraindicated in the presence of AV block, bronchial asthma, and severe heart failure. The most common side effects with tocainide or mexiletine are gastrointestinal and neurologic. Hypoxia, hypotension and electrolyte abnormalities should be corrected.

Ventricular Tachycardia

Ventricular tachycardia was present in 18% of our first 100 patients.[199] The incidence is usually reported as approximately 10%. Bursts of three or more consecutive PVBs that usually occur at a rate of 120 to 250 per minute (Fig 4–18) constitute paroxysmal ventricular tachycardia according to the criteria of the American Heart Association. This arrhythmia is usually intermittent and nonsustained in acute myocardial infarction, and the initial and maintenance therapy is the same as for PVBs.

A small group of patients have sustained attacks of ventricular tachycardia. A single, sharp blow over the precordium may terminate an attack, but it is best not to do this because it may produce ventricular fibrillation. If the pa-

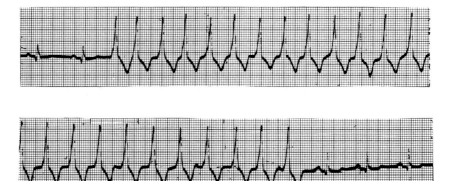

Fig 4–18.   Usual type of ventricular tachycardia, which responded to lidocaine. (From Gazes P.C.: Treatment of acute myocardial infarction. *Postgrad. Med.* 48:168, 1970.)

tient is hemodynamically stable and lidocaine, 1 mg/kg or procainamide, 50 mg/min up to 500 mg given I.V. fail to reverse the arrhythmia, we proceed with synchronized dc precordial shock. If the latter treatment is not available, we suggest that after a few minutes a second dose of lidocaine 1 mg/kg be given, followed by 50 mg of procainamide given I.V. every minute, the total dosage not to exceed 0.5 g. If reversion occurs before the total dosage is reached, injections are discontinued; if it does not occur, bretylium tosylate 5 mg/kg I.V. or 0.5 to 1 mg of propranolol I.V. every 3 minutes for not more than three doses, or 100 mg of diphenylhydantoin (Dilantin) I.V. can be tried. If congestive heart failure, shock, chest pain, or hypotension is present, dc cardioversion (if available) should be used immediately rather than antiarrhythmic drugs, which can cause further myocardial depression. Quinidine, procainamide, disopyramide, tocainide, or mexiletine can be given to prevent recurrent attacks of sustained ventricular tachycardia. If these drugs do not prevent these life-threatening attacks, amiodarone, encainide, or flecainide can be tried. Amiodarone has many adverse effects on the liver, lungs and other organs. Encainide and flecainide can be pro-arrhythmic when used for ventricular tachycardia, especially if they prolong the QRS greater than 50%; the dosages are high, and there is severe ventricular dysfunction. A recent unpublished report from the NHLBI cardiac arrhythmia suppression trial on postmyocardial infarction patients with asymptomatic ventricular arrhythmias showed that significantly greater mortality and nonfatal cardiac arrest occurred in patients receiving these drugs as compared to those in the placebo group. The rate for encainide was 40 of 415 patients (9.6%) and for the matched placebo group, 15 of 416 (3.6%). The rate for flecainide was 16 of 315 patients (5.1%) and for its matched placebo group, 7 of 309 patients (2.3%). These findings were consistent across a variety of subgroups. Thus it was recommended that these drugs be used only in patients with life-threatening arrhythmias such as sustained ventricular tachycardia.

Accelerated Idioventricular Rhythm

This generally benign paroxysmal ventricular arrhythmia, with rates ranging from 60 to 100 beats per minute, occurred in 10% of our patients.[199] It has been noted in up to 20% of cases since the advent of continuous monitoring and has been given a variety of names, such as slow ventricular tachycardia, paroxysmal ventricular tachycardia, nonparoxysmal ventricular tachycardia, and accelerated idioventricular rhythm. It often appears with an inferior infarction with sinus bradycardia and sinus arrhythmia, especially when the ectopic escape rhythm exceeds the sinus rate. However, it can occur almost as frequently with anterior infarcts.[217] It is frequently seen during sleep, when the sinus rate is even slower. Accelerated idioventricular rhythm usually begins as a late end-diastolic ventricular ectopic beat rather than a premature beat near the preceding, normally conducted sinus beat, as is often seen with the conventional type of ventricular tachycardia. It disappears as the rate of the sinus rhythm exceeds the rate of the ectopic rhythm; if both occur at the same rate, fusion complexes result (Fig 4–19). The paroxysms are usually only 4 to 30 beats. It is usually benign, does not lead to ventricular fibrillation, often clears with no medications, and will respond to atropine, which should be given if hypotension or heart failure develops. Cardiac pacing is seldom necessary. At times this arrhythmia may coexist with ventricular tachycardia in the same patient,[218] or it may represent ventricular tachycardia with an exit block (Fig 4–20). In the latter instance a slow ventricular rate can increase, suddenly double, or become a multiple of a more rapid rate, or the exit block can present as a Wenckebach grouping. A study considered the arrhythmia to be slow ventricular tachycardia if it started with a PVB, the rhythm was irregular, and it terminated suddenly.[219] These variations should be treated in the same manner as was described for ventricular tachycardia.

Ventricular Fibrillation

Ventricular fibrillation can occur suddenly and unexpectedly, often in the patient who seems to be doing well with no evidence of pump failure (primary

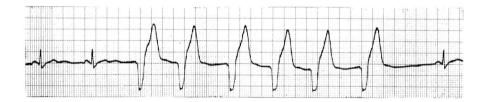

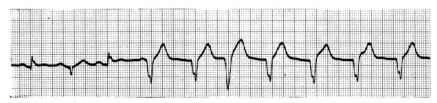

Fig 4–19. Two cases of accelerated idioventricular rhythm. Note that the paroxysms began with late ventricular ectopic beats rather than premature beats near the normal sinus impulse. The second complex in the bottom strip is a fusion beat (simultaneous activation of the ventricle by the sinus and ectopic impulse). (From Gazes P.C.: Treatment of acute myocardial infarction. *Postgrad. Med.* 48:168, 1970.)

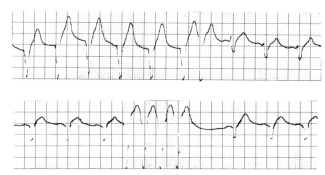

Fig 4–20. Ventricular tachycardia with probable 2:1 exit block (rate 100, *top*), since at the end of the paroxysm, the rate suddenly doubled (rate 200) and continued the same in the ventricular ectopic paroxysm (*bottom*). (From Gazes P.C.: Treatment of acute myocardial infarction. *Postgrad. Med.* 48:168, 1970.)

type). Unless there is underlying heart block, ventricular fibrillation is seldom self-limiting. Cardiopulmonary resuscitation should be started immediately until defibrillation can be done. Usually reversion to sinus rhythm is successful (Fig 4–21) unless the patient has the secondary type of ventricular fibrillation with circulatory failure (intractable heart failure or shock). If cardiac arrest persists after several DC shocks, epinephrine, lidocaine, and bretylium are given in this sequence with DC shock administered after each drug. The value of sodium bicarbonate is questionable and is considered only if the above fails. The details in the management of ventricular fibrillation are discussed in Chapter 15. After reversion to a sinus rhythm, continuous infusion with lidocaine should be given for maintenance antiarrhythmic therapy, and later procainamide, quinidine sulfate, propranolol, tocainide, mexiletine, disopyramide, amiodarone, flecainide, or encainide therapy, such as that described for ventricular tachycardia, can be administered. Besides the primary and secondary types of ventricular fibrillation, there is the late type that occurs 1 to 6 weeks after the onset of the infarction and is noted more often with anteroseptal infarctions with intraventricular conduction abnormalities.

BRADYARRHYTHMIAS

Sinus Bradycardia

Sinus bradycardia (22% of our first 100 patients) is most commonly observed in patients with inferior and posterior myocardial infarction.[199,220] The aver-

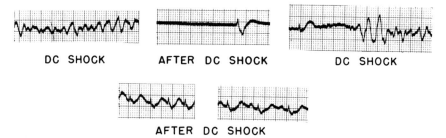

DC SHOCK   AFTER DC SHOCK   DC SHOCK

AFTER DC SHOCK

Fig 4–21. Unexpected primary ventricular fibrillation in acute myocardial infarction. After direct-current shock, asystole occurred, followed by a return of ventricular fibrillation that required a second shock to restore a regular sinus rhythm. (From Gazes P.C.: Treatment of acute myocardial infarction. *Postgrad. Med.* 48:168, 1970.)

age incidence reported is approximately 15%. However, during the first hour after the onset of symptoms, it may occur in up to 40% of patients. The heart rate is under 60 beats per minute, and the slowness may be followed by escape beats and slow junctional (nodal) rhythms or even cardiac standstill. The long diastolic pauses favor the development of ventricular arrhythmias (premature ventricular contractions, ventricular tachycardia, or ventricular fibrillation). In addition, these patients are prone to vasovagal (Bezold-Jarisch reflex) attacks characterized by pallor and nausea, and at times confusion, slow heart rate, and fall in BP. Morphine can precipitate or aggravate such attacks.

At one time atropine was given to all patients with sinus bradycardia secondary to acute myocardial infarction to prevent such complications. However, Epstein et al.[221] showed that in dogs sinus tachycardia may precipitate serious ventricular arrhythmias and that slow rates may be protective. Therefore, if the patient has a moderate level of bradycardia and is stable, it is best not to give atropine. Other studies, with which we agree, have shown that if the heart rate is below 50, or if ventricular arrhythmias, heart failure, or hypotension are present, atropine can be of benefit.[222,223] The usual dose initially is 0.5 or 0.6 mg I.V. (Fig 4–22). The total cumulative dose should not exceed 2.5 mg over 2.5 hours. Doses smaller than 0.4 mg may produce a paradoxical slowing of the rate.[224] In the event of excessive sinus tachycardia (more than 100 beats per minute) or ventricular arrhythmia, the rate can be slowed by the use of propranolol. In addition, atropine can produce urinary retention, glaucoma, and mental confusion. Raising the legs may also aid in alleviating the vasovagal attacks by increasing venous return and stretching the right atrium and by increasing the arterial pressure. Thus, the sinus rate is increased (Bainbridge reflex) by reducing vagal tone. Occasionally, temporary noninvasive external (Zoll type) or transvenous pacing of the right atrium may be necessary, especially if there is circulatory collapse.

Atrioventricular Conduction Disturbances

Atrioventricular conduction disturbances also were seen most often in patients with inferior myocardial infarction, usually due to a vagal component and reversible ischemia. First-degree AV block occurred in 18%, second-degree block in 14%, and third-degree block in 16% of our first 100 patients.[199] The incidence varies in many studies and is usually lower. We do not treat first-degree AV blocks. It remains controversial whether a transvenous pacer

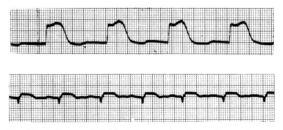

Fig 4–22. *Upper strip.* First-degree AV block, sinus bradycardia, and marked ST segment elevation in a patient with acute inferior myocardial infarction with hypotension. *Lower strip:* After atropine, there was an increase in the sinus rate and a shorter P-R interval. Both strips taken in lead II. (From Gazes P.C.: Treatment of acute myocardial infarction. *Postgrad. Med.* 48:141, 1970.)

should be inserted if second- or third-degree AV block occurs with an inferior infarction.

The overall mortality for inferior infarction and third-degree AV block is 20 to 40%. However, Rotman et al.[225] showed that if heart failure and shock are absent, the mortality is only 11% and this group was at no higher risk of mortality than were others without block. We do not insert a temporary pacing catheter in patients with an inferior infarction and second- or third-degree AV block unless the patient's ventricular rate is below 50, his condition is deteriorating (hypotension, heart failure, ventricular arrhythmias), dizziness or syncope occurs, or complete heart block exists with a wide QRS complex (Fig 4–23). One study[226] showed that lidocaine caused severe bradycardia or asystole when given I.V. to patients with inferior infarction and complete AV block proximal to the His bundle and who had an AV junctional escape rhythm. Lidocaine selectively depresses conduction in ischemic or partly depolarized myocardium and so blocks the impulse from the escape focus. Without prior insertion of a pacemaker, lidocaine is unsafe in patients with acute infarction and complete AV block proximal to the His bundle. Before the pacing catheter is removed, sinus rhythm should be present for several days. Seldom can it be removed sooner than 1 week. Corticosteroids are of questionable value but are used.

Heart block due to extensive septal infarction is usually associated with an anterior myocardial infarction and has a mortality up to 75%. Most often in such cases, the level of the block is infranodal. This type of block is often preceded by conduction impairments in various combinations involving the right bundle and the two fascicles of the left bundle. Table 4–16 compares the features of third-degree AV block in anterior and inferior infarctions.

Trifascicular block is impending if right bundle-branch block occurs with extreme left axis (about −60 degrees) or right axis (about +120 degrees), especially if such axes occur intermittently in the same patient. The left axis indicates block of the left anterior superior branch of the left bundle (left anterior hemiblock), and the right axis indicates block of the left posterior inferior branch of the left bundle (left posterior hemiblock; Fig 4–24). Also,

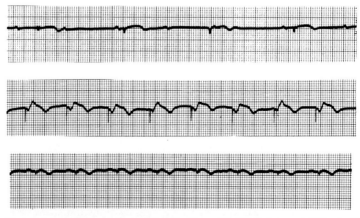

Fig 4–23. *Upper strip:* Inferior myocardial infarction with third-degree AV block. *Middle strip:* Paced rhythm. *Lower strip:* One week later. Regular sinus rhythm. All strips taken in lead II. (From Gazes P.C.: Treatment of acute myocardial infarction. *Postgrad. Med.* 48:141, 1970.)

Table 4–16. Comparison of Features of Third-Degree AV Block in Inferior and Anterior Infarctions

Feature	Inferior	Anterior
Pathology	Edema of AV node or His bundle	Infarction of septum involving bundle branches
Onset	Slow	Sudden
QRS width	Narrow	Wide
Ventricular rate, beats/min	≥45	<45
Associated with Mobitz type II	Rare	Common
Adams-Stokes	Rare	Common
Mortality	20%–40%	75%
Hemodynamic effects	Usually none	Circulatory failure

any type of bundle-branch block with first degree AV block or alternating right and left bundle-branch block can precede trifascicular block. These various combinations can progress to complete AV block in an average of about 45% of cases.[227] This progression can be sudden and often unheralded. Somewhat unexpected is the incidence of progression of pure right bundle branch to complete block in 43% of patients and of left bundle-branch block in only 20% of patients. A recent collaborative study by Hindman et al.[228,229] described the clinical significance of bundle-branch block complicating acute myocardial infarctions and the indication for temporary and permanent pacemaker insertion. Table 4–17 lists our present indications for insertion of a transvenous pacemaker if bundle-branch block or heart block occurs in a patient with an anterior infarction. If the patient is unstable, external non-invasive pacing can be done until a transvenous type is inserted. The high mortality has not been significantly changed by temporary pacing, but as mentioned by Hindman et al., "A strictly statistical argument ignores the mechanism of dying for patients with and without prophylactic temporary pacing." Bifascicular block progresses to complete heart block at a rather high rate. In the collaborative study, nine patients died as a result of sudden development of complete heart block in the hospital. Standby pacing in bifascicular block must prevent some

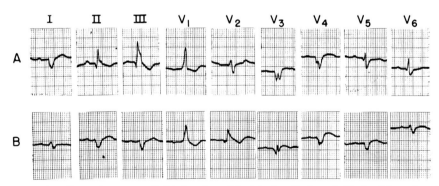

Fig 4–24. **A,** midanterior myocardial infarction with right bundle-branch block, right axis +120 degrees (left posterior hemiblock), and first-degree AV tricular block. **B,** midanterior myocardial infarction with right bundle-branch block, and left axis −90 degrees (left anterior hemiblock). Complete heart block requiring transvenous pacing developed subsequently in both patients. (From Gazes P.C.: Treatment of acute myocardial infarction. *Postgrad. Med.* 48:141, 1970.)

Table 4–17.   Indications for Temporary Pacemaker Insertion in Patients with Anterior Infarctions*

Usual
Second-degree or complete AVB
New RBBB + LAH
New RBBB + LPH
New alternating RBBB and LBBB
New BBB with first-degree AVB
Possible
New RBBB
New LBBB
Old RBBB + LAH + first-degree AVB
Old RBBB + LPH + first-degree AVB
Old alternating RBBB and LBBB + first-degree AVB
No
Old LBBB ⎫
Old RBBB ⎭   Regardless of PR interval
Old RBBB + LAH
Old RBBB + LPH
Old alternating RBBB and LBBB

*AVB = atrioventricular block; RBBB = right bundle-branch block; LAH = left anterior hemiblock; LPH = left posterior hemiblock; LBBB = left bundle-branch block.

of the mortality due to sudden development of complete heart block, even though death from pump failure will continue to be high. In addition, temporary pacing may be of value in treating the frequent ventricular arrhythmias observed in such cases by the use of continuous Holter monitoring.[230]

Patients with inferior infarction and AV block seldom require a permanent pacer; however, among those with anterior infarction and its low level of block, a few have permanent block and require a permanent pacer. Some studies advocate permanent pacemakers in all patients with anterior infarctions who develop high-degree AV block (Mobitz type II AV block or third-degree AV block), even though the high-degree block may be transient, since sudden late deaths are common in such patients.[227,228] At present we agree with this policy.

Ventricular Asystole

Ventricular asystole or slow idioventricular rhythm (agonal) occurred in 10% of our first 100 patients.[220] Reported incidences vary. Asystole is usually associated with pump failure. At times it may actually be fine ventricular fibrillation, and when there is doubt electric countershock should be used. If the heartbeat is not restored after a sharp blow to the chest, closed-chest cardiac massage should be started along with adequate pulmonary ventilation. Next, 5 ml of a 1:10,000 solution of epinephrine is injected I.V. and repeated every 5 minutes if necessary. Atropine, 1.0 mg I.V. is given and repeated in 5 minutes. Following this sequence, sodium bicarbonate (1 mEq/kg) can be administered, though its value is questionable (see Chap. 15). External pacing, transvenous pacing, or direct percutaneous puncture of the heart with a needle electrode may be tried, although it is usually ineffective unless the ventricular asystole is intermittent with underlying complete AV heart block.

Table 4–18 outlines the treatment of arrhythmias associated with acute myocardial infarction.

HEMODYNAMIC AND MECHANICAL COMPLICATIONS

The recognition and proper treatment of hemodynamic and mechanical complications of acute myocardial infarction has become an area of increasing importance. Improvements in arrhythmia detection and treatment have allowed more patients to survive the early hours of an infarction, only to later develop a hemodynamic or mechanical complication. However, as yet it is not known if thrombolytic therapy will decrease their incidence. For the most part, these patients require therapy that can be delivered only in a large medical center with readily available cardiovascular surgery. Recognition and initial therapy are critical, however, and remain the responsibility of the primary physician.

The Killip classification of patients with acute myocardial infarction gives a clinical assessment of patients.[231] Class I patients have no clinical signs of cardiac decompensation; Class II patients have rales, S_3 gallop and venous hypertension; Class III patients have frank pulmonary edema; and Class IV patients have cardiogenic shock. Forrester et al.[232] divided patients into four classes based on hemodynamic data monitored by a Swan-Ganz catheter. Class I patients had no pulmonary congestion or peripheral hypoperfusion and the cardiac index and pulmonary capillary wedge pressure (PCW) are normal. Class II patients have pulmonary congestion with elevated PCW pressure (>18 mmHg). Class III patients have peripheral hypoperfusion with a decreased cardiac index (<2.2 L/min/m^2) and a PCW pressure less than 18 mm Hg. Class IV patients have pulmonary congestion and hypoperfusion with a low cardiac index (<2.2 L/min/m^2) and elevated PCW pressure (>18 mm Hg).

HEART FAILURE

Left ventricular failure of varying degrees is common in the majority of patients during the first week after the onset of infarction. However, clinically the degree is difficult to evaluate. Left heart failure may occur with a normal-sized heart, with normal pulse rate, and in the presence of a normal CVP and a lack of hypervolemia as is noted with chronic failure. A balloon-tipped, flow-directed venous Swan-Ganz catheter can measure pulmonary artery end-diastolic and pulmonary wedge pressures, which give a better evaluation of the function of the left ventricle. With left ventricular failure, these can be elevated, yet the CVP will be normal. Subtle symptoms and signs are often present before overt evidence of congestive heart failure. Some of these subtle findings are a positive hepatojugular reflux, ventricular (S_3) gallop, paradoxical splitting of the second sound, pulsus alternans, sinus tachycardia more than 110 beats per minute, weakness, coughing (especially on lying flat), Cheyne-Stokes respiration, wheezing instead of rales, and pulmonary interstitial edema on x ray. A portable chest x ray has limitations, yet it may demonstrate early evidence of left ventricular failure. It should be made in the upright position, since the recumbent position may give false suggestions of pulmonary venous hypertension. The x ray may show dilatation of upper lobe vessels due to increasing shunting of blood, loss of normal sharp hilar markings, increased interstitial density of lungs, and confluent areas of edema. Less

Table 4–18.   Outline of Treatment of Arrhythmias Associated With Acute Myocardial Infarction

Type of Arrhythmia	Recommended Therapy
Supraventricular	
Premature atrial or junctional beats (nodal)—6 or more per minute	Quinidine 200–300 mg orally every 6 hr. If there is associated heart failure or hypotension, digitalis.
Supraventricular (reentrant or ectopic) tachycardia, atrial flutter, atrial fibrillation	Digitalis and/or propranolol, verapamil, or dc shock. If condition is deteriorating, dc shock should be tried first. Atrial overdrive (except for atrial fibrillation).
Sinus tachycardia	Digitalis if in failure. If patient is not in overt failure, propranolol, 10–20 mg orally every 6 hr.
Ventricular	
Ventricular ectopic beats	Lidocaine, 100 mg bolus IV, then 50 mg every 5 min for 3 doses; or initially give 200–250 mg IV, over a 20-min period.
Ventricular tachycardia (sustained)	Lidocaine, 1 mg/kg bolus IV; repeat in 2 min. If ineffective, dc shock (first therapy if hypotension, angina, or heart failure present). If latter is unavailable, procainamide, 50 mg I.V. every minute up to 0.5 gm, or propranolol 0.5 mg to 1 mg every 3 min up to 3 doses, or dilantin, 100 mg I.V., or bretylium tosylate, 5 mg/kg I.V.
Prevention of recurrences of ventricular arrhythmias	Drip of 2–4 gm of lidocaine per L of 5% glucose in water, 1 ml/min for 48 hr. Then procainamide, 375–500 mg orally every 4 to 6 hr; quinidine, 300 mg orally every 6 hr; propranolol, 10–40 mg orally every 6 hr; disopyramide, 150–200 mg every 6 hr orally; Tocainide, 400–600 mg orally every 8 to 12 hr; mexiletine, 150–300 mg orally every 6 to 8 hr; or Bretylium tosylate, 5 mg/kg IM every 6–8 hr. If response to these drugs is inadequate and arrhythmias are life-threatening, then amiodarone, loading 800–1600 mg orally for 2 weeks, then 200–600 mg daily; flecainide, 100–200 mg orally every 12 hr; or encainide, 25–75 mg orally every 6 to 8 hr.

Table 4–18. *Continued*

Type of Arrhythmia	Recommended Therapy
Drug-resistant ventricular arrhythmias	Check antiarrhythmic blood levels, electrolytes, and magnesium levels. Electrophysiologic studies, antitachycardia electrical devices, or surgery.
Accelerated idioventricular rhythm	None, or atropine, 0.6 to 0.8 mg IV, as needed. Rarely, cardiac pacing.
Bradyarrhythmias Sinus bradycardia	Atropine, 0.6 to 0.8 mg IV, as needed, if rate below 50/min, hypotension, heart failure or ventricular arrhythmias occur. Rarely, external, atrial, or ventricular pacing for atropine-resistant bradycardia.
Inferior infarction First-degree AV block	None.
Second- and third-degree AV block	None if patient is stable. If rate below 50, QRS wide, hypotension, ventricular arrhythmias, syncope, or heart failure is present, atropine, 0.6 mg IV, then insert standby transvenous pacer.
Anterior infarction with bundle-branch block and AV block	See Table 4–17.
Cardiac arrest Ventricular fibrillation	Adequate ventilation. External cardiac massage. Immediate dc shock. Epinephrine, 5 ml of 1:10,000 solution IV. Lidocaine, 1 mg/kg I.V. Bretylium tosylate, 5 mg/kg IV. Consider bicarbonate, 1 mEq/kg. After each drug repeat DC shock.
Ventricular standstill or slow idioventricular (agonal) rhythm	Thump chest. Adequate ventilation. External cardiac massage. Epinephrine, 5 ml of 1:10,000 solution IV. Atropine, 1.0 mg I.V. Consider sodium bicarbonate, 1 mEq/kg IV. Rarely, percutaneous or transvenous pacing.

often, one may note thickening of the interlobar fissures, dilatation of the right descending branch of the pulmonary artery, and interlobar or mild pleural effusions. Dyspnea, rales, deep jugular vein pulsations, and external jugular distention, hepatomegaly, and edema are late findings of heart failure.

Patients with a normal-sized heart and evidence of mild failure during the initial few days of infarction usually require no therapy or only oxygen to avoid hypoxemia. Diuretics may be given in small doses (20 to 40 mg of furosemide I.V., repeated at intervals if needed) to avoid a brisk diuresis, which can rapidly lower the left ventricular filling pressure, with a fall in cardiac output and the development of hypotension. The use of digitalis in patients with sinus rhythm and myocardial infarction remains controversial. Patients (Killip class 2) in heart failure with cardiomegaly, congestion that does not respond to diuretics and a vasodilator, and an S_3 gallop should be given digitalis.[233] It should be administered cautiously, since these patients are more sensitive to the drug and prone to intoxication, especially arrhythmias. We would prescribe two thirds of the usual loading dose. The clinical state dictates the method, rate, and route of administration. We often begin with 0.5 mg of digoxin orally, and then give 0.25 mg every 4 hours for one or two more doses, maintaining the patient on 0.25 mg daily provided that renal function is adequate. If necessary, this can be given slowly I.V. as mentioned in Chapter 16. In the absence of monitoring of the pulmonary arterial and wedge pressures by use of the Swan-Ganz catheter, one must exhibit good clinical judgment as to the response of the patient to digitalis, diuretics, and vasodilators. Studies have shown that pulmonary congestion is rare when the pulmonary capillary wedge pressure is below 18 mm Hg. McHugh et al.[234] reported that x-ray changes correlate reasonably well with hemodynamics, but there may be abnormal wedge pressure elevation initially in the absence of x-ray changes, and there may be a posttherapeutic lag of x-ray findings.

Patients with an acute infarction and moderate or severe failure may respond well to vasodilator therapy, especially if they are normotensive or hypertensive. Intravenous nitroglycerin (initially 5 to 10 µg/min) or sodium nitroprusside (0.5 µg/kg/min initially) are most often used. Nitroglycerin has a greater effect on reducing the preload (venous capacitance vessels) and sodium nitroprusside has a greater effect on reducing the afterload (arteriolar resistance). Vasodilator therapy is especially useful if there is associated mitral insufficiency or septal rupture. The advantage vasodilators have over digitalis and diuretics is that they avoid the side reactions of these drugs, namely, arrhythmias and electrolyte disturbances. The systemic arterial pressure, the pulmonary capillary wedge pressure, and the cardiac output should be monitored to avoid excessive reduction of arterial pressure and ventricular filling pressure. Therapy with diuretics and vasodilators is often contraindicated in patients with right ventricular infarction.

Dobutamine (initial dose 2 µg/kg/min) improves hemodynamics, increases coronary blood flow, relieves pulmonary congestion, and is considered by many the inotropic agent of choice in patients with an acute myocardial infarction and cardiac failure.[235]

PULMONARY EDEMA

Pulmonary edema is often associated with hypotension or shock and is often fatal. The patient should be in the Fowler position, and oxygen should be administered. Intramuscular or, at times, I.V. administration of 6–12 mg of morphine sulfate is useful to slow exaggerated respirations, produce venous pooling of blood, and allay apprehension. In the event of an inferior infarction, one should be cautious, since the vagomimetic effect of morphine may precipitate or aggravate heart block. We administer digitalis immediately if an S_3 gallop is present, although some consider this useful initially only if supraventricular arrhythmias are also present. Immediate increase in venous capacitance and later diuresis can be produced by administering 40 mg I.V. of furo-semide (Lasix). Electrolyte levels should be checked often, since potassium loss may be significant. If the patient does not respond to these measures and is not hypotensive, vasodilator therapy may be tried in an attempt to reduce preload (left ventricular filling pressure) and afterload (systemic impedance), which are important determinants of myocardial oxygen consumption.[236,237] Initially, sublingual or I.V. nitroglycerin can be started, which predominantly cause venodilation and reduce preload and pulmonary congestion but have less effect on systemic impedance and, therefore, produce minimal alterations of cardiac output. If improvement is not achieved, sodium nitroprusside, which affects both preload and afterload, can be given I.V.[238] However, it is preferable not to give I.V. nitroglycerin or nitroprusside unless the patient's pressures can be monitored by a Swan-Ganz catheter. The dosage should be titrated to lower the pulmonary capillary wedge pressure to an optimal level (14 to 18 mm Hg) without lowering the systemic arterial pressure below 95 mm Hg.

CARDIOGENIC SHOCK

This complication is usually associated with extensive myocardial infarctions in which at least 40% of the left ventricular myocardium has been destroyed.[239] Cardiogenic shock should be correctly defined. Often the BP may fall below 90 mm Hg, yet the patient is warm, has adequate urinary output, and is not in shock. A patient with an inferior infarction may be hypotensive and warm because of peripheral vasodilatation secondary to vagal effect. The patient in myocardiogenic shock usually is cold and clammy and has a narrow pulse pressure, and the urine output is less than 0.5 ml per minute. Pulmonary congestion is often present, and if it is absent, one should suspect hypovolemia or right ventricular infarction and failure. Until recently this complication was associated with a survival rate of no more than 10%. However, with the use of hemodynamic monitoring, improved medical and surgical therapy, and, most important, intraaortic balloon counterpulsation, the prognosis is not as dismal. It is important that the primary physician not equate a low BP with cardiogenic shock. Patients with infarction frequently have volume depletion due to poor oral intake, nausea and vomiting, and diuretic use. A Swan-Ganz catheter should be placed for diagnosis and management of therapy, since hemodynamic changes will precede by several hours changes notable by physical examination and by chest x-ray. The Swan-Ganz catheter can be inserted at the bedside via a vein to measure pulmonary artery and pulmonary capillary wedge pressure and cardiac output (thermodilution technique). The pulmonary artery end-diastolic and wedge pressures usually reflect left ventricular filling pressure, whereas the CVP reflects right ventricular filling pressure. With the cardiac output and mean systemic and right atrial pressures, the systemic vascular resistance can be calculated. Although we occasionally try a fluid challenge without monitoring filling pressure with a Swan-Ganz catheter, we feel that pulmonary artery pressure monitoring should always precede the use of vasopressors and vasodilators to avoid their inappropriate use in a volume-depleted patient. We use the criteria set forth by Forrester et al.[240] in diagnosing cardiogenic shock, which is defined by a pulmonary capillary wedge pressure of greater than 18 mm Hg and a cardiac index of less than 2.2 L/min/m^2. Once this diagnosis is made, we attempt to increase the cardiac output by direct effect on the myocardium, using inotropic agents such as dopamine (Intropin) or dobutamine (Dobutrex), and to decrease preload and afterload with nitroprusside (Nipride). Dopamine is a naturally occurring catecholamine and is preferably used in patients whose systolic BP is 80 mm Hg or above. Administration is begun I.V. at doses of 2 to 5 μg/kg/min. At these low doses, dopaminergic receptors are stimulated, resulting in renal and mesenteric blood vessel vasodilatation. At higher doses, however, dopamine's α-adrenergic actions predominate, in which case BP is maintained at the expense of increased cardiac afterload. Therefore, it is frequently given with sodium nitroprusside, which reduces preload and afterload. Usually we begin with 0.5 μg/kg/min of nitroprusside IV and increase the dosage according to clinical and hemodynamic response. Dobutamine,[241] a synthetic derivative of isoproterenol, has been used because it has a positive inotropic effect and decreases the systemic vascular resistance, giving an effect similar to that of a combination of dopamine and nitroprusside. In addition, left ventricular filling pressure increases with dopamine in high doses and tends to decrease with dobutamine. We usually begin with 2 to 5 μg/kg/min of dobutamine I.V. Levarterenol bitartrate (norepinephrine; Levophed) and metaraminol (Aramine) have both α- and β-adrenergic agonist properties and so increase contractility and peripheral vascular resistance. Such vasopressor therapy is begun initially if the BP is unobtainable or the systolic BP is extremely low, in an attempt to raise it above 80 mm Hg. Two to 4 mg of norepinephrine or 100 mg of metaraminol in 500 ml of glucose in water is given slowly I.V. It should be recognized that their vasoconstrictor action can unduly increase the afterload, therefore, these drugs are used initially for BP support until other measures can be started. Most patients will not respond to this medical regimen, in which case intra-aortic balloon counterpulsation (IABP) is instituted. Vasodilators and inotropic agents are usually more useful in combination with IABP. Percutaneous double-lumen intra-aortic balloon insertion has simplified the procedure, but is not applicable to all cases. The inflated balloon during diastole allows for better coronary perfusion. It also reduces afterload, with resultant decrease in myocardial oxygen requirement. The aim is to maintain systolic blood flow, reduce the load on the heart, and improve myocardial contraction. Patients who fail to improve with this measure or who show indications of pump dependence are advised to have cardiac catheterization to assess the possibility of cardiac surgery. Hutter and associates[242] have accumulated a large experience using this approach with results superior to medical management or intra-aortic balloon counterpulsation alone. Of 106 patients with cardiogenic shock, 80 lived long enough to undergo angiography. Forty-eight patients were ultimately operated upon, 50% of whom were alive at 1 year. The operation most often performed was coronary artery bypass grafting, with correction of mechanical abnormalities (rupture of ventricular septum or papillary muscle).

Reperfusion with thrombolytic agents, PTCA, or a combination has been reported to reverse cardiogenic shock.[243] The GISSI study showed a high mortality in patients with cardiogenic shock treated with intravenous streptokinase alone. Streptokinase has a hypotensive effect. Most studies in the United States with thrombolytic agents excluded patients with shock. A retrospective study[244] compared conventional therapy (59 patients) and angioplasty (24 patients) in myocardial infarction with cardiogenic shock. The 30-day survival for the angioplasty group was 50% and for the conventional group 17%. If the angioplasty was successful, the survival was 77% (10 of 13 patients) versus 18% (2 of 11 patients) if unsuccessful. Randomized controlled studies will be required to fully determine the value of thrombolytic agents, angioplasty, or a combination in cardiogenic shock.

These sophisticated methods should be limited primarily to research medical centers or to larger community hospitals that have appropriate equipment and specially trained personnel. The practicing physician, however, can help stabilize the patient prior to transfer to a center by giving oxygen, opiates for pain relief, atropine for bradyarrhythmias, cardioversion for supraventricular tachyarrhythmias (digitalis if cardioversion is not available or if arrhythmia is recurrent), and lidocaine for ventricular arrhythmias. If the patient cannot be transported to such centers, one can measure the CVP (or observe the neck veins), BP, and urinary output and use clinical judgment in therapy for shock. Even though most infarctions involve the left ventricle, taking the CVP, which reflects the right ventricular filling pressure, may be of value. If the CVP is normal or below, the patient may be hypovolemic and can be challenged with I.V. low molecular weight dextran, but one must realize that the pulmonary wedge pressure may be high, and the patient's condition may worsen. Sudden elevation of the CVP (over 5 cm of H_2O) or dyspnea should alert one to this latter problem. If the CVP is elevated, most often the pulmonary wedge pressure will be above the optimal range (except in some instances of right ventricular infarction), and therefore therapy should be the same as mentioned previously for cardiogenic shock. However, vasodilator therapy should not be given without monitoring of pulmonary capillary pressure and cardiac output. There have been conflicting reports of the value of large doses of steroids in cardiogenic shock. Arterial pH should be monitored, since metabolic acidosis develops rapidly in shock and should be corrected by the use of sodium bicarbonate. In the future, if studies confirm the value of thrombolytic agents in patients with acute myocardial infarction and shock, all community hospitals should use these as first-line therapy.

EMBOLISM

Pulmonary embolism has become a rather uncommon complication of acute myocardial infarction, probably because of the use of anticoagulants in complicated cases and the institution of early ambulation. Early recognition of pulmonary emboli can be difficult. Often one waits for classic lung findings or evidence of phlebitis. One should be suspicious of pulmonary emboli if a patient has periods of hypotension, tachypnea, tachycardia, fever, or low arterial O_2 oxygen tension. On the other hand, massive pulmonary embolism can occur in the absence of dyspnea, cyanosis, or hypotension.[245] If pulmonary emboli occur, heparin should be started and later replaced with oral anticoagulants. Anticoagulant therapy and thrombolytic (streptokinase and urokinase) therapy will be discussed in Chapter 9. The source of the emboli is usually the veins in the legs or lower abdomen. Ligation or clipping of the inferior vena cava or transvenous insertion of an umbrella filter is seldom required in acute myocardial infarction. Mural thrombi, as discussed earlier, occur more often in patients with anterior infarction and an akinetic or dyskinetic area. The reported incidence of systemic emboli is about 2 to 6%. Peripheral arterial emboli can be extracted by the use of a Fogarty catheter (balloon catheter) through remote arteriotomy incisions with local anesthesia.

HEART MURMURS

The most common causes of heart murmurs in myocardial infarction are papillary muscle dysfunction or rupture, rupture of the interventricular septum, or, rarely, rupture of chordae tendinae.

Papillary muscle dysfunction. The murmur of papillary muscle dysfunction occurs too commonly to be regarded as a true complication of infarction. Its importance lies in its recognition as a functional rather than mechanical disorder. The papillary muscles make up part of the complex mitral valve apparatus and are prone to ischemic dysfunction because of their relatively poor blood supply and their location, which is quite distal to the origin of the coronary arteries.[246] The posteromedial papillary muscle is supplied by the right coronary artery, the anterolateral papillary muscle is supplied by the left anterior descending coronary artery, and the circumflex coronary artery contributes to both papillary muscles. The murmur produced by papillary muscle dysfunction may be holosystolic, but often is limited to early systole, midsystole, or, more classically, late systole. For unknown reasons the first heart sound is often loud. The murmur of papillary muscle dysfunction is most often heard during transient ischemic episodes. Its major clinical implication is its suggestion of an imbalance between myocardial oxygen supply and demand.

Papillary muscle rupture. This includes rupture of the belly of the papillary muscle, papillary muscle head, or chordae tendinae. This is a rare complication of a transmural myocardial infarction. Rupture of the belly of the papillary muscle results in fulminant cardiovascular decompensation, and death occurs within hours. More commonly, a single head of the papillary muscle ruptures, the clinical presentation being acute and severe pulmonary edema due to regurgitation of blood into a small, unprepared left atrium and pulmonary vascular bed. The overall mortality for rupture of the papillary muscle is 50% within the first day and 80% in the first 2 weeks.[247] It is more often seen in the setting of right coronary artery occlusion with acute inferior myocardial infarction involving the postero-medial papillary muscle. In about 50% of the cases the infarct is relatively small. Physical examination classically reveals pulmonary edema and a holosystolic murmur loudest at the apex of the heart. A diastolic murmur may be heard, reflecting increased transmitral blood flow secondary to the left ventricular volume overload; however, tachycardia often shortens diastole sufficiently to mask this murmur. At times the murmur occurs only in early systole, or no murmur is heard due to the severity of regurgitation, resulting in early equilibration of left ventricular and left atrial pressures. When this complication is suspected, a Swan-Ganz catheter should be inserted. The presence of a large V wave (actually a regurgitant C-V wave) on the pulmonary capillary wedge and pulmonary artery pressure tracings suggests the diagnosis. It may also be seen with septal rupture. Two-D echocardiography and Doppler studies (including color) establish the diagnosis. Vasodilator therapy with sodium nitroprusside during intra-arterial and pulmonary artery pressure monitoring should be immediately instituted in an attempt to lower systemic vascular resistance, improve subvalvular left ventricular function, and consequently reduce mitral regurgitation. Vasodilator therapy should be started even in the presence of hypotension, since a reduction in aortic impedance and improved left ventricular function should result in an elevation of systemic arterial pressure. Occasionally this complication results in cardiogenic shock, but with a better than expected survival because a limited amount of myocardium is involved. Wei et al.[248] described autopsy findings of 13 patients with papillary muscle ruptures complicating myocardial infarction. The infarctions involved on the average only 19% of the left ventricle, which would represent a very treatable form of cardiogenic shock with current techniques. Echocardiography in this case would reveal preservation of left ventricular contractility, small left atrium, and a left ventricular volume overload. Patients whose conditions do not stabilize with vasodilator therapy should be treated with intra-aortic balloon counterpulsation. Early cardiac catheterization with surgical repair including aortocoronary bypass grafting to suitable arteries should be done.

Ventricular septal rupture. This is a rare and frequently fatal complication found in 1 to 2% of all patients dying of an acute myocardial infarction. The overall mortality for rupture of the ventricular septum is 24% within the first day and 65% in the first 2 weeks.[247,249] This complication usually occurs within the first week after the infarction, and the most common location is in the lower apical septum.[250] It may be seen with anterior or inferior infarctions, since both the left and right coronary arteries supply the septum through perforating septal branches. Rupture of the septum is virtually always associated with transmural infarction in contrast to papillary muscle rupture, which may complicate subendocardial infarction.[251] Differentiating ventricular septal rupture from papillary muscle rupture by clinical examination is often not possible. The murmur due to a ventricular septal rupture is classically loudest at the lower left sternal border and associated with a thrill in this location. Sudden neck vein distention is also a clue to this complication. Biventricular failure usually occurs and varies depending on the size of the defect and the degree of left-to-right shunt. A Swan-Ganz catheter should be placed, and the complication suspected if there is a step-up of oxygen saturation at the ventricular or pulmonary artery level. Two-D echocardiography and Doppler, especially color (Fig 4–25), can detect the defect. Medical therapy would include vasodilators and positive inotropic agents (dopamine or dobutamine), but failure to achieve stabilization indicates a need for intra-aortic balloon counterpulsation. Although with any complication of myocardial infarction a delay in surgery of at least 6 weeks is ideal, early operative closure of postinfarction ventricular septal defect can be accomplished with encouraging survival rates, the major determinant of success being the function of the uninvolved myocardium.[252] In fact, Montaya et al.[253] reported that surgical results were better in patients operated on less than 2 days after ventricular septal rupture (72% survival rate) and that ventricular septal rupture can occur with single-vessel disease (8 of 27 patients). Experience has now shown that the defect should be closed surgically as soon as possible. The earlier the closure, the less the mortality which still approaches about 40%.[254] Often such patients in addition need coronary revascularization. A catheter placement device to close the defect in critically ill patients is being evaluated.

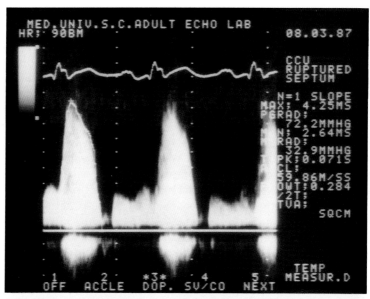

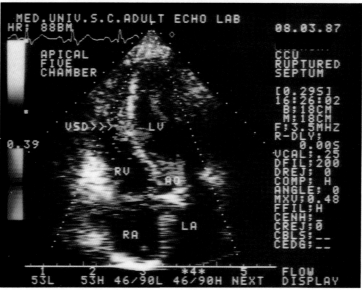

Fig 4–25. Two-D echocardiography and color Doppler showing a ventricular septal (VSD) rupture in the mid-septum secondary to an acute myocardial infarction. At top, continuous-wave Doppler recording of the jet from the left ventricle into the right ventricle (peak gradient 72 mm Hg). At the bottom (apical five-chamber view), color flow Doppler shows the VSD. The abnormal flow can be seen as a mosaic color high velocity shift from the left to right ventricle (arrow) at the level of the VSD. (Courtesy of Dr. Bruce Usher.)

FREE WALL RUPTURE

This is almost always a lethal complication of acute myocardial infarction, contributing to death in 5 to 10% of patients.[255] It most commonly occurs in the first week following the acute event, and is said to be more common in women and the elderly, patients with hypertension, patients with continued activity after the infarction, and those with no prior myocardial infarction. It usually occurs in the anterior or lateral walls of the left ventricle. Rarely, it may occur without any symptoms of myocardial infarction (silent infarction). The clinical presentation is one of severe congestive heart failure, shock, or cardiac tamponade. The ECG may reveal electromechanical dissociation, severe bradycardia, unexplained peaked T waves, or evidence for acute extension of the infarction. Immediate pericardiocentesis to relieve tamponade and surgical closure has been performed successfully in the proper circumstances. This complication can occasionally occur as a subacute event and may be treatable with pericardial drainage, surgical repair, or both.[256] Incomplete rupture may lead to a pseudoaneurysm or diverticulum whose wall is made up of organized thrombus, hematoma, and pericardium. These can become very large and communicate with the left ventricle through a narrow neck. Since rupture of these can occur frequently, they should be surgically repaired.

VENTRICULAR ANEURYSM

A ventricular aneurysm can develop either early or months to years after the infarction (Fig 4–26). It usually occurs with total occlusion of the left anterior descending coronary artery. Often it is the only vessel involved and there are few or any collaterals present. Surprisingly, this is rarely a source of cardiac rupture. It may, however, cause intractable congestive heart failure, ventricular tachycardia resistant to drug therapy, or continuing angina, and may be a source for thromboembolic events. Two-dimensional echocardiography and radionuclear angiograms make the noninvasive recognition of this complication more reliable. Persistent ST elevation as late as 6 weeks following the acute event may also suggest this complication. Individuals have lived for many years with ventricular aneurysms. Surgical resection is indicated if heart failure, angina, systemic emboli, or medically uncontrolled ventricular tachyarrhythmias are present, but before surgery coronary arteriography and

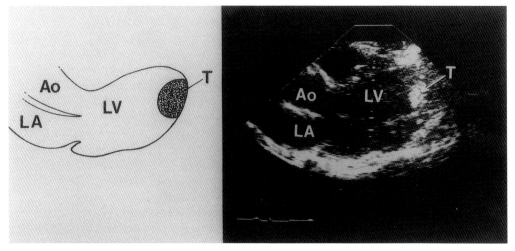

Fig 4–26. Two-dimensional echocardiogram (long-axis view) of a patient with a ventricular aneurysm and mural thrombus secondary to a myocardial infarction. Ao = aortic; LA = left atrium; LV = left ventricle; T = thrombus. (From Usher B.W.: Role of echocardiography in evaluating patients with congestive heart failure. Reprinted by permission of *Medical Times*, vol. 110, no. 6, 1982.)

ventriculography should be performed. The criteria for selection of patients for operation should be based on the extent of reversible ischemia and the amount of mechanical dysfunction. Hemodynamic and radionuclide angiography studies at rest and during exercise can be of value in this assessment.[257,258] Froehlich et al.[257] showed that surgery can be accomplished with relatively small risk and that functional improvement is common but is not related to substantial improvement in global left ventricular function.

POSTMYOCARDIAL INFARCTION SYNDROME

The postmyocardial infarction syndrome (Dressler's syndrome) is a recurrent febrile illness with pericarditis, pleuritis, and pneumonitis. It probably results from an autoimmune antibody reaction to myocardial antigens. It should not be mistaken for pulmonary embolism or recurrent myocardial infarction. It can occur any time after the first week[259] following an acute myocardial infarction and may be recurrent up to 1 year. A pericardial rub is often present with a transmural infarction within 36 to 48 hours and usually clears in 3 to 5 days. If it persists longer, the Dressler syndrome may be developing. Anticoagulants should be discontinued in the presence of this syndrome, since pericardial hemorrhage and even cardiac tamponade can occur. The treatment is symptomatic, giving aspirin, unless the syndrome persists or recurs, in which case steroids may be tried. Indomethacin (Indocin) should not be used in patients with severe coronary artery disease because it can produce coronary vasoconstriction.[260] Rarely, after recurrent attacks in spite of therapy, the pericardium should be resected.

RIGHT VENTRICULAR INFARCTION

In a study of 2000 patients with transmural infarctions of the left ventricle, Wartman and Hellerstein[261] found an associated right ventricular infarction in 14% of cases. Isner and Roberts[262] emphasized that right ventricular infarction occurred exclusively with transmural inferior infarctions of the left ventricle and infarction of the posterior ventricular septum. Wackers and associates[263] found an incidence of right ventricular infarction of 38% in 64 patients with acute inferior infarction who underwent dual imaging with thallium 201 and ^{99m}Tc Pyp. A clinical study, however, by Lorell et al.[264] described only 12 patients with a clinical diagnosis of right ventricular infarction among 306 patients with acute inferior wall infarction. Those authors emphasized the similarity in the physical findings of right ventricular infarction with pericardial disease. In their study, 4 of the 12 patients had received erroneous diagnoses of acute pericardial tamponade. The diagnosis of right ventricular infarction is important because these patients frequently have electric instability as well as a low-output state due to reduced left ventricular volume with hypotension. Clinically, these patients may have findings of right heart failure and Kussmaul's sign. Findings of tricuspid insufficiency may occur and, rarely, myocardial rupture (usually posterior septal rupture). The electrocardiogram may show ST elevation in lead V_4R (right precordial lead V_4 position). Echocardiography and radionuclide angiography can demonstrate right ventricular dysfunction. Right heart catheterization reveals right heart filling pressures to be elevated and left ventricular filling pressure to be normal or slightly elevated. Volume expansion under the guide of a Swan-Ganz catheter is usually all that is needed. Inotropic agents and vasodilators (to decrease afterload) may be helpful, depending on the degree of associated left ventricular dysfunction.[265,266] Atrioventricular sequential pacing rather than ventricular pacing may be necessary if right ventricular infarction is complicated by third-degree AV block, for atrial contraction may be necessary to maintain hemodynamic stability. For bradyarrhythmias without AV block, atrial pacing may be sufficient.

Atrial Infarction

Atrial infarction can rarely occur in the absence of ventricular infarction. Most often its findings are overshadowed by changes of the concomitant ventricular involvement. Abnormalities in P wave morphology, PR (T of P) segment depression or elevation, AV conduction disturbances, and supraventricular arrhythmias can occur. Other complications are atrial mural thrombi, pulmonary embolism, and rupture of the atrium. Electrocardiographic changes of atrial infarction may give the clue to concomitant ventricular infarction in the presence of left bundle-branch block. Atrial infarctions should be observed carefully for supraventricular arrhythmias, which should be immediately treated. Anticoagulants can be of value because of the high incidence of intramural thrombosis and pulmonary emboli; however, this therapy should be weighed in light of possible atrial rupture. The importance of diagnosis and localization of atrial infarction has been reviewed by Gardin and Singer.[267]

Postinfarction Management

Uncomplicated patients are now being discharged at approximately 7 to 10 days postinfarction when they are ambulatory. The prognosis of patients recovering from infarction depends primarily on ventricular function and ongoing evidence of ischemia and ventricular arrhythmias. Therefore, usually at discharge, patients should have an echocardiogram, radionuclide angiogram (Muga), exercise stress test, and 24-hour Holter monitoring. If the patient has no complications, a submaximal treadmill stress test is performed at a low level of exercise prior to discharge.[102,268,269] Various protocols are used, but the majority prefer a modified Naughton treadmill exercise protocol (Table 4–19). The exercise is continued on the treadmill until the patient reaches the target rate of 70% of maximal heart rate predicted on the basis of age. The test is stopped if the patient has angina, severe fatigue or dyspnea, frequent (more than 5 beats per minute), multifocal, or paired PVBs, horizontal or downslop-

Table 4–19. Modified Naughton Protocol

Stage	Duration (min)	Speed (mph)	Grade (%)	METS (unit)	VO$_2$ (ml/kg/min)
1	3	2	0	2	7.0
2	3	2	3.5	3	10.5
3	3	2	7.0	4	14.0
4	3	2	10.5	5	17.5
5	3	2	14.0	6	21.0
6	3	2	17.5	7	24.5

ing ST depression greater than 2 mm compared with the resting tracing, a fall in BP prior to attaining the predicted target heart rate or until a load corresponding to 17.5 ml of oxygen per kg of body weight per minute (5 metabolic equivalents) was performed. At times it is preferable to do a thallium stress test, especially for those with marked resting ECG abnormalities. In addition, a 24-hour Holter recording is performed for arrhythmias. Also, radionuclide ventricular function studies and echocardiography are often done prior to discharge for evaluating prognosis. One study showed that an ejection fraction of less than 40% indicated a poor prognosis and even worse if complex ventricular arrhythmias were also present.[270] If coronary arteriography has not been performed, this should be done if the patient has symptoms of ischemia, positive stress test, or an ejection fraction less than 40% and then, depending on the findings, angioplasty or bypass surgery should be considered. In addition, depending on the results of these tests, the patient's activities are outlined and these activities are explained and given to him in writing at the time of discharge.

DRUGS TO PREVENT MORBIDITY AND MORTALITY

Beta-Blockers

Earlier in this chapter, the use of β-blockers in the initial management of acute myocardial infarction was discussed. There have been many clinical trials evaluating β-adrenergic blockers for reducing morbidity and mortality several days after the onset of acute myocardial infarction. A large study[271,272] showing favorable results used practolol, which later was taken off the British market because of side effects on the eyes and retroperitoneal fibrosis. Wilhelmsson et al.[273] found a statistically significant difference in sudden death between patients treated with alprenolol and those treated with placebo. However, the total mortality difference was not statistically significant, and the study did not show any effects on reinfarction. The Norwegian Multicenter Study Group carried out a double-blind, randomized study with timolol, a noncardioselective β-blocker, and a placebo in patients surviving acute myocardial infarction.[274] Treatment was begun 7 to 28 days after infarction, and the patients were followed up for 12 to 33 months (mean, 17 months). There were 152 deaths in the placebo group and 98 in the timolol group. Cumulated mortality rates for 33 months were 17.5% with placebo and 10.6% with timolol (a reduction of 39.4%), and cumulated reinfarction rates were 20.1% with placebo and 14.4% with timolol (a reduction of 28.4%). The 6-year follow-up of this study has shown that beneficial effects are maintained for up to 6 years. The group concluded that long-term treatment with timolol reduces mortality and rate of reinfarction. Soon after this report, the results of two other double-blind, randomized trials were released. The β-blocker heart attack trial (BHAT)[275] was a randomized, double-blind, multicenter clinical trial of propranolol vs. placebo in patients enrolled 5 to 21 days after the onset of an acute myocardial infarction. Prior to discharge, patients were taking 40 mg of propranolol or placebo three times per day. Depending on serum propranolol levels, a maintenance dose of 60 mg or 80 mg three times per day was prescribed at the one-month follow-up visit. Initial data at the 30-months follow-up show a mortality of 9.5% in the placebo group (183 deaths) and 7.0% in the propranolol group (135 deaths), a reduction of 26%. The greatest reduction in mortality was in patients over age 65. In the Swedish study[276] metoprolol was compared with placebo, started soon after the patients arrived in the hospital and continued for 90 days. Metoprolol was given initially as 15 mg I.V., followed with oral medication 100 mg twice per day. There were 62 deaths in the placebo group (8.9%) and 40 deaths in the metoprolol group (5.7%), a reduction of 36%. Studies have suggested that high-risk patients (those with large infarcts, over age 65, and with complex arrhythmias) benefit the most from β-blockers.[277]

In most of the trials of β-blockade following infarction, patients have been kept on these for 2 to 3 years. One major consideration is the effect of these when given long-term on serum lipids. Nonselective β-blockers have been shown to increase serum triglycerides and decrease high-density lipoproteins (HDL). Variable effects have been reported on the total cholesterol. The selective types of β-blockers have a less adverse effect and those with intrinsic sympathetic activity (ISA) may be neutral or can decrease cholesterol and increase HDL. However, agents with ISA are less beneficial regarding mortality than those that lack this effect.[278] The deleterious effect of nonselective types on lipids may be offset by the beneficial effects of β-blockers on long-term mortality.

Although the exact mechanism by which β-blockers improve survival is not known, several factors may be important, such as controlling ischemia, hypertension, arrhythmias, and an antiplatelet effect. In summary, in view of reduction in mortality and reinfarction found in all major trials in patients on β-blockers after infarction, it appears wise to give them to all postinfarction patients unless there is a contraindication. This should be continued for at least 2 to 3 years and even longer if, on withdrawal, patients have symptoms or findings such as hypertension, angina, or ventricular arrhythmias.

ANTIPLATELET AGENTS

The use of antiplatelet agents such as aspirin, dipyridamole (Persantine), or sulfinpyrazone (Anturane) is still under discussion. Such drugs are known to prevent platelet aggregation, which plays a fundamental role in initiating thrombus formation in arteries. Aspirin inhibits the enzyme cyclooxygenase and thus inhibits platelet production of thromboxane A_2 and thereby platelet activation and aggregation. Dipyridamole raises the intracellular concentration of cyclic AMP by inhibiting the enzyme phosphodiesterase and thus prevents platelet aggregation. The Amis study,[279] which compared aspirin with placebo after an acute myocardial infarction, showed no differences in the three-year mortality between the two groups. Eighty-five percent of these patients were enrolled more than 6 months after their myocardial infarction. The Anturane study[280] showed that patients taking this drug within 25 to 35 days after infarction had a significantly lower death rate than patients taking a placebo. Difference between the two groups was due mostly to a low incidence of sudden cardiac death in the second to seventh month after a myocardial infarction. However, some patients who entered into the trial and subsequently died were excluded from the analysis of the results. This factor and others have produced debate, and the evidence favoring the drug is now in question. At this point it is best to wait for more information before adding the drug as standard treatment. The "PARIS" study[281] (our group participated in this collaborative study) compared the results of using Persantine plus aspirin,

aspirin alone, and placebo. Persantine and aspirin or aspirin alone showed favorable effects for coronary incidence (coronary death or definite nonfatal myocardial infarction) from 8 to 24 months. In addition, patients receiving Persantine and aspirin or aspirin alone within 6 months of their last myocardial infarction had the least mortality. However, only 20% of patients were in this category, and the results were not statistically significant. Because of these results, the PARIS-II Study[282] was done in which patients were recruited within 4 months of their acute myocardial infarction. Patients were randomized into two groups, dipyridamole (Persantine) plus aspirin (1563 patients) and placebo (1565 patients). This study did not include an aspirin-alone group. Coronary incidence (definite nonfatal myocardial infarction plus death due to recent or acute cardiac event) in the Persantine plus aspirin group was significantly lower than in the placebo group at 1 year, showing a 30% reduction, and at 23.4 months at the end of study, the reduction was 24%. The dosage used was 75 mg of dipyridamole and 330 mg of aspirin three times per day. A review by Fitzgerald[283] concluded that, in the majority of prospective clinical trials designed to assess the efficacy of dipyridamole, it was combined with aspirin and not compared directly with placebo. Therefore, it appears that aspirin alone is useful for coronary artery disease. The dosage of aspirin has been debated because, in larger amounts, it may inhibit prostacyclin (PGI_2), a vasodilator, generated by normal vascular endothelial cells, which may offset its beneficial effect. Enteric-coated aspirin may prevent gastric complications, but in addition is absorbed slowly and nearly completely deacetylated to salicylate during its passage through the liver. Salicylate is not capable of inhibiting production of prostacyclin, which is a vasodilator. Yet platelets flowing through the portal system encounter unaltered acetylsalicylic acid, which will block their thromboxane activity.[283a] In summary, I agree with Fuster,[284] who recommends 325 mg daily based on the present observations until clinical trials are done to assess the efficacy of low-dose aspirin between 60 and 325 mg. I recommend aspirin in all patients who have had any of the coronary syndromes (angina, infarction) and those who have had angioplasty or bypass surgery) unless there is a contraindication. In addition, it is important to periodically check one's hematocrit since occult blood lost may not otherwise be detected.

The use of aspirin in healthy persons is a matter of considerable importance. A recent study[285] randomized male physicians 40 to 84 years of age into one of four treatment groups: active aspirin (325 mg) and active β-carotene; active aspirin and β-carotene placebo; aspirin placebo and active β-carotene; or aspirin placebo and β-carotene placebo. Thus, 11,037 physicians were assigned to receive 325 mg active aspirin every other day and 11,034 to receive aspirin placebo. β-carotene was included to determine if it decreases the incidence of cancer. There was a 47% reduction (statistically significant) in the risk of myocardial infarction in the aspirin group, which included a significant benefit on both nonfatal and fatal events after an average of 4.8 years. There was a nonsignificant increase in strokes in the aspirin group with an increase in the hemorrhagic type (but numbers were small). A recent final report of this study indicated that aspirin was most beneficial in the prevention of a first myocardial infarction in men over age 50 and had its largest effect in those with uncontrolled risk factors for the development of coronary events.[285a] The low cardiovascular mortality rate among participants who entered the study raised some important questions. For example, what would have been the results if those who were unwilling or ineligible or who were nonphysicians had entered the study? Therefore, at present, the decision to prescribe aspirin for primary prevention of cardiovascular disease must be based on individual judgment as to its benefit weighed against its side reactions (namely, hemorrhage, strokes).[286]

ANTIARRHYTHMIC AGENTS

Ventricular arrhythmias encountered within the first few days in the coronary care unit fail to predict which patients are likely to have them at the time of discharge,[287] and in some studies have not been important in predicting long-term survival.[288] However, Conley et al.[289] reported an excess mortality after hospital discharge in patients with acute myocardial infarction complicated by ventricular fibrillation in the coronary care unit. Other reports suggested that ventricular arrhythmias present at discharge appeared to have a worse prognosis than those occurring during the first few days after admission.[290,291] In view of these findings, predischarge Holter recordings should be made. At present there is no agreement on how long a patient should be monitored. Ruberman et al.[292] monitored their patients 1 hour for ectopic activity. Others have suggested 6 to 24 hours. Currently some patients (New York Heart Association Functional class I or II) are being stressed at a low level of exercise prior to discharge (see Table 4–19).[268,269] The exercise ECG provides a small increase in the detection of serious arrhythmias. All studies agree that the presence of complex premature beats (R on T, runs of two or more, multiform, bigeminal, more than five per minute) at the time of discharge is associated with an increased risk of sudden coronary death at least three times that of patients free of these arrhythmias. Schulze and coworkers[270] reported the relationship between ventricular arrhythmias in the late hospital phase of acute infarction and left ventricular function as determined by radionuclide studies (MUGA), showing a striking association between depressed left ventricular function (ejection fraction 40% or less) and complex PVBs. They concluded that the low ejection fraction indicates a poor prognosis and that the presence of complex PVBs increases the risk of sudden death. In addition, Schulze et al.[293] further complemented the radionuclide studies by showing the patients 10 to 24 days after infarction with complex PVBs on angiography had a greater number of proximally obstructed coronary vessels, greater incidence of prior infarction, and a lower ejection fraction and greater percentage of abnormal left ventricular segments. Kotler et al.[294] noted that 16.8% of patients after infarction on Holter monitoring had parasystole and that none died in the follow-up period. Myeburg et al.[295] studied the long-term effect of procainamide and quinidine on chronic complex ventricular arrhythmias in patients who survived prehospital cardiac arrest. Although these drugs did not suppress the complex ventricular arrhythmias, the group with therapeutic blood levels had lower incidence of recurrent cardiac arrest. This apparent dissociation suggests that the effectiveness of these agents may be best measured not by their effect on chronic ventricular ectopies, but rather by their therapeutic blood levels. These two studies need further confirmation and indicate that distinguishing types of PVBs and blood levels of antiarrhythmic agents may be very important with regard to long-term therapy.

In summary, it has been shown that left ventricular dysfunction and complex ventricular arrhythmias are independent predictors of both total mortality and sudden cardiac death. However, this does not indicate a cause-and-effect relationship with the ventricular arrhythmias and sudden cardiac death. As of this date, antiarrhythmic therapy has made no impact on the incidence of sudden death. However, such studies were nonrandomized. Because complex ventricular arrhythmias, (although frequently associated with left ventricular dysfunction) carry a poor prognosis even when left ventricular function is normal, I feel that, until further data are available, they should be treated. Prior to discharge, patients postinfarction should have Holter monitoring for at least 24 hours without receiving antiarrhythmic drugs. If complex PVBs are present, then they should be treated for at least 1 year. At the end of the third month postinfarction, the Holter monitoring should be repeated. The 1-year mortality of patients surviving 30 days is nearly twice that of any subsequent year through the fifth year.[296] At present, there is no agreement with regard to the type of therapy. Because most of these patients are on a β-blocker, this may be sufficient. Otherwise, if this is not effective, I still prefer quinidine, and if it cannot be tolerated or is ineffective, other type 1A drugs as procainamide, disopyramide, type 1B drugs as tocainide or mexiletine, or a combination of 1A and 1B types, can be given with the considerations discussed in Chapter 15. Amiodarone and type 1C drugs such as flecainide or encainide should be considered only if other drugs fail and the ventricular arrhythmias are considered life-threatening. The NHLBI conducted a large multicenter cardiac arrhythmic pilot study (CAPS),[297] which showed that it was feasible to conduct a cardiac arrhythmic suppression trial (CAST) in postinfarction patients. Recently, it was announced that the encainide and flecainide arms of the CAST trial were prematurely terminated due to the high mortality rate of patients taking these agents.

CARDIAC REHABILITATION

At our institution, the cardiac rehabilitation program is divided into four phases: Phase 1: In-patient treatment during the time the patient is in the hospital; Phase II: Early therapeutic exercise phase that begins when the patient is discharged from the hospital and continues until the patient is ready to return to work, usually 8 to 12 weeks; Phase III: Progressive therapeutic exercise that may begin as early as 6 to 12 weeks following hospital discharge and lasts until the patient has reached an optimal level of fitness, in most cases 1 year; and Phase IV: Fitness maintenance designed to meet the long-term needs of those previously rehabilitated. It involves flexible scheduling and reduced monitoring, and emphasizes recreational pursuits. Patients in this phase should still follow an exercise prescription design and have periodic follow-up examinations. In the future, the time intervals for each phase may be pushed up earlier because of the new modalities of therapy such as thrombolytic treatment.

Phase I

This in-hospital phase was discussed earlier in this chapter.

Phase II

Phase II takes place from discharge until the patient returns to work, usually 8 to 12 weeks. During the hospital stay, the patient and his family should be given a clear understanding of the disease. It should be emphasized that, most often, the patient can return to his former occupation and activities. In fact, many patients will be required to be more active than before their attack. Often the patient thinks he will be totally disabled, and if this impression is given it may be difficult to change.

Activities should be gradually increased until the patient has returned to his usual level. Emphasis should be placed on avoiding strenuous activities, such as lifting heavy objects, and avoiding emotional problems. It is permissible to climb stairs slowly, go for a car ride, and begin a walking program. Some patients may return to the hospital three times per week for a structured monitored program of exercise (phase II). Usually, by 8 weeks, the patient is walking one mile daily. At this time the patient is allowed to return to work, depending on his occupation. This course may have to be altered if the patient experiences angina, congestive failure, or arrhythmias. Work should be resumed on a part-time basis for the first few weeks. Besides having the physical ability to return to work, the patient should also be psychologically fit. It is very important that work be enjoyable, not stressful. In some cases patients must change to a less demanding job. Often patients think they are totally disabled if they cannot pursue their usual occupations and must be convinced that they can perform some type of work. This can present a problem, because the patient may be disabled for his prior job, yet be unable to obtain some other type of work because he lacks training. It is important that he receive counseling and be directed to the proper agency for vocational rehabilitation. Work classification units are available for evaluating the working capacity of the patient. The physician must be interested in employment for the patient, if he hopes to motivate him. I fear that physicians are responsible for industry's shunning the cardiac patient. Often, because of the family's persuasion, we declare the patient totally disabled or we use vague terms, saying that he can return to mild, moderate, or heavy work. Industry needs more specific information. Specific details can be given according to caloric expenditure. It is necessary that the individual's physical capacity be matched to the demands of the job. The exercise stress test gives only an approximation of occupational caloric expenditure, since the job requirements often involve activation of muscles not used during stress testing. In addition, age, skill, and emotional and environmental factors should be considered. For an equivalent load, oxygen requirements are higher for arm-work than for leg-work. Many established tables list oxygen costs for most occupational activities (Table 4–20).The MET (energy expenditure at rest, equivalent to 3.5 to 4.0 ml of O_2/kg of body weight/ minute) is often used as a measure of external work rather than oxygen consumption. For example, 3 to 4 METS are required for such jobs as bricklaying, welding, or cleaning windows.

Sexual intercourse should be discussed with patient and spouse prior to the patient's discharge from the hospital. Often sex is resumed too soon, or fears develop which may lead to psychic impotence. Sex can usually be resumed 6 weeks after the attack. Hellerstein and Friedman[297a] have shown that the energy levels and demands on the heart of sexual intercourse are equal to walking briskly or climbing up a flight of stairs. However, the energy cost is much higher during extramarital sex. Patients should not have sex if they are tired, have just eaten a heavy meal, have been drinking, or are angry with their mate. If chest pain or shortness of breath develops during sexual relations, the

Table 4–20. Approximate Energy Requirements of Selected Activities

Category	Self-Care or Home	Occupational	Recreational	Physical Conditioning
Very light <3 METS <10 mL/kg† · min <4 kcal	Washing, shaving, dressing Desk work, writing Washing dishes Driving auto	Sitting (clerical, assembly) Standing (store clerk, bartender) Driving truck Operating crane	Shuffleboard Horseshoes Bait casting Billiards Archery Golf (cart)	Walking (2 mph) Stationary bicycle (very low resistance) Very light calisthenics
Light 3–5 METS 11–18 mL/kg · min 4–6 kcal	Cleaning windows Raking leaves Weeding Power lawn mowing Waxing floors (slowly) Painting Carrying objects (15–30 lb)	Stocking shelves (light objects) Light welding Light carpentry Machine assembly Auto repair Paper hanging	Dancing (social and square) Golf (walking) Sailing Horseback riding Volleyball (6 man) Tennis (doubles)	Walking (3–4 mph) Level bicycling (6–8 mph) Light calisthenics
Moderate 5–7 METS 18–25 mL/kg · min 6–8 kcal	Easy digging in garden Level hand lawn mowing Climbing f stairs (slowly) Carrying objects (30–60 lb)	Carpentry (exterior home building) Shoveling dirt Using pneumatic tools	Badminton (competitive) Tennis (singles) Snow skiing (downhill) Light backpacking	Walking (4.5–5 mph) Bicycling (9–10 mph) Swimming (breast stroke)

Intensity	Occupational		Recreational	
Heavy 7–9 METS 25–32 mL/kg · min 8–10 kcal	Sawing wood Heavy shoveling Climbing stairs (moderate speed) Carrying objects (60–90 lb)	Tending furnace Digging ditches Pick and shovel	Basketball Football Skating (ice and roller) Horseback riding (gallop) Canoeing Mountain climbing Fencing Paddleball Touch football	Jog (5 mph) Swim (crawl stroke) Rowing machine Heavy calisthenics Bicycling (12 mph)
Very heavy >9 METS >32 mL/kg · min >10 kcal	Carrying loads upstairs Carrying objects (>90 lb) Climbing stairs (quickly) Shoveling heavy snow Shoveling 10 min (16 lb)	Lumber jack Heavy laborer	Handball Squash Ski touring over hills Vigorous basketball	Running (≥6 mph) Bicycle (≥13 mph or up steep hill) Rope jumping

By permission of publisher and author, Haskell, W.L.: Rehabilitation of Coronary Patient. New York, John Wiley, 1978:214.

†A MET is a multiple of the resting energy expenditure; 1 MET = approximately 3.5 mL O_2/kg body weight min.

patient should stop and discuss this with his physician at the next examination. Patients who have angina can often prevent an attack by taking prophylactic nitroglycerin.

Car driving is allowed usually about 2 months after the attack. It is not the physical act of operating a vehicle that is harmful, but the emotional tension created when driving on busy streets. About this same time, the patient can fly on commercial airlines. Flights should be arranged to allow ample time for making connections in order to avoid rushing and its associated tension. The patient's progress will dictate when he can resume such activities as golfing, hunting, swimming, and tennis; generally, they can be started in a limited manner after three months. Table 4–21 summarizes the hospital and posthospital activities after an uncomplicated acute myocardial infarction.

Phase III

Phase III usually begins about 2 to 3 months postinfarction. It is also encouraged for patients with all types of coronary disease syndromes, postbypass surgical patients, and those who desire a prevention program (especially those at high risk for developing coronary disease). The mode of rehabilitation is aerobic exercise, and all sessions are held under the direct supervision of physicians, nurses, exercise physiologists, or other program personnel. Many such units are available. Guidelines have been proposed for physical conditioning programs for apparently healthy subjects, particularly those who are prone to coronary disease and those with heart disease. The patient should have a medical history, physical examination, resting ECG, and chest x-ray. Unless contraindicated, an exercise stress test should be performed using the treadmill, although some prefer to use the bicycle ergometer. The patient's exercise target zone should be determined. There are many protocols, and often the exercise prescription is based on work loads expressed in metabolic equiv-

Table 4–21. Hospital and Posthospital Activities After Uncomplicated Acute Myocardial Infarction

First week (phase I)	In coronary care unit
	Unrestricted motion in bed
	Passive exercise
	Bedside commode
	Feeding self
	Up in chair, shaving, bathroom privileges and bathing after 3–5 days
Second week (phase I)	Walking about room and hall if no complications
	Up in chair for longer periods
	Discharge home
Third to eighth week (phase II)	Progressive program of walking daily, toward a goal of 1 mile in 25 min on a flat surface
	Stair climbing
	Return to work
	Driving car
	Sexual intercourse
	Flying on commercial airlines
Eighth to twelfth week (phase III)	Evaluation for exercise program (phase III)

alents (METS). METS allow performance in different protocols to be compared. The patient may choose from a list of activities (such as swimming, jogging, or running) which are comparable to a given number of METS. The exercise target zone for the patient should be between 70% and 85% of his maximal heart rate (MHR). Another method of determining the exercise prescription is based on variability of the resting heart rate. In this method, the resting rate is subtracted from the MHR and 70 to 85% of this difference is added to the resting rate. This target heart rate should not produce symptoms, excessive BP rise, major arrhythmias, or more than 2 mm horizontal ST depression. For example, if an exercise test was stopped because of angina at a heart rate of 130 beats per minute, the patient should be advised to exercise to a heart rate of between 91 and 110 beats per minute (70 to 85% of his maximal rate). The training period should include a warm-up of 5 to 10 minutes, an exercise period of 30 to 60 minutes, and a cool-down period of 5 to 10 minutes. The patient should learn to count his pulse to determine if he is in the target zone. I prefer that the patient check his radial rather than carotid pulse rate for 10 seconds and multiply by six. A few minutes after the warm-up, the patient should check his pulse rate. If it is not within the target zone, he should increase or decrease the intensity of exercise. Kinetic exercises, such as walking, jogging, swimming, rope-jumping, and cycling are recommended over isometric exercises, such as weight lifting, which produce no improvement in cardiovascular function and may cause the BP to rise excessively. I usually have the patient walking until he is able to cover two miles in 30 minutes. Experts now agree that walking can be as effective an aerobic exercise as jogging, biking, or swimming. If the target heart rate cannot be achieved by a brisk walk, one can carry a weight or can go on to jogging and walking. Some may need to run, increase bicycle pedaling, or increase the number of laps that they swim. To be effective, the exercise should last for 30 to 60 minutes and be performed at least four to five times per week. If a program is discontinued or reduced, any progress made will be lost, and the patient will have to restart at a lower level. The patient should be reevaluated on development of such symptoms as chest pain, persistent fatigue, nausea or vomiting, dizziness or syncope, dyspnea, arrhythmias, intermittent claudication, or musculoskeletal problems.

Patients continue in such units indefinitely or until an optimal level of fitness is attained. Although many persons without cardiac disease begin on their own, without supervision, we prefer that the patient with a cardiac problem enter a supervised program for at least one year. At that time, depending on the patient's condition, he may graduate into a health maintenance program (phase IV).

CORONARY ARTERY DISEASE RISK FACTORS

A specific cause for coronary artery disease is not known, but many large-scale epidemiologic studies have identified risk factors (primarily hypercholesterolemia, hypertension, smoking and physical activity), especially the Framingham study.[298]

The Charleston Heart Study[299] was implemented in 1960 by the late Dr. Boyle and continued by Drs. Keil and Gazes to test the hypothesis that there are social, racial, and sex correlates of coronary heart disease. It is a prospective cohort study that has been observing the natural evolution of coronary disease in the study population over a period of 28 years. In 1960, the cohort numbered 2180 persons, 35 years of age and older, and represented an overall response rate of 84% to a population-based sampling plan. This study differs from the Framingham Heart Study in that blacks as well as whites are included. In 1964 the four primary race-sex groups were supplemented with 102 black men of high socioeconomic status (SES). Some of the important findings of the Charleston Heart Study have been that black men have the highest mortality rates, followed by white men, black women, white women and high SES black men with the lowest overall mortality rates. Coronary disease mortality was highest in black men and white men, who had comparable rates. High SES black men had the lowest rates. Systolic blood pressure, cigarette smoking, low education, and history of diabetes were consistent risk factors for all causes of mortality. For coronary mortality, elevated blood pressure and cigarette smoking were the most consistent risk factors. Diabetes was a risk factor for all groups except white men and serum cholesterol appeared to be a significant risk factor only in white and black women.

Regardless of whether the patient has had medical, angioplasty, or surgical therapy, risk factors such as elevated blood lipids (namely, cholesterol), hypertension, cigarette smoking, and a sedentary life-style should be actively monitored and managed. Susceptibility to coronary artery disease is greatly increased in an individual as the risk factors are combined. Other important risk factors are genetic predisposition, emotional stress, excess weight, diabetes, and hyperuricemia. Since coronary heart disease age-adjusted death rate has declined approximately 42% from 1963 to 1985, it appears that the public is aware of the risk factors. Studies have shown that, concomitant with this decline in mortality, there has been a 30% decline in levels of cholesterol and blood pressure and in smoking among adults.

Blood Lipids

Cholesterol and triglycerides do not circulate in the blood as such, but together in different amounts combine with protein to form lipoproteins. The major lipoproteins are chylomicrons (primarily exogenous triglycerides), very-low-density lipoproteins (VLDL, primarily endogenous triglycerides from the liver), low-density lipoproteins (LDL, primarily cholesterol), and high-density lipoproteins (HDL, contains relatively small amounts of both cholesterol and triglycerides and more protein). The protein carriers that are formed on the surface of the lipoprotein are called apolipoproteins. These have been studied extensively as markers for coronary artery disease. Apo A-1 is the major protein in HDL and is inversely related to coronary artery disease. Apo B-100 in LDL and Apo B-100 in VLDL are predictors of coronary artery disease. Other apolipoproteins are also being evaluated. It appears that the HDL cholesterol has an inverse relationship to coronary heart disease incidence. Apparently HDL transports cholesterol from the tissues to the liver for excretion and, in addition, seems to block the cellular deposition of LDL cholesterol. There are several subclasses (based on density), but HDL_2 and HDL_3 have been more extensively studied. Evidence suggests that the protective effect of HDL lies with the HDL_2 subclass.[300] Ratios of total cholesterol or LDL cholesterol to HDL cholesterol have been used as indicators of risk. A ratio of LDL to HDL of greater than 5 would place one at a high risk, 3 at average risk, and less than 2 at low risk. The relationship between plasma triglyceride levels and cardiovascular disease is still controversial. The plasma triglyceride level was found to be an independent predictor of coronary artery disease in women. High levels are usually associated with a low HDL cholesterol. Rather than a direct cause of coronary disease, it may reflect the presence of certain atherogenic lipoproteins. Diabetes, nephrotic syndrome, chronic renal disease, and other conditions may have elevated triglyceride levels. Patients who have severe hypertriglyceridemia with chylomicronemia and eruptive xanthomata are prone to abdominal pain and/or pancreatitis.

The National Cholesterol Education Program Committee recommends that total cholesterol level be measured in all adults 20 years of age and older at least once every 5 years.[301] This can be a nonfasting specimen because total cholesterol does not change significantly after a fat-containing meal. Rapid capillary blood (fingerstick) cholesterol measurements are currently being used for massive screening. Those who have a high cholesterol level, risk factors, or coronary artery disease should, in addition to cholesterol levels, have triglyceride and HDL levels checked after 12 hours fasting (except for water and black coffee). If the triglyceride level is below 400 mg dl, it can be divided by 5 to give an estimate of the VLDL cholesterol level. The LDL cholesterol can be estimated by this equation: LDL cholesterol = total cholesterol − HDL cholesterol − (triglyceride/5). If the triglyceride value is above 400 mg dl, this estimate is less accurate and ultracentrifugation should be done. It is important that lipid measurements be made in a laboratory that participates in a standardization program because there can be considerable variability in the accuracy of some laboratories.

The system of Fredrickson et al.[302,303] of phenotyping has given a clearer understanding of fat metabolism and its disorders. He and his associates have classified five types of disorders; each may be familial (primary) or acquired (secondary). The acquired types are often secondary to diabetes, alcoholism, nephrotic syndrome, biliary obstruction, oral contraceptives, hypothyroidism, and drugs such as the thiazides. Both types are exaggerated by diet intake. From a practical point of view, only type 2 and type 4 should be considered, since these make up the bulk of the disorders. Type 2 is divided into type A (hypercholesterolemia) and type B (hypercholesterolemia and hypertriglyceridemia). Type 4 shows primarily hypertriglyceridemia. Xanthomata are more common in the familial types. Type 2 may have xanthelasmas and early arcus senilis, xanthomata at the elbows and Achilles tendons, and less frequently the tuberous variety on the bony tubercles. The eruptive type over the trunk and buttocks is more frequently noted in types 1, 4, and 5. Xanthomas in the creases of the palms and fingers and the tuberoeruptive type on the extensor surfaces of the extremities are seen in type 3.

The National Cholesterol Education program report[301] recommends initial classification and follow-up of patients based on total cholesterol (Table 4−22). Patients with definite coronary heart disease, two other coronary artery disease risk factors (one of which can be male sex) or a total cholesterol equal to or greater than 240 mg dl should have lipoprotein analysis and further treatment decisions based on LDL-cholesterol levels (Table 4−23).

Dietary Treatment

Dietary therapy is now recommended in two steps, which progressively reduces intake of saturated fats and cholesterol and induces weight loss in the overweight by reducing calories. The step-one diet involves an intake of total

Table 4–22.   Initial Classification and Recommended Follow-up Based on Total Cholesterol

A. Classification	
<200 mg/dl	Desirable blood cholesterol
200–239 mg/dl	Borderline-high blood cholesterol
≥240 mg/dl	High blood cholesterol
B. Recommended Follow-up	
Total cholesterol <200 mg/dl	Repeat within 5 years
Total cholesterol 200–239 mg/dl	
Without definite CHD or two other CHD risk factors (one of which can be male sex)	Dietary information and recheck annually
With definite CHD or two other CHD risk factors (one of which can be male sex)	Lipoprotein analysis; further action based on LDL-cholesterol level
Total cholesterol ≥240 mg/dl	

Reference 303, reprinted by permission by the National Cholesterol Education Program NIH publication No. 88-2925, Jan. 1988.

fat less than 30% of calories, saturated fatty acids less than 10% of calories, and cholesterol less than 300 mg per day. If the response to this diet is not adequate, then the saturated fatty acid intake is reduced to less than 7% of calories and the cholesterol to less than 200 mg/day (step-two diet). Substituting unsaturated fat facilitates cholesterol reduction to a lesser degree. The cholesterol level should be checked at 4 to 6 weeks after starting the step-one diet and at 3 months. Usually it can be expected that the cholesterol will decrease by 10 to 15%. If this response is not achieved or further response is needed, then one proceeds to step-two diet. Usually it is best that the patient be referred for counseling to a registered dietitian, since physicians are very busy and patients like to go into detail in their diet. Table 4–24 outlines the dietary therapy for high blood cholesterol and Table 4–25 lists some foods to

Table 4–23.   Classification and Treatment Decisions Based on LDL-Cholesterol

A. Classification		
<130 mg/dl	Desirable LDL-cholesterol	
130–159 mg/dl	Borderline-high-risk LDL-cholesterol	
≥160 mg/dl	High-risk LDL-cholesterol	
B. Dietary Treatment	Initiation Level	Minimal Goal
Without CHD or two other risk factors*	≥160 mg/dl	<160 mg/dl†
With CHD or two other risk factors*	≥130 mg/dl	<130 mg/dl‡
C. Drug Treatment	Initiation Level	Minimal Goal
Without CHD or two other risk factors*	≥190 mg/dl	<160 mg/dl
With CHD or two other risk factors*	≥160 mg/dl	<130 mg/dl

*Patients have a lower initiation level and goal if they are at high risk because they already have definite CHD, or because they have any two of the following risk factors: male sex, family history of premature CHD, cigarette smoking, hypertension, low HDL cholesterol, diabetes mellitus, definite cerebrovascular or peripheral vascular disease, or severe obesity.
†‡Roughly equivalent to total cholesterol <240 mg/dl (†) or <200 mg/dl (‡) as goals for monitoring dietary treatment.
Reference 303, reprinted by permission by the National Cholesterol Education Program NIH publication No. 88-2925, Jan. 1988.

Table 4–24. Dietary Therapy of High Blood Cholesterol

Nutrient	Recommended Intake	
	Step-One Diet	Step-Two Diet
Total fat	Less than 30% of total calories	
Saturated fatty acids	Less than 10% of total calories	Less than 7% of total calories
Polyunsaturated fatty acids	Up to 10% of total calories	
Monounsaturated fatty acids	10 to 15% of total calories	
Carbohydrates	50 to 60% of total calories	
Protein	10 to 20% of total calories	
Cholesterol	Less than 300 mg/day	Less than 200 mg/day
Total calories	To achieve and maintain desirable weight	

Reference 303, reprinted by permission by the National Cholesterol Education Program, NIH publication No. 88-2925, Jan. 1988.

choose or decrease to lower blood cholesterol. Diets have to be modified depending on the lipid response and calorie level needed for proper weight control. Lean cuts of meats should have the fat trimmed from the outside and poultry should have the skin removed. Fish consumption has become popular in the past few years because its fatty acids belong to the "omega-3" family of polyunsaturated fatty acids consisting largely of eicosapentaenoic and docasahexaenoic acids rather than linoleic acid (omega-6), which is the predominant polyunsaturated fatty acid in vegetable oils, such as safflower and corn oil. It has been suggested that the low coronary artery disease death rate in Eskimos of Greenland may be due to high intake of marine animals (seal, whale, fish), which have large quantities of omega-3 fatty acids.[304] Kromhout et al.[305] studied the relationship between fish consumption and coronary artery disease in a group of Dutchmen. These patients were followed up to 20 years and the study concluded that consumption of as little as one or two fish meals per week may prevent coronary heart disease. Mortality from coronary heart disease was more than 50% lower among those who consumed 30 g of fish per day as compared to those who did not and this relation was independent of other risk factors. The mechanism of action of omega-3 fatty acids on atherothrombotic disease is not clear. Possible mechanisms are the following: may block thromboxane production, increase prostacyclin and inhibit platelet aggregation; inhibit production of leukotrienes (LTB_4), which influences the adherence of monocytes to the arterial endothelium; and reduce triglycerides.[306] The effect on cholesterol has been variable, but omega-3 fatty acids may qualitatively alter the LDL without causing a reduction, thus producing an antiatherogenic effect.[307] Omega-3 is found predominantly in fatty fish such as mackerel, trout, tuna, sardines, and salmon. Shellfish such as oysters, crabs, and shrimp have high cholesterol content but also have significant amounts of omega-3 fatty acids and therefore are now allowed in moderation. At present, I would not recommend fish oil supplements because there are potential adverse effects of fish oil such as increasing bleeding, especially if one is also taking aspirin. Prospective double-blind, placebo-controlled studies in the future may resolve this problem. I usually advise patients to begin by eating 3 fish meals per week, one of which can be shellfish. Monounsaturated fatty acids (mainly oleic acid) may decrease cholesterol. Oleic acid is found primarily in olive oil and rapeseed (canola oil). Soluble dietary fiber, present in oat products and beans,

Table 4-25. Recommended Diet Modifications to Lower Blood Cholesterol: The Step-One Diet

	Choose	Decrease
Fish, chicken, turkey, and lean meats	Fish, poultry without skin, lean cuts of beef, lamb, pork or veal, shellfish	Fatty cuts of beef, lamb, pork; spare ribs, organ meats, regular cold cuts, sausage, hot dogs, bacon, sardines, roe
Skim and low-fat milk, cheese, yogurt, and dairy substitutes	Skim or 1% fat milk (liquid, powdered, evaporated) Buttermilk	Whole milk (4% fat): regular, evaporated, condensed; cream, half and half, 2% milk, imitation milk products, most nondairy creamers, whipped toppings
	Nonfat (0% fat) or low-fat yogurt	Whole-milk yogurt
	Low-fat cottage cheese (1% or 2% fat)	Whole-milk cottage cheese (4% fat)
	Low-fat cheeses, farmer, or pot cheeses (all of these should be labeled no more than 2–6 g fat/ounce)	All natural cheeses (e.g. blue, roquefort, camembert, cheddar, swiss)
		Low-fat or "light" cream cheese, low-fat or "light" sour cream
		Cream cheeses, sour cream
	Sherbet Sorbet	Ice cream
Eggs	Egg whites (2 whites = 1 whole egg in recipes), cholesterol-free egg substitutes	Egg yolks

	Choose	Decrease
Fruits and vegetables	Fresh, frozen, canned, or dried fruits and vegetables	Vegetables prepared in butter, cream, or other sauces
Breads and cereals	Homemade baked goods using unsaturated oils sparingly, angel food cake, low-fat crackers, low-fat cookies	Commercial baked goods: pies, cakes, doughnuts, croissants, pastries, muffins, biscuits, high-fat crackers, high-fat cookies
	Rice, pasta	Egg noodles
	Whole-grain breads and cereals (oatmeal, whole wheat, rye, bran, multigrain, etc.)	Breads in which eggs are major ingredient
Fats and oils	Baking cocoa	Chocolate
	Unsaturated vegetable oils: corn, olive, rapeseed (canola oil), safflower, sesame, soybean, sunflower	Butter, coconut oil, palm oil, palm kernel oil, lard, bacon fat
	Margarine or shortening made from one of the unsaturated oils listed above	
	Diet margarine	
	Mayonnaise, salad dressings made with unsaturated oils listed above	Dressings made with egg yolk
	Low-fat dressings	
	Seeds and nuts	Coconut

Reference 303, reprinted by permission by the National Cholesterol Education Program NIH publication No. 88-2925, 1988.

has been reported to lower plasma cholesterol by 5 to 15%. One study showed that oat bran or beans selectively lowered the serum LDL cholesterol by approximately 24% in hypercholesterolemic men.[308] The oat bran diet provided 100 g of oat bran served as a bowl of hot cereal and 5 oat bran muffins per day and the bean dish contained 115 g of dried beans per day. Increased fecal loss of bile acids may be a factor in this reduction of cholesterol. Often the public is impressed with items labeled as having low or no cholesterol, not realizing that these may be high in saturated fats. For example, palm oil, palm kernel, and coconut oil contain significant amounts of saturated fat but little cholesterol. Therefore, these should not be used in a cholesterol-lowering diet. On the other hand, an item such as shellfish may have considerable cholesterol but little saturated fat, and is permissible in the diet.

Alcohol accounts for approximately 5% of the total calories that Americans consume. It may increase triglycerides and HDL cholesterol when taken in moderation. One study of men who died of coronary artery disease and an equal number of matched controls showed that daily consumption of small to moderate amounts of alcohol (2 oz or less daily) was inversely related to coronary death.[309] Beverage equivalents for 2 oz of alcohol daily were 40 oz of beer, 12 oz of wine, or 4 oz of liquor. Anything above this amount was considered heavy drinking and there was no association with coronary death in this group. In a prospective study among 85,000 health examinees giving an alcohol history at examination from 1978 through 1982, 756 were later found to have coronary artery disease in the same years.[310] Lifelong abstainers were used as the reference group. This study concluded that 1 to 2 drinks daily appear to give some protection against coronary disease. Other recent studies suggested that regular substantial alcohol intake raises both HDL_2 and HDL_3.[311] It appears that HDL_2 has a more protective effect against coronary artery disease. Excessive ethanol can depress myocardial function. Left ventricular end-diastolic pressure rises, while stroke volume and left ventricular ejection fraction falls. In addition, other hazards of alcohol should be considered such as the fact that patients may continue to exercise when they are having myocardial ischemia, if the cerebrum is dulled by alcohol and pain is not well perceived. Patients should be advised to refrain for at least 2 hours from activities that can precipitate angina after drinking, since alcohol is metabolized at a rate of about 1 oz of whiskey per hour.

Coffee consumption and its relation to coronary artery disease has been extensively studied. A prospective study in 1,130 male medical students who were followed for 1 to 35 years found the relative risk for coronary artery disease among men drinking 5 or more cups of coffee per day, as compared with nondrinkers, to be approximately 2.80.[312]

Drug Treatment

After 6 months of dietary therapy, if the response is not adequate, an antilipid drug should be considered with the diet as indicated in Table 4–23, based on LDL cholesterol. The major drugs used today are bile acid sequestrants (cholestyramine, colestipol), nicotinic acid, gemfibrozil, probucol and HMG COA reductase inhibitors (lovastatin). The drugs of first choice in patients with hypercholesterolemia without concurrent hypertriglyceridemia (triglyceride <250 mg dl) are the bile acid sequestrants and nicotinic acid. Bile acid sequestrants lower LDL cholesterol. These agents bind bile acids and interrupt the enterohepatic circulation of bile acids and in turn the hepatic synthesis of bile acids from cholesterol increase. The LDL receptor in the liver increases and so removes LDL from plasma, but the hepatic VLDL production may increase with a rise in triglycerides. Cholestyramine (Questran) and colestipol (Colestid) are powders that must be mixed with fluids (it is usually best to blend them with pineapple juice). The usual starting doses are 4 g of cholestyramine or 5 g of colestipol twice daily. These amounts can be increased, but patients often have gastrointestinal side effects (constipation, bloating, nausea, and flatulence). They can interfere with absorption of drugs such as digitoxin, warfarin, thiazides, diuretics, β-blockers, and others. Therefore these medications are best given 1 hour before or 4 hours after the bile sequestrant. They also interfere with absorption of fat-soluble vitamins and folic acid, but this is not a problem except in those with small bowel or liver disease. Nicotinic acid has been used for many years and was the only medication in the coronary drug project collaborative study that showed a reduction in recurrent myocardial infarction and longterm mortality. Nicotinic acid lowers both LDL and triglycerides and increases HDL. It is best to start with small doses (100 to 250 mg daily) after dinner to minimize side reactions, namely flushing. This is increased every 4 to 7 days with dosages between 1.5 to 3 g daily or more. Higher doses may produce liver function abnormalities, hyperuricemia, hyperglycemia, and gastrointestinal side effects. Pretreatment with aspirin can decrease the flushing, which is prostaglandin-mediated. Often tolerance develops to the flushing. Gemfibrozel (Lopid) is more effective for reducing triglycerides and may increase HDL. The usual dosage is 600 mg twice daily. It is well tolerated but can produce gastrointestinal symptoms and, rarely, hematologic and liver changes. Clofibrate (Atromid-S) is a fibric acid derivative like gemfibrozil and primarily decreases triglycerides. The usual dosage is 500 mg four times per day. It is seldom used today because of its toxic effects. Probucol (Lorelco) may inhibit the oxidation and tissue deposition of LDL and increases the rate of LDL catabolism. It may decrease HDL. The significance of this reduction is unknown. It has been shown that Probucol produces smaller active HDL particles, which may be advantageous even though the HDL level is low.[312a] Probucol is also an antioxidant agent and may exert an antiatherogenic effect by other mechanisms than its lipid effects. The usual dosage is 500 mg twice daily. It is well tolerated but may produce gastrointestinal symptoms such as flatulence, nausea, and diarrhea. It may prolong the QT interval. The newest antilipid agents available are the inhibitors of HMG COA Reductase. Such drugs increase the LDL receptor activity in the liver, increase the rate of receptor-mediated removal of LDL from the plasma, and reduce the production of LDL. Apolipoprotein B, VLDL, and triglycerides decrease with treatment and HDL increases. At present, the only drug available in this group is lovastatin (Mevacor). The starting dose is 20 mg once daily with the evening meal; this may be increased to 80 mg daily if necessary. Side effects include gastrointestinal symptoms, headaches, insomnia, skin rashes, myositis, and liver changes. The serum transaminase increases occurred in 1.9% of patients who received lovastatin for 1 year (more than three times normal levels) but fall to normal when the drug is discontinued. Therefore, it is recommended that liver function tests be performed every 4 to 6 weeks during the first 15 months of therapy and thereafter periodically. The CPK levels should also be checked. Lenticular opacities have been noted, but the causal relationship to lovastatin has not been established. However, slit lamp examination is recommended before treatment and annually thereafter. Mean reduction in LDL cholesterol of 25 to 45% has been noted with lovastatin, whereas the reduction with cholestyramine, colestipol, or nicotinic acid has been 15 to 30%. Probucol reduces LDL to about 8 to 15%, but may reduce HDL up to 25%.

If the patient does not respond to a single drug, combined therapy can be used. The combination of a bile acid sequestrant with either nicotinic acid or lovastatin is effective in lowering LDL (up to 45 to 60%) in patients without concurrent hypertriglyceridemia. Nicotinic acid or lovastatin can be used as initial drugs for patients with increased LDL and triglycerides, or a combination of lovastatin and nicotinic acid or either of these alone can be combined with a bile acid sequestrant. Gemfibrozil added to a bile acid sequestrant, lovastatin, or nicotinic acid can produce additional lowering of triglycerides.

With good compliance, maximum lowering of lipids should occur within 4 to 6 weeks, at which time a follow-up LDL cholesterol should be done and repeated in 3 months. After this, total cholesterol should be monitored every 4 months and a complete lipid profile performed yearly.

It has been known for years that elevated cholesterol levels are associated with coronary artery disease, but not until recently has it been shown that if the level is reduced, mortality and morbidity can also be reduced. Each 1% reduction in serum cholesterol levels yields approximately a 2% reduction in coronary heart disease.[312b] The lipid research clinics coronary primary prevention trial (a multicenter, randomized, double-blind study) compared cholestyramine and a placebo in a group of middle-aged men with primary hypercholesterolemia for an average of 7.4 years.[313] The cholestyramine group had a significantly greater reduction in total and LDL cholesterol, and a 19% reduction in risk of definite coronary disease death and/or definite nonfatal myocardial infarction (reflecting a 24% reduction in definite CHD death and 19% reduction in nonfatal myocardial infarction). The cholesterol-lowering atherosclerosis study (CLAS) was a randomized placebo-controlled trial involving 162 nonsmoking men aged 40 to 59 years with previous coronary bypass surgery.[314] The drug group received a combination of colestipol and niacin therapy and both groups had coronary arteriograms before and after 2 years of therapy. The drug group had a 26% reduction in total cholesterol, a 43% reduction in LDL and a 37% elevation of HDL. In addition, the treatment group had a significant reduction in the average number of lesions per subject that progressed and in the percentage of subjects with new atheroma in the native vessels. The percentage of subjects with new lesions or any adverse change in bypass grafts was also significantly reduced. In 16.2% of the treated group, there was an improvement in overall coronary status, compared to only 2.4% in the placebo-treated group. A third study (Helsinki Heart Study)[315] was also a double-blind trial in middle-aged males with primary dyslipedemia (non-HDL cholesterol ≥200 mg dl) comparing a group on gemfibrozil (600 mg twice daily) and a placebo-treated group. Gemfibrozel produced a marked increase in HDL and reduction in total cholesterol, LDL, and triglycerides. At 5 years the gemfibrozil group had a 34% reduction in the incidence of coronary heart disease, but there was no difference between the groups in the total death rate.

High density lipoprotein (HDL) can be elevated by exercise, no smoking, reducing obesity, and moderate intake of alcohol. One must be careful in advising the use of alcohol because in some this may encourage excessive intake. Nicotinic acid, gemfibrozil, cholestyramine, colestipol, and lovastatin also increase HDL. Several drugs may adversely affect lipids such as the thiazides, β-blockers, progestins, and anabolic steroids.

Hypertension

Hypertension is a treatable condition. There is a continuous increase in risk of cardiovascular complications with increasing levels of both systolic and diastolic blood pressure. Hypertension detection and follow-up study[316] have revealed that mortality and complications of hypertension can be reduced even when mild hypertension (diastolic pressures between 90 and 104 mm Hg) is treated. Chapter 5 discusses hypertension in detail.

Smoking

Epidemiologic studies indicate that the mortality and morbidity related to coronary heart disease increase proportionately with the amount of cigarettes smoked.[317] If one smokes 20 or more cigarettes per day, the risk of myocardial infarction is almost three times greater than in nonsmokers, former smokers, or pipe or cigar smokers. Also, cigarette smokers have almost a threefold greater risk for sudden death than nonsmokers.[318] A study by Auerbach et al.[319] revealed that not only are the epicardial coronary arteries more involved with atherosclerosis in heavy smokers, but in addition there is advanced hyaline thickening in the myocardial arterioles. Macroscopically, atherosclerosis occurred 4.4 times more frequently in men smoking two or more packs per day, with gradations proportional to the amount smoked. Most interesting was their finding that 90.7% of smokers of two packs or more daily showed advanced hyaline thickening of myocardial arterioles, whereas this was found in 48.4% of those smoking less than one pack per day and in none of those who never smoked regularly. Debate continues as to whether it is the inhaled nicotine or the carbon monoxide of cigarette smoking that is more responsible. Both are probably significant. Carbon monoxide can produce high levels of carboxyhemoglobin, which can lower the partial pressure of oxygen, especially in the presence of coronary disease. It also may reduce the oxygen affinity of hemoglobin and may produce intimal hypoxia and endothelial injury. Some of the acute circulatory effects (increase in heart rate, BP, and cardiac output) can be due to the absorption of nicotine with resultant mobilization of catecholamines. Nicotine may also exert a toxic effect on endothelial cells and produce a reduction in vascular endothelial prostacyclin (a potent vasodilator). In addition, one study showed that nicotine may produce platelet thrombus formation in dogs that had stenosed coronary arteries.[320] Cigarette smoking has untoward effects on plasma lipoproteins and enhances platelet aggregation. Pipe and cigar smokers apparently do not face the same risks, because they inhale less nicotine and other substances. Cigarette smokers who change to cigars or pipes and continue to inhale may have no decrease in CHD risk, however. Wald[321] reported a decrease in death from lung cancer in men who smoke filter-tipped cigarettes, but an increase in coronary disease mortality. He mentioned that the filter tips do not mix as much air with smoke, and so more carbon monoxide passes through (28% more) than in the nonfilter-tipped types. The risk of CHD has not been shown to be reduced by using cigarettes which have been shown to give lower yields of carbon monoxide, tar, and nicotine.[322] Nonsmokers may be exposed to passive smoking. Mainstream smoke is exhaled by a smoker and sidestream smoke arises from the burning end of the cigarette. Sidestream smoke contains a higher concentration of the potentially dangerous substances, carbon monoxide and nicotine.[323] Carbon monoxide and nicotine concentrations in nonsmokers in smoking environments (over 4 to 8 hours) can be equivalent to those in voluntary smokers consuming about 5 cigarettes.[324,325] Smoking cessation results in a decreased mortality from CHD. This decrease is related to the amount smoked, the duration of smoking prior to quitting, and the length of time after cessation. One year after cessation, the risk of CHD due to smoking decreased by about 50%. It may take up to 10 years or more of cessation to approach the less risk that a patient has who never smoked.

We advise patients with coronary disease to stop smoking. The emotional problems and weight gain that can result should be discussed with patients. It is better for them to stop smoking abruptly than to taper off; tapering may produce guilt feelings because they often cheat or lie. However, we as physicians should motivate our patients and be very emphatic. Often the physician is smoking while trying to advise the patient to stop. Some patients may need to attend cessation programs, which include education, behavior modification, and drug therapy.

Exercise

Epidemiologic studies also suggest that exercise aids both in preventing coronary disease and in rehabilitating patients with known coronary artery disease. However, the protective effect of exercise against coronary heart disease is circumstantial in the human. One study[326] showed that moderate exercise may prevent or retard coronary heart disease in primates receiving an atherogenic diet. The conditioned monkeys had less atherosclerosis in wider coronary arteries (shown by coronary angiography and postmortem studies). The level of exercise in the conditioned monkeys was comparable to jogging in human beings (one hour three times per week). Exercise in the human does decrease peripheral vascular resistance and BP, slows the heart rate, and thus lowers myocardial oxygen requirements for a given workload. Physical exercise can be expected to increase a patient's maximal exercise capacity after myocardial infarction, angina, or in patients recovering from coronary bypass surgery by an average of 15 to 20% over that which would occur spontaneously.[327] Patients frequently improve in psychologic well-being. Many randomized trials have shown a trend toward reduced morbidity and mortality secondary to cardiac rehabilitation compared to usual care, but sample sizes have been small. Paffenbarger found that activity in Harvard alumni that could burn 2,000 or more kilocalories a week could prolong their lives by 2½ years.[328] Short-term studies have not shown that exercise improves myocardial perfusion or performance. Exercise may modify risk factors, such as increasing HDL, lowering triglycerides and cholesterol, and lowering blood pressure. A recent study showed that fat loss through dieting or exercising produces comparable and favorable changes in plasma lipoprotein concentrations as compared with the control group.[329] The total cholesterol and LDL cholesterol did not change, but there were decreases in triglyceride levels and increases in HDL_2 and HDL_3 levels. There is evidence that the protective effect of HDL lies with the HDL_2 subclass. The ratio of HDL_2/HDL_3 is higher in sedentary women than in men and increases in runners of both sexes.[330] Another study showed that prolonged exercise training of sedentary men results in modest changes in HDL and triglycerides that are qualitatively similar to those observed in elite endurance athletes.[331] The exercise size prescription and types of exercise have been discussed earlier in this chapter in the section on cardiac rehabilitation, phase III. A careful medical assessment of all patients should be done prior to cardiac rehabilitation to exclude patients such as those with unstable angina, uncontrolled arrhythmias, symptomatic congestive heart failure and uncontrolled hypertension. Adverse events with exercise are infrequent as noted in large surveys of supervised cardiac exercise programs. Camp and Peterson[332] surveyed by questionnaire 167 randomly selected cardiac rehabilitation programs (51,303 patients) and found that cardiac arrests occurred at a rate of 8.9 per million patient-hours of exercise (1 per 111,996 patients hours), myocardial infarction occurred at a rate of 3.4 per million hours (1 per 293,990 patient-hours), and fatalities were reported at a rate of 1.3 per million hours (1 per 783,972 patient-hours).

Genetic Factors

Coronary artery disease is often noted to run in families. The risk appears to be greater for relatives of younger patients with myocardial infarction. In addition, concordance rates are higher in monozygotic than in dizygotic twins. Coronary artery disease does not often manifest a classic Mendelian pattern of inheritance. More than one type of gene may be required to manifest the disease, and environmental factors may enhance or inhibit gene expression. First-degree relatives of individuals with early onset of coronary heart disease (onset in men before age 55 and in women before age 65) have on the average six times the usual risk of being affected.[333] Occasionally a Mendelian pattern is observed such as that the most frequently implicated major gene is that for familial hypercholesterolemia (0.1 to 0.5% frequency). A case-controlled study indicated that the familial aggregation of coronary artery disease is not entirely explained by the familial clustering of known risk factors such as cholesterol, triglycerides, fasting blood sugar levels, blood pressure, and smoking history.[334]

Personality Types

Data have more firmly established emotional stress as an important risk factor in coronary heart disease.[335] Many of the patients have the type A personality characteristics, such as aggressiveness, ambitiousness, competitive drive, and accepting unreasonable deadlines for jobs. Persons with type B behavior have relative absence of these characteristics. Friedman and Rosenman, beginning in the 1950s, considered type A personality to be at higher risk for the development of coronary disease. The Western Collaborative Group

Study (WCGS) followed 3154 healthy men for 8.5 years and demonstrated that persons with type A behavior had about twice the chance of having coronary artery disease and that the risk was independent of other risk factors.[336] Several studies have found, by coronary arteriography, that type A individuals had more extensive coronary artery disease. Other studies failed to show that type A behavior related to coronary disease. Ragland, using the WCGS data base, found that subsequent coronary mortality in patients who had suffered a first coronary event was lower among type A than type B patients.[337] This, along with other studies, presents some doubt that type A behavior may be a significant risk factor.[338] Many factors need re-evaluation, such as the methods of diagnosis of type A behavior, its response to stressors, and its relationship to other factors such as hostility. Hostility appears to be a significant component of type A behavior as a predictor of coronary events.[339] It appears that personality types are a more complex situation than originally thought and more study of their various components is indicated.

Because stress does produce high levels of catecholamines, cortisol, and cholesterol and can trigger a myocardial infarction in susceptible subjects or accelerate atherosclerosis, patients with coronary disease should be counseled. Family relationships, job insecurity, and other emotional problems should be openly discussed. Actually, many patients want the physician to be firm and help them eliminate excessive and unnecessary activities and reestablish their goals. Periods of relaxation and leisurely vacations should be encouraged. Life-styles cannot be changed overnight. Counseling over several months may be necessary to help these patients develop insight into problems and ways to cope with stress and tension.

Other Factors

Associated aggravating risk factors, such as diabetes, hyperuricemia, excess weight, and use of oral contraceptives must be recognized and appropriately treated. Epidemiologic studies[340] show an increased risk of venous thromboembolic disease, myocardial infarction, and stroke for women 35 years of age or older who are taking oral contraceptives, especially if they also smoke cigarettes or have hypertension. Oral contraceptives appear to multiply the effects of age and other risk factors for myocardial infarction and stroke rather than simply adding to them. The effects of HDL are related in part to the relative proportions of estrogens and progesterone. Estrogen raises HDL and progesterone lowers it.[341] The relationship between exogenous estrogen use and cardiovascular disease is controversial. The Framingham study reported that in postmenopausal women the use of noncontraceptive estrogens increases the risk of cardiovascular disease.[342] Other studies such as that by Colditz et al. suggest that bilateral oophorectomy increases the risk of coronary artery disease in contrast to natural menopause and that this increase appears to be prevented by estrogen replacement.[343] In addition, in another study, this group found that those with natural menopause taking estrogen may have a lower risk of coronary heart disease.[344] The Lipid Research Clinics program followed a cohort of 2270 white women, aged 40 to 69 years at baseline, for an average of 8.5 years. After multivariable analysis, this study concluded that estrogen users have less cardiovascular mortality and that this protective effect of estrogen is substantially mediated through the increase of HDL levels.[345]

REFERENCES

1. Gazes P.C., Mobley E.M., Jr., Faris H.M., Jr., et al.: Preinfarctional (unstable) angina—A prospective study—Ten year follow-up. *Circulation* 48:331, 1973.
2. Sherman C.T., Litvack M.D., Grundfest W., et al.: Coronary angioscopy in patients with unstable angina pectoris. *N. Engl. J. Med.* 315:913, 1986.
3. Maseri A.: Role of coronary artery spasm in symptomatic and silent myocardial ischemia. *J. Am. Coll. Cardiol.* 9:249, 1987.
4. Cohn P.F.: Silent myocardial ischemia: Present status. *Mod. Concepts Cardiovasc. Dis.* 56:1, 1987.
5. Kubler W., Opherk D., Tillmanns H.: Syndrome X: Diagnostic criteria and long term prognosis. *Can. J. Cardiol*/Suppl. 219A, 1986.
6. Picano E., Lattanzi F., Masini M., et al.: Usefulness of high-dose dipyridamole-echocardiography test for diagnosis of syndrome X. *Am. J. Cardiol.* 60:508, 1987.
7. Cannon R.O., Leon M.B., Watson R.M., et al.: Chest pain and "normal" coronary arteries—role of small coronary arteries. *Am. J. Cardiol.* 55:50B, 1985.
8. Prinzmetal M., Kennamer R., Merliss R., et al.: Angina pectoris: I. The variant form of angina pectoris. *Am. J. Med.* 27:375, 1959.
9. Yasue H., Nagao M., Omote S., et al.: Coronary arterial spasm and Prinzmetal's variant form of angina induced by hyperventilation and tris-buffer infusion. *Circulation* 58:56, 1978.
10. Conti C.R., Pepine C.J., Curry J.C.: Coronary artery spasm: An important mechanism in the pathophysiology of ischemic heart disease. *Curr. Probl. Cardiol.* 4:1–70, 1979.
11. Fontana M.E., Wooley C.F., Leighton R.F., et al.: Postural changes in left ventricular and mitral valvular dynamics in the systolic click-late systolic murmur syndrome. *Circulation* 51:165, 1975.
12. Irvin R.G.: The antiographic prevalence of myocardial bridging in man. *Chest* 81:198, 1982.
13. Betriu A., Tubau J., Sanz G., et al.: Relief of angina by periarterial muscle resection of myocardial bridges. *Am. Heart J.* 100:223, 1980.
14. Wigle E.D.: Hypertrophic cardiomyopathy 1988. *Mod. Concepts Cardiovasc. Dis.* 57:1, 1988.
15. O'Gara P.T., Bonow R.O., Maron B.J., et al.: Myocardial perfusion abnormalities in patients with hypertrophic cardiomyopathy: Assessment with thallium-201 emission computed tomography. *Circulation* 76:1214, 1987.
16. Dunn F.G., Pringle, S.D.: Left ventricular hypertrophy and myocardial ischemia in systemic hypertension. *Am. J. Cardiol.* 60:191, 1987.
17. Heberden W.: Some account of a disorder of the heart. *Med. Trans. R. Coll. Physicians* 2:59, 1772.
18. Faerman I, Faccio E., Milei J., et al.: Autonomic neuropathy and painless myocardial infarction in diabetic patients: Histologic evidence of their relationship. *Diabetes* 26:1147, 1977.
19. Rocco M.B., Barry J., Campbell S., et al.: Circadian variation of transient myocardial ischemia in patients with coronary artery disease. *Circulation* 75:395, 1987.
20. Frank S.T.: Aural sign of coronary-artery disease. *N. Engl. J. Med.* 289:327, 1973.
21. Elliott W.J.: Ear lobe crease and coronary artery disease. *Am. J. Med.* 75:1024, 1983.
22. Brady P.M., Zive M.A., Goldberg R.J., et al.: A new wrinkle to the earlobe crease. *Arch. Intern. Med.* 147:65, 1987.
23. Levine S.A.: Carotid sinus massage: The new diagnostic test for angina pectoris. *JAMA* 182:1332, 1962.
24. Sheffield T., Roitman D., Reeves T.J.: Submaximal exercise testing. *J. S.C. Med. Assoc.* 65:18, 1969.
25. Doan A.E., Peterson D.R., Blackmon J.R., Bruce R.A.: Myocardial ischemia after maximal exercise in healthy men. *Am. Heart J.* 69:11, 1965.
26. Gazes P.C., Culler M.R., Stokes J.K.: The diagnosis of angina pectoris. *Am. Heart J.* 67:830, 1964.
27. Goldschlager N., Seltzer A., Cohn K.: Treadmill stress tests as indicators of presence and severity of coronary artery disease. *Ann. Intern. Med.* 85:277, 1976.
28. Weiner D.A., McCabe C.H., Ryan T.J.: Identification of patients with left main and three vessel coronary disease with clinical and exercise test variables. *Am. J. Cardiol.* 46:21, 1980.
29. Kligfield P., Okin P.M., Ameisen O., et al.: Correlation of the exercise ST/HR slope in stable angina pectoris with anatomic and radionuclide cineangiographic findings. *Am. J. Cardiol.* 56:418, 1985.
30. Detrano R., Salcedo E., Passalacqua M., et al.: Exercise electrocardiographic variables: A critical appraisal. *J. Am. Coll. Cardiol.* 8:836, 1986.

31. Gerson M.C., Phillips J.F., Morris S.N., et al.: Exercise induced U-wave inversion as a marker of stenosis of the left anterior descending coronary artery. *Circulation* 60:1014, 1977.
32. Bonoris P.E., Greenberg P.S., Christison G.W., et al.: Evaluation of R wave amplitude changes versus ST segment depression in stress testing. *Circulation* 57:904, 1978.
33. Battler A., Froelicher V., Slutsky R., et al.: Relationship of QRS amplitude changes during exercise to left ventricular function and volumes and the diagnosis of coronary artery disease. *Circulation* 60:1004, 1979.
34. Morales-Ballejo H., Greenberg P.J., Ellestad M.H., et al.: Septal Q wave in exercise testing: Angiographic correlation. *Am. J. Cardiol.* 48:247, 1981.
35. Furuse T., Mashiba H., Jordan J.W., et al.: Usefulness of Q-wave response to exercise as a predictor of coronary artery disease. *Am. J. Cardiol.* 57:57, 1986.
36. Chaitman B.R.: The changing role of the exercise electrocardiogram as a diagnostic and prognostic test for chronic ischemic heart disease. *J. Am. Coll. Cardiol.* 8:1195, 1986.
37. Goldschlager N., Cohn K., Goldschlager A.: Exercise-related ventricular arrhythmias. *Mod. Concepts Cardiovasc. Dis.* 48:67, 1979.
38. Kurita A., Chaitman B.R., Bourassa M.G.: Significance of exercise-induced junctional S-T depression in evaluation of coronary artery disease. *Am. J. Cardiol.* 40:492, 1977.
39. Rijneke R.D., Ascoop C.A., Talmon J.L.: Clinical significance of upsloping ST segments in exercise electrocardiography. *Circulation* 6:671, 1980.
40. Gazes P.C.: False-positive exercise test in the presence of the Wolff-Parkinson-White syndrome. *Am. Heart J.* 78:13, 1969.
41. Whinnery J.E., Froelicher V.F., Jr., Stewart A.J.: The electrocardiographic response to maximal treadmill exercise of asymptomatic men with left bundle branch block. *Am. Heart J.* 94:316, 1977.
42. Tanaka T., Friedman M.J., Okada R.D., et al.: Diagnostic value of exercise-induced S-T segment depression in patients with right bundle branch block. *Am. J. Cardiol.* 41:670, 1978.
43. Weiner D.A., Ryan T.J., McCabe C.H., et al.: Exercise stress testing: Correlations among history of angina, ST-segment response and prevalence of coronary-artery disease in the coronary artery surgery study (CASS). *N. Engl. J. Med.* 301:230, 1979.
44. Rifkin R.D., Hood W.B., Jr.: Bayesian analysis of electrocardiographic exercise stress testing. *N. Engl. J. Med.* 297:681, 1977.
45. Friesinger G.C., Page E.E., Ross R.S.: Prognostic significance of coronary arteriography. *Trans. Assoc. Am. Phys.* 83:78, 1970.
46. Sanmarco M.E., Pontius S., Selvester R.H.: Abnormal blood pressure response and marked ischemic ST-segment depression as predictors of severe coronary artery disease. *Circulation* 61:572, 1980.
47. Sheps D.S., Ernst J.C., Briese F.W., et al.: Exercise-induced increase in diastolic pressure: Indicators of severe coronary artery disease. *Am. J. Cardiol.* 43:708, 1979.
48. Beller G.: Nuclear cardiology: Current indications and clinical usefulness. *Curr. Probl. Cardiol.* 10:4, 1985.
49. Iskandrian A.S., Heo J., Askenase A., et al.: Thallium imaging with single photon emission computed tomography. *Am. Heart J.* 114:852, 1987.
50. Proudfit W.L., Shirey E.K., Sones F.M., Jr.: Selective cine coronary arteriography: correlation with clinical findings in 1,000 patients. *Circulation* 33:901, 1966.
51. Henderson R.D., Wigle E.D., Sample K., et al.: Atypical chest pain of cardiac and esophageal origin. *Chest* 73:24, 1978.
52. Chobanian S.J., Benjamin S.B., Curtis D.J., Cattau E.L.: Systematic esophageal evaluation of patients with noncardiac chest pain. *Arch. Intern Med.* 146:1505, 1986.
53. Murad F.: Cyclic guanosine monophosphate as a mediator of vasodilation. *J. Clin. Invest.* 78:1, 1986.
54. Markis J.E., Gorlin R., Mills R.M., et al.: Sustained effect of orally administered isosorbide dinitrate on exercise performance of patients with angina pectoris. *Am. J. Cardiol.* 43:265, 1979.
55. Thadani U., Whitsett T., Hamilton S.F.: Nitrate therapy for myocardial ischemic syndrome: Current perspectives including tolerance. *Curr. Probl. Cardiol.* 13:731, 1988.
55a. Background Information on Nitrate Therapy and the Cooperative Study. Distributed by Ciba, Division of Ciba-Geigy Corporation, Summit, New Jersey.
55b. Demots H. and Glasser S.P.: Intermittent transdermal nitroglycerin therapy in the treatment of chronic stable angina. *JACC* 13:786, 1989.
56. Parker J.O.: Nitrate Therapy in Stable Angina Pectoris. *N. Engl. J. Med.* 316:1635, 1987.
57. Luke R., Sharpe N., Coxon R.: Transdermal nitroglycerin in angina pectoris: Efficacy of intermittent application. *JACC* 10:642, 1987.
58. Frishman W.H.: B-adrenoceptor antagonists. New drugs and new indications. *N. Engl. J. Med.* 305:500, 1981.
59. Brown M.J., Brown D.C., Murphy M.B.: Hypokalemia from $beta_2$-receptor stimulation by circulatory epinephrine. *N. Engl. J. Med.* 309:1414, 1983.

60. Vincent H.H., Boomsma F., Veld A.J., et al.: Effects of selective and nonselective B-agonists on plasma potassium and norepinephrine. *J. Cardiovasc. Pharmacol.* 6:107, 1984.

61. Cruickshank J.M.: The clinical importance of cardioselectivity and lipophilicity in beta blockers. *Am. Heart J.* 100:160, 1980.

62. Goldman L.: Noncardiac surgery in patients receiving propranolol. *Arch. Intern. Med.* 141:193, 1981.

63. Samuel P., Chin B., Fenderson R.W., et al.: Improvement of the lipid profile during long-term administration of pindolol and hydrochlorothiazide in patients with hypertension. *Am. J. Cardiol.* 57:24C, 1986.

64. Crawford M.H.: The role of triple therapy in patients with chronic stable angina pectoris. *Circulation* 75:V-122, 1987.

65. Rocco M.B., Barry J., Campbell S., et al.: Circadian variation of transient myocardial ischemia in patients with coronary artery disease. *Circulation* 75:395, 1987.

66. Muller J.E., Stone P.H., Turi Z.G., et al.: Circadian variation in the frequency of onset of acute myocardial infarction. *N. Engl. J. Med.* 313:1315, 1985.

67. Muller J.E., Ludmer P.L., Willich S.N., et al.: Circadian variation in the frequency of sudden cardiac death. *Circulation* 75:131, 1987.

68. Lewis H.D., Davis J.W., Archibald D.G., et al.: Protective effects of aspirin against acute myocardial infarction and death in men with unstable angina. *N. Engl. J. Med.* 309:396, 1983.

69. Cairns J.A., Gent M., Singer J., et al.: Aspirin, sulfinpyrazone, or both in unstable angina. Result of a Canadian multicenter trial. *N. Engl. J. Med.* 313:1369, 1985.

70. Theroux P., Ouimet H., McCans J., et al.: Aspirin, heparin, or both to treat acute unstable angina. *N. Engl. J. Med.* 319:1105, 1988.

71. Gold H.K., Johns J.A., Leinbach R.C., et al: Thrombolytic therapy for unstable angina pectoris: Rationale and results. *JACC* 10:91B, 1987.

72. Brown B.G.: Coronary vasospasm: Observations linking the clinical spectrum of ischemic heart disease to the dynamic pathology of coronary atherosclerosis. *Arch. Intern. Med.* 141:716, 1981.

73. Maseri A., Severi S., DeNes M., et al.: Variant angina: One aspect of a continuous spectrum of vasospastic myocardial ischemia: Pathogenic mechanisms, estimated incidence and clinical and coronary arteriographic findings in 138 patients. *Am. J. Cardiol.* 42:1019, 1978.

74. Murphy E.S., Rosch J., Boicourt O.W., et al.: Left main coronary artery spasm: A potential cause for angiographic misdiagnosis of severe coronary artery disease. *Arch. Intern. Med.* 136:350, 1976.

75. Theroux P., Waters D.D., Affaki G.S., et al.: Provocative testing with ergonovine to evaluate the efficacy of treatment with calcium antagonists in variant angina. *Circulation* 60:504, 1979.

76. Dotter C.T., Judkins M.P.: Transluminal treatment of arteriosclerotic obstruction: Description of a new technique and a preliminary result of its application. *Circulation* 30:654, 1964.

77. Grüntzig A.R., Myler R., Stertzer S., et al.: Coronary percutaneous transluminal angioplasty: preliminary results. *Circulation* 58(Suppl.):56, 1978.

78. Grüntzig A.R., Senning A., Seigenthaler W.E.: Nonoperative dilatation of coronary-artery stenosis: Percutaneous transluminal coronary angioplasty. *N. Engl. J. Med.* 301:61, 1979.

78a. Manyari D.E., Knudtson M., Kloiber R.: Sequential thallium-201 myocardial perfusion studies after successful percutaneous transluminal coronary artery angioplasty: delayed resolution of exercise-induced scintigraphic abnormalities. *Circulation* 77:86, 1988.

79. Dehmer G.J., Popma J.J., van den Berg, E.K., et al.: Reduction in the rate of early restenosis after coronary angioplasty by a diet supplemented with n-3 fatty acids. *N. Engl. J. Med.* 319:733, 1988.

80. Schwartz L., Bourassa M.G., Lesperance J., et al.: Aspirin and dipyridamole in the prevention of restenosis after percutaneous transluminal coronary angioplasty. *N. Engl. J. Med.* 318:1714, 1988.

81. Roubin G.S., Robinson K.A., King S.B., et al.: Early and late results of intracoronary arterial stenting after coronary angioplasty in dogs. *Circulation* 76:891, 1987.

82. Detre K., Holubkov R., Kelsey S., et al.: Percutaneous transluminal coronary angioplasty in 1985–1986 and 1977–1981. *N. Engl. J. Med.* 318:265, 1988.

83. Gruentzig A.R., King S.B., Schlumph M., et al.: Long-term follow-up after percutaneous transluminal coronary angioplasty. The Early Zurich Experience. *N. Engl. J. Med.* 316:1127, 1987.

84. Abela G.S.: Laser Recanalization: Preliminary clinical experience. *Cardiovas Dis Chest Pain* 3:3, 1987.

85. Mock M.B., Ringqvist I., Fisher L.D., et al.: Survival of medically treated patients in the coronary artery surgery study (CASS) registry. *Circulation* 66:562, 1982.

86. VA Cooperative Study Group: Eleven-year survival in the veterans administration randomized trial of coronary bypass surgery for stable angina. *N. Engl. J. Med.* 311:1333, 1984.
87. European Coronary Surgery Study Group: Prospective randomized study of coronary artery bypass surgery in stable angina pectoris. *Lancet* 2:491, 1980.
88. Varnauskas E. European Coronary Surgery Study Group: Survival, myocardial infarction and employment status in a prospective randomized study of coronary bypass surgery. *Circulation* 72:V-90, 1985.
89. Kumpuris A.G., Quinones M.A., Kanon D., et al.: Isolated stenosis of left anterior descending or right coronary artery: Relation between site of stenosis and ventricular dysfunction and therapeutic implications. *Am. J. Cardiol.* 46:13, 1980.
90. Spray T.L., Roberts W.C.: Changes in saphenous veins used as aortocoronary bypass grafts. *Am. Heart J.* 94:500, 1977.
91. Campeau S.L., Nielsen S.L., Amtorp O., et al.: The relation of risk factors to the development of atherosclerosis in saphenous-vein bypass grafts and the progression of disease in the native circulation. A study ten years after aortocoronary bypass surgery. *N. Engl. J. Med.* 311:1329, 1984.
92. Fuster V., Chesebro J.H.: Role of platelets and platelet inhibitors in aortocoronary artery vein-graft disease. *Circulation* 73:227, 1986.
93. Lytle B.W., Loop F.D., Cosgrove D.M., et al.: Long-term (5 to 12 years) serial studies of internal mammary artery and saphenous vein coronary bypass grafts. *J. Thorac. Cardiovasc. Surg.* 89:248, 1985.
94. Loop F.D., Lytle B.W., Cosgrove D.M., et al.: Influence of the internal-mammary-artery graft on 10-year survival and other cardiac events. *N. Engl. J. Med.* 314:1, 1986.
95. Chesebro J.H., Fuster V., Elveback L.R., et al.: Effect of dipyridamole and aspirin on late vein-graft patency after coronary bypass operations. *N. Engl. J. Med.* 310:209, 1984.
96. Reed G.L., Singer D.E., Picard E.H., et al.: Stroke following coronary-artery bypass surgery: A case-control estimate of the risk from carotid bruits. *N. Engl. J. Med.* 319:1246, 1988.
97. Chambers B.R., Norris J.W.: Outcome in patients with asymptomatic neck bruits. *N. Engl. J. Med.* 315:860, 1986.
98. Meissner I., Wiebers D.O., Whisnant J.P., et al.: The natural history of asymptomatic carotid artery occlusive lesions. *JAMA* 258:2704, 1987.
99. Graor R.A. Hetzer N.R.: Management of coexistent carotid artery and coronary artery disease. *Current Concepts of Cerebrovasc. Dis. and Stroke* 23:19, 1988.
100. Cohn P.F.: Silent myocardial ischemia: Present status. *Mod. Conc. Cardiovas. Dis.* 56:1, 1987.
101. Erikssen J., Thaulow E.: Follow-up of patients with asymptomatic myocardial ischemia, in Rutishauser W., Roskamm H. (eds): *Silent Myocardial Ischemia*. Berlin, Springer-Verlag, 1984, pp 156–164.
102. Theroux P., Waters D.D., Halphen C., et al.: Prognostic value of exercise testing soon after myocardial infarction. *N. Engl. J. Med.* 301:341, 1979.
103. Gottlieb S.O., Gottlieb S.H., Achuff S.C., et al.: Silent ischemia on holter monitoring predicts mortality in high-risk postinfarction patients. *JAMA* 259:1028, 1988.
104. Selwyn A.P., Shea M., Deanfield J.E., et al.: Character of transient ischemia in angina pectoris. *Am. J. Cardiol.* 58:21B, 1986.
105. Weidinger F., Hammerle A., Sochor H., et al.: Role of beta-endorphins in silent myocardial ischemia. *Am. J. Cardiol.* 58:428, 1986.
106. Gottlieb S.O., Weisfeldt M.L., Ouyang P., et al.: Silent ischemia as a marker for early unfavorable outcomes in patients with unstable angina. *N. Engl. J. Med.* 314:1214, 1986.
107. Assey M.E., Walters G.L., Hendrix G.H., et al.: Incidence of acute myocardial infarction in patients with exercise-induced silent myocardial ischemia. *Am. J. Cardiol.* 59:497, 1987.
108. Rozanski A., Bairey C.N., Krantz D.S., et al.: Mental stress and the induction of silent myocardial ischemia in patients with coronary artery disease. *N. Engl. J. Med.* 318:1005, 1988.
109. DeWood M.A., Spores J., Notske R., et al.: Prevalence of total coronary occlusion during the early hours of transmural myocardial infarction. *N. Engl. J. Med.* 303:898, 1980.
110. American Heart Association: Fact sheet on heart attack, stroke and risk factors. 1986.
111. Feinleib M., Davidson M.J.: Coronary heart disease mortality: A community perspective. JAMA 222:1129, 1972.
112. Liberthson R.R., Nagel E.L., Hirschman J.C., et al.: Pathophysiologic observations in prehospital ventricular fibrillation and sudden cardiac death. *Circulation* 49:790, 1974.
113. Moss A.J., Goldstein S.: The prehospital phase of acute myocardial infarction. *Circulation* 41:737, 1970.
114. Gillum R.F., Feinleib M., Margolis J.R., et al.: Delay in the prehospital phase of acute myocardial infarction. *Arch. Intern. Med.* 136:649, 1976.

115. Goldstein S., Moss A.J., Greene W.: Sudden death in acute myocardial infarction. *Arch. Intern Med.* 129:720, 1972.
116. Solomon H.A., Edwards A.L., Killip T.: Prodromata in acute myocardial infarction. *Circulation* 45:463, 1969.
117. Medalie J.H., Goldbourt U.: Unrecognized myocardial infarction: Five-year incidence, mortality and risk factors. *Ann. Intern. Med.* 84:526, 1976.
118. Margolis J.R., Kannel W.B., Feinleib M., et al.: Clinical features of unrecognized myocardial infarction: 18 year follow-up, The Framingham Study. *Am. J. Cardiol.* 32:1, 1973.
119. Cintron G.B., Hernandez E., Linares E., et al.: Bedside recognition, incidence and clinical course of right ventricular infarction. *Am. J. Cardiol.* 47:224, 1981.
120. Coodley E.L.: Prognostic value of enzymes in myocardial infarction. *JAMA* 225:597, 1973.
121. Yusuf S., Collins R., Lin L., et al.: Significance of elevated MB isoenzyme with normal creatine kinase in acute myocardial infarction. *Am. J. Cardiol.* 59:245, 1987.
122. Sharkey S.W., Apple F.S., Elsperger J., et al.: Early peak of creatine kinase-MB in acute myocardial infarction with a nondiagnostic electrocardiogram. *Am. Heart J.* 116:1207, 1988.
123. Irvin R.G., Cobb F.E., Roe C.R.: Acute myocardial infarction and MB creatine phosphokinase: Relationship between onset of symptoms of infarction and appearance and disappearance of enzyme. *Arch. Intern. Med.* 140:329, 1980.
124. Navin T.R., Hager D.W.: Creatine kinase MB isoenzyme in the evaluation of myocardial infarction. *Curr. Probl. Cardiol.* 3:7–32, 1979.
125. Becker R.C., Alpert J.S.: Electrocardiographic ST segment depression in coronary heart disease. *Am. Heart J.* 115:862, 1988.
126. Reid D.S., Pelides L.J., Shillingford J.P.: Surface mapping of RS-T segment in acute myocardial infarction. *Br. Heart J.* 33:370, 1971.
127. Dymond D.S., Jarritt P.N., Britton K.E., et al.: Positive myocardial scintigraphy at the bedside: Evaluation using a portable gamma camera. *Postgrad. Med. J.* 54:641, 1978.
128. Walsh W., Lessem J., Fill H., et al.: Value of ^{99m}Tc-pyrophosphate myocardial scintigraphy in patients with suspected myocardial infarction. *Am. J. Cardiol.* 37:180, 1976.
129. Pugh B.R., Buja L.M., Parkey R.W., et al.: Cardioversion and "false positive" technetium-99m stannous pyrophosphate myocardial scintigrams. *Circulation* 54:399, 1976.
130. Saranchak H.J., Bernstein S.H.: A new diagnostic test for acute myocardial infarction: The detection of myoglobinuria by radioimmunodiffusion assay. *JAMA* 228:1251, 1974.
131. Kagen L., Scheidt S., Butt A.: Serum myoglobin in myocardial infarction: The "Staccato phenomenon." Is acute myocardial infarction in man an intermittent event? *Am. J. Med.* 62:86, 1977.
132. Grace W.J.: The mobile coronary care unit and the intermediate coronary care unit in the total systems approach to coronary care. *Chest* 58:363, 1970.
133. Pantridge J.F., Webb S.W., Adgey A.A.J., et al.: The first hour after the onset of acute myocardial infarction, in Yu P.N., Goodwin J.F. (eds.): *Progress in Cardiology.* Philadelphia, Lea & Febiger, 1974, vol 3, p 173.
134. Lee G., DeMaria A.N., Amsterdam E.N.: Comparative effects of morphine, meperidine and pentazocine on circulatory dynamics in patients with acute myocardial infarction. *Am. J. Cardiol.* 60:949, 1976.
135. Filmore S.J., Shapiro M., Killip T.: Arterial oxygen tension in acute myocardial infarction. Serial analysis of clinical state and blood gas changes. *Am. Heart J.* 76:620, 1970.
136. Madias J.E., Madias N.E., Hood W.B., Jr.: Precordial ST-segment mapping: 2. Effects of oxygen inhalation on ischemic injury in patients with acute myocardial infarction. *Circulation* 53:411, 1976.
137. Yusuf S., Wittes J., Friedman L.: Overview of results of randomized clinical trials in heart disease. I. Treatments following myocardial infarction. *JAMA* 260:2088, 1988.
138. McAllister R.G.: Kinetics and dynamics of nifedipine after oral and sublingual doses. *Am. J. Med.* 81:2, 1986.
139. Gibson R.S., Boden W.E., Theroux P., et al.: Diltiazem and reinfarction in patients with non-Q-wave myocardial infarction. Results of a double-blind, randomized multicenter trial. *N. Engl. J. Med.* 315:423, 1986.
140. The Multicenter Diltiazem Postinfarction Trial Research Group: The effect of diltiazem on mortality and reinfarction after myocardial infarction. *N. Engl. J. Med.* 319:385, 1988.
141. Frishman W.H., Furberg C.D., Friedewald W.T.: The use of β-adrenergic blocking drugs in patients with myocardial infarction. *Curr. Probl. Cardiol.* 9:1, 1984.
142. The International Collaborative Study Group: Reduction of infarct size with the early use of timolol in acute myocardial infarction. *N. Engl. J. Med.* 310:9, 1984.
143. The MIAMI Trial Research Group: Metoprolol in acute myocardial infarction (MIAMI): A randomized placebo-controlled international trial. *Eur. Heart J.* 6:199, 1985.
144. ISIS-1 Collaborative Group: A randomized trial of intravenous atenolol among 16,027 cases of suspected acute myocardial infarction. *Lancet* 2:57, 1986.

145. Roberts R., Croft C., Gold H.K., et al.: Effect of propranolol on myocardial-infarct size in a randomized blinded multicenter trial. *N. Engl. J. Med.* 311:218, 1984.
146. Hearse D.J., Yellon D.M., Downey J.M.: Can beta blockers limit myocardial infarct size? *Eur. Heart J.* 7:925, 1986.
147. Croft C.H., Rude R.E., Gustafson N., et al.: Abrupt withdrawal of β-blockade therapy in patients with myocardial infarction: Effects on infarct size, left ventricular function, and hospital course. *Circulation* 73:1281, 1986.
148. McMahon S., Yusuf S.: Effects of lidocaine on ventricular fibrillation, asystole, and early death in patients with suspected acute myocardial infarction. In Califf R.M., Wagner G.S. (eds.) *Acute Coronary Care,* Boston, Martinus Nijhoff Publishing, 1987, pp. 51–60.
149. Volpi A., Maggioni A., Franzosi M.G., et al.: In-hospital prognosis of patients with acute myocardial infarction complicated by primary ventricular fibrillation. *N. Engl. J. Med.* 317:257, 1987.
150. Wyman M.G., Slaughter R.L., Farolino D.A., et al.: Multiple bolus technique for lidocaine administration in acute ischemic heart disease. II. Treatment of refractory ventricular arrhythmias and the pharmacokinetic significance of severe left ventricular failure. *J. Am. Coll. Cardiol.* 2:764, 1983.
151. Woosley R.L.: Lidocaine Therapy: Application of clinical pharmacokinetic principles. *Cardiac Impulse* 8:1, 1987.
152. DeWood M.A., Spores J., Notske R., et al.: Prevalence of total coronary occlusion during the early hours of transmural myocardial infarction. *N. Engl. J. Med.* 303:897, 1980.
153. Braunwald E.: Symposium on modern thrombolytic therapy. *JACC* 10:1B, 1987.
154. Sherry S.: Recombinant tissue plasminogen activator (rt-PA): Is it the thrombolytic agent of choice for an evolving acute myocardial infarction? *Am. J. Cardiol.* 59:984, 1987.
155. Lew A.S., Laramee P., Cercek B., et al.: The hypotension effect of intravenous streptokinase in patients with acute myocardial infarction. *Circulation* 72:1321, 1985.
156. Habbab M.A., Haft J.I.: Heparin resistance induced by intravenous nitroglycerin. A word of caution when both drugs are used concomitantly. *Arch. Intern Med.* 147:857, 1987.
157. Chesebro J.H., Knatterud G., Roberts R., et al.: Thrombolysis in myocardial infarction (TIMI) trial, phase I: A comparison between intravenous tissue plasminogen activator and intravenous streptokinase. Clinical findings through hospital discharge. *Circulation* 76:142, 1987.
158. Mueller H.S., Rao A.K., Forman S.A., et al.: Thrombolysis in myocardial infarction (TIMI): Comparative studies of coronary reperfusion and systemic fibrinogenolysis with two forms of recombinant tissue-type plasminogen activator. *J. Am. Coll. Cardiol.* 10:479, 1987.
159. TIMI Operations Committee—Braunwald E., Knatterud G.L., Passamani E., Robertson T.L., Solomon R., Maryland Medical Research Institute: Update from the thrombolysis in myocardial infarction trial. *JACC* 10:970, 1987.
160. Loscalzo J., Braunwald E.: Tissue plasminogen activator. *N. Engl. J. Med.* 319:925, 1988.
161. Gruppo Italiano per lo Studio della Streptochinasi nell'Infarto Miocardico (GISSI). Effectiveness of intravenous thrombolytic treatment in acute myocardial infarction. *Lancet* 1:397, 1986.
162. ISIS-2 Collaborative Group. Randomized trial of intravenous streptokinase, oral aspirin, both, or neither among 17187 cases of suspected acute myocardial infarction: ISIS-2. *Lancet* 2:349, 1988.
163. Wilcox R.G., von der Lippe G., Olsson C.G., et al.: Trial of tissue plasminogen activator for mortality reduction in acute myocardial infarction. Anglo-Scandinavian Study of Early Thrombolysis (ASSET). *Lancet* 2:525, 1988.
164. Laffel G.L., Fineberg H.V., Braunwald E.: A cost-effectiveness model for coronary thrombolysis/reperfusion therapy. *JACC* 10:79B, 1987.
165. Cheitlin M.D.: The aggressive war on acute myocardial infarction: Is the blitzkrieg strategy changing? *JAMA* 260:2894, 1988.
166. Fine D.G., Weiss A.T., Sapoznikov D., et al.: Importance of early initiation of intravenous streptokinase therapy for acute myocardial infarction. *Am. J. Cardiol.* 58:411, 1986.
167. Topol E.J., Bates E.R., Walton J.A., et al.: Community hospital administration of intravenous tissue plasminogen activator in acute myocardial infarction: Improved timing, thrombolytic efficacy and ventricular function. *JACC* 10:1173, 1987.
168. White H.D., Norris R.M., Brown M.A., et al.: Effect of intravenous streptokinase on left ventricular function and early survival after acute myocardial infarction. *N. Engl. J. Med.* 317:850, 1987.
169. Bassand J.P., Faivre R., Becque O., et al.: Effects of early high-dose streptokinase intravenously on left ventricular function in acute myocardial infarction. *Am. J. Cardiol.* 60:435, 1987.
170. Neuhaus K.L., Tebbe U., Gottwik M., et al.: Intravenous recombinant tissue plasminogen activator (rt-PA) and urokinase in acute myocardial infarction: Results of the German activator urokinase study (GAUS). *JACC* 12:581, 1988.

171. Bates E.R.: Acute thrombolysis for inferior infarction? *Cardiol.* (November):57, 1988.
172. Bates E.R.: Reperfusion therapy in inferior myocardial infarction. *J. Am. Coll. Cardiol.* 12:44A, 1988.
173. Timmis A.D., Griffin B., Crick J.C., et al.: Anisoylated plasminogen streptokinase activator complex in acute myocardial infarction: A placebo-controlled arteriographic coronary recanalization study. *J. Am. Coll. Cardiol.* 10:205, 1987.
174. Anderson J.L., Rothbard R.L., Hackworthy R.A., et al.: Multicenter reperfusion trial of intravenous anisoylated plasminogen streptokinase activator complex (APSAC) in acute myocardial infarction: Controlled comparison with intracoronary streptokinase. *J. Am. Coll. Cardiol.* 11:1153, 1988.
175. ISIS-2 (Second International Study of Infarct Survival) Collaborative Group: Randomized trial of intravenous streptokinase, oral aspirin, both, or neither among 17,187 cases of suscepted acute myocardial infarction: ISIS-2. *J. Am. Coll. Cardiol.* 12:3A, 1988.
176. Topol E.J., George B.S., Kereiakes D.J., et al.: A multicenter randomized, controlled trial of intravenous tissue plasminogen activator and early intravenous heparin in acute myocardial infarction (abstr). *J. Am. Coll. Cardiol.* 11:232A, 1988.
177. Hackett D., Davies G., Chierchia S. et al.: Intermittent coronary occlusion in acute myocardial infarction. Value of combined thrombolytic and vasodilator therapy. *N. Engl. J. Med.* 317:1055, 1987.
178. Maza S.R., Fishman W.H.: Therapeutic options to minimize free radical damage and thrombogenicity in ischemic/reperfused myocardium. *Am. Heart J.* 114:1206, 1987.
179. Patel B., Zhu W.Z., O'Neill P.G., et al.: The iron chelator desferrioxamine attenuates post ischemic myocardial dysfunction (suppl). *Circulation* 76:IV-229, 1987.
180. Topol E.J., Califf R.M., George B.S., et al.: Coronary arterial thrombolysis with combined infusion of recombinant tissue-type plasminogen activator and urokinase in patients with acute myocardial infarction. *Circulation* 77:1100, 1988.
181. Schaer D.H., Ross A.M., Wasserman A.G.: Reinfarction, recurrent angina, and reocclusion after thrombolytic therapy. *Circulation* 76 (Suppl) 2:57, 1987.
182. Kircher B.J., Topol E.J., O'Neill W.W., et al.: Prediction of infarct coronary artery recanalization after intravenous thrombolytic therapy. *Am. J. Cardiol.* 59:513, 1987.
183. Topol E.J., Califf R.M., George B.S., et al.: A randomized trial of immediate versus delayed elective angioplasty after intravenous tissue plasminogen activator in acute myocardial infarction. *N. Engl. J. Med.* 317:581, 1987.
184. Simoons M.L., Betriu A., Col J., et al.: Thrombolysis with tissue plasminogen activator in acute myocardial infarction: No additional benefit from immediate percutaneous coronary angioplasty. *Lancet* (January), 1988.
185. The TIMI Research Group: Immediate vs delayed catheterization and angioplasty following thrombolytic therapy for acute myocardial infarction. *JAMA* 260:2849, 1988.
186. Guerci A.D., Gerstenblith G., Brinker J.A., et al.: A randomized trial of intravenous tissue plasminogen activator for acute myocardial infarction with subsequent randomization to elective coronary angioplasty. *N. Engl. J. Med.* 317:1613, 1987.
187. The TIMI-IIB trial report at the American Heart Association meeting, November 1988.
187a. The TIMI Study Group: Comparison of Invasive and Conservative Strategies after Treatment with Intravenous Tissue Plasminogen Activator in Acute Myocardial Infarction. Results of the Thrombolysis in Myocardial Infarction (TIMI) Phase II Trial. *N. Engl. J. Med.* 320:618, 1989.
188. Nakagawa A., Hanada Y., Koiwaya Y., et al.: Angiographic features in the infarct-related artery after intracoronary urokinase followed by prolonged anticoagulation. Role of ruptured atheromatous plaque and adherent thrombus in acute myocardial infarction in vivo. *Circulation* 78:1335, 1988.
189. Penny W.J., Chesebro J.H., Heras M., et al.: Antithrombotic therapy for patients with cardiac disease. *Curr. Probl. Cardiol.* 13:433, 1988.
190. Ezekowitz M.D.: Acute infarction, left ventricular thrombus and systemic embolization: An approach to management. (Editorial) *J. Am. Coll. Cardiol.* 5:1281, 1985.
191. Fuster V., Cohen M., Chesebro J.H.: Antithrombotic therapy in cardiac disease: Approach for the selection of agents. *Learning Center Highlights* 3:1, 1988.
192. Asinger R.W., Mikell F.L., Elsperger J., et al.: Incidence of left-ventricular thrombosis after acute transmural myocardial infarction. Serial evaluation by two-dimensional echocardiography. *N. Engl. J. Med.* 305:297, 1981.
193. Nordrehaug J.E., Johannessen K.A., von der Lippe G.: Usefulness of high-dose anticoagulants in preventing left ventricular thrombus in acute myocardial infarction. *Am. J. Cardiol.* 55:1491, 1985.
194. Visser C.A., Kan G., Meltzer R.S., et al.: Embolic potential of left ventricular thrombus after myocardial infarction: A two-dimensional echocardiographic study of 119 patients. *JACC* 5:1276, 1985.

194a. Turpie A.G.G., Robinson J.G., Doyle D.J., et al.: Comparison of high-dose with low-dose subcutaneous heparin to prevent left ventricular mural thrombosis in patients with acute transmural anterior myocardial infarction. *N. Engl. J. Med.* 320:352, 1989.

195. Levine S.A., Lown B.: Armchair treatment of acute coronary thrombosis. *JAMA* 148:1365, 1952.

196. McNeer J.F., Wagner G.S., Ginsburg P.B., et al.: Hospital discharge one week after acute myocardial infarction. *N. Engl. J. Med.* 298:229, 1978.

197. Fyfe T., Baxter R.A., Cochran K.M., et al.: Plasma lipid changes after myocardial infarction. *Lancet* 2:997, 1971.

198. Cohen I.M., Alpert J.S., Francis G.S., et al.: Safety of hot and cold liquids in patients with acute myocardial infarction. *Chest* 71:450, 1977.

199. Gazes P.C.: Treatment of acute myocardial infarction: I. General management. *Postgrad. Med.* 47:143, 1970.

200. Meltzer L.E., Cohen H.E.: The incidence of arrhythmias associated with acute myocardial infarction, in Meltzer L.E., Dunning A.J. (eds.): *Textbook of Coronary Care*. Philadelphia, Charles Press, 1972.

201. Koch-Weser J., Klein S.W., Foo-Canton, et al.: Antiarrhythmic prophylaxis with procainamide in acute myocardial infarction. *N. Engl. J. Med.* 281:1253, 1969.

202. Bloomfield S.S., Romhilt D.W., Chou T., et al.: Quinidine for prophylaxis of arrhythmias in acute myocardial infarction. *N. Engl. J. Med.* 285:979, 1971.

203. Zainal N., Carmichael D.J.S., Griffiths J.W., et al.: Oral disopyramide for the prevention of arrhythmias in patients with acute myocardial infarction admitted to open wards. *Lancet* 2:887, 1977.

204. Pitt A., Lipp H., Anderson S.T.: Lignocaine given prophylactically to patients with acute myocardial infarction. *Lancet* 1:612, 1971.

205. Wyman M.C., Hammersmith L.: Comprehensive treatment plan for the prevention of primary ventricular fibrillation in acute myocardial infarction. *Am. J. Cardiol.* 33:661, 1974.

206. Lie K.I., Wellens H.J., vanCapelle F.J., et al.: Lidocaine in the prevention of primary ventricular fibrillation: A double-blind, randomized study of 212 consecutive patients. *N. Engl. J. Med.* 291:1324, 1974.

207. DeSilva R.A., Lown B., Hennekens C.H., et al.: Lignocaine prophylaxis in acute myocardial infarction: An evaluation of randomized trials. *Lancet* 2:855, 1981.

208. Cristal N., Szwarcberg J., Gueron M.: Supraventricular arrhythmia in acute myocardial infarction: Prognostic importance of clinical setting: Mechanism of production. *Ann. Intern. Med.* 82:35, 1975.

209. Shell W.E., Sobel B.E.: Deleterious effects of increased heart rate on infarct size in the conscious dog. *Am. J. Cardiol.* 31:474, 1973.

210. Gazes P.C.: Treatment of acute myocardial infarction: 2. Ventricular ectopic arrhythmias. *Postgrad. Med.* 48:168, 1970.

211. Engel T.R., Meister S.G., Frankl W.S.: The "R-on-T" phenomenon: An update and critical review. *Ann. Intern. Med.* 88:221, 1978.

212. Te-Chuan C., Wenzke F.: The importance of R on T phenomenon. *Am. Heart J.* 96:191, 1978.

213. Roberts R., Ambos H.D., Loh C.W., et al.: Initiation of repetitive ventricular depolarizations by relatively late premature complexes in patients with acute myocardial infarction. *Am. J. Cardiol.* 41:678, 1978.

214. Lie K.I., Wellen H.J.J., Downar E., et al.: Observations on patients with primary ventricular fibrillation complicating acute myocardial infarction. *Circulation* 52:755, 1975.

215. Harrison D.C.: Should lidocaine be administered routinely to all patients after acute myocardial infarction? *Circulation* 58:581, 1978.

216. Rowland M., Thompson P.D., Guichard A., et al.: Disposition kinetics of lidocaine in normal subjects. *Ann. NY Acad. Sci.* 179:383, 1971.

217. Lichstein E., Ribas-Meneclier C., Gupta P.K., et al.: Incidence and description of accelerated ventricular rhythm complicating acute myocardial infarction. *Am. J. Med.* 58:192, 1975.

218. Talbot S., Greaves M.: Association of ventricular extrasystoles and ventricular tachycardia with idioventricular rhythm. *Br. Heart J.* 38:457, 1976.

219. Sclarovsky S., Strasberg B., Martonovich G., et al.: Ventricular rhythms with intermediate rates in acute myocardial infarction. *Chest* 74:180, 1978.

220. Gazes P.C.: Treatment of acute myocardial infarction: 3. Bradyarrhythmias. *Postgrad. Med.* 48:141, 1970.

221. Epstein S.E., Goldstein R.E., Redwood D.R., et al.: The early phase of acute myocardial infarction: Pharmacologic aspects of therapy. *Ann. Intern. Med.* 78:918, 1973.

222. Warren T.V., Lewis R.P.: Beneficial effects of atropine in the pre-hospital phase of coronary care. *Am. J. Cardiol.* 37:68, 1976.

223. Scheinman M.M., Thorburn D., Abbott J.A.: Use of atropine in patients with acute myocardial infarction and sinus bradycardia. *Circulation* 52:627, 1975.

224. Das G., Talmers F.N., Weissler A.M.: New observations on the effects of atropine on the sinoatrial and atrioventricular nodes in man. *Am. J. Cardiol.* 36:281, 1975.
225. Rotman M., Wagner G.S., Waugh R.A.: Significance of high degree atrioventricular block in acute posterior myocardial infarction. *Circulation* 47:257, 1973.
226. Kuo C., Reddy C.P.: Effect of lidocaine on escape rate in patients with complete atrioventricular block: B. Proximal His bundle block. *Am. J. Cardiol.* 47:1315, 1981.
227. Mullins C.B., Atkins J.M.: Prognoses and management of ventricular conduction blocks in acute myocardial infarction. *Mod. Concepts Cardiovasc. Dis.* 45:129, 1976.
228. Hindman M.C., Wagner G.S., JaRo M., et al.: The clinical significance of bundle branch block complicating acute myocardial infarction: 1. Clinical characteristics, hospital mortality, and one-year follow-up. *Circulation* 58:679, 1978.
229. Hindman M.C., Wagner G.S., JaRo M., et al.: The clinical significance of bundle branch block complicating acute myocardial infarction: 2. Indications for temporary and permanent pacemaker insertion. *Circulation* 58:689, 1978.
230. Lichstein E., Letafati A., Gupta P.K., et al.: Continuous Holter monitoring of patients with bifascicular block complicating anterior wall myocardial infarction. *Am. J. Cardiol.* 40:860, 1977.
231. Killip, T., Kimball J.T.: Treatment of myocardial infarction in a coronary care unit. A two year experience with 250 patients. *Am. J. Cardiol.* 20:457, 1967.
232. Forrester J.S., Waters D.D.: Hospital treatment of congestive heart failure. Management according to hemodynamic profile. *Am. J. Med.* 65:173, 1978.
233. Morrison J., Caromilas J., Robbins M., et al.: Digitalis and myocardial infarction in man. *Circulation* 62:8, 1980.
234. McHugh T.J., Forrester J.S., Adler L., et al.: Pulmonary vascular congestion in acute myocardial infarction: Hemodynamic and radiologic correlations. *Ann. Intern. Med.* 76:29, 1972.
235. Roberts R.: Inotropic therapy for cardiac failure associated with acute myocardial infarction. *Chest* 93:22S, 1988.
236. Chatterjee K., Swan H.J.C.: Vasodilator therapy in acute myocardial infarction. *Mod. Concepts Cardiovasc. Dis.* 43:119, 1974.
237. Chatterjee J., Parmley W.W.: Vasodilator treatment of acute and chronic heart failure. *Br. Heart J.* 39:706, 1977.
238. Armstrong P.W, Walker D.C., Burton J.R., et al.: Vasodilator therapy in acute myocardial infarction: A comparison of sodium nitroprusside and nitroglycerin. *Circulation* 52:1118, 1975.
239. Alonso D.R., Sheidt S., Post M., et al.: Pathophysiology of cardiogenic shock: Quantification of myocardial necrosis, clinical, pathologic, and electrocardiographic correlations. *Circulation* 48:588, 1973.
240. Forrester J.S., Diamond G.A., Swan H.J.C.: Correlative classification of clinical and hemodynamic function after an acute myocardial infarction. *Am. J. Cardiol.* 39:137, 1977.
241. Leier C.V., Heban P.T., Huss P., et al.: Comparative systemic and regional hemodynamic effects of dopamine and dobutamine in patients with cardiomyopathic heart failure. *Circulation* 58:466, 1978.
242. Hutter A.M., Gold H.K., Leinbach R.C., et al.: Various uses of intra-aortic balloon pump in acute myocardial infarction, in *Acute Myocardial Infarction—First 25 Hours.* New York, Verlag Gerbard Witzstrock, 1977, p. 169.
243. Ayres S.M.: The prevention and treatment of shock in acute myocardial infarction. *Chest* 93:17S, 1988.
244. Lee L., Bates E.R., Pitt B., et al.: Percutaneous transluminal coronary angioplasty improves survival in acute myocardial infarction complicated by cardiogenic shock. *Circulation* 78:1345, 1988.
245. Wenger N.K., Stein P.D., and Willis P.W. III: Massive acute pulmonary embolism: Deceivingly non-specific manifestations. *Am. J. Cardiol.* 29:296, 1972.
246. Roberts W.C., Perloff J.K.: Mitral valvular disease—a clinico-pathologic survey of the conditions causing the mitral valve to function abnormally. *Ann. Intern. Med.* 77:939, 1972.
247. Kleiger R., Shaw R., Avioli L.V.: Postmyocardial infarction complications requiring surgery. *Arch. Intern. Med.* 137:1580, 1977.
248. Wei J.T., Hutchins G.M., Bulkley B.H.: Papillary muscle rupture in fatal acute myocardial infarction—A potentially treatable form of cardiogenic shock. *Ann. Intern. Med.* 90:149, 1979.
249. Donahoo J.S., Brawley R.K., Taylor D., et al.: Factors influencing survival following postinfarction ventricular septal defects. *Ann. Thorac. Surg.* 19:648, 1975.
250. Swithinbank J.M.: Perforation of the interventricular septum in myocardial infarction. *Br. Heart J.* 21:562, 1959.
251. Vlodaver Z., Edwards J.E.: Rupture of ventricular septum or papillary muscle complicating myocardial infarction. *Circulation* 55:815, 1977.

252. Graham A.F., Stinson E.B., Daily P.O., et al.: Ventricular septal defects after myocardial infarction—early operative treatment. *JAMA* 225:708, 1973.
253. Montaya A., McKeever L., Scanlon P., et al.: Early repair of ventricular septal rupture after infarction. *Am. J. Cardiol.* 45:345, 1980.
254. Cohn L.H.: Surgical treatment of acute myocardial infarction. *Chest* 93:13S, 1988.
255. London R.E., London S.B.: Rupture of the heart: A critical analysis of forty-seven consecutive autopsy cases. *Circulation* 31:202, 1965.
256. O'Rourke M.F.: Subacute heart rupture following myocardial infarction. Clinical features of a correctable condition. *Lancet* 2:124, 1973.
257. Froehlich R.T., Falsetti H.L., Doty D.B., et al.: Prospective study of surgery for left ventricular aneurysm. *Am. J. Cardiol.* 45:923, 1980.
258. Stephens J.D., Dymond D.S., Stone D.L., et al.: Left ventricular aneurysm and congestive heart failure: Value of exercise stress and isosorbide dinitrate in predicting hemodynamic results of aneurysmectomy. *Am. J. Cardiol.* 45:932, 1980.
259. Kossowsky W.A., Epstein P.J., Levine R.S.: Postmyocardial infarction syndrome: An early complication of acute myocardial infarction. *Chest* 63:35, 1973.
260. Friedman P.L., Brown E.J. Jr., Gunther S., et al.: Coronary vasoconstrictor effect of indomethacin in patients with coronary artery disease. *N. Engl. J. Med.* 305:1171, 1981.
261. Wartman W.B., Hellerstein H.K.: The incidence of heart disease in 2,000 consecutive autopsies. *Ann. Intern. Med.* 28:41, 1948.
262. Isner J.M., Roberts W.C.: Right ventricular infarction complicating left ventricular infarction secondary to coronary artery disease. *Am. J. Cardiol.* 42:885, 1978.
263. Wackers F.J., Lie K.I., Sokole E.B., et al.: Prevalence of right ventricular involvement in inferior wall infarction assessed with myocardial imaging with thallium-201 and technetium-99m pyrophosphate. *Am. J. Cardiol.* 42:358, 1978.
264. Lorell B., Leinbach R.C., Pohost G.M., et al.: Right ventricular infarction—clinical diagnosis and differentiation from cardiac tamponade and pericardial constriction. *Am. J. Cardiol.* 43:465, 1979.
265. Kulbertus H.E., Rigo P., Legrand V.: Right ventricular infarction: Pathophysiology, diagnosis, clinical course, and treatment. *Modern Concepts Cardiovasc. Dis.* 54:1, 1985.
266. Shah P.K., Berman D.S., Maddahi J., et al.: Postinfarction predominant right ventricular dysfunction: Clinical implications. *Cardiology Board Review* 3:17, 1986.
267. Gardin J.M., Singer D.H.: Atrial infarction: Importance, diagnosis and localization. *Arch. Intern. Med.* 141:1345, 1981.
268. Granath A., Sodermark T., Winge T., et al.: Early work load tests for evaluation of long-term prognosis of acute myocardial infarction. *Br. Heart J.* 39:758, 1977.
269. Markiewicz W., Houston N., DeBusk R.F.: Exercise testing soon after myocardial infarction. *Circulation* 56:26, 1977.
270. Schulze R., Strauss H., Pitt B.: Sudden death in the year following myocardial infarction. *Am. J. Med.* 62:192, 1977.
271. Multicenter International Study. Improvement of prognosis of myocardial infarction by long-term beta-adrenoreceptor blockade using practolol: A multicenter international study. *Br. Med. J.* 3:735, 1975.
272. Multicenter International Study. Reduction in mortality with long-term beta-adrenoreceptor blockade: A multicenter international study. *Br. Med. J.* 2:49, 1977.
273. Wilhelmsson C., Vedin J.A., Wilhelmsen L., et al.: Reduction of sudden death after myocardial infarction by treatment with alprenolol, preliminary results. *Lancet* 2:1157, 1974.
274. Timolol-induced reduction in mortality and reinfarction in patients surviving acute myocardial infarction. The Norwegian Multicenter Study Group. *N. Engl. J. Med.* 304:801, 1981.
275. The β-Blocker Heart Attack Trial: Cooperative trial—preliminary report. *JAMA* 246:2973, 1981.
276. Hjalmarson A., Herlitz J., Malek I., et al.: Effect on mortality of metoprolol in acute myocardial infarction. *Lancet* 2:823, 1981.
277. Pitt B.: Perspectives on the use of B-blockade in acute myocardial infarction. *Primary Cardiol.* Edition #1, 1986.
278. Yusuf S., Peto R., Lewis J., et al.: Beta blockade during and after myocardial infarction: An overview of the randomized trials. *Prog. Cardiovasc. Dis.* 27:335, 1985.
279. A randomized, controlled trial of aspirin in persons recovering from acute myocardial infarction. Aspirin-Myocardial Infarction Study Research Group. *JAMA* 243:661, 1980.
280. Sulfinpyrazone in the prevention of sudden death after myocardial infarction. The Anturane Reinfarction Trial Research Group. *JAMA* 302:250, 1980.
281. Persantine and aspirin in coronary heart disease. The Persantin-Aspirin Reinfarction Study Research Group. *Circulation* 62:449, 1980.
282. Klimt C.R., Knatterud G.L., Stamler J., Meier P.: Persantine-aspirin reinfarction study. Part II. Secondary coronary prevention with persantine and aspirin. *JACC* 7:251, 1986.

283. Fitzgerald G.A.: Dipyridamole. *N. Engl. J. Med.* 316:1247, 1987.
283a. Cerletti, C., Latini, R., Dejana, E., et al: Inhibition of human platelet thromboxane generation by aspirin in the absence of measurable drug levels in peripheral blood. *Biochem. Pharmacol.* 34:1839, 1985.
284. Fuster V., Cohen M., Chesebro J.H.: Usefulness of aspirin for coronary artery disease. *Am. J. Cardiol.* 61:637, 1988.
285. The Steering Committee of the Physicians' Health Study Group. Preliminary report: Findings from the aspirin component of the ongoing physicians' health study. *N. Engl. J. Med.* 318:262, 1988.
285a. Steering committee of the Physician's Health Study Research Group. Final report on the aspirin component of the ongoing Physician's Health Study. *N. Engl. J. Med.* 321:129, 1989.
286. Young F.E., Nightingale S.L., Temple R.A.: The preliminary report of the findings of the aspirin component of the ongoing physicians' health study. The FDA perspective on aspirin for the primary prevention of myocardial infarction. *JAMA* 259:3158, 1988.
287. Moss A.J., Schnitzler R., Green R., et al.: Ventricular arrhythmias three weeks after acute myocardial infarction. *Ann. Intern. Med.* 75:837, 1971.
288. Vismara L.A., Amsterdam E.A., Mason D.T.: Relation of ventricular arrhythmias in the late hospital phase of acute myocardial infarction to sudden death after hospital discharge. *Am. J. Med.* 59:6, 1975.
289. Conley M.J., McNeer J.F., Lee K.L., et al.: Cardiac arrest complicating acute myocardial infarction: Predictability and prognosis. *Am. J. Cardiol.* 39:7, 1977.
290. Oliver G.C., Nolle F.M., Tiefenbrunn A.J., et al.: Ventricular arrhythmias associated with sudden death in survivors of acute myocardial infarction. *Am. J. Cardiol.* 33:160, 1974.
291. Geddes J.A., Adgey A.A.J., Pantridge J.F.: Prognosis after recovery from ventricular fibrillation complicating ischemic heart disease. *Lancet* 2:273, 1967.
292. Ruberman W., Weinblatt E., Goldberg J.D., et al.: Ventricular premature beats and mortality after myocardial infarction. *N. Engl. J. Med.* 297:750, 1977.
293. Schulze R., Humphries J., Griffith L., et al.: Left ventricular and coronary angiographic anatomy. *Circulation* 55:839, 1977.
294. Kotler M.N., Tabatnik B., Mower M.M., et al.: Prognostic significance of ventricular ectopic beats with respect to sudden death in the late postinfarction period. *Circulation* 47:595, 1973.
295. Myeburg R.J., Conde C., Sheps D.S., et al.: Antiarrhythmic drug therapy in survivors of prehospital cardiac arrest: Comparison of effects on chronic ventricular arrhythmias and recurrent cardiac arrest. *Circulation* 59:855, 1979.
296. Weinblatt E., Shapiro S., Frank C.W., et al.: Prognosis of men after first myocardial infarction: Mortality and first recurrence in relation to selected parameters. *Am. J. Public Health* 58:1329, 1968.
297. Caps Investigators: The cardiac arrhythmia pilot study. *Am. J. Cardiol.* 57:91, 1986.
297a. Hellerstein, H.K., Friedman, E.H.: Sexual activity and the post-coronary patient. *Arch. Intern. Med.* 125:987, 1970.
298. Kannel W.B., Castelli W.P., McNamara P.M.: The Coronary Profile: 12-Year follow-up in the Framingham Study. *J. Occup. Med.* 9:611, 1967.
299. Keil J.E., Gazes P.C., Loadholt C.B., et al.: Coronary heart disease mortality and its predictors among women in Charleston, South Carolina, in Eaker E., Packard B., Wanger N., Clarkson T., Tyrolar H.A. (eds): *Coronary Heart Disease in Women.* Haymarket Doyma Inc., New York, 1987, pp 90–98.
300. Anderson D.W.: HDL cholesterol: The variable components. *Lancet* 1:819, April 15, 1978.
301. National Cholesterol Education Program: Report of the Expert Panel on Detection, Evaluation, and Treatment of High Blood Cholesterol in Adults. NIH Publication No. 88-2925 (January), 1988.
302. Fredrickson D.S., Lees R.S.: A system for phenotyping hyperlipoproteinemia. *Circulation* 31:321, 1965.
303. Fredrickson D.S., Levy R.I.: Familial hyperlipoproteinemia, in Stanbury J.B., Wyngaarden J.B., Fredrickson D.S. (eds.): *The Metabolic Basis of Inherited Diseases,* ed. 3. New York, McGraw-Hill Book Co., 1972.
304. Bang H.O., Dyerberg J., Hjorne N.: The composition of food consumed by Greenland Eskimos. *Acta Med. Scand.* 200:69, 1976.
305. Kromhout D., Bosschieter E.B., Coulander C.: The inverse relation between fish consumption and 20-year mortality from coronary heart disease. *N. Engl. J. Med.* 312:1205, 1985.
306. Glomset J.A.: Fish, fatty acids, and human health. *N. Engl. J. Med.* 312:1253, 1985.
307. Leaf A., Weber P.C.: Omega-3 fatty acids and cardiovascular disease. *Heart Disease Update* 3:49, 1988.
308. Anderson J.W., Story L., Sieling B., et al.: Hypocholesterolemic effects of oat-bran or bean intake for hypercholesterolemic men. *Am. J. Clin. Nutrit.* 40:1146, 1984.

309. Hennekens C.H., Willett W., Rosner B., et al.: Effects of beer, wine, and liquor in coronary deaths. *JAMA* 242:1973, 1979.
310. Klatsky A.L., Armstrong M.A., Friedman G.D.: Relations of alcoholic beverage use to subsequent coronary artery disease hospitalization. *Am. J. Cardiol.* 58:710, 1986.
311. Dai W.S., LaPorte R.E., Hom D.L., et al.: Alcohol consumption and high density lipoprotein cholesterol concentration among alcoholics. *Am. J. Epidemiol.* 122:620, 1985.
312. LaCroix A.Z., Mead L.A., Liang K.Y., et al.: Coffee consumption and the incidence of coronary heart disease. *N. Engl. J. Med.* 315:977, 1986.
312a. Yamamoto A., Matsuzawa Y., Yokoyama S., et al.: Effects of Probucol on xanthomta regression in familial hypercholesterolemia. *Am. J. Cardiol.* 57:29H, 1986.
312b. Lipid Research Clinics Program: The Lipid Research Clinics Coronary Primary Prevention Trial Results: II. The relationship of reduction in incidence of coronary heart disease to cholesterol lowering. *JAMA* 251:365, 1984.
313. Lipid Research Clinics Program: The lipid research clinics coronary primary prevention trial results. I. Reduction in incidence of coronary heart disease. *JAMA* 251:351, 1984.
314. Blankenhorn D.H., Nessim S.A., Johnson R.L., et al.: Beneficial effects of combined colestipol-niacin therapy on coronary atherosclerosis and coronary venous bypass grafts. *JAMA* 257:3233, 1987.
315. Frick M.H., Elo O., Haapa K., et al.: Helsinki Heart Study: Primary-prevention trial with gemfibrozil in middle-aged men with dyslipidemia. Safety of treatment, changes in risk factors, and incidence of coronary heart disease. *N. Engl. J. Med.* 317:1237, 1987.
316. Hypertension Detecting and Follow-Up Program Cooperative Group: Five-year findings of the Hypertension Detection and Follow-Up Program. *JAMA* 242:2562, 1979.
317. Willett W.C., Green A., Stampfer M.J., et al.: Relative and absolute excess risks of coronary heart disease among women who smoke cigarettes. *N. Engl. J. Med.* 317:1303, 1987.
318. Holbrook J.H., Grundy S.M., Hennekens C.H., et al.: Cigarette smoking and cardiovascular diseases. A statement for health professionals by a Task Force appointed by the Steering Committee of the American Heart Association. *Circulation* 70:1114A, 1984.
319. Auerbach O., Carter H.W., Garfinkel L., et al.: Cigarette smoking and coronary artery disease. *Chest* 70:697, 1976.
320. Folts J.D., Bonebrake F.C.: The effects of cigarette smoke and nicotine on platelet thrombus formation in stenosed dog coronary arteries: Inhibition with phentolamine. *Circulation* 65:465, 1982.
321. Wald N.J.: Mortality from lung cancer and coronary heart-disease in relation to changes in smoking habits. *Lancet* 1:136, 1976.
322. Benowitz N.L., Jacob P., Yu L., et al.: Reduced tar, nicotine, and carbon monoxide exposure while smoking ultralow—but not low–yield cigarettes. *JAMA* 256:241, 1986.
323. Fielding J.E.: Smoking: Health effects and control. *N. Engl. J. Med.* 313:491, 1985.
324. Seppanen A.: Smoking in closed space and its effect on carboxyhaemoglobin saturation of smoking and nonsmoking subjects. *Ann. Clin. Res.* 9:281, 1977.
325. Feyerabend C., Higenbottam T., Russell M.A.H.: Nicotine concentrations in urine and saliva of smokers and non-smokers. *Br. Med. J.* 284:1002, 1982.
326. Kramsch D.M., Aspen A.J., Abramowitz B.M.: Reduction of coronary atherosclerosis by moderate conditioning exercise in monkeys on an atherogenic diet. *N. Engl. J. Med.* 305:1483, 1981.
327. Greenland P. Chu J.S.: Efficacy of cardiac rehabilitation services with emphasis on patients after myocardial infarction. *Ann. Intern. Med.* 109:650, 1988.
328. Paffenbarger R.S., Hyde R.T., Wing A.L., et al.: Physical activity, all-cause mortality, and longevity of college alumni. *N. Engl. J. Med.* 314:605, 1986.
329. Wood P.D., Stefanick M.L., Dreon D.M., et al.: Changes in plasma lipids and lipoproteins in overweight men during weight loss through dieting as compared with exercise. *N. Engl. J. Med.* 319:1173, 1988.
330. Witztum J., Schonfeld G.: High density lipoproteins. *Diabetes* 28:326, 1979.
331. Thompson P.D., Cullinane E.M., Sady S.P., et al.: Modest changes in high-density lipoprotein concentration and metabolism with prolonged exercise training. *Circulation* 78:25, 1988.
332. Van Camp S.P., Peterson R.A.: Cardiovascular complications of out-patient cardiac rehabilitation programs. *JAMA* 256:1160, 1986.
333. Rowley P.T.: Genetics for the cardiologist: Parts I and II. *Mod. Concepts Cardiovasc. Dis.* 47:63, 1978.
334. Kate L.P., Boman H., Daiger S.P., et al.: Familial aggregation of coronary heart disease and its relation to known genetic risk factors. *Am. J. Cardiol.* 50:945, 1982.
335. Brand R.J., Rosenman R.H., Sholtz R.T., et al.: Multivariate prediction of coronary heart disease in the Western Collaborative Study compared to the findings of The Framingham Study. *Circulation* 53:348, 1976.

336. Rosenman R.H., Brand R.J., Jenkins C.D., et al.: Coronary heart disease in the Western Collaborative Group Study: final follow-up experience of 8½ years. *JAMA* 233:872, 1975.
337. Ragland D.R., Brand R.J.: Type A behavior and mortality from coronary heart disease. *N. Engl. J. Med.* 318:65, 1988.
338. Dimsdale J.E.: A perspective on Type A behavior and coronary disease. *N. Engl. J. Med.* 318:110, 1988.
339. MacDougall J.M., Dembroski T.M., Dimsdale J.B., et al.: Components of type A, hostility, and anger-in: further relationships to angiographic findings. *Health Psychol.* 4:137, 1985.
340. Stadel B.V.: Oral contraceptives and cardiovascular disease, Parts 1 and 2. *N. Engl. J. Med.* 305:612;672, 1981.
341. Bradley D.D., Wingerd J., Petitti D.B., et al.: Serum high density lipoprotein cholesterol in women using oral contraceptives, estrogens and progestins. *N. Engl. J. Med.* 299:17, 1978.
342. Wilson P.W.F., Garrison R.J., Castelli W.P.: Postmenopausal estrogen use, cigarette smoking, and cardiovascular morbidity in women over 50: the Framingham Study. *N. Engl. J. Med.* 313:1038, 1985.
343. Colditz G.A., Willett W.C., Stampfer M.J., et al.: Menopause and the risk of coronary heart disease in women. *N. Engl. J. Med.* 316:1105, 1987.
344. Stampfer M.J., Willett W.C., Colditz G.A., et al.: A prospective study of postmenopausal estrogen therapy and coronary heart disease. *N. Engl. J. Med.* 313:1044, 1985.
345. Bush T.L., Barrett-Connor E., Cowan L.D., et al.: Cardiovascular mortality and noncontraceptive use of estrogen in women: results from the Lipid Research Clinics Program Follow-up Study. *Circulation* 75:1102, 1987.

Chapter 5

SYSTEMIC HYPERTENSION AND HYPERTENSIVE HEART DISEASE

It has been estimated that as many as 58 million people in the United States have hypertension (systolic blood pressure ≥140 mm Hg or diastolic ≥90 mm Hg). The prevalence of hypertension increases with age and is more prevalent in blacks, especially those living in the southeastern United States.[1] Table 5–1 depicts a scheme based on risk level for the classification of systolic and diastolic blood pressure for persons aged 18 years and older.[2] Elevated levels should be confirmed on at least two subsequent visits and hypertension not diagnosed on a single measurement. At each visit, two or more readings should be averaged.

Blood pressures should routinely be checked in both arms and legs, especially in the young. The standard 12-cm cuff can indicate an erroneously high BP in arms with a large diameter and too low pressure in thin arms. The same cuff often indicates a pressure in the legs 30 mm Hg or more higher than in the arms. A cuff of about 16 cm is generally preferable for the legs. The width of the compression cuff should be about 20% greater than the diameter of the extremity (the rubber bladder should encircle at least two-thirds of the arm). Frequently, patients may not have any symptoms, and the BP elevation is found during a routine examination.

The medical history should include known duration of hypertension and response to therapy; history of cerebrovascular, cardiac, renal disease or diabetes; family history of hypertension; salt intake, usual diet and alcohol use; symptoms that may indicate secondary hypertension; history of emotional problems; other cardiovascular risk factors such as smoking and abnormal lipids; and other medications that may interfere or can raise the blood pressure, such as steroids, amphetamines, tricyclic antidepressants, and oral contraceptives.

Although headaches may occur as a result of hypertension, most headaches are not due to this. Beside the elevated BP, the funduscopic changes may be the only initial abnormal physical finding. The arterioles may become narrow and tortuous, and arteriovenous nicking can develop. With increasing arteriosclerosis, the arteriole may completely obstruct the vein, giving a clear area between it and the vein at the crossing. Hemorrhages and exudates can appear, and papilledema is the hallmark of accelerated or malignant hyperten-

Table 5–1. Classification of BP in Adults Age 18 Years or Older

Range, mm Hg	Category
Diastolic	
<85	Normal BP
85–89	High Normal BP
90–104	Mild Hypertension
105–114	Moderate Hypertension
≥115	Severe Hypertension
Systolic, when Diastolic BP is <90	
<140	Normal BP
140–159	Borderline ISH
≥160	ISH

BP = Blood pressure
ISH = Isolated Systolic Hypertension.
From the 1988 report of the Joint National Committee on Detection, Evaluation and Treatment of High Blood Pressure. *Arch. Intern. Med.* 148:May, 1988.

sion. When other symptoms and abnormal physical findings develop, they are usually due to cardiac, cerebral, or kidney involvement, or to a secondary form of hypertension (which will be discussed later).

Initially, left ventricular enlargement can occur, as demonstrated by physical examination, x ray of the chest, or the ECG. Frequently an S_4 gallop is noted. With left ventricular enlargement, an apical systolic murmur can develop. If the aorta becomes widened, an aortic systolic ejection murmur may be heard, and at times a murmur of aortic insufficiency is present. Later a patient may progress and have symptoms of left heart failure characterized by exertional dyspnea, orthopnea, paroxysmal nocturnal dyspnea, and bouts of pulmonary edema; eventually, the findings of right heart failure can develop. Often when the heart failure is chronic or the patient sustains a myocardial infarction, the BP, especially the systolic level, may return to normal. Coronary artery disease is frequently associated with hypertension, and, in addition, there is an increased incidence of dissecting aneurysms. Cerebral findings are variable and may range from hypertensive encephalopathy with confusion, headaches, vomiting, and convulsions or localized lesions due to thrombosis or hemorrhage with hemiparesis. Renal findings initially may be only abnormal renal studies (proteinuria, red cells, and casts, and decreased clearance studies). Later the patient can develop symptoms of uremia.

CAUSES OF HYPERTENSION

A cause can be found in up to 5% of cases; the remainder have no demonstrable cause or underlying condition that can be identified at present. Patients without a known cause may have a chronic or a malignant-accelerated course. This "essential" hypertension is usually detected after age 40, and often the patient gives a family history of hypertension. One may find out how long the hypertension has been present by carefully questioning the patient, especially males, about their BP during military service examinations or during an insurance examination or blood donation. Females should be questioned to determine if hypertension was present during their pregnancies. Hypertension may be present for years before cardiac, brain, or kidney changes occur. It appears that white women tolerate hypertension best and black men fare worst. Patients with comparable levels of hypertension tolerate it differently, some being more prone to complications. Patients with malignant or accelerated hypertension usually have a diastolic pressure over 120 mm Hg, papilledema, cardiomegaly, and renal findings. In the past, 80% of these patients had a rapid downhill course and died in uremia within 1 to 2 years. However, with proper therapy the prognosis has markedly improved.

MECHANISMS OF ESSENTIAL HYPERTENSION

Many factors affect the BP, especially cardiac output and peripheral vascular resistance (BP equals cardiac output times the peripheral vascular resistance). Increased vascular smooth muscle tone increases arteriolar resistance and reduces venular capacitance. Cardiac output is affected by heart rate, stroke volume, contractility, and blood volume (sodium and mineralocorticoids), and peripheral vascular resistance is affected by local effects and overactivity of the sympathetic nervous system. Humoral factors, such as prostaglandins and kinins (vasodilators) and angiotensin, vasopressin, and catecholamines (vasoconstrictors), also are important factors that regulate peripheral vascular resistance. The renin-angiotensin-aldosterone system not only produces constriction of blood vessels by its angiotensin effect, but also, through aldosterone, increases retention of salt and water. Renal excretion of sodium is increased when plasma volume is expanded, partly because of natriuretic hormones. The role of these hormones in hypertension is unclear.[3] Patients with essential hypertension have been classified according to the level of plasma renin activity into those with a normal level, low, or high level under conditions that normally stimulate renin release. It has been estimated that 30% of patients with essential hypertension have low plasma renin activity, 60% normal, and 10% high values.[4] The difference between Conn's syndrome and the low renin essential hypertension is the inappropriate increase in aldosterone that is seen in Conn's syndrome at a given level of sodium intake. Some studies[5] have shown that there are more complications (myocardial infarction, renal damage, and stroke) in patients with essential hypertension and high renin activity (vasoconstriction) than in those with low renin activity (volume expansion). The so-called volume hypertension (low renin) may respond to diuretics alone, and the "vasoconstrictor" hypertension (high renin) may respond to antirenin drugs such as propranolol and converting enzyme inhibitors. Those with normal levels may respond to both, since according to Laragh[5] these patients express inappropriate volume-vasoconstrictor interaction. However, these findings have not been confirmed by several studies.[6,7] In fact, these studies have shown that the peripheral vascular resistance progressively decreased as the renin increased. At present, it appears that routine determination of renin is not necessary for management of essential hypertension.

However, the hemodynamic sequence of events varies in the young and elderly, and there are also differences related to gender and race.[8] In the young, the main hemodynamic abnormality is an increase in cardiac output. Total peripheral vascular resistance is usually normal. In addition, in the young, the plasma norepinephrine levels, plasma renin activity, renal blood flow, and heart rate are increased, and there is a shift of the intravascular volume from the capacitance (venoconstriction) to cardiopulmonary vessels.

Thus the young have a hyperadrenergic state with increased left ventricular contractility. By middle age, the cardiac output returns to normal and peripheral vascular resistance begins to increase and target-organ disease may develop. In the elderly, cardiac output is decreased, peripheral resistance is increased, and the intravascular volume contracts. Target-organ change in these untreated patients can become severe. Premenopausal women have a higher cardiac output and a lower peripheral vascular resistance than men of the same age. In blacks, intravascular volume is not as contracted and thus the plasma volume is more expanded than in whites. The volume changes are associated with lower levels of plasma renin activity. Blacks have a greater degree of left ventricular hypertrophy, total peripheral vascular resistance, and intrarenal vascular resistance than whites with comparable levels of blood pressure. In the obese, cardiac output is increased and intravascular volume is expanded, which leads to increased ventricular preload. This preload increase, along with the increased blood pressure (afterload), causes left ventricular hypertrophy. In view of these various hemodynamic changes, young, elderly, black, and obese patients with hypertension are treated somewhat differently.

Table 5–2 outlines the studies that are usually performed in evaluating hypertension before treatment is begun. There has been much discussion of the value of many laboratory studies. However, since there are now automated tests, a blood biochemical profile can be obtained at a reasonable cost. One can begin with a complete blood cell count, urinalysis, automated blood biochemical profile, and an ECG, and then add the other studies included in Table 5–2 depending on findings and response to therapy. Depending on these studies or the history and physical examination, specific tests for secondary causes can be done (Table 5–3). Usually the younger the patient, the more comprehensive should be the evaluation. Among the specific causes of hypertension are renal

Table 5–2.   Routine Hypertensive Evaluation

1. Complete history (emphasis on family history, date of onset, and genitourinary tract disease)

2. Physical examination (emphasis on funduscopic, BP in arms and legs, abdominal bruit, and cardiac findings)

3. PA and lateral x-ray views of chest

4. Electrocardiogram

5. Complete blood cell count

6. Careful urinalysis; 24-hr urine for volume, protein, creatinine, urea, uric acid, sodium, potassium, and chloride; urine culture

7. Renal function tests (BUN, creatinine)

8. Serum electrolytes (Na, K, Cl, CO_2)

9. Fasting and 2-hr Pc blood sugar

10. Total serum proteins, A:G ratio and liver function tests (bilirubin, alkaline phosphatase, serum enzymes)

11. Plasma cholesterol, triglycerides, and lipid electrophoresis

12. Calcium and phosphate

13. Uric acid

Table 5–3. Tests for Secondary Causes of Hypertension*

1. Creatinine, endogenous creatinine clearance
2. T_3, T_4
3. Minute sequence hypertensive pyelogram
4. Radioisotope studies
5. Serum and 24-hr urine catecholamines, vanillylmandelic acid, or metanephrines (pheochromocytoma)
6. Oral captopril test (renovascular hypertension)
7. Plasma renin activity and bilateral renal vein renin (renovascular hypertension)
8. Serum and/or urine aldosterone (primary aldosteronism)
9. Dexamethasone suppression test (Cushing's syndrome)
10. Aortography (aorta and renal arteries)

*To be added if necessary to routine tests in Table 5–2.

(arterial stenosis or parenchymal disease), adrenal (pheochromocytoma, primary aldosteronism, or Cushing's syndrome), hyperthyroidism, coarctation of the aorta, and drug use (oral contraceptives, steroids, or licorice).

Renal Disease

Renal disease is responsible for 2 to 4% of the secondary forms of hypertension. This may be suspected if there is a history of nephritis, repeated urinary tract infections, or renal colic. Chronic glomerulonephritis or pyelonephritis may cause hypertension, especially if progressive renal abnormalities have been known to be present prior to the development of cardiac or cerebral findings. The urine should be tested for protein, and the sediment should be carefully examined and urine cultures obtained. Twenty-four–hour urine collections for protein and creatinine and an intravenous pyelogram (IVP) should be performed.

Renovascular Hypertension

This occurs in about 2% of referred patients. Renal artery obstruction may be due to atherosclerosis, fibromuscular hyperplasia, or an aneurysm. This diagnosis should be entertained if the hypertension occurs in a young person, has sudden onset (especially after age 50), occurs after trauma (back pain and hematuria), or increases in severity in spite of adequate therapy. A systolic bruit, especially if a diastolic component is present, over the upper abdomen or flanks far enough from the aorta may suggest renal artery stenosis. In addition, the renal function deteriorates during therapy with a converting enzyme inhibitor.[9] Until recently, many noninvasive studies were done in such suspicious patients prior to considering direct arteriography of the renal arteries. However, hypertensive intravenous pyelograms, radioisotope studies, and peripheral plasma renin activity (PRA) assays are nonspecific, are not highly sensitive, and have many false-positives and negatives. The captopril test appears to be a good noninvasive screening test in those who have clinical features suggesting renovascular hypertension.[10] In addition, it helps establish the functional significance of a lesion. The patient should be on a normal sodium diet and off diuretics. After the patient sits for 30 minutes, 50 mg captopril is given orally and venous blood is obtained for a basal PRA. Blood for stimulated PRA is drawn at 60 minutes later. The test is considered positive if the stimulated PRA is 12 ng/ml/h or more, an absolute increase in PRA of 10 ng/ml/h or greater, or a 150% increase or greater of PRA (if the baseline PRA is less than 3 ng/ml/h then the increase should be 400%). This report included 112 patients with essential hypertension. Only 2 had false-positive results and, among the 40 with renovascular hypertension, there were no false-negatives. This test is more accurate if renal function is good. It should be considered before direct arteriography, although if the clinical picture is suspicious, one could go directly to arteriography. Because many patients requiring coronary arteriography have hypertension, I routinely advise, during such a study, that the renal arteries also be injected unless there is a contraindication. Renal vein renin assays can confirm the functional significance of the lesions noted on arteriography. A ratio greater than 1.5 to 2.0 between the abnormal and the uninvolved kidney suggests that the renal stenosis is producing the hypertension.[11] There is still much discussion about whether such patients should first have a trial of medical therapy because converting enzyme inhibitors are available. However, such drugs can control the hypertension, but may cause deterioration of the function of the already ischemic kidney.[9] Therefore, these drugs can be used to control the blood pressure before surgery, observing carefully that renal function is maintained, or they may be used on a continuous long-term basis if the patient is unsuitable for surgery. Angioplasty has been shown to be more effective in fibromuscular lesions than in atherosclerotic lesions (especially if the lesion is ostial). It should be done as the first procedure in patients who are poor surgical risks.[12]

Pheochromocytomas

These are tumors arising in the majority of instances from the adrenal medulla (chromaffin cells) and rarely from extramedullary chromaffin tissue in the chest, along the aorta (organ of Zuckerkandl) and the urinary bladder. About 10% within the adrenal glands are bilateral. Patients with neurofibromatosis have a high incidence of such tumors. There also is a high association with thyroid carcinoma and parathyroid adenoma. The majority are benign tumors and secrete the catecholamines epinephrine and norepinephrine. With excess epinephrine, patients have paroxysms of headache, flushing, sweating, palpitations, facial pallor, nausea, anxiety, hyperglycemia, and hypertension. Pulmonary edema or a cerebrovascular accident can occur. The extramedullary types secrete more norepinephrine and have fewer symptoms and hypertension. When the hypertension is sustained, these patients are often overlooked as having essential hypertension. Such patients often present with a thin habitus, and when they stand, the heart rate increases and orthostatic hypotension may be demonstrable. Rarely a tumor is palpable or an attack can be produced by massaging the flanks. Crises can be precipitated by such drugs as tricyclic antidepressants,[13] saralasin (a selective angiotensin antagonist),[14] nicotine, β-blockers, histamine, caffeine, and glucocorticoids. During general anesthesia or manipulations at abdominal surgery, a sudden rise in BP should suggest a pheochromocytoma. Similar paroxysms may occur during radiographic contrast studies. Plasma, 24-hour urine catecholamine, or a metabolite level are diagnostic. Reserpine, guanethidine, methyldopa, monoamine oxidase inhibitors, decongestive nose drops, aminophylline, clofibrate, tetracycline, quinidine, isoproterenol, theophylline, chlorpromazine, and x-ray contrast material may alter the results of these tests. Twenty-four–hour urinary metanephrines are less affected by these agents than catecholamines and vanillylmandelic acid (VMA). In fact, one study showed significantly fewer false negative results with metanephrine levels.[15] Urine should be collected prior to performing an IVP or any other study using contrast media. Plasma catecholamine assays may be used to confirm the diagnosis. Pharmacologic tests such as the histamine provocative test and phentolamine (Regitine), an α-adrenergic blocker, are seldom used today. Clonidine has been used as a test for pheochromocytoma.[16] The plasma norepinephrine level 3 hours after a 0.3 mg oral dose of clonidine will not be suppressed in a patient with a pheochromocytoma, whereas in a normal subject, suppression does occur. However, hypotension can occur during this test.

Chest x ray, IVP, nephrotomography, ultrasound of abdomen, computerized axial tomography (CT) scan, arteriography, adrenal venography, and regional venous sampling for catecholamine determination have been used for localization of the tumor. However, today CT scan is used more often and radioisotopes may help in the few that are not localized by CT. Fortunately, 98% of pheochromocytomas are located in the abdominal area (diaphragm to pelvic floor). Multiple pheochromocytomas occur in about 20% of patients. There is a remote possibility that a tumor may be in the neck, chest, or bladder. Actually, preoperative localization of the tumor is not absolutely necessary because the surgeon should explore both adrenal glands and the entire abdomen. Pheochromocytoma crisis can occur preoperatively or during surgery. For such a crisis, 2 to 5 mg of phentolamine (Regitine) should be given I.V. every 5 minutes until the BP is normal. One to 2 mg of propranolol should be given I.V. every 5 to 10 minutes for tachycardia or tachyarrhythmia. Phenoxybenzamine (Dibenzyline), an α-adrenergic blocker, 40 to 80 mg daily, is given for long-term therapy. This drug can produce sedation, orthostatic hypotension, nasal congestion, and xerostomia. Propranolol given orally can control the tachyarrhythmias. However, propranolol should not be given without an α-adrenergic blocker, for the α-adrenergic (vasoconstrictor) activity becomes predominant after β-blockage, producing a paradoxical rise in BP. Prazosin, a postsynaptic α-adrenergic blocker, has been used and has fewer side effects than phenoxybenzamine. Alpha-methyltyrosine, an inhibitor of catecholamine synthesis, has been used in patients with malignant pheochromocytoma.[16,17] The preferred therapy is surgical excision in most cases. Careful preoperative thought should be given to medical therapy, blood volume, and the anesthetic agent. During surgery, the tumors must be handled carefully because release of catecholamines can produce a severe rise in BP. After the tumor is removed, there may be a marked fall in BP due to shrunken blood volume, which is no longer compensated by intense vasoconstriction. Preoperative use of volume-expanding fluids (plasma, 5% albumin, saline) and whole blood has reduced the need for pressor agents postoperatively.

Primary Aldosteronism (Conn's Syndrome)

This is usually associated with a benign adenoma of the adrenal cortex or bilateral hyperplasia of the adrenal cortex, which secretes an increased amount of aldosterone. There is an increased aldosterone concentration in the urine or plasma and an abnormally depressed renin level in the peripheral blood. The elevated aldosterone produces retention of sodium and water, with a resulting increase in the plasma volume, and blocks renin release by a feedback mechanism. Clinically, primary aldosteronism can be suspected when there is hypokalemia and metabolic alkalosis associated with muscle weakness and hypertension. These patients can have headaches out of proportion to the hypertension.

It must be remembered that the diuretics used in the treatment of hypertension may produce hypokalemia and confuse the picture, or, rarely, hypokalemia may be due to excessive use of licorice, which contains the mineralocorticoid glycyrrhizinic acid.[18] If the serum potassium is less than 3.8 mEq/L and hypertension is present, a 24-hour urine level for sodium and potassium should be collected while the patient is taking no supplemental potassium or diuretic. If adequate intake of sodium is indicated by the urinary sodium excretion's being greater than 100 mEq/L and if the potassium is less than 40 mEq/L, the hypokalemia is most likely not due to adrenal cortical hormone excretion, and no further work-up is necessary. However, if the 24-hour urine potassium is above 40 mEq/L, the laboratory should be instructed to measure the urinary aldosterone. If aldosterone is increased, the patient could have hyperaldosteronism, and further documentation should be pursued. The diagnosis of primary aldosteronism is supported by the finding of a suppressed release of renin under controlled conditions. Renin plasma activity is measured in the patient on a high-sodium diet in the recumbent and upright postures and repeated on a low-sodium diet in both positions and after diuretic-induced volume and sodium depletion in the upright posture. In the upright posture with a low-sodium diet or diuretic-induced volume depletion, plasma renin activity is low in the patient with primary aldosteronism. If a solitary adenoma is found, surgery is indicated, especially if preoperative treatment with spironolactone reduces BP to near normal. Bilateral hyperplasia responds better to medical therapy with spironolactone.[19] It may be difficult to differentiate an adenoma from bilateral hyperplasia. Isotope scanning, adrenal venography, adrenal venous sampling, and computerized tomography have been used to differentiate these two.

Cushing's Syndrome

This may be of pituitary or adrenocortical origin and is mostly secondary to bilateral adrenal hyperplasia. Clinically, these patients have central obesity, moon facies, a buffalo hump, striae, thin skin, muscle wasting, hirsutism, osteoporosis, polycythemia, hypertension, and cardiomegaly. The diagnosis depends on demonstrating cortisol excess. The dexamethasone suppression test is specific. One mg of dexamethasone is given at bedtime, and the next morning plasma cortisol is measured between 7 and 10 a.m. The level in the normal is less than 5 µg/dl. If this test is abnormal, a longer dexamethasone test should be done. Pituitary adenomas or adrenal tumors can be surgically removed.

Coarctation of the Aorta

This is a cause of hypertension and will be presented in Chapter 7.

Oral Contraceptives

Five percent of contraceptive pill users will become hypertensive in 5 years.[20] The incidence increases with longer use and is more likely to develop in those over age 35. Hypertension is caused by the pill renin-aldosterone–mediated volume expansion. When the pill is discontinued, the BP returns to normal within 3 to 6 months in about 50% of cases. It is not known whether the pill uncovered essential hypertension or produced permanent hypertension in those in whom it did not clear. It is probably judicious while controlling the BP to withdraw these estrogen-containing compounds for at least 3 months before attempting definitive evaluation of these patients.

Table 5–4 lists clues for some of the causes of hypertension. Naturally, there are many other findings, and some of these are not specific. For example, the absence of a strong family history does not exclude the diagnosis of essential hypertension.

SYSTOLIC HYPERTENSION

In certain conditions there may be systolic hypertension out of proportion to the diastolic level. The most frequent cause is aortic arteriosclerosis that is seen in the elderly associated with diminished arterial elasticity. High-output states such as anemia, thyrotoxicosis, beriberi, arteriovenous fistula, and the hyperdynamic β-adrenergic circulatory state can produce systolic hypertension. The hyperdynamic β-adrenergic circulatory state is a syndrome characterized by cardiac awareness, increased heart rate, and a hyperkinetic circulation. In addition, conditions with a slow heart rate (such as sinus bradycardia or heart block) and aortic insufficiency can increase the cardiac stroke volume with a rise in systolic BP. The underlying conditions producing the systolic hypertension should be treated. In the absence of any cause and in the younger individual, the Framingham study[24] has shown that there is an increased risk in such patients even when correction for the diastolic pressure is made.

TREATMENT OF HYPERTENSION

Therapy for those patients with definable causes of hypertension, such as coarctation of the aorta or pheochromocytoma, is usually good. However, since a cause can be found in only 5% of subjects, most essential hypertension pa-

Table 5–4.   Clues for Some of the Causes of Hypertension

Type of Hypertension	Features
Essential	Strong family history
Coarctation of aorta	Blood pressure higher in arms than legs
Conn's syndrome	Hypokalemia, metabolic alkalosis, muscle weakness
Pheochromocytoma	Paroxysmal hypertension with symptoms of excess catecholamines
Cushing's syndrome	Central obesity, buffalo hump, thin skin, muscle weakness, osteoporosis
Renovascular	Sudden onset or worsening, abdominal bruit, youth, after trauma, severe and uncontrolled hypertension

tients must rely on a drug regimen to achieve control of their hypertension. Evidence is accumulating that these drugs can delay and prevent complications and prolong life. Studies from the Veterans Administration, Public Health Service, and from England have shown a reduction in mortality and morbidity in patients treated who have a fixed diastolic pressure of 105 mm Hg or higher.[21-23] First, a decision has to be made about when to begin therapy. The Framingham study[24] has shown that as BP rises, complications increase. That study has shown that even systolic pressure rises to more than 160 mm Hg have a four times greater risk for coronary attacks than if the BP is below 120 mm Hg. Diastolic pressures over 90 mm Hg have an increased risk of events associated with coronary occlusion.

Most studies agree that drug therapy is indicated if the diastolic pressure is sustained over 105 mm Hg or at any level if there is evidence of cerebral or cardiac damage. Until recently, good evidence for treating mild hypertension was not available. However, the Hypertension Detection and Follow-up Program (HDFP Study) has given further support for the value of treating patients with diastolic pressures between 90 and 104 mm Hg.[25] This randomized, controlled trial involved 10,940 persons with hypertension and compared the effect of a systematic antihypertensive treatment program (stepped-care) and referral with usual community medical therapy (referred care). Five-year mortality from all causes was 17% lower for the stepped-care group and 20% lower for this group in those with an entry BP of 90 to 104 mm Hg (70% of the total). This study has also given clearer evidence that coronary events are reduced, in addition to strokes, heart failure, and renal damage. The stepped-care group had 26% fewer deaths from acute myocardial infarction, and among those with diastolic pressure between 90 and 104 mm Hg this was 46%. A 7-year study showed that therapy with the β-blocker metoprolol produced regression of cardiovascular structural changes in 13 hypertensive men.[26] MacMahon et al. have reviewed the benefits of drug therapy for hypertension as shown in several randomized controlled trials.[27]

Patients who have occasional high readings should be followed up closely because some of them may develop sustained hypertension in later life. Formerly this was called "labile" hypertension, but now it is termed "borderline." In all instances of hypertension, excess salt intake should be avoided, maintenance of normal weight urged, and smoking stopped. Excessive alcohol use should be avoided, and a regular aerobic exercise program should be encouraged. Other risk factors such as abnormal lipids should be corrected. Patients with mild hypertension should not be overtreated and those with severe hypertension not undertreated. During therapy, the BP should be checked in both the supine and standing positions. The patient should be motivated and advised that it may take several months to control the BP and that therapy often is lifelong. It is difficult to convince asymptomatic patients that they need such long-term therapy. For better compliance, it is best not to change the patient's life-style drastically and to avoid drug therapy that produces undue reactions. Patients should be made aware of how the drugs work and what reactions can occur. The physician should convince the patient that he really is concerned about his welfare. In certain instances, for better control and compliance, a member of the family should be shown how to take the patient's BP. Twenty-four–hour ambulatory blood pressure recording devices are available, but are not recommended for the majority of patients. It may be of value in cases of marked lability in blood pressure, where it may help in therapeutic decisions.[28]

Despite the fact that studies have shown less morbidity and mortality if mild hypertension (diastolic pressure between 90 and 104 mm Hg) is treated pharmacologically, there is still concern among many of us using drug therapy as a first step and committing the patient to such long-term therapy. Our policy at present (unless the patient has some target organ damage) is to advise such patients to lose weight (if overweight), modify behavior, stop smoking, limit salt and saturated fat intake, control diabetes, and get a regular amount of exercise.[2] If the pressure is not reduced on such a program within 6 months, pharmacologic therapy is begun.

The stepped-care approach, as recommended by the 1984 report of the joint National Committee on Detection, Evaluation, and Treatment of High Blood Pressure, is still consistent with current treatment[29] (Table 5–5). However, there have been modifications since then, though the basic concept of progressing from nondrug therapy to drugs, then to drugs with few side effects, then to those with more significant risks has been retained. Initial therapy that was recommended was either a thiazide-type diuretic or a β-blocker, but recent evidence shows that in some cases angiotensin-converting enzymes (ACE) inhibitors and calcium blockers may be the best initial therapy. Such changes have come about because of the better understanding of the hemodynamic abnormalities associated with hypertension in different age groups, races, obese, and associated diseases. Now therapy can be better tailored to the individual patient. Young patients with a hyperadrenergic state (cardiac output increased, total peripheral resistance normal, plasma renin activity and norepinephrine levels increased) respond better to an alpha or β-blocker and ACE inhibitors. In older patients, cardiac output is decreased, peripheral vascular resistance is increased, and intravascular volume is contracted. In such patients, the response is better to diuretics and calcium blockers. Blacks respond like older patients except that their intravascular volume is not as contracted. Obese patients have an increase in cardiac output, greater intravascular volume, and lower total peripheral resistance than lean patients with the same level of blood pressure. Such patients respond to diuretics, but adrenergic inhibitors, calcium blockers, and ACE inhibitors are also effective.

The antihypertensive agents which are used today are the diuretics, adren-

Table 5–5. Individualized Stepped-Care Approach to Drug Therapy of Hypertension*

Step 1. Diuretic, β-blocker, calcium blocker, or ACE inhibitor. Begin with less than full dose.
Step 2. Increase dose of first drug or substitute another drug or Add a second drug of different class
Step 3. Substitute second drug or Add third drug of different class
Step 4. Add third or fourth drug

*See Table 5–6 for specific classes and dosages
Modified from the 1984 report of the joint National Committee on Detection, Evaluation, and Treatment of High Blood Pressure. *Arch. Intern. Med.* 144:1045, 1984.

ergic-blocking drugs, and vasodilators. The commonly used diuretics can be classified as thiazides, loop diuretics, and potassium-sparing diuretics (see Chap. 16). Their mechanism of antihypertensive action is due to sodium excretion with reduction in intravascular volume and lowering of the cardiac output. After a few weeks, the peripheral vascular resistance falls and cardiac output returns to normal. The fall in peripheral vascular resistance may be a direct effect or due to a reduction of sodium and water in the vessel wall. Plasma renin activity increases in response to the volume depletion that retards sodium diuresis, but the fall in peripheral vascular resistance continues. The side effects of the diuretics are similar; e.g., electrolyte depletion, hyperlipidemia, hyperuricemia, hyperglycemia, skin rashes, and blood dyscrasias. Potassium-sparing diuretics increase sodium excretion and retain potassium. These should be avoided in the presence of renal disease or when supplemental potassium is given because hyperkalemia may develop. Spironolactone (Aldactone) also can produce gynecomastia.

Adrenergic-blocking drugs can be classified depending on their site of action, which may be centrally upon receptors in the vasomotor centers, or peripherally upon the neurons or α- or β-receptors. Some may have multiple sites of action.

Alpha-methyldopa (Aldomet), clonidine (Catapres), and guanabenz are predominantly central agonists. Methyldopa probably lowers BP by means of releasing α-methyl-norepinephrine within the CNS, which by its alpha-adrenoreceptor stimulation, reduces the sympathetic outflow,[30] and thus peripheral resistance falls with little effect on the cardiac output. Clonidine acts at similar central sites.[31] Both of these drugs also lower plasma renin activity and renal perfusion is well maintained. Sedation, dryness of the mouth, orthostatic hypotension, and impotence are the most common side effects. Methyldopa can produce a positive ANA test in about 10%, a positive direct Coombs test in 10 to 20% of patients, and rarely associated hemolytic anemia. It also can cause fever, abnormal liver function tests, and hepatitis. Clonidine can produce a withdrawal reaction if it is stopped abruptly. Withdrawal symptoms are restlessness, insomnia, tremors, tachycardia, headache, abdominal pain, and rebound hypertension. Clonidine may also be a factor in producing high-grade AV block, especially if the patient is receiving digitalis.[32] Methyldopa and clonidine are best used with a diuretic, since they are associated with sodium and water retention. Guanabenz differs from the other drugs in this group by not causing fluid retention. It may reduce cholesterol.

Reserpine, guanethidine (Ismelin) and guanadrel (Hylorel) inhibit the release of norepinephrine from peripheral adrenergic neurons. Reserpine, to a less extent, depletes brain catecholamines, producing its major side effects of sedation and depression. Since the advent of more effective and better tolerated adrenergic-blocking drugs and a possible association with cancer[33] (although not proved), reserpine has lost much of its popularity. Tricyclic antidepressants, ephedrine, and amphetamines competitively block the uptake of guanethidine. Guanethidine does not enter the brain and it does not suppress renin activity (which other adrenergic blockers do). Its most common side effect is postural hypotension, since compensatory sympathetic vasoconstriction is blocked.[34] Its use has declined since the advent of β-blockers and vasodilator drugs. Guanadrel is similar to guanethidine but has a shorter duration of action and fewer side effects.

Prazosin (Minipress) is a selective antagonist of the postsynaptic α-receptors.[35] Since prazosin does not block the presynaptic α-receptors, the feedback for the inhibition of norepinephrine release is present and accounts for the absence of tachycardia and renin release. After the first dose, postural hypotension has been noted because of increased alpha tone or blunted renin reactivity.[36] Usually this can be avoided by giving less than 1 mg for the first dose and at bedtime. It also can produce dizziness, fatigue, and headache. Prazosin does not alter the lipids, an effect noted with diuretics and β-blockers.

Beta-blockers have been used extensively for hypertension, and there is a great variety of these agents available.[37] The BP falls in those without intrinsic sypathomimetic activity (ISA) because of the fall in cardiac output, renin release is reduced, and CNS β-blockade reduces sympathetic discharge. Initially, since α-adrenergic vasoconstriction is unopposed, the peripheral vascular resistance increases. Acebutolol and pindolol, ISA-β-blockers, have little effect on cardiac output and decrease total peripheral resistance and so reduce blood pressure. The β-blockers can be divided into the lipophilic types (propranolol, metoprolol, timolol, and pindolol) and the hydrophilic types (nadolol, acebutolol, and atenolol). The lipophilic types are absorbed well and cross the brain barrier. They are metabolized by the liver and have a plasma half-life of about 6 hours. The hydrophilic types are not absorbed well, do not cross the brain barrier, are excreted by the kidney, and have a half-life up to 24 hours. Metoprolol, atenolol, and acebutolol are cardioselective (affinity for β_1-adrenergic receptors); however, in high doses this selectivity is lost, and β_2-receptors can also be blocked. Pindolol and acebutolol have ISA and produce low levels of beta stimulation when sympathetic activity is low, whereas during stress and exercise, they act the same as the conventional beta blockers. With the patient at rest, these drugs cause little slowing of the heart rate. The β-blockers should not be given in the presence of congestive heart failure, greater than first-degree AV block, or in patients with chronic lung disease with asthmatic bronchitis. Beta-blockers can also mask and prolong hypoglycemia in diabetics and aggravate peripheral vascular disease. Metoprolol (Lopressor) and atenolol (Tenormin) have been used with some success in lower doses in patients with chronic lung disease, diabetes, or peripheral vascular disease. Sudden withdrawal of β-blockers, especially in patients with known coronary disease, can produce exaggerated cardiac β-adrenergic responsiveness with an increase in angina, precipitation of arrhythmias, or even acute myocardial infarction. The hydrophilic types may produce less fatigue and fewer cerebral symptoms, since they do not cross the brain barrier. However, because these are excreted by the kidney, their half-life can be prolonged in the presence of renal failure, and the dosage must be decreased and the interval of dosage increased. Beta-blockers rarely produce postural hypotension, but can produce impotence.

Labetalol has α- and β-blocking activity. Its α effect is greater. Blood pressure decrease is due to lowering of peripheral vascular resistance. It can produce postural hypotension, bronchospasm, and peripheral vascular insufficiency.

Vasodilators, because they reverse elevated peripheral vascular resistance, should be the ideal drugs for hypertension; however, their effects are limited because of the increased sympathetic activity (increased heart rate and cardiac output) and increased plasma renin activity (increased sodium and water retention). For these reasons they are best given with a β-blocker and a diuretic. Hydralazine (Apresoline) acts by direct relaxation of arteriolar smooth muscle and has little effect on venous capacitance.[38] Doses of this drug exceeding 300 to 400 mg can produce a syndrome resembling lupus erythematosus, especially more common in the slow acetylators of hydralazine. Minoxidil[39] has a similar action to hydralazine, but is more potent and is particularly effective in the treatment of accelerated or malignant hypertension in patients with renal failure. Hirsutism can occur with prolonged use. Initially reported cases of right atrial lesions in dogs and pulmonary hypertension in humans have not been confirmed.

Angiotensin-converting enzyme inhibitors (captopril, enalapril, lisinopril) have been found to be effective in hypertension and are well tolerated.[40-42] They inhibit the enzyme responsible for conversion of angiotensin I to the potent vasopressor angiotensin II and for breakdown of bradykinin (vasodepressor). They reduce filling pressures and systemic vascular resistance with little effect on heart rate, fluid volume, or cardiac output. Enalapril does not have a sulfhydryl group and is hydrolyzed to form the active enalaprilat; thus its onset of action is slower, but its duration of action longer. Lisinopril is not a prodrug like enalapril and has a long half-life up to 13 hours, which is longer than that of either enalapril or captopril. It can be given once per day. Side effects reported with ACE inhibitors have been proteinuria, hypotension (in severely volume-depleted persons), neutropenia, maculopapular skin rash, and alteration in taste. They can cause reversible acute renal failure in patients with bilateral renal artery stenosis or unilateral stenosis in a solitary kidney. Hyperkalemia can develop especially in patients with renal insufficiency and in patients also taking potassium-sparing agents. However, all of the side effects are rare, and these drugs have significantly fewer side effects than the other antihypertensive agents.

Calcium channel blockers (diltiazem, nifedipine, verapamil) are now being widely used for hypertension.[43] They reduce blood pressure by reducing arteriolar smooth muscle tone with resulting decrease in total peripheral resistance. These drugs do not produce expansion of the blood volume, thus obviating the need for diuretics, and are effective in elderly and black hypertensives. Their side reactions are few. Headache, constipation (namely with verapamil), and ankle edema and tachycardia (with nifedipine). Diltiazem and verapamil should not be used in the presence of heart block.

Table 5–6 lists the commonly used antihypertensive drugs with their dosages.

SPECIAL THERAPEUTIC CONSIDERATIONS

The stepped-care approach has been broadened to include other drugs for the initial step. Formerly, a diuretic or a β-blocker was the first choice, but now ACE inhibitors and calcium blockers are often used initially. As mentioned earlier in this chapter, therapy can be varied according to the hemodynamic differences noted in different age groups, races, the obese, and those with other

Table 5–6. Commonly Used Antihypertensive Drugs and Doses

Agents	Usual Dosage Range (mg/day)
Diuretics	
Thiazide and related diuretics	
Hydrochlorothiazide (Hydrodiuril, Oretic, Esidrix)	12.5–50
Chlorthalidone (Hygroton)	12.5–50
Metolazone (Zaroxolyn, Diulo)	1.25–10
Loop diuretics	
Furosemide (Lasix)	20–320
Bumetanide (Bumex)	0.5–5
Potassium-sparing diuretics	
Spironolactone (Aldactone)	25–100
Triamterene (Dyrenium)	50–150
Amioloride (Midamor)	5–10
Adrenergic Inhibitors	
Centrally acting α-blockers	
Clonidine (Catapres)	0.1–1.2
Clonidine TTS (Patch)	0.1–0.3
Guanabenz (Wytensin)	4–64
Methyldopa (Aldomet)	250–2000
Peripheral-acting adrenergic antagonists	
Guanadrel (Hylorel)	10–100
Guanethidine (Ismelin)	10–150
Reserpine (Serpasil)	0.1–0.25
α-1 adrenergic blockers	
Prazosin (Minipress)	1–20
Terazosin	1–20
β-adrenergic blockers	
Acebutolol (Sectral)	200–1200
Atenolol (Tenormin)	25–150
Metoprolol (Lopressor)	50–200
Nadolol (Corgard)	40–320
Pindolol (Visken)	10–60
Propranolol (Inderal)	40–320
Propanolol Long-Acting	60–320
Timolol (Blocadren)	20–80
Combined α and β-adrenergic blockers	
Labetalol (Normodyne, Trandate)	200–1800
Vasodilators	
Hydralazine (Apresoline)	50–300
Minoxidil (Loniten)	2.5–80
Ace inhibitors	
Captopril (Capoten)	25–300
Enalapril (Vasotec)	2.5–40
Lisinopril (Zestril)	5–40
Calcium antagonists	
Diltiazem (Cardizem)	60–360
Diltiazem SR	180–360
Nifedipine (Procardia)	30–180
Verapamil (Calan, Isoptin)	120–480
Verapamil SR	120–480

associated diseases. Younger patients respond better to β-blockers and ACE inhibitors. Older patients, blacks, and the obese respond better to diuretics and calcium blockers. If congestive heart failure occurs in the hypertensive, the ACE inhibitors are the drugs of choice. β-blockers or calcium blockers may be best in those who have hypertension and angina. β-blockers should be avoided if possible in patients with peripheral vascular disease, calcium blockers and ACE inhibitors being preferable. They should also be avoided in patients with asthma and chronic obstructive lung disease. β-blockers with ISA (pindolol, acebutolol) and the cardioselective types[44] (metoprolol, atenolol), have no or little adverse effects on the lipids. In fact, a study by Samuel et al.[45] showed improvement in the lipid profile during long-term treatment with pindolol and hydrochlorothiazide in patients with hypertension. β-blockers that do not have these activities (nonselective types such as propranolol) and diuretics adversely effect the lipids. Calcium blockers do not adversely effect the lipids. Alpha-1-blocker (prazosin) and central adrenergic agonists (clonidine, guanabenz, methyldopa) may decrease serum cholesterol. ACE inhibitors may become the first-line drugs for the hypertensive diabetic because of the renal protective effect and the lack of aggravation of glucose control and lipids.

Isolated systolic hypertension occurs more frequently in the elderly. If the systolic pressure remains consistently 160 mm/Hg or greater, and the diastolic is less than 90 mm Hg despite nonpharmacologic therapy, antihypertensive drugs should be given.[46] Some elderly hypertensive patients with severe concentric cardiac hypertrophy, excellent systolic function, and abnormal diastolic function as noted by echocardiography respond better to either β-blockers or calcium blockers.[46a]

There are many drug interactions with antihypertensive agents. Diuretics can raise lithium blood levels; aspirin may antagonize the effects of diuretics and magnify the potassium retaining effects of ACE inhibitors; ACE inhibitors may increase potassium with the potassium-sparing drugs; ephedrine, amphetamine, tricyclic antidepressants, and cocaine may reduce the action of guanithidine and guanadrel; tricyclic antidepressants may reduce the effects of clonidine; cimetidine may reduce the bioavailability of β-blockers that are metabolized by the liver and increase blood levels of nifedipine; hydralazine may increase the plasma concentration of β-blockers; and calcium antagonists may increase plasma digoxin levels.

After 1 to 3 months of therapy, if the response to the initial drug is inadequate, one has three choices: increase the dose of the first drug to the maximum, add another agent, or discontinue the first choice and substitute another drug. Combining drugs with different actions may allow smaller doses of each to control the blood pressure and thus minimize side effects. After blood pressure is controlled, comparable combination tablets can be substituted to simplify the regimens, promote adherence, and reduce cost.

HYPERTENSIVE EMERGENCIES

A hypertensive crisis is characterized by a sudden rise in both systolic and diastolic blood pressure (usually diastolic over 140 mm Hg). Hypertensive emergencies can occur in patients who have either essential or malignant hypertension as well as in patients who have previously been normotensive. In

Table 5–7.   Dosage of Drugs Used in Hypertensive Emergencies

Drug	Dosage
Sodium nitroprusside	0.5–10 mg/kg/min I.V. infusion
Diazoxide	50–150 mg I.V. bolus, repeated, or 15–30 mg/min I.V. infusion
Hydralazine	10–20 mg I.V. 10–50 mg I.M.
Nitroglycerin	5–100 µg/min I.V. infusion
Phentolamine	5–15 mg I.V.
Trimethaphan	1–4 mg I.V. infusion
Labetalol	20–80 mg I.V. bolus q 10 min, 2 mg/min I.V. infusion
Methyldopa	250–500 mg I.V. infusion

addition, it has been noted in patients with renal disease (acute or chronic glomerulonephritis, renal vascular hypertension, and pyelonephritis), collagen diseases, toxemia of pregnancy, pheochromocytoma, dissecting aneurysm, and patients taking monoamine oxidase inhibitors who are also consuming tyramine-containing foods (aged cheese, beer, wine, chicken livers) or taking sympathomimetic drugs or amphetamines. Pargyline (Eutonyl), phenelzine (Nardil), isocarboxazid (Marplan), and tranylcypromine (Parnate) are some of the monoamine oxidase inhibitors. The hypertensive crisis may present with cerebral findings (encephalopathy, intracranial hemorrhage), cardiac findings (acute pulmonary edema), renal findings (oliguria, uremia), or GI tract findings (nausea, vomiting).

The aim of therapy is to reduce the BP as quickly as possible without compromising any organ function, especially if there is associated renal or cardiac disease. The BP should be monitored with an intra-arterial line. The following drugs are used: diazoxide (Hyperstat), trimethaphan (Arfonad), sodium nitroprusside (Nipride), methyldopa, hydralazine, nitroglycerin, and labetalol. Sodium nitroprusside is a most effective agent. The antihypertensive effect is noted within minutes, and the BP usually rises immediately when it is stopped. Diazoxide can produce tachycardia, hypotension, and cerebral or myocardial ischemia. Table 5–7 outlines the usual dosage of these drugs. The choice of therapy may vary depending on the etiology of the hypertensive crisis, e.g., phentolamine (Regitine) is given for pheochromocytoma crises and for crises associated with monoamine oxidase inhibitors. Fifty percent magnesium sulfate is often used I.M. in repeated doses for the convulsions of toxemia of pregnancy along with the antihypertensive therapy (hydralazine is often preferred). After the treatment of hypertensive crises, long-term therapy should be started. With all types of emergency therapy (vasodilators or antiadrenergic) there is associated sodium and water retention, and diuretics are necessary.

The hypertensive emergency of dissecting aneurysm will be discussed in Chapter 10.

REFERENCES

1. Hypertension prevalence and the Status of Awareness, Treatment, and Control in the United States: Final report of the subcommittee on definition and prevalence of the 1984 Joint National Committee. *Hypertension* 7:457, 1985.
2. The 1988 Report of the Joint National Committee on Detection, Evaluation, and Treatment of High Blood Pressure. *Arch. Intern. Med.* 148:May, 1988.
3. Sagnella G.A., Shore A.C., Markandu N.D., et al.: Raised level of atrial natriuretic peptides in essential hypertension. *Lancet* 1:179, 1986.
4. Helmer O.M.: Renin activity in blood from patients with hypertension. *Can. Med. Assoc. J.* 90:221, 1964.
5. Laragh J.H.: Vasoconstriction-volume analysis for understanding and treating hypertension: The use of renin and aldosterone profiles. *Am. J. Med.* 55:261, 1973.
6. Fagard R., Amery A., Reybrouck T., et al.: Plasma renin levels and systemic hemodynamics in essential hypertension. *Clin. Sci. Mol. Med.* 52:591, 1977.
7. London G.M., Safer M.E., Weiss Y.A., et al.: Relationship of plasma renin activity and aldosterone level with hemodynamic functions in essential hypertension. *Arch. Intern. Med.* 137:1042, 1977.
8. Frohlich E.D.: Hypertension in the elderly. *Curr. Prob. Cardiol.* 13:319, 1988.
9. Wenting G.J., Tan-Tsiong H.L., Derkx F.H.M., et al.: Split renal function after captopril in unilateral renal artery stenosis. *Br. Med. J.* 288:886, 1984.
10. Muller F.B., Sealey J.E., Case D.B., et al.: The captopril test for identifying renovascular disease in hypertension patients. *Am. J. Med.* 80:633, 1986.
11. Marks L.S., Maxwell M.H., Varady P.D., et al.: Renovascular hypertension: Does the renal vein ratio predict operative results? *J. Urol.* 115:365, 1976.
12. Weinberger M.H., Yune H.Y., Grim C.E., et al.: Percutaneous transluminal angioplasty for renal artery stenosis in a solitary functioning kidney. *Ann. Intern. Med.* 91:684, 1979.
13. Kaufman J.S.: Pheochromocytoma and tricyclic antidepressants. *JAMA* 229:1282, 1974.
14. Dunn F.G., DeCarvalho J.G.R., Kem D.C., et al.: Pheochromocytoma crisis induced by saralasin: Relation of angiotensin analogue to catecholamine release. *N. Engl. J. Med.* 295:605, 1976.
15. Remine W.H., Chong G.C., VanHeerden J.A., et al.: Current management of pheochromocytoma. *Ann. Surg.* 179:740, 1974.
16. Bravo E.L., Gifford R.W.: Pheochromocytoma: Diagnosis, localization, and management. *N. Engl. J. Med.* 311:1298, 1984.
17. Engleman K., Horwitz D., Jequiere E., et al.: Biochemical and pharmacologic effects of alpha-methyl-tyrosine in man. *J. Clin. Invest.* 47:577, 1968.
18. Epstein M.T., Espiner E.A., Donald R.A., et al.: Effect of eating liquorice on the renin-angiotensin aldosterone axis in normal subjects. *Br. Med. J.* 1:488, 1977.
19. Ferris J.B., Beevers D.G., Boddy K., et al.: The treatment of low-renin (primary) hyperaldosteronism. *Am. Heart. J.* 96:97, 1978.
20. Oral Contraceptive Study of the Royal College of General Practitioners: Hypertension, in *Oral Contraceptives and Health.* New York, Pitman Publishing Corp., 1974, p. 37.
21. Effects of treatment on morbidity in hypertension: I. Results in patients with diastolic blood pressure averaging 115 through 129 mm Hg. Veterans Administration Cooperative Study Group on Antihypertensive Agents. *JAMA* 202:1028, 1967.
22. Effects of treatment on morbidity in hypertension: II. Results in patients with diastolic blood pressure averaging 90 through 114 mm Hg. Veterans Administration Cooperative Study Group on Antihypertensive Agents. *JAMA* 213:1143, 1970.
23. *Professional Education: Report of Task Force II to the Hypertension Information and Education Advisory Committee.* National High Blood Pressure Education Program, National Heart and Lung Institute. Sept. 1, 1973.
24. Kannel W.B.: Systolic versus diastolic blood pressure and risk of coronary heart disease: The Framingham Study. *Am. J. Cardiol.* 27:335, 1971.
25. Five-year findings of the hypertension detection and follow-up program: 1. Reduction in mortality of persons with high blood pressure, including mild hypertension. *JAMA* 242:2562, 1979.
26. Hartford M., Wendelhag I., Berglund G., et al.: Cardiovascular and renal effects of long-term antihypertensive treatment. *JAMA* 259:2553, 1988.
27. MacMahon S.W., Cutler J.A., Furberg C.D., et al.: The effects of drug treatment for hypertension on morbidity and mortality from cardiovascular disease. A review of randomized controlled trials. *Progress Cardiovasc. Dis.* 24(3, Suppl. 1):99, 1986.
28. Hunt J.C., Frolich E.D., Moser M., et al.: Devices used for self-measurement of blood pressure: Revised statement of the National High Blood Pressure Education Program. *Arch. Intern. Med.* 145:2231, 1985.

29. The 1984 Report of the Joint National Committee on Detection, Evaluation, and Treatment of High Blood Pressure. *Arch. Intern. Med.* 144:1045, 1984.
30. Haeusler G.: Cardiovascular regulation by central adrenergic mechanisms and its alteration by hypotensive drugs. *Circ. Res.* 37(suppl. 1):1, 1975.
31. Pettinger W.A.: Clonidine, a new antihypertensive drug. *N. Engl. J. Med.* 293:1179, 1975.
32. Kibler L.E., Gazes P.C.: Effect of clonidine on atrioventricular conduction. *JAMA* 238:1930, 1977.
33. Reserpine and breast cancer. Report from the Boston Collaborative Drug Surveillance Program. *Lancet* 2:669, 1974.
34. Boura A.L., Green A.F.: Adrenergic neurone blocking agents. *Ann. Rev. Pharmacol. Toxicol.* 5:183, 1965.
35. Graham R.M., Oates H.F., Stoker L.M., et al.: Alpha-blocking action of the antihypertensive agent, prazosin. *J. Pharmacol. Exp. Ther.* 201:747, 1977.
36. Nicholson J.P., Resnick L.M., Pickering T.G., et al.: Relationship of blood pressure response and the renin-angiotension system to first-dose prazosin. *Am. J. Med.* 78:241, 1985.
37. Frishman W.H.: Recent advances in beta-adrenoceptor blocker pharmacology. *Council Clin. Cardiol. Newsletter* 9:1, 1983.
38. Koch-Weser J.: The vasodilator antihypertensives. *Drug Ther.* 5:67, 1975.
39. Mitchell H.C., Pettinger W.A.: A long-term treatment of refractory hypertensive patients with minoxidil. *JAMA* 239:2131, 1978.
40. Frohlich E.D., Cooper R.A., Lewis E.J.: Review of the overall experience of captopril in hypertension. *Arch. Intern. Med.* 144:1441, 1984.
41. Todd P.A., Heel R.C.: Enalapril. A review of the pharmacodynamic and pharmacokinetic properties, and therapeutic use in hypertension and congestive heart failure. *Drugs* 31:198, 1986.
42. Gomez H.J., Cirillo V.J., Moncloa F.: The clinical pharmacology of lisinopril. *J. Cardiovasc. Pharmacol.* 9:S27, 1987.
43. Agabiti-Rosei A, Muiesan M.L., Romanelli G., et al.: Similarities and differences in the antihypertensive effect of two calcium antagonist drugs, verapamil and nifedipine. *J. Am. Coll. Cardiol.* 7:916, 1986.
44. Wikstrand J., Warnold I., Olsson G., et al.: Primary prevention with metoprolol in patients with hypertension. *JAMA* 259:1976, 1988.
45. Samuel P., Chin B., Fenderson R.W., et al.: Improvement of the lipid profile during long-term administration of Pindolol and hydrochlorothiazide in patients with hypertension. *Am. J. Cardiol.* 57:24C, 1986.
46. Working group on hypertension in the elderly. National Blood Pressure Education Program, Statement on Hypertension in the elderly. *JAMA* 256:70, 1986.
46a. Topol E.J., Traill T.A., and Fortuin N.J.: Hypertensive hypertrophic cardiomyopathy of the elderly. *N. Engl. J. Med.* 312:277, 1985.

Chapter 6

RHEUMATIC FEVER AND VALVULAR HEART DISEASE

ACUTE RHEUMATIC FEVER

Rheumatic fever, although the incidence has decreased, is still responsible for most acquired heart disease in childhood. It occurs most frequently between the ages of 5 and 15 years, is uncommon under 5, and rarely occurs under age 2. However, it can also occur in the adult population. It is related to prior infection with group A β-hemolytic streptococci,[1] but the exact mechanism has not been clarified. A hyperimmune reaction due to bacterial allergy or to autoimmunity is probably a factor. However, the dilemma is whether the myocardial lesions are the result of autoimmunity induced by streptococcal antigens or the myocardial damage produced the immunologic reaction. In addition, the surface structure of the streptococcal cell (such as the M proteins) is a virulence factor. The M proteins also form the basis for the system of classification of group A streptococci into types. Group A streptococci must infect the pharynx, for other sites of infection will not cause rheumatic fever.

A typical history of a preceding streptococcal infection occurring 1 to 4 weeks before the onset of rheumatic fever may be obtained. Streptococcal throat infections may be asymptomatic, and many sore throats have other causes. However, asymptomatic streptococcal infections are not likely to produce rheumatic fever. In epidemics of β-hemolytic streptococcal throat infections, 3% develop acute rheumatic fever, and with endemic infections, only 0.3% occur.[2,3] An individual's susceptibility is probably an important factor in accounting for the low percentage.

There has been a further decrease in the incidence of rheumatic fever during the past several years, probably due to early recognition and treatment of streptococcal infections and to better living conditions. Usually an attack of rheumatic fever can be aborted if the streptococcal throat infection is treated with penicillin during the first 10 days after the onset of symptoms.

Diffuse exudative and proliferative inflammatory reactions occur in the heart, joints, and skin during the acute phase of rheumatic fever. As a result, the clinical syndrome of acute rheumatic fever is characterized by major and minor manifestations as originally proposed by Jones and subsequently revised by a committee of the American Heart Association.[4] The major manifestations are polyarthritis, carditis, chorea, subcutaneous nodules and erythema marginatum. The minor manifestations are fever, arthralgia, prior rheumatic fever or rheumatic heart disease, first-degree AV block, and elevation of phase reactants (sedimentation rate, C-reactive protein). In addition, there must be supporting evidence of preceding group A streptococcal infection (increased antistreptolysin-O, other streptococcal antibodies, positive throat culture for group A streptococcus, or recent scarlet fever). Fulminating acute rheumatic fever with high fever, severe carditis, and prominent migratory arthritis is infrequent.

MAJOR MANIFESTATIONS

Arthritis

The polyarthritis is often migratory. One or more joints (usually the larger ones) may be red, tender, and swollen and often show improvement within 24 hours and leave no sequelae. Migratory polyarthralgia (a minor criterion) is more common and should not be mistaken for a major criterion.

Carditis

Carditis can be characterized by a significant murmur, cardiomegaly, pericarditis, or congestive heart failure. It usually occurs in 40 to 50% of first attacks and within the first 3 weeks of an attack. Severe polyarthritis and severe cardiac involvement are usually not seen in the same patient.[5] Severe carditis is rare in the adult. Carditis is a most important finding, with many pitfalls in its recognition. Young children often have a short, early, or midsystolic vibratory innocent murmur heard best between the sternum and apex, and teenagers often have a short ejection, scratchy-type innocent systolic murmur in the pulmonic area. Because of these functional murmurs, a child with a history of sore throat is often erroneously suspected of having rheumatic fever.

The most common murmur of acute rheumatic fever is an apical pansystolic murmur, regardless of the intensity. This significant apical systolic murmur of mitral insufficiency may be accompanied by a short, low-pitched, mid-diastolic rumbling murmur at the apex (Carey-Coombs murmur) presumably due to "relative" mitral stenosis caused by dilatation of the left ventricle. The presence of this latter murmur aids in confirming the significance of the organic nature of the systolic murmur and suggests active carditis. This diastolic murmur often is transient but may be the forerunner of later mitral stenosis. A basal diastolic high-pitched murmur of aortic insufficiency, although less common, also is diagnostic of carditis. At times during the active stage the murmurs from the mitral and aortic valves may be cooing or very high-pitched, simulating a "sea gull" cry. Murmurs during the acute phase of rheumatic fever may clear and do not necessarily indicate permanent damage. This is especially true for the apical mitral systolic murmur but is less likely for the aortic diastolic murmur. Systolic murmurs in the region of the outflow tract of the pulmonic area or in the aortic area are not usually attributable to acute rheumatic fever. Children and young adults with hyperkinetic circulations often have a systolic bruit over the carotid, subclavian, or innominate arteries which may radiate to the upper chest. These often are mistaken for significant murmurs.

Pericarditis is unusual as the sole manifestation of acute rheumatic carditis and is usually associated with endocarditis and myocarditis. A pericardial effusion may mask the endocarditis. The murmurs of mitral insufficiency or aortic insufficiency may become audible only after the effusion clears.

Chorea

Chorea (Sydenham's) produces involuntary movements and facial grimaces. Today it occurs rarely. It may be the only manifestation of rheumatic fever and usually occurs long after the streptococcal throat infection has subsided. In such cases fever may be absent and the phase reactants may be normal, unless there is associated arthritis or carditis. Chorea is often first recognized by the parents. They note that the child begins dropping articles and shows a lack of coordination, especially on being asked to perform a specific act. Chorea is seldom seen in adults except during pregnancy. Patients who apparently had chorea as an isolated entity often have rheumatic heart disease in later years.[6]

Subcutaneous Nodules

Subcutaneous nodules are rarely seen today. They develop on the extensor surface of the elbows, knees, or wrists, or on any bony prominence, and vary in size from the diameter of a pinhead to about 2 cm. The olecranon area is most frequently involved. The skin moves freely over these nodules, and they are nontender. They eventually disappear, often in less than 1 month.

Erythema Marginatum

Erythema marginatum is confined primarily to the trunk and arms and is not on the face. It is often transient and can recur long after the acute phase of rheumatic fever has subsided. The lesions expand centrifugally while the skin in their centers returns to normal. It occurs in about 2 to 10% of patients and appears only in those with carditis.

MINOR MANIFESTATIONS PLUS EVIDENCE OF STREPTOCOCCAL INFECTION

The minor manifestations are nonspecific. Fever, prolonged P-R interval, and elevated sedimentation rate are seen in many diseases. A high titer of antibody to one or more streptococcal antigens (antistreptolysin-O, antistreptokinase, antihyaluronidase, anti-DPNase, and anti-DNase) is indicative of an antecedent streptococcal infection. In recent years the antistreptozyme test (ASTZ) has been used as a screening test before doing the ASO study. It is a hemagglutination reaction to extracellular streptococcal antigens absorbed to red cells and is a sensitive indicator of streptococcal infection. Patients with acute rheumatic fever usually have a level over 200 Todd units per ml.[7] The sore throat may be severe and the cultures positive for the streptococcus; however, acute rheumatic fever occurs only if the antistreptococcal antibody titers rise. A significant titer of ASO is usually 250 or more Todd units in adults and 333 in children over 5 years of age.[4] It begins to rise in about 1 week after the streptococcal infection, reaches a peak in 3 to 4 weeks, and returns to normal in 2 to 4 months. Other antistreptococcal titers reach peak levels at various times, with the anti-DNase remaining positive the longest. Antistreptolysin-O titer will rise in 80 to 85% of patients with acute rheumatic fever. Streptococcal antibodies should always be increased with acute rheumatic fever, unless the fever is noted many months after the pharyngeal infection. This can occur when chorea is the only manifestation or with chronic rheumatic carditis. The degree of rheumatic activity is not related to the increased streptococcal antibodies, and the course of the rheumatic attack is not related to their decline.[8]

The presence of two major criteria or one major and two minor criteria is considered to indicate a high probability of the presence of rheumatic fever, especially if there is evidence of a preceding streptococcal infection. These criteria have been important in directing attention to the diagnosis of acute rheumatic fever. However, on occasion they are inadequate, since certain minor criteria are almost a prerequisite to making a diagnosis. For example, fever is a minor criterion, yet it is essential for the diagnosis because rarely is it absent. Likewise, an elevated sedimentation rate or a positive C-reactive protein (CRP) are important adjuncts to the diagnosis. Combinations of polyarthritis (major), fever, and elevated sedimentation rate (two minor criteria) are rather weak diagnostic findings, since these can occur with many conditions, such as rheumatoid arthritis, streptococcal arthritis, and many others. Subcutaneous nodules and erythema marginatum are most specific for acute rheumatic fever but are uncommon. Overdiagnosis occurs most often because of the misinterpretation of the signs and symptoms of carditis and arthritis. Functional systolic murmurs are considered organic, P-R-interval prolongation is overemphasized, and arthralgia is mistaken for arthritis. Also, because streptococcal infections are so common, they often occur by chance with an unrelated disease. However, if two clear-cut major or one major and two minor criteria and evidence of a preceding streptococcal infection are present, acute rheumatic fever should be high on the diagnostic list.

DIFFERENTIAL DIAGNOSIS

Rheumatoid arthritis, systemic lupus erythematosus (SLE), gonococcal arthritis, viral carditis, infective endocarditis, atrial myxoma, and sickle cell anemia are some of the conditions that may be confused with acute rheumatic fever. Polyarthritis as the only major criterion causes the greatest difficulty in diagnosis. If the time interval is not too long and streptococccal antibodies have not increased, rheumatic fever is unlikely. Initially the arthritis of rheumatoid arthritis can resemble that of rheumatic fever; however, the rheumatoid arthritis will not clear rapidly, and often deformities of the joints develop. A trial of therapy may help to clear the diagnosis; e.g., gonococcal arthritis responds rapidly to penicillin. Viral carditis may present with cardiomegaly, pericarditis, murmurs, and heart failure and may resemble rheumatic fever, yet the streptococcal antibodies should not rise unless it happens coincidentally. Viral antibodies may be helpful. Blood cultures and hemoglobin electrophoresis should indicate whether the problem is infective endocarditis or sickle cell anemia. Echocardiography has made the determination of atrial myxoma easy.

TREATMENT

Chemoprophylaxis

Streptococcal throat infections should be treated. A beefy red throat with an exudate, tender anterior cervical nodes, and fever are the usual features.

Other suggestive signs are excoriated nares and a scarlatiniform rash (scarlet fever). A throat culture should be taken for identification of the organism. The perplexing problem is that a streptococcal infection at times may be asymptomatic, and, in addition, there are many other causes for sore throat. In the absence of a throat culture, it is often difficult to decide whether an antibiotic should be given. Some contend that an antibiotic, especially penicillin, should be given for all upper respiratory infections in the event that any of these are due to streptococcus. Therefore, eradication would prevent attacks of rheumatic fever.

Naturally, this brings up the problem of the many side reactions which are caused by the indiscriminate use of antibiotics. Most authorities agree that throat cultures should be taken prior to treatment. However, there are occasions when the practicing physician may not be able to obtain a culture and may have to use his clinical judgment and begin treatment if the picture is typical of streptococcal pharyngitis, especially if the patient is in a toxic state. One can wait several days for cultures if the cases are mild, for short delays prior to treatment do not interfere with rheumatic fever prevention. Once a streptococcal throat infection has been identified, penicillin is the drug of choice. The recommended schedule by the Rheumatic Fever Committee of the Council on Rheumatic Fever of the American Heart Association[9] is as follows: (1) for children weighing less than 60 lb: one I.M. injection of 600,000 units of benzathine penicillin; (2) for those weighing over 60 lb: one I.M. injection of 1.2 million units of benzathine penicillin. Oral therapy with penicillin V can also be used. The dosage for both children and adults is 125 to 250 mg three or four times daily for a full 10 days. If the patient is noncompliant or is in a family unit where rheumatic fever has occurred or is at a substantial risk, the preferred treatment should be by the intramuscular route. Combinations of oral and I.M. penicillin should be effective, provided adequate coverage is continued for 10 days. If patients are sensitive to penicillin, erythromycin (1 g daily) is the second best choice. This should be given for 10 days. Tetracyclines are not recommended because of the high prevalence of strains resistant to this antibiotic. In addition, antibiotic troches and lozenges also are inadequate for the treatment of streptococcal infections. Prophylaxis is recommended for patients who have well-documented rheumatic fever (including those with only chorea) and for those who have evidence of rheumatic heart disease. Prophylaxis after the first attack of rheumatic fever is essential, since more than half of those who have recurrences develop heart disease. Monthly benzathine penicillin injections of 1.2 million units usually are recommended. This is the most efficient and effective regimen. Alternatives are penicillin V, 125 to 250 mg orally twice per day, or 1 g of oral sulfadiazine daily for patients weighing over 60 lb, and 0.5 g once a day for patients under 60 lb. Patients taking sulfadiazine should have a CBC after 2 weeks or if a rash develops, because if the white blood cell count falls below 4,000/cu mm, the drug should be discontinued. Prophylaxis with sulfonamides is contraindicated in late pregnancy. These agents may cross the placenta and compete with bilirubin for neonatal albumin-binding sites. If the patient is sensitive to both penicillin and the sulfa drugs, erythromycin (250 mg twice daily) can be given. Authorities' opinions vary as to the length of time chemoprophylaxis should be continued. Generally, if there is no heart involvement, it should be given for a minimum of 5 years or up to 18 years of age. Thereafter, all throat infections should be cultured and treated appropriately. Most agree that prophylaxis should be given indefinitely, or certainly for the period of highest risk, if rheumatic heart disease is present. The decision as to the duration of prophylaxis should include the patient's risk of acquiring streptococcal infections (high-risk patients include young children, teachers, physicians, nurses, and others living in crowded situations). Prophylaxis should also be given to patients with rheumatic heart disease even after prosthetic valve replacement, for such patients remain at risk of developing recurrence of rheumatic fever.

There have been many attempts to develop an antistreptococcal vaccine. M proteins, the only streptococcal components that elicit protective antibodies, have been extensively studied. However, attempts to obtain preparations that are both highly antigenic and well tolerated have failed. Such studies continue and eventually should lead to a nontoxic streptococcal vaccine.[10]

Treatment of Acute Rheumatic Fever

Even though there have been several studies comparing salicylate therapy with that of steroids, there is still no agreement as to the best type of therapy. The majority agree that salicylates are satisfactory for those who have no clear evidence of carditis and that steroids should be given if there is severe carditis (cardiomegaly or failure). Patients with mild carditis are also often given steroids, but there is no evidence that they are superior to salicylates. Steroids reduce fever and suppress symptoms and also eliminate subcutaneous nodules. There is no evidence that steroids lessen the degree of cardiac damage. However, prednisone is usually given in fairly large doses in the severely ill patient. Generally 40 to 60 mg of prednisone is given daily for the first 2 to 3 weeks. Subsequently, the dosage is reduced by 5 to 10 mg every 2 or 3 days until eliminated. Some physicians also prefer to combine the prednisone with salicylates. Standard doses of aspirin can be added as the prednisone is being tapered. In the absence of severe carditis (marked cardiomegaly or failure), salicylates can be given initially. For children, one can start with a dose of 100 to 150 mg/kg and for adults 6 to 8 g daily in divided doses. Therapy with salicylates is usually continued for 6 to 12 weeks. The sedimentation rate is used by many as a guide to the length of therapy. When doses are reduced, if relapse occurs, it may be necessary to return to the previous higher dosage. Bed and chair rest are recommended. However, once the severe signs of arthritis and carditis have disappeared, the patient is allowed up. Bathroom privileges are given as early as possible. Generally the patients are confined until the acute phase reactants return to normal. This occurs most often in 2 to 3 months. Sedatives and tranquilizers are used during the active phase of chorea.

The cardiac manifestations of acute rheumatic fever are important and will be described in detail with the subsequent clinical sequelae. The mitral and aortic valves most often are involved. The tricuspid valve is rarely involved, and the pulmonic valve almost never. Other nonrheumatic valvular lesions will be presented in this chapter so that these may be compared with those produced by rheumatic fever.

MITRAL VALVE DISEASE

Mitral Insufficiency

Etiology. Rheumatic fever until recently was considered almost the sole cause of mitral insufficiency. However, more sophisticated studies and pathologic disorders found at surgery have disclosed a number of other important causes depending on the portion of the mitral valve apparatus (leaflets, anulus, chordae, and papillary muscle) involved.[11] In addition, these can produce acute mitral insufficiency, chronic mitral insufficiency, or a combination and so vary the clinical picture. Other causes of chronic mitral insufficiency are mitral valve prolapse, coronary artery disease, calcified mitral anulus, connective tissue diseases, cardiomyopathies, congenital lesions, and any causes for left ventricular enlargement. Acute mitral insufficiency can occur because of rupture of the chordae or papillary muscle or perforation of the mitral valve.

Rheumatic mitral insufficiency. It is difficult to make a diagnosis of rheumatic mitral insufficiency without having associated aortic valve involvement or a good history of acute rheumatic fever. Rheumatic fever most commonly involves the mitral valve, with resultant residual insufficiency, stenosis, or both. Diffuse exudative, fibrinoid degeneration and proliferative inflammatory reactions occur in the heart during the acute phase of rheumatic fever. Fibrinoid degeneration occurs in the collagen of the connective tissues. This, along with the exudative phase, lasts about 2 to 3 weeks and is followed by the development of the myocardial Aschoff nodules. The proliferative and healing phase follows and continues for months. Aschoff nodules persist for many years after all clinical and laboratory evidence of acute rheumatic activity subsides. They have been demonstrated in biopsies of the left atrial appendage during mitral valve surgery. In rheumatic mitral insufficiency scarring, there is calcification, and retraction of the valve leaflets and shortening and fusion of the papillary muscles and chordae tendineae. When mitral valve closure is incomplete, mitral regurgitation develops. Therefore, the left ventricle has to eject blood into the aorta and also through the insufficient mitral valve into the left atrium. The volume of blood regurgitated will determine the clinical picture.[12] A small leak may produce a loud murmur but no change in heart size or any ECG changes. If the regurgitation volume is great, the left atrium and left ventricle enlarge. Eventually, there may be total heart enlargement. The left atrium may become huge; in fact, it can become larger than the rest of the heart. Clinically, with moderate or severe degrees of regurgitation, beside the high-pitched, blowing, usually holosystolic apical murmur radiating over the precordium into the left axilla and back, there is a marked lift in the left parasternal region[13] (left atrial lift) and a prominent hyperdynamic apical impulse with a left ventricular lift. The atrial lift is more delayed in systole than that of right ventricular enlargement and falls off more rapidly. The murmur does not vary significantly during respiration. It also does not change with variations in the cardiac cycles. The first heart sound may be diminished, and because the duration of systole may be shortened, there can be splitting of the second sound due to the early aortic valve closure. In addition, a prominent third heart sound may be present because of rapid filling of the left ventricle in early diastole. This filling wave may be palpable in early diastole.

Atrial fibrillation usually develops in the later stages. The murmur of tricuspid insufficiency may be confused with mitral insufficiency, but is usually best heard at the lower left sternal border and does not radiate well to the left. It is louder with inspiration and is often associated with other findings of tricuspid insufficiency, such as prominent systolic neck vein pulsations and a prominent systolic liver pulsation. Tricuspid insufficiency most often is secondary to lesions that produce pulmonary hypertension.

Mild or moderate mitral insufficiency may not produce symptoms for many years. However, the development of ruptured chordae or bacterial endocarditis may change the picture suddenly into a more severe type with prominent symptoms. Usually, unless these two hazards develop, the patient will remain asymptomatic until the left ventricle begins to decompensate. Once this occurs, symptoms of fatigue, exertional dyspnea, and at times orthopnea develop. The onset of atrial fibrillation may aggravate the failure and make the patient aware of palpitation. The ECG will show left atrial enlargement until atrial fibrillation develops. The fibrillatory waves may be coarse in the atrial fibrillation of mitral insufficiency. Subsequently left ventricular hypertrophy will be evident. Chest x rays confirm a prominent left atrium, which produces a long indentation on the barium-filled esophagus. Biventricular enlargement is present, and the pulmonary arteries are slightly prominent. An echocardiogram will show an enlarged left atrium and an enlarged left ventricle with increased systolic motion of these chambers (Fig 6–1). Doppler echocardiography shows a high-velocity jet into the left atrium during systole. The distance of the jet into the left atrium cannot be used to estimate degree of mitral regurgitation. This method has been known to both underestimate and overestimate the severity. A study by Helmcke et al.[14] using color flow Doppler to assess mitral regurgitation as compared to angiographic studies showed a sensitivity and specificity of color Doppler detecting mitral regurgitation of 100%. This study also concluded that color Doppler provides an accurate estimation of the severity of mitral regurgitation. The regurgitation jet area expressed as a percentage of the left atrial area (a maximum obtained from three orthogonal planes) indicated that under 20% was consistent with mild regurgitation, between 20% and 40% moderate, and greater than 40% severe. A pulsed Doppler flow study of the patient in Figure 6–2 detected mitral regurgitation to the posterior left atrial wall. Color flow Doppler of another patient (Fig 6–3) was consistent with significant regurgitation with a ratio of the left atrial regurgitant jet area to the left atrial area of 50%. This ratio was obtained from the average of three orthogonal views. In this same patient (Fig 6–4), there was tricuspid regurgitation from which the right ventricular systolic pressure was estimated to be 35 mm Hg. The following equation can be used to estimate the peak right ventricular systolic pressure (RVSP) when tricuspid regurgitation is present: $RVSP = 4 (Vmax)^2 + 10$ (estimated right atrial pressure) where the Vmax is the maximal velocity of the tricuspid regurgitant jet in systole as demonstrated by continuous wave Doppler. In the absence of pulmonic stenosis, this estimated RVSP is equal to the pulmonary artery systolic pressure. Because mitral regurgitation may be markedly affected by systolic pressure, serial studies used to compare the severity of regurgitation at different dates should be obtained at similar systolic blood pressures. Because of this and other hemodynamic and technical factors, at present quantitations of regur-

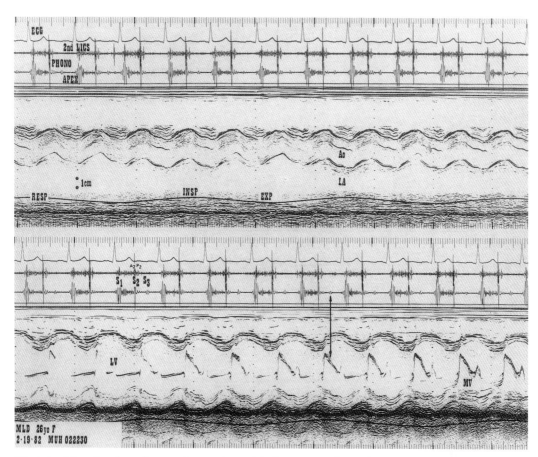

Fig 6–1. M-mode echocardiogram in a patient with chronic mitral insufficiency. The left atrium and left ventricle are dilated, and there is hyperkinetic motion of the septum and posterior ventricular wall. Note the systolic murmur and third heart sound (*arrow*) on the phonocardiogram taken at the apex. The third sound (S_3) occurs after the mitral leaflet has begun its posterior descent. ECG = electrocardiogram; Phono = phonocardiogram; RESP = respiration; INSP = inspiration; EXP = expiration; Ao = aorta; LA = left atrium; LV = left ventricle; MV = mitral valve. (Courtesy of Dr. Bruce W. Usher.)

gitant lesions by Doppler should be considered reasonable estimates until further investigation can be done. Radionuclide studies can measure the left ventricular ejection fraction at rest and after exercise. Such studies aid in determining the optimal time for valve replacement and in following the progress of such patients.

Heart catheterization studies reveal a high mean left atrial pressure and prominent V waves. The V wave, the phasic rise in left atrial pressure, in mitral insufficiency is related to the volume of regurgitation and to the size and elasticity of the left atrium. If the left atrium is dilated, there may be a small rise in left atrial pressure even though there is a large regurgitant volume. A small regurgitant stream can produce a large rise of left atrial pressure if there is a small, nondistensible left atrium. The height of the V wave in patients with mitral insufficiency may also be affected by the afterload (systemic vascular resistance). Reducing the afterload can make the V wave fall, at times dramatically. Injection of contrast material into the left ventricle

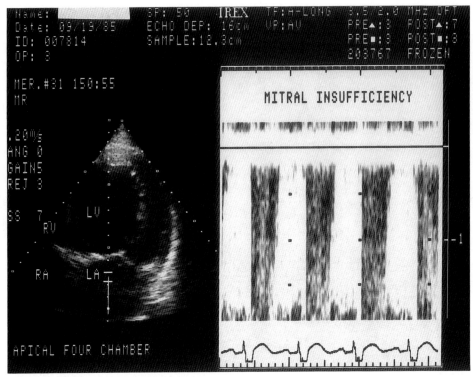

Fig 6–2. Pulsed Doppler recording of the left atrium showing mitral regurgitation which was recorded well back into the left atrium. (Courtesy of Dr. Bruce W. Usher.)

can demonstrate the systolic regurgitation of this material into the left atrium. If the regurgitation is cleared with each heartbeat, it is 1 + ; in 2 + it does not clear with one beat and opacifies the entire left atrium after several beats, but its opacification does not equal that of the left ventricle; in 3 + the left atrium

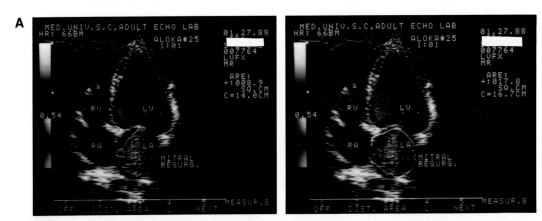

Fig 6–3. A, Color flow Doppler showing outline of mitral regurgitant jet (arrow points to blue-mosaic signals) into the left atrium during systole which has a planimetry area of 8.9 sq cm. B, Outline of left atrium which has a planimetry area of 17.8 sq cm. The regurgitation ratio is calculated to be 50% indicating significant mitral regurgitation. The left ventricle and left atrium are dilated. RV = right ventricle, LV = left ventricle, RA = right atrium, LA = left atrium. (Courtesy of Dr. Bruce W. Usher.)

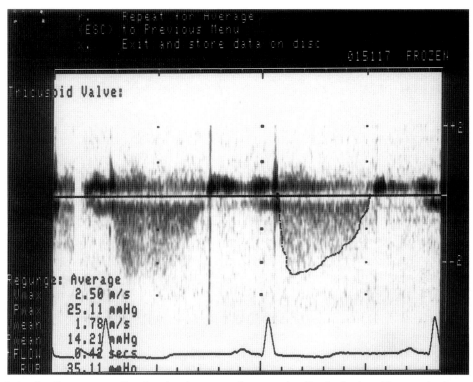

Fig 6–4. Continuous wave Doppler showing spectral pattern (outlined) of tricuspid regurgitation with a maximal velocity of 2.50 m/sec. The estimated right ventricular pressure is 35 mm Hg. (RVSP = 4(2.50)^2 + 10). RVSP = right ventricular systolic pressure. (Courtesy of Dr. Bruce W. Usher.)

opacification equals that of the left ventricle; in 4+ the entire left atrium opacifies with one beat and becomes more dense with each beat and even refluxes into the pulmonary veins during systole. Angiographic left ventricular ejection fraction and left ventricular stroke volume can be determined. If the effective forward stroke volume, as measured by the Fick or indicator dilution method, is subtracted from the angiographic left ventricular stroke volume, the regurgitant volume can be estimated and the regurgitant fraction can be calculated. Figure 6–5 summarizes the main features of mitral insufficiency.

Mitral valve prolapse. The mitral valve prolapse syndrome has been presented under many different names, such as the systolic click-murmur syndrome, prolapsing mitral leaflet syndrome, billowing mitral valve syndrome, floppy valve syndrome, Barlow's syndrome, and others. This syndrome is characterized by middle or late systolic clicks followed by a late systolic murmur. Originally the clicks were thought to be extracardiac in origin, such as from the pericardium. Reid[15] in 1961 postulated that the findings were associated with the mitral valve, but Barlow et al.[16] in 1963 confirmed this by left ventricular cineangiography. Recent surveys using clinical and echocardiographic criteria indicate that mitral valve prolapse occurs in about 5% of the population.[17] Most studies show a greater prevalence in women than in men.

The exact cause is not known. Studies[18] have shown an increased familial

MITRAL INSUFFICIENCY

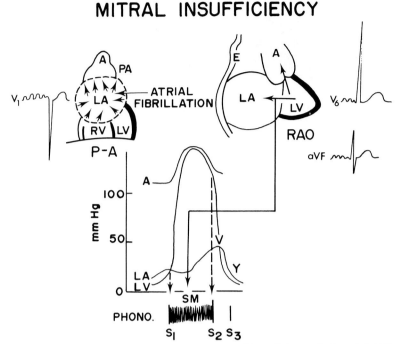

Fig 6–5. Main findings in chronic rheumatic mitral insufficiency. Left atrial (LA) and left ventricular (LV) enlargement producing anterior precordial and apical lifts. High-pitched apical holosystolic murmur (SM) and early diastolic third heart filling sound (S_3). PA view of chest shows biventricular enlargement and left atrial enlargement. Right anterior oblique (RAO) view of chest shows a diffuse posterior sweep of the barium-filled esophagus (E) due to the large left atrium. ECG reveals atrial fibrillation and left ventricular hypertrophy. Left ventricular cineangiography in the RAO position reveals a regurgitant jet into the large left atrium during systole. Prominent V wave in left atrial pressure curve with rapid Y descent.

incidence that suggests a genetic basis (autosomal dominant). It may occur as a primary entity or result from or be associated with other conditions, such as connective tissue disorders (such as Marfan's syndrome and osteogenesis imperfecta), atrial septal defects, rheumatic heart disease, ischemic heart disease, and cardiomyopathies. Abnormal left ventricular contraction patterns demonstrated by cineangiography and right ventricular endomyocardial biopsies have prompted some to consider this syndrome a primary cardiomyopathy with secondary mitral valve changes.[19]

The primary lesion described in mitral valve prolapse is an increase in the spongiosa (myxomatous tissue in middle layer of the mitral valve) which encroaches upon the fibrosa (ventricular aspect of valve).[20] This allows abnormal degrees of interchordal hooding or prolapse of elements of the valve toward the left atrium. The valve becomes grossly redundant and voluminous (appearing like a parachute), the chordae are elongated and thin, and fibrosis and calcification can occur in the anulus. At times the chordae can rupture. The posterior leaflet is most often involved.

Patients with mitral valve prolapse may be asymptomatic or complain of chest pain, dyspnea and fatigue, palpitations, dizziness, and syncope. These patients have more chest pain than the average population. The chest pain is variable and can be incapacitating. It can be a sharp sticking, or a pressure sensation, usually occurring at rest and often almost constant. Rarely it suggests angina. It has been postulated that excessive stretching and tension on the papillary muscles during prolapse may produce papillary muscle and subendocardial ischemia.[21] These patients' dyspnea is rather vague and occurs usually at rest. Many have extreme fatigue and are anxious, suggesting DaCosta's syndrome or neurocirculatory asthenia.[22,23] Perhaps many of these latter cases described years ago were actually the mitral valve prolapse syndrome. Patients with mitral valve prolapse may have a hyperadrenergic state, increased vagal activity and panic disorders. Data suggest an autonomic dysfunction in this syndrome, with increased level of circulating catecholamines.[24] Palpitations often prompt such patients to see a physician, and many have arrhythmias. Dizziness and syncope can occur, but these symptoms may not correlate with arrhythmias.

Patients with mitral valve prolapse often have pectus excavatum or carinatum, straight spine, or scoliosis as noted with Marfan's syndrome. Women often have small breasts. Middle or late systolic clicks alone or followed by a systolic murmur are often noted. This mitral regurgitation is due to the loss of coaptation produced by prolapse of a part of the mitral leaflets. There may be one isolated click or multiple clicks which reach their peak intensity at the time of maximal leaflet prolapse. The murmur is often crescendo or crescendodecrescendo and may extend through the aortic second sound. The murmur may be musical, sounding like a "whoop" or a "honk." The clicks and murmurs can be variable because they depend on several hemodynamic factors; namely, left ventricular volume, contractility, and systemic BP. Altering these factors can change the auscultatory findings. Any maneuver that makes the left ventricular cavity smaller will accentuate the degree of prolapse. One should listen to the patient lying, standing, and squatting. Left ventricular volume is reduced on standing and leaflet redundancy is more prominent and prolapse occurs earlier in systole, so that the click and murmur occur earlier, toward the first heart sound. In fact, occasionally the auscultatory findings can be noted only on standing. Squatting will increase venous return, systemic vascular resistance, abdominal pressure, systolic blood pressure, and left ventricular end-diastolic volume, delaying the onset of prolapse, and the click and murmur move toward the second heart sound. The loudness of the auscultatory events depends on left ventricular systolic pressure. Standing maintains left ventricular pressure and myocardial contractility is increased due to catecholamine secretion; therefore, the systolic murmur in addition to being earlier is usually louder and may become pansystolic. On the other hand, amyl nitrite decreases the systemic BP and may diminish the intensity of the murmur even though it occurs earlier in systole. Figure 6–6 shows the effect of various interventions on left ventricular volume, which in turn can change the auscultatory events.[25]

The ECG in approximately one third of patients will show inverted T waves in the inferolateral leads and at times mild ST depression. In one study of 43 patients exercised, 12 (28%) had significant ST depression during or following treadmill exercise.[26] The majority of these patients demonstrated ST-T changes on standing, ST depression during early and middle portion of the exercise, and absence of ST segment depression during peak exercise and immediate recovery, which may return during late recovery. Such changes have

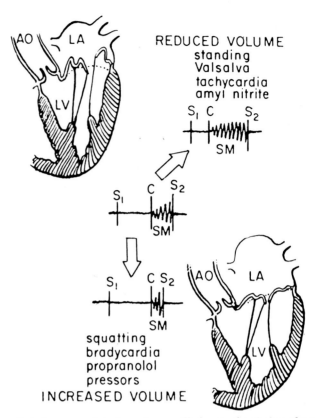

Fig 6–6. Interventions that change ventricular volume will change the timing of auscultatory events in mitral valve prolapse. AO = aorta; LA = left atrium; LV = left ventricle. (Devereux R.B., et al.: Mitral valve prolapse. *Circulation* 54:3, 1976, by permission of the American Heart Association, Inc.)

been noted with vasoregulatory abnormalities. Q-T interval prolongation has been reported.[24] The majority of patients have some arrhythmias with tread-mill exercise or 24-hour ambulatory ECG monitoring. Various arrhythmias have been detected, such as atrial and ventricular premature beats, supraventricular tachycardia, atrial fibrillation and flutter, ventricular tachycardia and fibrillation, and SA and AV node conduction disturbances. Premature ventricular beats are the most common arrhythmias; they may be unifocal or multifocal and are often precipitated or aggravated by exercise and emotion. Mechanical factors such as abnormal tension on the papillary muscles or stretching of the mitral leaflets are thought to be a factor in production of the arrhythmias.

Chest x rays are often normal unless the mitral insufficiency is moderate or severe, when left atrial and left ventricular enlargement may be noted. Calcification of the anulus is rare and should suggest Marfan's syndrome or a forme fruste of this syndrome. Bony abnormalities may also be detected.

Echocardiography has become a valuable noninvasive method of detecting mitral valve prolapse. The most specific pattern is the abrupt movement of one or both mitral leaflets posteriorly in middle or late systole or even pansystolic (Fig 6–7). M-mode may at times not detect prolapse or even give a false-positive diagnosis, depending on the angle of the beam. Two-dimensional echo-

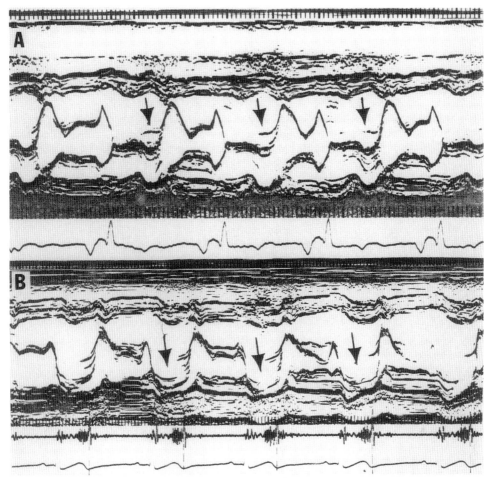

Fig 6–7. M-mode echocardiogram showing mitral valve prolapse. **A,** arrow points to late systolic prolapse. **B,** arrow points to holosystolic prolapse. (Courtesy of Dr. Bruce W. Usher.)

cardiography may detect prolapse that was missed by M-mode. Doppler (conventional and color) echocardiography can detect mitral regurgitation. Auscultatory findings have been noted in the absence of echo findings and vice versa. Tricuspid valve prolapse has also been noted in some patients with mitral valve prolapse.

Cardiac catheterization and angiographic studies are seldom performed unless complications occur that warrant them. It has been suggested that such patients have more frequently tortuous or "corkscrew" coronary arteries. However, this needs further confirmation. Left ventricular cineangiograms have revealed unusual contraction patterns referred to as "ballerina foot," "hourglass," and others.[27]

A problem today is overdiagnosis of mitral valve prolapse. There is a spectrum of mitral valve prolapse. The mitral valve normally billows slightly in the left atrium, and at the other end of the spectrum is a "floppy" valve with extreme billowing with mitral regurgitation. Perloff et al.[28] have proposed criteria for the diagnosis which they have divided into three groups—major, minor, and nonspecific (Table 6–1). The presence of one or more of the major

criteria establishes the diagnosis beyond reasonable doubt; minor criteria indicate suspicion but are not definitely diagnostic; and nonspecific features,
individually or collectively, do not provide a basis for the diagnosis. Such
criteria may aid in preventing overdiagnosis.

Table 6–1.   Diagnostic Criteria and Nonspecific Findings in Mitral Valve Prolapse

MAJOR CRITERIA

Auscultation
  Mid to late systolic clicks and a late systolic murmur at the cardiac apex
  Mobile mid to late systolic clicks at the cardiac apex
  Late systolic murmur at the cardiac apex in the young patient

Auscultation plus echocardiography
  Apical holosystolic murmur of mitral regurgitation plus echocardiographic
    criteria (below)

Two-dimensional/Doppler echocardiography
  Marked systolic displacement of mitral leaflets with coaptation point at or on the
    left atrial side of the anulus
  Moderate systolic displacement of the leaflets with at least moderate mitral
    regurgitation, chordal rupture, and anular dilatation

Two-dimensionally targeted M-mode echocardiography
  Marked ($\geqslant$3 mm) late systolic buckling posterior to the C-D line

MINOR CRITERIA

History
  Focal neurologic attacks or amaurosis fugax in the young patient
  First-degree relatives with major criteria
  Recurrent supraventricular tachycardia (documented)

Auscultation
  Soft, inconstant, or equivocal mid to late systolic sounds at the cardiac apex

Other physical signs
  Low body weight, asthenic habitus
  Low blood pressure
  Thoracic bony abnormalities

Two-dimensional/Doppler/color flow echocardiography
  Moderate superior systolic displacement of mitral leaflets with Doppler mitral
    regurgitation

Two-dimensionally targeted M-mode echocardiography
  Moderate (2 mm) late systolic buckling posterior to the C-D line
  Holosystolic displacement (3 mm) posterior to the C-D line

NONSPECIFIC FINDINGS

Symptoms
  Chest pain, fatigue, lassitude, dyspnea, light-headedness, dizziness, anxiety
    attacks

Scalar electrocardiogram
  T wave inversions in inferior limb leads or lateral precordial leads

Ambulatory electrocardiography
  Atrial premature beats, ventricular premature beats (simple or complex)

Two-dimensional echocardiography
  Isolated mild to moderate superior systolic displacement of mitral leaflets,
    especially in the apical four-chamber view

From Perloff J.K., Child J.S.: Clinical and epidemiologic issues in mitral valve prolapse: Overview and perspective. Am. Heart J.
113:1324, 1987.

Although the prognosis is good,[29] with a mean survival of 13.7 years for 85% as noted in one study,[30] the following complications can occur: sudden death, progressive mitral regurgitation, ruptured chordae, endocarditis, and transient cerebral ischemic attacks. The severity of the mitral regurgitation is of central importance in all of these complications.[31] One study showed that these complications were more frequent in patients who had thickening and redundancy of the mitral-valve leaflets as noted by 2-D echocardiography.[31a] Sudden death is rare and most often occurs in the familial variety (see Chap. 15). Mitral insufficiency can become progressive, with a final picture resembling that described earlier for chronic mitral insufficiency of rheumatic origin. This is the most frequent of the major complications. We have followed up several patients who initially had only an isolated click, later developed a systolic murmur, and then progressively demonstrated left atrial and left ventricular enlargement and failure requiring valve replacement. In about 75% of such patients there is sudden deterioration due to chordal rupture.[32] In one study, severe mitral regurgitation requiring surgery was shown to rise sharply after age 50, more so in men.[33] About 4% of men and 1.5% of women with mitral valve prolapse require mitral valve surgery by age 70. Endocarditis has been noted, primarily in those with mitral insufficiency and infrequently in those with only clicks.[34] The risks of endocarditis have been calculated annually to be in the range of 1 in 5000 to 7000 among all adults with mitral valve prolapse and equal or greater than 1 in 2000 among those with mitral regurgitation.[35] In addition, it is noted more frequently in males and in older age groups. The majority agree that patients with the typical murmur should receive prophylaxis; it is debatable for the click only, although we do advise it. Several studies have reported cerebral emboli in this syndrome producing transient ischemic attacks, retinal arteriolar occlusions, and amaurosis fugáx. In fact, Barnett et al.[36] found prolapse in 40% of 60 patients who had transient ischemia or partial stroke and were under 45 years of age. Prolapse was found in only 6.8% of 60 age-matched controls, in 5.7% of 141 patients over 45 years old who had transient ischemia or partial stroke, and in 7.1% of 141 age-matched controls. Platelet aggregation on myxomatous valves have been considered to produce thrombi which can be the major source of the emboli. In fact, atrial thrombi have been detected by two-dimensional echo studies in patients with mitral valve prolapse and strokes.[37] At present it is not known whether the use of aspirin or other drugs which inhibit platelet aggregation or anticoagulants are of benefit. Mitral valve prolapse has been noted in patients who have had an acute myocardial infarction with normal coronary arteries. Such patients have been suspected of having a coronary artery embolism or spasm. It has already been mentioned that arrhythmias are common in mitral valve prolapse, especially ventricular, and that sudden death is rare. Duren et al.[38] in a long-term follow-up of 300 patients with mitral valve prolapse reported that one-third developed a serious complication. However, these were patients referred for further cardiology assessment, so the results do not reflect the natural history of mitral valve prolapse in the general population. Several studies suggest that the prevalence of symptoms in patients with mitral valve prolapse and the incidence of complications occur with similar frequency in the general population.[39,40]

Patients with mitral valve prolapse often do not require any specific therapy. Chest pain is a major problem, but unless it is typical angina, it does not require therapy. A β-adrenergic blocker is the drug of choice for angina. Nitrates should be used cautiously, for they may increase the prolapse by reducing the left ventricular volume and increase the tension on the papillary muscle. If there is typical angina and a positive ECG or thallium stress test, coronary arteriography should be performed, and if coronary disease is found, it should be treated appropriately (see Chap. 4). Tachyarrhythmias are managed with β-blockers. A β-blocker should also be used if there are complex PVBs (more than five per minute, couplets, multiform, or R on T types) or malignant ventricular arrhythmias (bouts of ventricular tachycardia or ventricular fibrillation). Quinidine and procainamide have been used, but should be avoided if the Q-T interval is long, in which situation a β-blocker, tocainide, or mexiletine would be more appropriate. Digoxin may increase contractility and worsen the prolapse; however, it can be helpful in certain instances of a supraventricular tachycardia and if there is cardiomegaly with heart failure. Progressive or acute mitral insufficiency is managed the same as for other causes of these conditions, with medical therapy, surgery, or both.

One should suspect mitral valve prolapse in any young person complaining of an undue amount of chest pain, palpitations, dizziness, or syncope whose ECG shows PVBs or nonspecific ST-T changes or both. A major question is "To what extent should these patients be studied?" If the patient is asymptomatic and there is no evidence of arrhythmias or severe mitral regurgitation, a follow-up study every 2 years should include an echo and Doppler study. Holter monitoring should be done if arrhythmias are noted or the patient complains of syncope or palpitations. A stress test should be included if symptoms suggest angina. Significant mitral regurgitation requires more frequent follow-ups.

Coronary artery disease. Papillary muscle dysfunction can occur secondary to ischemia, producing permanent or transient mitral insufficiency. This murmur is often mid to late systolic and resembles that of mitral valve prolapse. Usually this in itself does not require specific therapy. Acute myocardial infarction can produce papillary muscle necrosis and severe mitral insufficiency that often requires surgery (see Chap. 4).

Calcified mitral anulus. Calcification of the mitral anulus can cause mitral insufficiency in the elderly, especially in women. It can invade the conducting system and produce AV block or bundle-branch block. In Marfan's and Hurler's syndromes, the anulus can be calcified and dilated. The calcified anulus appears on x ray as a curved shadow forming a U-shaped density. It is easily detected by echocardiography. Patients with mitral insufficiency due to calcified anulus should have endocarditis prophylaxis.

Connective tissue diseases. Marfan's syndrome, Ehlers-Danlos syndrome, Hurler's syndrome, SLE, osteogenesis imperfecta, and others can produce mitral insufficiency. Marfan's syndrome may have primary mitral valve involvement with the findings noted with mitral valve prolapse. Ruptured chordae and anulus calcification can occur. Ehlers-Danlos syndrome is characterized by hyperelasticity of the skin, hyperextensibility of the joints, and sometimes involvement of the cardiac connective tissue and mitral valve prolapse. Hurler's syndrome is associated with abnormal metabolism of mucopolysaccharides which can involve the connective tissue of the valves. Verrucous valvular lesions (Libman-Sacks disease) may produce mitral insufficiency as a part of the clinical picture of SLE. Osteogenesis imperfecta can also affect the mitral valve and even produce chordal rupture.

Congenital mitral insufficiency. Congenital mitral insufficiency as an isolated abnormality is rare. Most often it is associated with other lesions, such as endocardial cushion defects, anomalous origin of coronary artery from the pulmonary artery, and idiopathic hypertrophic subaortic stenosis (IHSS).

Left ventricular enlargement. Left ventricular enlargement from any cause can produce mitral insufficiency by altering the spatial relationship between the chordae and papillary muscle.

Treatment of Chronic Mitral Insufficiency

Regardless of the etiology, chronic mitral insufficiency is treated according to its severity. The usual measures for arrhythmias and heart failure are instituted. Afterload reduction has become important for reducing the amount of regurgitation by decreasing impedance to left ventricular ejection. Oral hydralazine, converting enzyme inhibitors, or prazosin can be given until surgery is indicated, or if surgery is contraindicated, these can be given indefinitely depending on the response. The most difficult decision the physician has to make is to determine the optimal time for mitral valve replacement. In spite of our many sophisticated studies, we still lack specific data for determining the time when there will be serious irreversible left ventricular dysfunction if the valve is not removed. In addition, no tissue or prosthetic valve is without problems. The majority agree that the valve should be replaced if the patient has cardiomegaly and progressive symptoms despite medical therapy. Braunwald and his group[41] emphasize the importance of end-systolic volume in evaluating mitral insufficiency. Patients with severe mitral regurgitation and a normal preoperative end-systolic volume (<30 ml/m^2) maintained normal ventricular function postoperatively, whereas those with end-systolic volume >90 ml/m^2 had a high perioperative mortality and residual left ventricular dysfunction. Between 30 and 90 ml/m^2, surgery can be tolerated well, but there may be some reduction in left ventricular function postoperatively. Many other studies have looked at heart catheterization parameters, echocardiography, radionuclide studies, exercise testing, and combinations of these for determining optimal time for surgery prior to deterioration of left ventricular function. Ejection fraction is the most commonly used index of left ventricular function. However, it is affected by muscle function and by preload and afterload abnormalities. For example, in mitral insufficiency the afterload is reduced because of the regurgitant jet, and therefore patients may have a good preoperative ejection fraction. Once the valve is replaced and this afterload is removed, the ejection fraction often drops. Therefore, an index of function that is not influenced by loading conditions would be a better method of predicting surgical outcome. End-systolic volume is not related to preload, but it is affected by afterload. With a correction of end-systolic volume for afterload and body size, an index of ventricular function may be obtained which is less affected by loading. Carabello demonstrated in patients with mitral regurgitation that the ratio of end-systolic wall stress to end-systolic volume index is useful in predicting a patient's surgical outcome.[42] If this ratio is more than 2.5, the patient usually has a satisfactory outcome. Cardiac volumes and pressures for these studies were obtained from ventriculograms and pressure measurements made during preoperative catheterization. The surgical mortality is now between 2 and 7% in most centers. There are many different types of artificial valves. The incidence of thromboembolism is much higher with mechanical prosthetic valves (Starr-Edwards caged-ball valve, Smeloff-Cutter, Bjork-Shiley, Lillehei-Kaster, St. Jude) than with tissue valves (Carpentier-Edwards and Hancock porcine valves). We advise the use of tissue valves in patients in whom there is a contraindication to anticoagulants, in those of child-bearing age, and in the elderly.

Managing the pregnant patient taking anticoagulants can be difficult, and there is a risk of a teratogenic effect from warfarin and fetal bleeding, since the warfarin crosses the placenta.[43,44] Coumarin derivatives are contraindicated from the 6th to the 12th week of gestation. Such patients with mechanical prosthetic valves should be given heparin (which does not cross the placental barrier) during the first trimester; then oral anticoagulants, until the 37th week of gestation; then the oral agent is stopped and heparin is restarted until the onset of labor; and then the heparin is stopped until after delivery, when it is restarted with the oral anticoagulant until the oral anticoagulant has an adequate effect.[43] Some have advocated the use of self-administered heparin subcutaneously throughout pregnancy except for the period before onset of labor (time of increased coagulation factors), when it should be given intravenously. The appropriate heparin dosage, regardless of the above regimens, has not been worked out. The range of dosage usually is 150 to 250 u/kg every 12 hours subcutaneously with the dose adjusted to maintain the activated partial thromboplastin time at 1.5 times control when it is determined 4 to 6 hours after injection. This type of program requires close management. Although it can be avoided by using a tissue valve in the patient of child-bearing age, it should be understood by the patient that such valves have developed calcification and breakdown in increasing numbers (follow-up to 13 years) and must be replaced.[45] The incidence of breakdown is higher in children than adults. All mechanical prosthetic valves require long-term anticoagulation therapy with warfarin. Anticoagulants are given postoperatively for tissue valves for about 3 months (risk of thromboembolism is greatest during this time), then gradually stopped unless there is chronic atrial fibrillation and a large dilated left atrium. In some instances drugs such as aspirin and persantine to inhibit platelet aggregation have been given to patients with mechanical prostheses, especially those who have a problem with compliance.

Reconstructive procedures have been done on the mitral valve with some success. This repair would be ideal because it would eliminate the use of anticoagulants and risk of failure of the prosthesis. In addition, with preservation of the mitral valve apparatus, ventricular function would be less affected.

Acute Mitral Insufficiency

Acute mitral insufficiency can occur because of rupture of the chordae or papillary muscle, perforation of the mitral valve, or prosthetic valve malfunction. Ruptured chordae can occur in patients with known heart disease (rheumatic, mitral valve prolapse, and others) or spontaneously in a person with no known heart disease.

The acute and chronic types present differently. In some instances a combination picture can be noted, as when an acute situation such as ruptured chordae occurs in a patient with chronic mitral insufficiency.

The picture of acute mitral insufficiency is one with sudden onset of heart failure (even pulmonary edema), S_4 gallop, normal-sized heart, and sinus rhythm rather than atrial fibrillation. The left atrium may be of normal size or moderately enlarged, since the insufficiency is acute, whereas the chronic types produce a huge left atrium. The systolic apical murmur, instead of being the blowing pansystolic type, may be rather harsh and of the ejection type. The murmur may be decrescendo and stop before the second sound because the pressure gradient between the left ventricle and atrium declines at the end of systole in view of the very high V wave. If the chordae of the posterior leaflet are involved, the murmur may be referred to the aortic area simulating aortic stenosis.[46] If there is rupture of the chordae of the anterior leaflet, the murmur can be transmitted posteriorly to the spine and can be heard on the top of the head.[47] A systolic thrill may be palpated at the apex, and the apical impulse can be hyperactive. Echocardiography may show abnormal echoes due to ruptured chordae or papillary muscle, a perforated valve, or vegetations. Conventional and color flow Doppler can assess the mitral insufficiency. The left atrium and left ventricle may be of normal size but have increased systolic motion. Catheterization studies will reveal an increase in left ventricular end-diastolic pressure and mean left atrial pressure, with a very high V wave and also elevated pulmonary artery pressure. In fact, the left atrial V wave may be transmitted retrograde into the main pulmonary artery.[48] The giant V wave is due to the regurgitation of blood into a relatively small and noncompliant left atrium. Afterload reduction with sodium nitroprusside (starting dose, 0.5 µg/kg/min) will reduce the left ventricular end-diastolic pressure and the left atrial pressure and the V wave and reduce the regurgitant fraction. This type of therapy can be lifesaving and aids in reducing pulmonary congestion and stabilizing the patient until surgery can be performed.

Valve replacement is usually necessary, although in some instances a ruptured chordae may produce only a murmur without acute symptoms or any significant hemodynamic changes. A low-profile prosthetic valve is preferable in a small left ventricular cavity to avoid hemodynamic obstruction in the left ventricular outflow tract. The rupture of chordae produces a lesser degree of mitral insufficiency than rupture of a papillary muscle. Rupture of a papillary muscle is most often due to an acute myocardial infarction.

Mitral Stenosis

Rheumatic fever is still the most common cause of mitral stenosis. Infrequently it can be congenital or due to an atrial myxoma or calcified anulus. The incidence is slightly higher in patients with atrial septal defect (Lutembacher's syndrome). I suspect that in the past the higher incidence reported with atrial septal defect was actually the misinterpretation of the tricuspid flow murmur associated with the shunt as mitral stenosis. A history of rheumatic fever is present in only about 50% of patients, which has caused some to consider a viral etiology.[49] Mitral stenosis is more common in females.

Mitral stenosis blocks the inflow of blood to the left ventricle. The fibrotic changes of rheumatic mitral stenosis cause fusion of the cusp at the commissures, and the chordae become fused, shortened, and thickened, producing a funnel-shaped valve. Significant mitral stenosis after an acute attack of rheumatic fever may occur in a few years but usually has a latent interval up to 15 to 20 years. The patient may have the mitral facies, pinkish-purple cheeks.

This type of patient usually has a low cardiac output and systemic vasoconstriction secondary to severe mitral stenosis. The arterial pulse is usually normal and the jugular venous pulse may show a prominent "A" wave, if there is sinus rhythm and elevated pulmonary vascular resistance. A right ventricular lift may be present, and a diastolic thrill may be palpable at the apex. A very large right ventricle can produce an apical impulse that may be interpreted as a left ventricular lift. In such cases the left ventricle is small and is displaced posteriorly. The second sound is usually loudest in the pulmonic area, and the first sound is loud at the apex (when the mitral valve is flexible). The loud first sound is thought to be due to the wide closing of the valve leaflets after being depressed by the diastolic gradient across the valve and the sudden stoppage of its upward motion.[50] However, Criley et al.[51] consider it to be due to a more rapid rate of left ventricular pressure rise at the time of closure. An opening snap, related to abnormal mitral valve with its abrupt recoil, may be audible along the left sternal border (0.03 to 0.12 seconds from the second heart sound). The closer the opening snap is to the second heart sound, the tighter is the stenosis and the more elevated is the left atrial pressure. This does vary with the heart rate. Standing decreases venous return and left atrial pressure and increases the time from the aortic second sound to the opening snap. This time interval may also increase when the mitral valve is calcified and there is tight stenosis. This can prolong the time interval between opening of the mitral valve and the opening snap. The thickened valve leaflets at the peak of opening are suddenly tense and produce the popping opening snap[52] which coincides with the E point on the anterior leaflet echocardiogram (Fig 6–8). At times the opening snap can be heard at the base of the heart and must be distinguished from splitting of the second heart sound, but it does not vary with respirations, occurs later than P_2, and is well heard at the apex. An S_3 gallop is low-pitched and should not be mistaken for the high-pitched opening snap.

The diastolic murmur is a low-pitched, rumbling murmur and is often heard best in the left lateral position at the apex with the bell of the stethoscope applied lightly to the chest. It begins after the opening snap. If regular sinus rhythm is present, there is presystolic accentuation of the murmur due to atrial contraction. With severe stenosis the murmur may be long. Atrial fibrillation will cause the murmur to be shorter and in mid-diastole; however, there can be presystolic accentuation. Progressive narrowing of the mitral valve opening after the onset of left ventricular contraction, with resulting increased velocity of flow as the valve closes, can produce the presystolic murmur even though atrial fibrillation is present.[51] If the valve becomes severely calcified and fixed, the opening snap disappears and the intensity of the murmur may be much reduced. Pulmonary hypertension secondary to mitral stenosis rarely produces pulmonary valvular regurgitation (Graham Steell murmur). This was thought to be common years ago, but studies have shown that the faint, high-pitched diastolic murmur was due to aortic insufficiency. Likewise, secondary tricuspid insufficiency rarely occurs. The latter murmur may be mistaken for mitral insufficiency; however, it is heard best with inspiration. By the time atrial fibrillation develops, there is usually a significant diastolic gradient across the mitral valve. However, atrial fibrillation can occur with mild mitral stenosis when rheumatic Aschoff's nodules are in the atrial walls.

The ECG will vary depending upon the degree of mitral stenosis. Early left

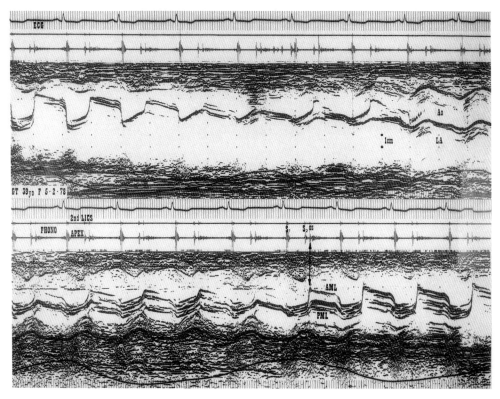

Fig 6–8. M-mode echocardiogram in mitral stenosis. Note slow velocity of descent of the anterior mitral leaflet (AML) and abnormal motion of the posterior mitral leaflet (PML). Left atrium is enlarged. Phonocardiogram at the apex reveals an opening snap (OS) followed by a low-pitched diastolic murmur. Opening snap occurring (*arrow*) at the time of maximum opening of the mitral valve. ECG = electrocardiogram; Ao = aorta; LA = left atrium; Phono = phonocardiogram; OS = opening snap; AML = anterior mitral leaflet; PML = posterior mitral leaflet. (Courtesy of Dr. Bruce W. Usher.)

atrial enlargement will be noted, and, later, right ventricular hypertrophy and atrial fibrillation. Chest x rays usually reveal prominent pulmonary arteries, large left atrium (demonstrated easily by barium swallow), right ventricular enlargement, and prominence of the superior pulmonary veins. The left border of the heart is often referred to as having four knobs; beginning from above the aortic, pulmonary artery, left atrial appendage, and left ventricle knobs. The prominent superior pulmonary veins are often referred to as antlers because they resemble those on a deer. At times there may be thickened interstitial lines at the bases, referred to as Kerley-B lines. As pulmonary hypertension becomes more severe, the central pulmonary arteries become more prominent and straight lines at the hilum (Kerley-A lines) can develop. Hemosiderosis can occur and rarely parenchymal ossification.

M-mode echocardiography shows that the anterior leaflet during diastole has a diminished velocity of descent of the E-to-F slope. However, this can occur in any condition in which left ventricular compliance is reduced or in which there is right ventricular pressure overload. The posterior leaflet in diastole moves in the same direction as the anterior leaflet instead of having its normal posterior movement (see Fig 6–8). Left atrial and right ventricular enlargement, left atrial thrombus (Fig 6–9), and valvular calcification can be detected. Two-dimensional echocardiography has become superior for the de-

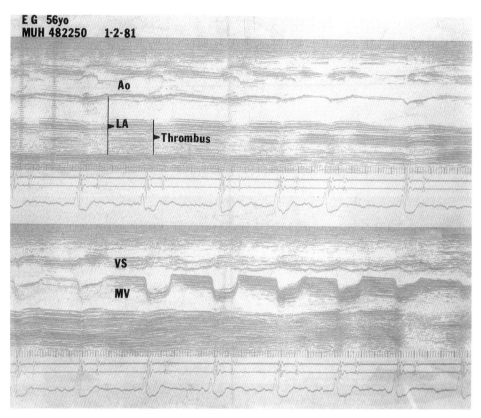

Fig 6–9. M-mode echocardiogram revealing mitral stenosis and a thrombus in the left atrium (LA). Ao = aorta; LA = left atrium; VS = ventricular septum; MV = mitral valve. (From Usher B.W.: Role of echocardiography in evaluating patients with congestive heart failure. Reprinted by permission of *Medical Times,* vol. 110, no. 6, 1982.)

tection of mitral stenosis and also for giving some idea of the mitral orifice size. It can show the doming and restricted motion of the valve and the orifice can be measured directly to give the area of the valve (Fig 6–10A). There are limitations to this method because patients with low cardiac output have a reduced mitral orifice. This and technical errors can occur. Despite the limitations, it correlates well with the hemodynamic data and the surgeon's or pathologist's findings. Doppler echocardiography of mitral valve flow is another method of assessing the mitral valve. The pressure half-time can be used for calculating the valve area. The time taken by the atrioventricular pressure gradient to decrease to half its initial level is the atrioventricular pressure half-time. Hatle and Angelsen[53] showed that with a pressure half-time of more than 220 m/sec, the valve area was less than 1 cm^2 and the formula was derived: MVA (cm^2) = 220/pressure half-time (msec). Pressure half-time may be estimated by plotting the instantaneous pressure gradients calculated from Doppler measurements, and it is the time taken for the gradient to decrease by half (Fig 6–10B). Color flow Doppler is useful for detecting associated lesions.

Right heart catheterization reveals an elevated pulmonary wedge pressure which is above that of the left ventricular end-diastolic pressure, giving a diastolic gradient across the mitral valve. The pulmonary artery pressure and the right atrial pressure may be elevated, depending upon the degree of mitral

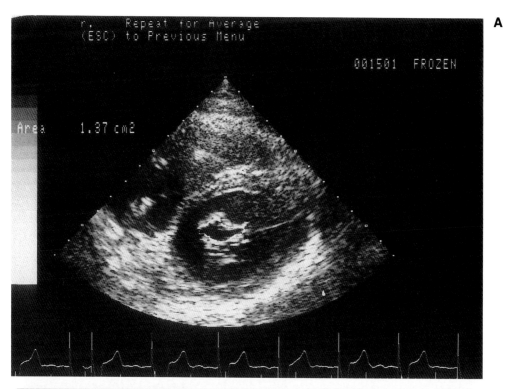

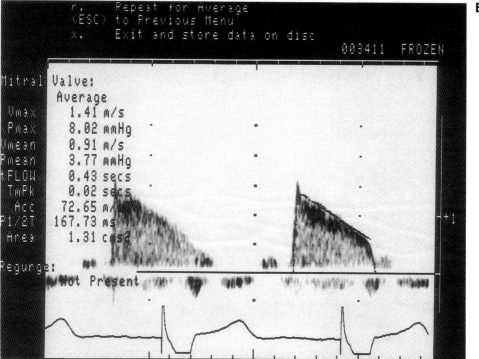

Fig 6–10. A, Two dimensional short axis view of patient with mitral stenosis (orifice outlined). The mitral valve area by planimetry is 1.37 cm². B, Continuous wave Doppler of mitral valve. Note that velocity decreases gradually through diastole. The estimated mitral valve area by pressure half-time is 1.31 cm² [MVA (cm²) = 220/167.7]. (Courtesy of Dr. Bruce W. Usher.)

stenosis. Cardiac output can be determined by the indicator dilution or Fick method at the time the mitral valve gradient is obtained, and by the Gorlin formula the mitral orifice size can be calculated.[54] The capillary wedge pressure is usually greater than 15 to 20 mm Hg when the patient is symptomatic.[55] If the wedge is not at this level, the hemodynamic data should be repeated after exercise, for a poor cardiac output response to exercise can indicate significant mitral stenosis. Pulmonary congestion develops when the valve orifice area is 1.1 to 1.5 cm^2 (normal, 4 to 6 cm^2), and cardiac output can be normal. When the stenosis is critical (less than 1 cm^2) pulmonary hypertension and reduced cardiac output are present. Braunwald[56] corrects valve area for body surface area (valve area index) and considers moderate or severe stenosis to be present if the mitral valve orifice size is <1.0 cm^2/m^2 BSA. Figure 6–11 summarizes the main features noted in mitral stenosis.

Surgery is usually considered for mitral stenosis if the patients are symptomatic.

Hemoptysis usually indicates beginning pulmonary venous hypertension. Later, with increasing venous hypertension, the bronchial veins become thickened and less likely to break and produce hemoptysis. Pulmonary alveolar congestion or interstitial edema of the lungs produce dyspnea. At the beginning the dyspnea may be exertional. This gradually increases to the point where it occurs with little activity. Orthopnea may develop later. In addition, nocturnal cough becomes a prominent feature. At times the patient may have

MITRAL STENOSIS

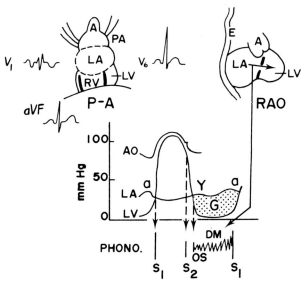

Fig 6–11. Main findings in mitral stenosis. Right ventricular (RV) lift due to right ventricular enlargement. Loud S$_1$ at apex and S$_2$ at pulmonic area. Opening snap (OS) along left sternal border. Low-pitched, rumbling apical diastolic murmur (DM) often associated with thrill. PA view of chest reveals prominent superior pulmonary veins (antlers) and four knobs of the left border of the heart—from above downward aorta (A), pulmonary artery (PA), left atrial appendage, and left ventricle (LV). Right anterior oblique (RAO) view shows the discrete indentation produced by the large left atrium (LA) on the barium-filled esophagus (E). ECG shows right ventricular and left atrial hypertrophy. Hatched area G represents the diastolic pressure gradient (25 mm Hg) between the elevated left atrial pressure (LA) and the normal left ventricular (LV) diastolic pressure.

pulmonary edema, and the diagnosis is overlooked because the murmur is obscured by the wheezing. One should suspect mitral stenosis in a young person who develops sudden pulmonary edema associated with pregnancy, intercourse, physical exertion, or emotional trauma. In the past many patients with mitral stenosis have been treated for chronic bronchitis and pulmonary infections. These latter findings are often associated with the chronic venous hypertension of mitral stenosis. The dilated left atrium and pulmonary artery can compress the left recurrent laryngeal nerve and cause hoarseness (Ortner syndrome). Atrial arrhythmias may make the patient aware of palpitations. A systemic embolism may produce the first symptoms. Rarely, a ball valve thrombus can develop and produce syncope.

Surgery is indicated when any of the above symptoms are noted and the valve orifice area is <1.0 cm^2. Areas between 1.0 and 1.5 cm^2 need individual attention; surgery is indicated depending on the patient's symptoms and findings (pulmonary hypertension, systemic emboli) and necessary activities. Mitral commissurotomy is still a good procedure unless mitral insufficiency, valvular calcification, or an atrial thrombus is present. However, most patients require valve replacement with the same considerations as mentioned for mitral insufficiency. A low-profile valve should be used, because the left ventricle can be of normal size and the valve may produce left ventricular outflow tract obstruction. Mitral stenosis with severe pulmonary hypertension is not a contraindication to surgery, for valve replacement reduces pulmonary vascular pressure and resistance.[57] We usually advise heart catheterization studies in all patients with mitral stenosis prior to surgery, even though some have considered it feasible to operate without this procedure if the noninvasive studies indicate isolated mitral stenosis in a patient under age 50 with no history of angina.

Balloon mitral valvuloplasty has been developed as an alternative procedure to surgery.[58,59] After trans-septal puncture, a small balloon flotation catheter is passed across the interatrial septum enlarging the opening and then a single 23 to 25 mm balloon (or two smaller 18 to 20 mm balloons) is advanced across the mitral orifice and inflated. Repeated inflations may be necessary. Recently 70 patients had this procedure done at Boston's Beth Israel Hospital.[59] The mitral valve area was improved (0.9 ± 0.3 to 1.8 ± 0.7 cm^2). In 5 patients, the dilatation could not be performed because of the technical problems. Only one death occurred during the procedure. Complications reported by this group and others include left atrial perforation, severe vagal reaction, small atrial septal defects, transient arrhythmias, cerebrovascular accident due to emboli, and severe mitral regurgitation. This procedure at present should be offered to those who are at high risk or unsuitable for surgery or refuse surgery, those with advanced age and those who have associated conditions such as pulmonary, renal, or malignancies. It can be considered for women of child-bearing age who are not ideal candidates for long-term anticoagulation or a tissue bioprosthesis.

AORTIC VALVE DISEASE

Aortic Insufficiency

An incompetent aortic valve, allowing backflow of blood into the left ventricle during diastole, produces an aortic diastolic murmur. The cause should be considered rheumatic (murmur usually heard best at the left side of the sternum) if such a history can be obtained or if this lesion is associated with mitral valve disease. Otherwise, it may be due to lesions that produce predominantly aortic root dilatation (murmur usually heard best at the right side of the sternum) such as Marfan's syndrome, aortic aneurysm, dissecting aneurysm, aneurysm of the sinus of Valsalva, hypertension, arteriosclerosis, cystic medionecrosis, trauma, syphilis, idiopathic osteogenesis imperfecta, psoriatic arthritis, giant cell arteritis, relapsing polychondritis, or rheumatoid spondylitis. Aortic root disease now accounts for more than one-third of patients with aortic regurgitation.[60] Deformities of the aortic valve other than rheumatic can be due to congenital bicuspid valve with or without coarctation, a high ventricular septal defect with aortic insufficiency, infective endocarditis, Reiter's disease, myxomatous degeneration of valve, rheumatoid arthritis, trauma, Ehlers-Danlos syndrome, and, rarely, SLE. Although the lesions are divided into those that produce valvular deformities and those that produce aortic root dilatation, there is overlapping such as with rheumatoid arthritis. Marfan and Reiter's syndromes, and others. Rheumatic fever can produce fibrosis and contracture of the cusps so that they cannot close in diastole. Often the valve cannot open well, and there is associated aortic stenosis. Eventually any cause can produce dilatation and hypertrophy of the left ventricle and even of the left atrium.

The murmur of aortic incompetence is usually high-pitched, blowing, and begins almost with the second sound and is decrescendo. It is usually best heard with the diaphragm at the end of expiration in the primary aortic area or at the right or left sternal border (Erb's area) with the patient sitting and leaning forward. It can radiate to the apex and occasionally may be heard only in that area. The longer duration in diastole the murmur occupies, the more severe is the aortic insufficiency. However, congestive heart failure with decrease in left ventricular stroke volume can result in a decrease in intensity and length of the diastolic murmur as well as attenuation of the peripheral pulses, so that the degree of aortic regurgitation will be underestimated. As mentioned previously, when the murmur is associated with primary valvular involvement, it usually is heard best along the left sternal border, and when associated with dilatation of the ascending aorta, it is best heard along the right sternal border. Any intervention that raises the BP will accentuate the murmur. An aortic ejection sound may be audible if the valve is not severely calcified. Because of the increased stroke volume, most patients will have a systolic flow murmur in the primary aortic area, with radiation into the neck. This murmur can produce a systolic thrill in the supraclavicular area without the patient having any degree of aortic stenosis. A thrill may be associated with the aortic diastolic murmur if there is prolapse, eversion, or perforation of the leaflets. Eversion of the leaflets can produce a "cooing" or musical murmur. A venticular gallop may be present. A low-pitched, mid-diastolic rumbling murmur may be heard at the apex with severe aortic insufficiency (Austin Flint murmur). The regurgitant jet of aortic insufficiency against the anteromedial mitral valve leaflet impedes the flow from the left atrium into the left ventricle, and also the rapidly rising left ventricular diastolic pressure impedes the opening of the mitral valve,[61] producing this functional diastolic murmur. These patients usually have large left ventricles and are in failure. The Austin Flint murmur may simulate mitral stenosis. Unless there is marked left atrial enlargement, loud first sound, or an opening snap, it may be difficult to differentiate these. Increasing the BP can augment the Austin Flint murmur, and amyl nitrite can reduce it. The murmur of mitral stenosis will increase in intensity after giving amyl nitrite. The echocardiogram is valuable in this differentiation, because it demonstrates classic findings in mitral stenosis (see Fig 6–8) and certain suggestive findings in aortic insufficiency. An S_3 gallop can indicate severe aortic regurgitation or depressed left ventricular function. A hyperactive left ventricular apical lift is present due to the over-filled left ventricle. The pulse pressure is wide and correlates well with the degree of aortic insufficiency unless advanced heart failure is present. The peripheral pulses are classically bounding with a brisk upstroke and rapid decline (water-hammer or Corrigan's pulse). This can best be detected by clasping the patient's wrist over the radial pulsation and raising the patient's arm high. Carotid pulsations can produce bobbing of the head (deMusset's sign) and pistol-shot sounds (Traube's sign). Capillary pulsations in the nail beds with pressure on the nail or capillary pulsations by pressing a glass slide on the patient's lip (Quincke's sign) and a systolic and diastolic murmur heard over the femoral artery with pressure of the stethoscope (Duroziez's sign) are other findings noted with aortic insufficiency. At times, the uvula can pulsate during systole (Müller's sign). The BP in the legs may be excessively elevated as compared with the arms (Hill's sign). At times, the carotid and peripheral pulses may be bifid (bisferiens pulse).

The ECG reveals increased voltage of the R waves over the left ventricle. Initially the T waves may be upright (volume overload), and later ST-T changes occur. Chest x ray usually shows a widened ascending aorta and left ventricular enlargement (boot-shaped heart). With syphilitic aortic insufficiency, a thin layer of calcification may be seen in the aortic wall. The echocardiogram reveals fluttering of the anterior mitral valve leaflet and septum and left ventricular volume overload with increased chamber size (Fig 6–12A). However, eventually the left ventricle can become hypokinetic (Fig 6–12B). Two-dimensional echocardiography shows the changes better, especially prolapse of the valve, flail leaflets, vegetations and aortic root dilatation. Doppler echocardiography is more sensitive in detecting aortic regurgitation (AR) and may detect mild AR that is not audible. In addition, the degree of aortic regurgitation may be quantitated from the slope of the aortic velocities as recorded by continuous wave Doppler. The more severe the regurgitation, the steeper the slope and the shorter the pressure half-time. Slopes greater than 3 m/sec^2 are usually seen only in patients with advanced (3 or 4+) aortic regurgitation.[62] Figure 6–13 shows a pressure half-time of 286 msec of the Doppler tracing of aortic regurgitation, indicating a significant degree of aortic regurgitation. Pressure half-time of 400 msec or less indicates significant aortic regurgitation.[63] Perry et al.[64] have shown by Doppler color flow mapping that the thickness of the regurgitant stream at its origin relative to the size of the left venticular outflow tract is a better predictor of the severity of AR (as judged by angiographic grading) than is the area of the regurgitant jet or depth to which the jet extends in the left ventricle. Doppler grading of AR using the jet short axis area (JSAA) divided by left ventricular outflow tract short axis area (LVOA) is as follows: less than 25% mild AR, between 25 to 60% moderate and greater than 60% severe. Figure 6–14 of the same patient in Figure 6–13 shows aortic insufficiency as detected and quantitated by the use of color flow

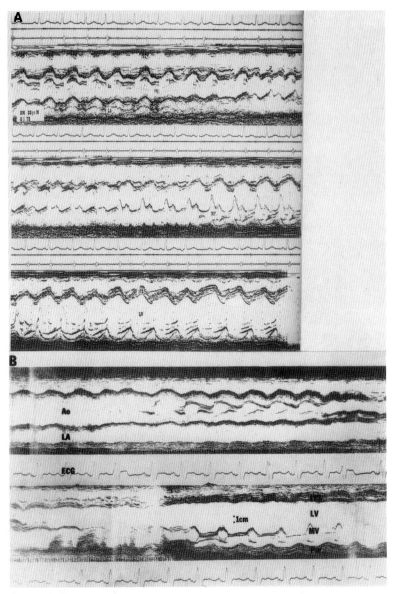

Fig 6–12. M-mode echocardiographic spectrum of volume overload of the left ventricle in aortic insufficiency. **A,** acute aortic insufficiency secondary to infective endocarditis. Note the vegetations (veg) on the aortic valve which protrude into the left ventricle outflow tract. Left ventricle (LV) is hyperkinetic. **B,** chronic end-stage aortic valvular insufficiency. Note dilated hypokinetic left ventricle (LV) and fluttering of the anterior mitral valve (MV) leaflet. Ao = aorta; IVS = interventricular septum; LA = left atrium; LV = left ventricle; MV = mitral valve; PW = posterior wall of left ventricle; veg = vegetation. (From Usher B.W.: Role of echocardiography in evaluating patients with congestive heart failure. Reprinted by permission of *Medical Times,* vol. 110, no. 6, 1982.)

Doppler. Such quantitation can be affected by hemodynamic and technical factors. Therefore, for the present, it should be considered along with other clinical data as a reasonable estimate until further investigation can be done. Cardiac catheterization should be performed prior to surgical consideration to assess the degree of aortic insufficiency, evaluate left ventricular function, and

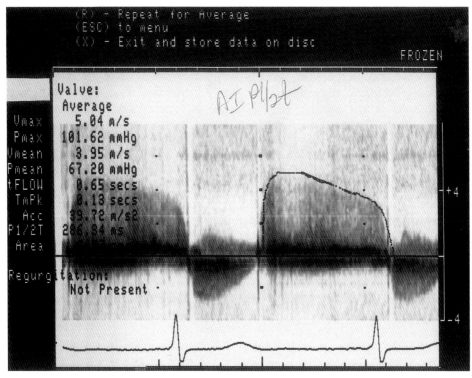

Fig 6–13. Continuous-wave Doppler showing the slope of the aortic regurgitation velocity curve. The pressure half-time is 286 msec, indicating significant aortic regurgitation. (Courtesy of Dr. Bruce W. Usher.)

detect any mitral or coronary abnormalities. The left ventricle dilates with chronic aortic insufficiency, allowing a larger ejection fraction with each beat; this results in an improved stroke volume through the Frank-Starling mechanism. In addition, the left atrial pressure is often normal but eventually, in advanced stages, increases to fill the dilated left ventricle, and the capillary

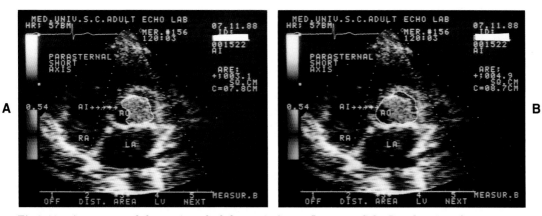

Fig 6–14. A, parasternal short axis at the left ventricular outflow tract. Color Doppler view of same patient as in Figure 6–13 with significant aortic regurgitation. Note blue-mosaic regurgitant jet (outlined) with area of 3.1 cm². B, Note aortic root (outlined) with area of 4.9 cm². Ratio of regurgitant jet area to aortic root area is 63%, indicating significant aortic insufficiency. AI = aortic insufficiency, RA = right atrium, AO = aorta, LA = left atrium. (Courtesy of Dr. Bruce W. Usher.)

wedge pressure rises; if this reaches a level greater than 25 mm Hg, pulmonary congestion can develop. The degree of aortic regurgitation can be determined by cineangiography. Contrast material is injected into the aortic root, and the amount regurgitated into the left ventricle can be noted. After aortic root injection, if there is immediate opacification of the ventricle in the first cardiac cycle and the ventricle is more densely opacified than the aortic root, severe 4 + aortic regurgitation is present; if the ventricle and the aortic root are equally opacified, then moderately severe 3 + regurgitation is present; if there is faint opacification of the ventricle after aortic root injection, moderate 2 + regurgitation is present; and if there is a faint appearance of the opaque medium below the aortic valve without outlining the ventricle, mild 1 + regurgitation is present. This grading is not precise and should be considered as a semi-quantitative estimate of regurgitation severity. The end-diastolic and end-systolic volumes can be determined by angiography and forward stroke volume by the indicator dilution or Fick method, and the regurgitant fraction can be calculated. Figure 6–15 summarizes the main features seen with chronic aortic insufficiency.

Chronic aortic insufficiency may be present for many years and not be associated with any symptoms. However, once symptoms develop, the patient can deteriorate rapidly. Angina is less frequent than noted in aortic stenosis. Congestive symptoms can clear with the use of digitalis and diuretics, salt intake restriction, and vasodilator therapy. A randomized double-blind, placebo-controlled clinical trial showed that long-term 24-month treatment with

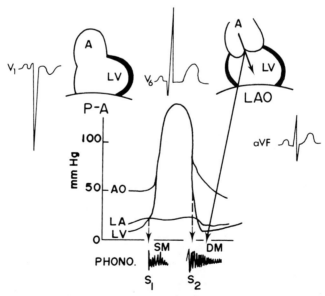

Fig 6–15. Main findings in aortic insufficiency. Hyperdynamic apical lift due to left ventricular (LV) volume load. Early systolic ejection murmur (SM) due to increased aortic outflow and high-pitched decrescendo diastolic murmur (DM) due to backflow into the left ventricle heard best in the primary aortic area or along the left sternal border. Wide pulse pressure (AO). Collapsing pulse. PA view of chest widened aorta (A) and left ventricular enlargement. ECG shows left ventricular hypertrophy. Supravalvular cineaortography in left anterior oblique view (LAO) reveals a regurgitant jet during diastole into left ventricle.

hydralazine (titrated up to a total of 3 mg/kg daily in divided doses) reduced the volume overload of aortic regurgitation and suggested that therapy may beneficially affect the natural history of the disease.[65] The best time for surgical intervention is still difficult to determine. It is ideal to intervene before there are irreversible changes in the left ventricle. However, there is still about 3 to 8% operative mortality, and the prosthetic valves, regardless of design, require continuing anticoagulation and are susceptible to many other problems. Tissue valves (porcine heterografts) do not usually require anticoagulation, although they may last for up to 7 to 9 years, they have been found to deteriorate, usually with calcification. Despite the many sophisticated procedures, there are still no clear-cut guidelines as to when surgery should be performed. The patient with aortic insufficiency may maintain his exercise tolerance for many years, because the peripheral resistance falls with exercise, and the aortic insufficiency produces less of a volume load on the ventricle. Surgery is usually offered when symptoms develop that are not easily controlled by the medical approach, the left ventricle is enlarging considerably, or there is evidence of increasing left ventricular hypertrophy by ECG. Other parameters in the asymptomatic patient that have been considered by some to favor surgery are systolic pressures above 140 or diastolic below 40 mm Hg, left ventricular end-diastolic pressure greater than 20 mm Hg, cardiac index at rest below 2.2 L/min/m^2, echocardiographic end-diastolic radius to wall thickness ratio[66] equal to or greater than 4, left ventricular end-systolic dimension by echo of 55 mm or greater,[67] and abnormal response to exercise using radionuclide cineangiography. Braunwald[41] considers the end-systolic volume (same as for mitral insufficiency) a good indicator of myocardial function; surgical results are good if the end-systolic volume is <30 ml/m^2; poor if >90 ml/m^2; and between these values, results are variable. A study by Dehmer et al.[68] using resting and exercise radionuclide ventriculography concluded that the end-systolic volume may be a better predictor of left ventricular function in patients with aortic regurgitation than the ejection fraction, which is preload-dependent. Ejection fraction of less than 0.50, shortening fraction of less than 0.27, and ratio of regurgitant to end-diastolic volume of less than 0.25 are other values that have been considered as predictors of a poor surgical outcome. Carabello et al. looked at these predictors of outcome for aortic valve replacement in patients with aortic regurgitation and left ventricular dysfunction.[68a] Preoperative end-systolic dimension by echocardiography correlated best with the postoperative ejection fraction. An end-systolic dimension of 60 mm correlated with a postoperative ejection fraction of 0.55. This study concluded that patients with moderate left ventricular dysfunction who have previously noted predictors of a poor outcome have a better prognosis after aortic valve replacement than was previously considered possible.

In summary, surgery should be advised if the patient has symptoms. Asymptomatic patients should be followed, and if there are definite findings of impaired or deteriorating left ventricular function, surgery should be offered.

Acute Aortic Insufficiency

Acute aortic insufficiency has emerged as an important clinical entity, since it gives a different picture than the chronic type. It can be produced by infective endocarditis, dissecting aneurysm, rupture or prolapse of aortic leaflets (trauma or spontaneous), and acute rheumatic fever. The sudden development of severe aortic insufficiency can produce a serious event, since a normal or mildly enlarged left ventricle from prior disease is presented with increased work and volume but without time for compensatory dilatation and hypertrophy. This can result in a high ventricular end-diastolic pressure, which may approximate the aortic diastolic pressure, and thus the aortic diastolic murmur may be short and soft. In addition, early mitral valve closure can occur when the ventricular end-diastolic pressure exceeds the left atrial pressure. The first heart sound can become soft or even absent.[69] An Austin Flint murmur and S_3 and S_4 sounds may be present. The pulse pressure will not widen, and the peripheral findings of chronic aortic insufficiency are not present. These patients often have sinus tachycardia, peripheral vasoconstriction, and at times cyanosis. Acute pulmonary edema can occur because of the pulmonary venous hypertension.

Electrocardiogram will reveal normal voltage, sometimes with ST-T changes. The left ventricle on x-ray examination can be normal or moderately increased, especially if the acute event was superimposed on a chronically diseased left ventricle. Pulmonary congestion and pulmonary edema are often noted. Echocardiogram may show essentially normal left ventricular dimensions and diastolic fluttering of the anterior leaflet of the mitral valve. Phonoechocardiographic tracings can determine early mitral valve closure (Fig 6–16). In addition, other echo findings may be noted depending on the underlying cause such as vegetations due to infective endocarditis (see Fig 6–12A). Doppler (including color flow) echocardiography gives a good estimate of the degree of aortic regurgitation.

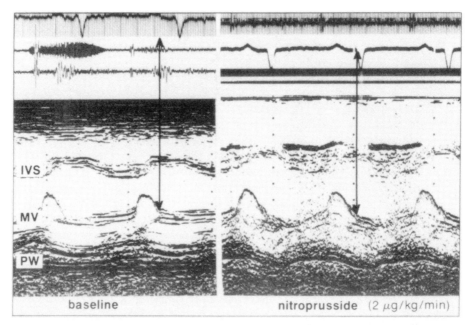

Fig 6–16. Premature closure of mitral valve (*arrow*) associated with severe acute aortic regurgitation secondary to endocarditis. With infusion of nitroprusside, the mitral valve closure point becomes less premature. IVS = interventricular septum; MV = mitral valve; PW = posterior wall. (From Usher B.W., Hendrix G.: Severe acute aortic regurgitation. Early recognition and management of life-threatening syndrome. *J. Cardiovasc. Med.* 5:169, 1980, by permission.)

Acute aortic insufficiency usually requires surgery and should be performed early if there is poorly controlled heart failure or premature mitral valve closure or both. Heart catheterization is not necessary in all cases prior to surgery. Vegetations on a flail aortic valve could be a potential risk of embolization, and large amounts of contrast material can produce adverse hemodynamic effects in a critically ill patient. Afterload reduction with sodium nitroprusside (beginning dose 0.5 μg/kg/min) can reduce the regurgitant fraction and stabilize the patient prior to surgery (see Fig 6–16). Dopamine or dobutamine may also be necessary. Excessive preload reduction should be avoided because it can adversely affect the hemodynamic status.

Aortic Stenosis

Valvular aortic stenosis was once considered rheumatic in origin in most instances. However, unless a history of rheumatic fever can be obtained or associated mitral valve disease is demonstrated, the diagnosis of rheumatic heart disease cannot be definite. Frequently a congenital bicuspid aortic valve (occurring in up to 2% of the general population) is the cause of stenosis. In patients under age 50, it is the most likely cause. Many of the mild degrees of aortic stenosis noted in childhood probably progress to a stage of calcific aortic stenosis in later life. A congenital valve may also be unicuspid, which produces obstruction during the first year of life, or tricuspid, which may produce obstruction in later years. In the elderly, calcific aortic stenosis may occur without a specific underlying cause.

Rheumatic fever can cause fibrosis and contracture of the cusps, fusion at the commissures, and, later, calcification. The bicuspid congenital valve can become calcified and is probably the most common cause of calcific aortic stenosis. Persons above 70 years of age can have degenerative changes, with calcific deposits on the aortic aspect of a tricuspid valve, and may develop significant aortic stenosis (senile type). Such patients often also have calcification of the mitral anulus. Concentric left ventricular hypertrophy occurs from any cause of aortic stenosis with significant valvular obstruction. Ventricular hypertrophy can result in diastolic stiffness, which requires greater intracavitary pressure for ventricular filling.

The obstruction caused by aortic stenosis produces a harsh ejection systolic murmur (simulating a bulldog's bark or somone clearing his throat), which gives a diamond-shaped appearance in the phonocardiogram. The longer the murmur and the later its peak, the more severe the stenosis. Severity is not usually related to intensity. The murmur is often maximum at the right second intercostal space in the primary aortic area and is usually well transmitted to the neck and also at times to the bony prominences, even to the elbows. It is often associated with a systolic thrill, which may first be felt in the sternal notch. Thrills in the primary aortic area are usually best felt while the patient is sitting up and leaning forward with his breath held at the end of expiration. At times this thrill is palpable over the carotids (carotid shudder). Frequently the murmur can be higher-pitched and musical as it radiates to the apex (Gallavardin phenomenon), making it difficult to exclude associated mitral insufficiency. Sometimes, especially in the patient with emphysema, the murmur of aortic stenosis may only be heard at the apex and must be differentiated from primary valvular mitral insufficiency. However, it is of the ejection type at the apex and is heard into the neck. If the rate varies, as it would following a premature beat, the murmur of aortic stenosis will become louder after the long cycle, whereas the murmur of mitral insufficiency will not change. The murmur of aortic stenosis can decrease in intensity with heart failure and a fall in cardiac output, but it usually will retain its length in systole. Often there will also be a murmur of aortic insufficiency, even though it has no hemodynamic significance. The aortic component of the second sound is often diminished because of fibrosis and calcification of the valve. The weak A_2 may be superimposed on the P_2 because of the delay in left ventricular ejection giving one sound, or it may be just P_2.

With severe aortic stenosis the second sound may be paradoxically split with expiration. If the value is not calcific, an aortic ejection sound is audible, which is usually best heard in the primary aortic area and at the apex. It is a high-frequency sound, occurring immediately after S_1, and coincides with the maximum opening or doming of the aortic leaflets. An S_4 gallop may be present early, and later, an S_3 gallop. At the apex there is a sustained left ventricular lift (felt to the last part of systole, whereas the normal apical impulse retracts from the chest wall during systole) and palpable S_4 gallop. The carotid pulse is of small amplitude, and the upstroke is delayed and gradually falls (pulsus parvus et tardus). A pulsus bisferiens (bifid carotid pulse) may be present when there is both aortic stenosis and insufficiency. The pulse pressure may become narrow, but this is usually a rather late sign of severe aortic stenosis. Patients can have hypertension and significant aortic stenosis. The ECG often will reveal left ventricular hypertrophy, but its relation to the severity of the disease may be deceiving. Heart size may appear normal by x ray because of the concentric (inward) hypertrophy of the left ventricle. There is often post-stenotic dilatation of the ascending aorta. Cardiac fluoroscopy will show valve calcification more often than on x ray. Echocardiography may reveal thickening or calcification of the valve and left ventricular hypertrophy (Fig 6–17). Whereas echocardiography can demonstrate the presence of aortic valve disease, it cannot demonstrate how severe the stenosis is because the thickening and calcification produce multiple ultrasonic reflectances which obscure the true aortic orifice. Doppler flow studies can confirm and quantitate the degree of stenosis by giving data for calculating the pressure gradient across the valve and its area. Transaortic gradient can be estimated by using a modification of the Bernoulli equation: gradient = 4 (velocity)^2 (Fig 6–18A). A maximum gradient greater than 50 mm Hg or a mean gradient greater than 35 mm Hg indicates significant aortic stenosis. The continuity equation[70] is used to calculate the aortic valve area. The equation is based on the fact that the volume of flow through the left ventricular outflow tract equals that through the stenotic aortic valve orifice. Volumetric flow is the product of velocity and cross-sectional area, and so the aortic valve area can be estimated from measurement of the other variables by the following equation: A_{AV} = ALVOT × VLVOT/VAV where ALVOT is the area of the left ventricular outflow tract and is calculated by A = $\pi(D/2)^2$; VLVOT is the mean left ventricular outflow tract velocity, and VAV is the mean transaortic velocity (Figs. 6–18, 6–19). Color flow Doppler is useful for detecting associated lesions. Heart catheterization studies will reveal a systolic gradient across the aortic valve, and a reduced valve area will be calculated. Figure 6–20 summarizes the main features noted in aortic valvular stenosis.

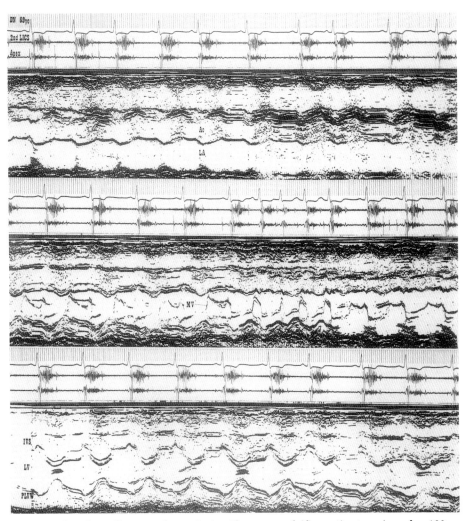

Fig 6–17. M-mode echocardiogram of a patient with severe calcific aortic stenosis and a 100 mm Hg gradient across the valve. Note in the aorta (Ao) that the aortic leaflet motion is not discernible because of the dense echoes from the calcified valve. The left ventricular cavity is small and there is concentric left ventricular hypertrophy. Phonocardiogram reveals the typical ejection murmur of aortic stenosis. Ao = aorta; IVS = interventricular septum; LA = left atrium; LV = left ventricle; PLVW = posterior left ventricular wall. (From Usher B.W.: Role of echocardiography in evaluating patients with congestive heart failure. Reprinted by permission of *Medical Times*, vol. 110, no. 6, 1982.)

Surgery is usually indicated if the patient is symptomatic and should be considered in any asymptomatic patient with evidence of progressive left ventricular hypertrophy. Symptoms usually develop when the valve orifice is reduced to 0.7 to 0.8 cm^2 (normal aortic valve is 2.5 to 3.5 cm^2). The three main symptoms that usually develop are dyspnea, angina, and syncope. There is usually a long latent period, depending on the etiology and degree of stenosis, prior to these symptoms developing. However, most often they occur later in the course of the disease at about the fifth or sixth decade. The frequency of angiodysplasia of the colon is increased in patients with calcific aortic stenosis and can produce gastrointestinal bleeding. Microthrombi or thickened valves or calcium may cause embolization.

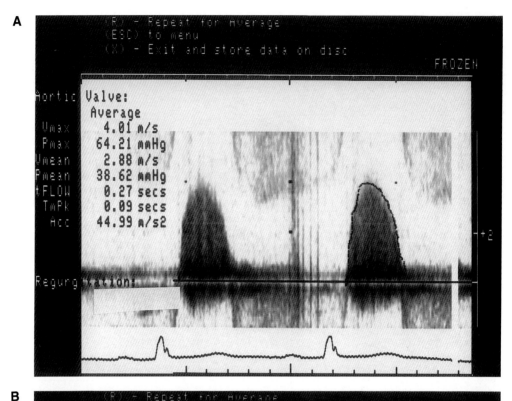

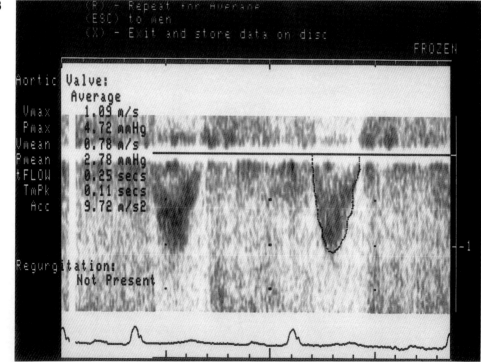

Fig 6–18. Doppler studies of a patient with calcific aortic stenosis. A, Continuous wave Doppler flow velocity recorded across the aortic valve from the right parasternal area. Note that peak gradient across the aortic valve is 64 mm Hg (Bernoulli equation = 4×4^2) and mean gradient is 38.6 mm Hg. B, Pulsed Doppler flow velocity of the left ventricular outflow tract. (Courtesy of Dr. Bruce W. Usher.)

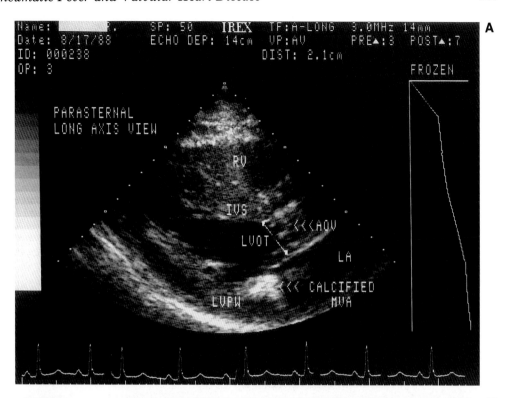

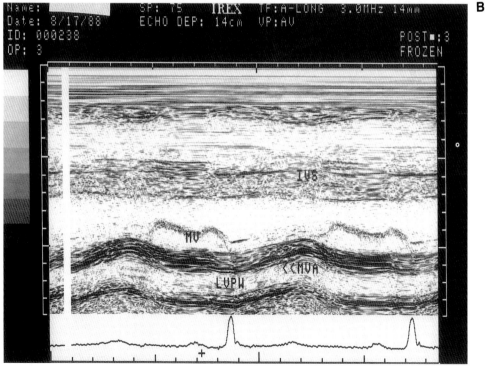

Fig 6–19. Two-dimensional and M-mode echocardiography of same patient with calcific aortic stenosis noted in Figure 6–18. A, Parasternal long axis view of 2-D echo. Note concentric hypertrophy of the left ventricle, calcification of the aortic valve (AOV), calcification of the mitral valve annulus (MVA) and diameter of the left ventricular outflow tract (LVOT). B, M-mode echo of left ventricle. Note hypertrophy of interventricular septum (IVS) and left ventricular posterior wall (LVPW), marked calcification of the mitral valve anulus (MVA) and diastolic shuttering of the anterior leaflet of the mitral valve (consistent with aortic regurgitation). Using the data from Figure 6–19A and Figure 6–18 into the continuity equation ($A_{AV} = 3.46 \times .78/2.88$) the area of the aortic valve is calculated as .94 cm^2. RV = Right ventricle, LA = Left atrium, A_{AV} = Aortic valve area. (Courtesy of Dr. Bruce W. Usher.)

AORTIC VALVE STENOSIS

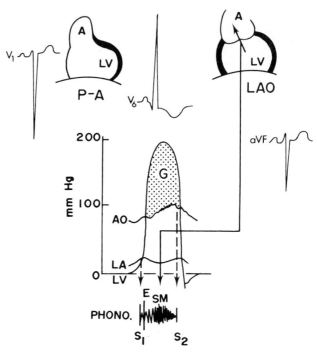

Fig 6–20. Main findings in aortic valvular stenosis. Slow, sustained apical lift due to left ventricular hypertrophy. Harsh ejection diamond-shaped systolic murmur (SM) best heard in the primary aortic area and often associated with a thrill. Aortic ejection (E) sound if valve is mobile. Intensity of aortic second sound (S$_2$) may be diminished especially if valve is calcified. Aortic pressure pulse (AO) shows small amplitude and delayed upstroke. PA of chest shows poststenotic dilatation of ascending aorta (A) and a rounded left ventricle (LV) due to concentric hypertrophy. ECG shows left ventricular hypertrophy. Hatched area (G) represents systolic gradient (100 mm Hg across aortic valve) due to increased systolic left ventricular (LV) pressure over that in the aorta (AO).

When overt heart failure develops, the prognosis is usually poor, and life expectancy is about 2 years. Once angina occurs, life expectancy is about 5 years and 3 years with syncope.[71,72] Often it is difficult to know whether there is coexistent coronary atherosclerosis (about 50% have significant coronary disease); therefore, during heart catheterization studies, these patients should have coronary arteriograms. Syncope or dizziness may occur at rest or on effort. Effort syncope is due to the decrease in BP secondary to peripheral vasodilation in the presence of a fixed cardiac output and may be associated with arrhythmias, such as heart block or ventricular fibrillation. Sudden death is a concern wih severe aortic stenosis, but in adults, it is rare in the presence of a normal ECG. By the time the patient is symptomatic and has critical stenosis, there is usually a peak-to-peak systolic gradient across the aortic valve of 50 mm Hg or more or a valve orifice area of 0.75 cm^2 or less or 0.4 cm^2/m^2 BSA or less. Naturally, a decline in cardiac output will reduce the gradient. Usually the orifice's size will be less than 0.8 cm^2 before there is significant obstruction to flow and forward cardiac output. Operation is advised in most centers in patients with aortic valve areas of 0.8 cm^2 or less. We advise surgery for valve orifice areas up to 1 cm^2 if the patient is symptomatic. Despite the presence of congestive heart failure and a reduced ejection fraction, patients have an exellent outcome with surgery with a significant increase in ejection fraction. Therefore, surgery is recommended even though patients may have poor left ventricular performance. A problem patient is the one with a low cardiac output, small transvalvular gradient, and a critical aortic valve area. Such patients may have only a mild aortic stenosis with concomitant cardiomyopathy and may not improve with surgery. Therefore, it is important in these patients that invasive and noninvasive studies confirm that the valve is really stenotic. Asymptomatic patients with a critically narrow valve present a problem because there has been no randomized controlled long-term study comparing those with and without surgery. Such patients should be followed carefully with clinical examinations, echocardiography, and Doppler at 6 to 12 months for signs of progression. If progressive left ventricular dysfunction or progressive cardiomegaly is noted, I would advise surgery even if the patient is totally asymptomatic and has a critical valve area. The selection of the type of valve (prosthetic or tissue) and the associated problems are the same as those mentioned for mitral valve replacement. The operative risk is usually about 2 to 8%. If significant coronary artery lesions are present, coronary bypass should also be performed. Oral anticoagulant therapy should be given indefinitely if the patient has a prosthetic valve, but is not necessary for a patient with a tissue valve. Valvulotomy can be performed at times in the young who have a noncalcified congenital valve.

Balloon valvuloplasty is a technique that can now be considered in children and adolescents as an alternative to valvulotomy and in adults (high-risk patients or those who refuse surgery) instead of valve replacement. Safian et al.[73] reported on 170 consecutive patients who had balloon aortic valvuloplasty for symptomatic aortic stenosis. The procedure was successful in 168 patients and resulted in an increase of mean aortic-valve area from 0.6 ± 0.2 to 0.9 ± 0.3 cm^2, an increase in cardiac output from 4.6 ± 3.4 to 4.8 ± 1.4 liters per minute, and a decrease in the peak-aortic valve pressure gradient from 71 ± 20 to 36 ± 14 mm Hg. Six in-hospital deaths occurred and 5 patients required aortic valve replacement. Twenty-five patients died out of hospital about 6.4 ± 5.3 months since discharge. Restenosis was found to be common, requiring repeat balloon dilation. Balloon aortic valvuloplasty is a palliative procedure that increases the valve area little but does improve symptoms and has a high rate of restenosis and significant mortality. Major complications include death, emboli, acute aortic regurgitation, and ventricular perforation.

Table 6–2 summarizes the indications for study and surgery in common valvular heart diseases.

Aortic Stenosis in the Elderly

Aortic stenosis is not uncommon in persons 65 years of age and older, and is usually due to degenerative changes rather than to congenital bicuspid aortic valve or rheumatic fever as seen in younger patients. With aging there is fibrous thickening, with calcium deposits at the base of the aortic cusps developing (so-called sclerotic valve).[74] If calcium progressively deposits, stenosis can occur without fusion of the commissures. Older patients also commonly have associated coronary artery disease, mitral anular calcification, and con-

Table 6–2.   Indications for Surgery in Common Valvular Heart Disease

Lesion	Indications for Study and Operation
Mitral stenosis	Symptomatic and valve area <1.0 cm^2; if between 1.0 and 1.5 cm^2, individualize, depending on other findings and patient's activities
Chronic mitral insufficiency	Progressive symptoms or progressive cardiomegaly despite medical therapy
Acute mitral insufficiency	Heart failure or hemodynamic instability
Aortic stenosis	Symptomatic with gradient of 50 mm Hg or greater and/or a valve area of 1 cm^2 or less; asymptomatic patients studied if there is progressive cardiomegaly or left ventricular dysfunction
Chronic aortic insufficiency	Symptomatic; asymptomatic with moderate or marked left ventricular enlargement and ECG evidence of left ventricular hypertrophy with ST-T changes or evidence of impaired or deteriorating left ventricular function
Acute aortic insufficiency	Heart failure or premature mitral valve closure by echo

duction defects. The severity of aortic stenosis in the elderly is frequently difficult to assess because the clinical findings may not be the same as in the younger patients. The elderly do not often have a slow carotid upstroke, narrow pulse pressure, decreased or absent aortic closure sound, and a left ventricular lift may not be detectable because of emphysema. The systolic pressure can be elevated because of the loss of arterial elasticity due to sclerosis. Often the systolic murmur is not intense in the aortic area, but there may be a loud systolic musical murmur along the left sternal border and at the apex.[75] The duration of the murmur (even though late peaking may be absent because of the absence of a jet lesion) may be helpful for suggesting significant stenosis, since many elderly patients (75% over 70 years of age[76]) have aortic systolic murmurs of short duration that are due to sclerosis or dilatation of the aorta rather than stenosis. Atrial fibrillation is more commonly noted in elderly patients with aortic stenosis compared with the younger group. Usually calcification in the aortic valve will be noted by fluoroscopy, and the ECG will show ST-T changes. Increased left ventricular voltage may be absent because of the emphysematous chest. Echocardiography and Doppler studies, as described earlier, are very useful for the diagnosis and quantitation of aortic stenosis.

These elderly patients should not be overlooked because aortic valve replacement or balloon valvuloplasty is indicated if they are symptomatic and have critical orifice stenosis as demonstrated by cardiac catheterization.

TRICUSPID VALVE DISEASE

Tricuspid Insufficiency

Tricuspid insufficiency is rarely a primary lesion, and more often is secondary to lesions that produce left ventricular failure with subsequent right heart failure, pulmonary hypertension (mitral valve disease, congenital heart lesions, primary pulmonary hypertension, cor pulmonale), or to right ventricular infarction. Rheumatic fever involves the tricuspid valve much less commonly (5 to 10% of patients) than the mitral and aortic valves. Tricuspid insufficiency can also be congenital (Ebstein's anomaly, endocardial cushion defects), due to myxomatous changes, as a part of the carcinoid syndrome, due to trauma, and due to cardiac tumors as right atrial myxomas. Infective endocarditis has become a more common cause with the increase in drug addiction.

One should suspect tricuspid insufficiency (especially in a patient with known left ventricular failure or mitral disease) if the patient notes increasing peripheral edema, abdominal swelling, and less dyspnea and orthopnea. The neck veins are often a clue to the diagnosis because of the prominent C-V deep jugular pulsation. In fact, at times this pulsation can even raise the lower portion of the ear lobe and may be mistaken for an arterial pulsation. When the patient lies down, the face has a cyanotic tinge, the frontal vein is prominent, and the patient complains of a throbbing fullness in the neck and head. A hyperdynamic right ventricular lift may be present. A holosystolic, high-pitched, blowing murmur can be present in the xiphoid area, along the left sternal border at the fourth intercostal space or because of a large right ventricle at the apex. Acute forms of tricuspid insufficiency may give only a short murmur or no murmur. In contrast to mitral insufficiency, the murmur of tricuspid insufficiency usually increases with inspiration (Carvallo's sign) unless there is marked right venticular dysfunction. A right ventricular S_3 gallop (louder with inspiration) may be present. The liver is enlarged (often painful) and may have systolic pulsations. Often a pulsatile liver cannot be distinguished from pulsations due to the abdominal aorta. One can be certain that the pulsation is from the liver if, by pressure on the liver anteriorly, a liver pulsation can be felt with the other hand posteriorly just below the ribs. Ascites can be present and at times there is jaundice. The ECG frequently shows atrial fibrillation. X ray reveals marked enlargement of the right atrium and ventricle and other features due to the primary lesion. Echocardiogram reveals right ventricular overload and paradoxical septal motion. It can also aid in the diagnosis; delayed closure of tricuspid valve in Ebstein's anomaly; diminished A wave in pulmonary hypertension; vegetations in infective endocarditis; and late systolic posterior displacement of leaflets in tricuspid valve prolapse. Cross-sectional echocardiography has been useful in detecting tricuspid insufficiency by using rapid injection of a bolus of saline in a peripheral vein and observing the "microcavities" go back and forth across the tricuspid valve.[77] Doppler echocardiography and color imaging are useful for diagnosing and assessing tricuspid regurgitation (Fig 6–4). The severity of tricuspid regurgitation will be affected by changes in right ventricular systolic pressure. Right heart catheterization will reveal elevated right atrial pressure and right ventricular end-diastolic pressure, and, if the regurgitation is severe, the right atrial pressure can resemble the right ventricular pressure recording.[78]

Secondary tricuspid insufficiency often requires no specific therapy other than that for the primary lesion, unless it is severe; then anuloplasty or valve replacement may be needed. Primary tricuspid lesions of sufficient severity usually require annuloplasty or valve replacement with a tissue valve (thromboembolism greater with prosthetic valves). If antibiotic therapy is not successful in infective tricuspid endocarditis, the infected valve may have to be removed and an artifical valve later inserted.

Tricuspid Stenosis

Tricuspid stenosis is rare as an isolated entity. It is most commonly due to rheumatic fever which has also involved the mitral and aortic valves.

Patients will have peripheral edema, abdominal swelling, and right upper quadrant pain and less evidence of pulmonary congestion (which is common with mitral stenosis). A large presystolic A wave may be noted in the jugular venous pulse if there is a sinus rhythm, or a high early diastolic V wave followed by a slow Y descent if atrial fibrillation is present. A right ventricular lift is absent, but a large right atrium may produce a lower right sternal pulsation. Auscultation may reveal an opening snap and a diastolic rumbling murmur heard best at the lower left sternal border. Both of these findings will be louder with inspiration. The lung fields are often clear, and the patient can lie flat without symptoms of congestion. A presystolic hepatic pulsation, ascites, peripheral edema, and jaundice can be present. Electrocardiogram may show atrial fibrillation or regular sinus rhythm with right atrial enlargement. A prominent right atrium without significant pulmonary hypertension or an enlarged pulmonary artery are common x-ray features, besides those chamber enlargements produced by the other associated valvular lesions. Echocardiography and Doppler show almost the same features in the tricuspid valve as noted in the mitral valve with mitral stenosis (Fig 6–21). The findings are best noted on two-dimensional echo study. Heart catheterization reveals a diastolic gradient between the right atrium and ventricle. Significant tricuspid stenosis can require commissurotomy or valve replacement at the same time that left chamber valvular lesions are managed. Thrombosis occurs more often in the tricuspid position, therefore it is preferable to use a tissue valve rather than a mechanical prosthesis.

PULMONARY VALVE DISEASE

Pulmonic valve disorders, other than those congenitally or surgically produced, are rare. Rheumatic involvement is usually associated with involvement of other valves. Carcinoid may affect the pulmonic valve with fibrous plaques. Both of these conditions can produce pulmonary stenosis. Pulmonary valvular insufficiency is usually secondary to pulmonary hypertension (Graham Steell murmur) from any cause. It can result as a primary lesion from infective endocarditis or from surgical procedures for pulmonic stenosis. It can also occur as an isolated congenital anomaly, but most often it is associated with other defects.

The findings of pulmonic valvular stenosis will be discussed in Chapter 7. Pulmonary valvular insufficiency secondary to pulmonary hypertension may produce a hyperdynamic right venticular lift and a palpable pulsation in the pulmonic area. The diastolic murmur often resembles that of aortic insufficiency, except that it is louder with inspiration and does not produce peripheral signs noted with aortic insufficiency. Pulmonic valvular insufficiency with low pulmonary artery pressure can be noted as a congenital abnormality, after surgical repair of pulmonic stenosis (as noted after tetralogy repair), or

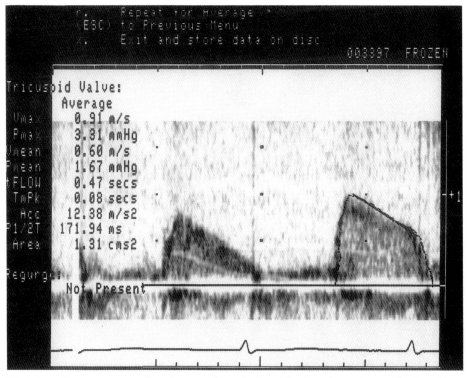

Fig 6–21. Continuous-wave Doppler recording of tricuspid valve of a patient with tricuspid stenosis. Note that velocity decreases gradually through diastole. The estimated tricuspid valve area by pressure half-time is 1.3 cm^2. (Courtesy of Dr. Bruce W. Usher.)

with infective endocarditis on a prior normal valve. The murmur of this low-pressure type differs from the high-pitched Graham Steell murmur in that it is of medium frequency, soft, and mid-diastolic.

Electrocardiogram shows right ventricular hypertrophy, and chest x ray usually depicts an enlarged pulmonary artery and right ventricle in the pulmonary insufficiency of the hypertensive type. The findings in the low-pressure type vary depending on the degree of pulmonary insufficiency and the underlying cause. Echocardiogram may reveal right ventricular dilatation and diastolic fluttering of the tricuspid valve leaflets when the pulmonary insufficiency is secondary to pulmonary hypertension. Vegetations on the pulmonic valve may be noted with infective endocarditis. Pulsed and colorflow Doppler can easily detect pulmonary regurgitation (Fig 6–22).

Pulmonic valvular insufficiency usually requires no therapy. The primary condition which produced pulmonary hypertension should be treated when possible. The surgical induced types often are mild and require no therapy.

MULTIVALVULAR DISEASE

Rheumatic heart disease accounts for the majority of cases with multivalve involvement. Various combinations can occur, such as mitral stenosis with aortic insufficiency or aortic stenosis or mitral insufficiency with aortic stenosis or insufficiency. One must listen carefully, for often one lesion may mask

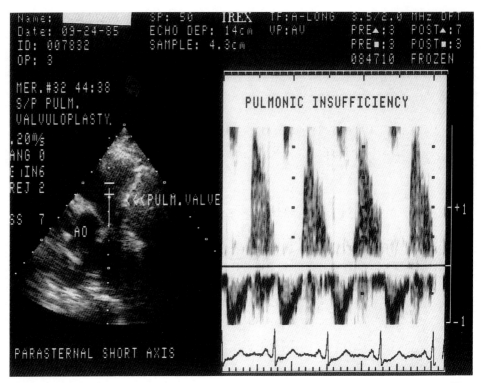

Fig 6–22. Pulsed Doppler recording of a patient with pulmonary regurgitation. (Courtesy of Dr. Bruce W. Usher.)

the other, aggravate it, or make it appear less important. A loud first sound at the apex may be the only clue that there may be mitral stenosis associated with aortic valvular disease. Tight mitral stenosis may mask significant aortic stenosis because of the reduced cardiac output. Aortic stenosis may increase associated mitral insufficiency, and combinations of severe aortic insufficiency and mitral insufficiency produce an excessive volume load and are tolerated poorly.

Multivalvular disease must be recognized preoperatively, for correcting one problem may place an undue burden on the heart because of the other uncorrected lesions. Mitral stenosis can be corrected, but may allow significant aortic valvular disease to add a sudden burden on the left ventricle and may precipitate pulmonary edema. At times, after repair of a severe aortic valve lesion, milder degrees of mitral insufficiency may regress. Echocardiography has been a valuable noninvasive method of recognizing multiple lesions. Color flow Doppler and other Doppler techniques are of great value in clarifying multivalvular lesions. Naturally, heart catheterization should be done in all such patients. Double- and triple-valve replacement increases the surgical mortality up to 10 to 15%, and even higher for functional class IV patients. Whenever possible, if mitral stenosis is present with an aortic valve lesion, a mitral commissurotomy should be attempted, with aortic valve replacement if the patient is a suitable candidate.

It should be recognized that even if the mechanical load (single or multiple valve) is removed by surgery, the course may eventually deteriorate because the ventricles were too damaged prior to surgery or there is an ongoing smoldering myocarditis, such as that associated with rheumatic carditis. In addition, some lesions respond better than others. Generally, the stenotic lesions have less ventricular damage, and after surgery the hemodynamics return closer to normal than with the volume overload insufficiency lesions.

REFERENCES

1. Stollerman G.H.: *Rheumatic Fever and Streptococcal Infection.* New York, Grune & Stratton, 1975.
2. Rammelkamp C.H., Denny F.W., Wannamaker L.W.: Studies on the epidemiology of rheumatic fever in the armed services, in Thomas L. (ed.): *Rheumatic Fever: A Symposium.* Minneapolis, University of Minnesota Press, 1952, p. 72.
3. Siegal A.C., Johnson E.F., Stollerman G.H.: Controlled studies of streptococcal pharyngitis in a pediatric population: I. Factors related to the attack rate of rheumatic fever. *N. Engl. J. Med.* 265:559, 1961.
4. Committee to Revise the Jones' Criteria. American Heart Association. Jones' Criteria (revised) for guidance in the diagnosis of rheumatic fever. *Circulation* 32:664, 1965.
5. Feinstein A.R., Spagnuolo M.: The clinical patterns of acute rheumatic fever: A reappraisal. *Medicine (Baltimore)* 41:279, 1962.
6. Bland E.F.: Chorea as a manifestation of rheumatic fever, a long-term perspective. *Trans. Am. Clin. Climatol. Assoc.* 73:209, 1961.
7. Bisno A.L., Ofek I.: Serological diagnosis of streptococcal infection: Comparison of a rapid hemagglutination technique with conventional antibody tests. *Am. J. Dis. Child.* 127:676, 1974.
8. Stollerman G.H., Lewis A.J., Schultz L., et al.: Relationship of immune response to group A streptococci to the cause of acute, chronic and recurrent rheumatic fever. *Am. J. Med.* 20:163, 1956.
9. American Heart Association Committee on Rheumatic Fever and Infective Endocarditis: Prevention of Rheumatic Fever. *Circulation* 70:1118A, 1984.
10. Beachey E.H., Grus-Masse T.A., Jolivet M., et al.: Opsonic antibodies evoked by hybrid peptide copies of types 5 and 24 streptococcal M proteins synthesized in tandem. *J. Exp. Med.* 163:1451, 1986.
11. Silverman M.E., Hurst W.J.: The mitral complex. *Am. Heart J.* 76:399, 1968.
12. Braunwald E.: Mitral regurgitation: Physiologic, clinical and surgical considerations. *N. Engl. J. Med.* 281:425, 1969.
13. Armstrong T.G., Meeran M.K., Gotsman M.S.: The left atrial lift. *Am. Heart J.* 82:764, 1971.
14. Helmcke F., Navin N.C., Hsiung M.C., et al.: Color Doppler assessment of mitral regurgitation with orthogonal planes. *Circulation* 75:175, 1987.
15. Reid J.V.: Mid-systolic clicks. *S. Afr. Med. J.* 35:353, 1961.
16. Barlow J.B., Pocock W.A., Marchand P., et al.: The significance of late systolic murmurs. *Am. Heart J.* 66:443, 1963.
17. Levy D., Savage D.: Prevalence and clinical features of mitral valve prolapse. *Am. Heart J.* 113:1281, 1987.
18. Shell W.E., Walton J.A., Clifford M.E., et al.: The familial occurrence of the syndrome of mid-late systolic click and late systolic murmur. *Circulation* 39:327, 1969.
19. Mason J.W., Koch F.H., Billingham M.E., et al.: Cardiac biopsy evidence for a cardiomyopathy associated with symptomatic mitral valve prolapse. *Am. J. Cardiol.* 42:557, 1978.
20. Shrivastava S., Guthrie R.B., Edwards J.E.: Prolapse of the mitral valve. *Mod. Concepts Cardiovasc. Dis.* 46:57, 1977.
21. Fontana M.E., Wooley C.F., Leighton R.F., et al.: Postural changes in left ventricular and mitral valvular dynamics in the systolic click-late systolic murmur syndrome. *Circulation* 51:165, 1975.
22. Wood P.: DaCosta's syndrome (or effort syndrome). *Br. Med. J.* 1:767, 1941.
23. Wolf E., Braun K., Stern S.: Effects of beta-receptor blocking agents propranolol and practolol on ST-T changes in neurocirculatory asthenia. *Br. Heart J.* 36:872, 1974.
24. Puddu P.E., Pasternac A., Tubau J.F., et al.: QT interval prolongation and increased plasma catecholamine levels in patients with mitral valve prolapse. *Am. Heart J.* 105:422, 1983.
25. Devereux R.B., Perloff J.K., Reichek N., et al.: Mitral valve prolapse. *Circulation* 54:3, 1976.
26. Engel P.J., Alpert B.L., Hickman J.R.: The nature and prevalence of the abnormal exercise electrocardiogram in mitral valve prolapse. *Am. Heart J.* 98:716, 1979.
27. Scampardonis G., Yang S.S., Maranhao V., et al.: Left ventricular abnormalities in prolapsed mitral leaflet syndrome. *Circulation* 48:287, 1973.

28. Perloff J.K., Child J.S.: Clinical and epidemiologic issues in mitral valve prolapse: Overview and perspective. *Am. Heart J.* 113:1324, 1987.
29. Belton D.C., Brear S.G., Edwards J.D., et al.: Mitral valve prolapse: An assessment of clinical features, associated conditions, and prognosis. *Q.J. Med.* 52:150, 1983.
30. Mills P., Rose J., Hollingsworth J., et al.: Long-term prognosis of mitral-valve prolapse. *N. Engl. J. Med.* 297:13, 1977.
31. Devereaux R.B.: Mitral valve prolapse and severe mitral regurgitation. *Circulation* 78:234, 1988.
31a. Marks A.R., Choong C.Y., Chir M.B.B., et al.: Identification of high-risk subgroups of patients with mitral-valve prolapse. *N. Engl. J. Med.* 320:1031, 1989.
32. Hickey A.J., Wilcken D.E.L., Wright J.S., Warren B.A.: Primary (spontaneous) chordal rupture: Relation to myxomatous valve disease and mitral valve prolapse. *J. Am. Coll. Cardiol.* 5:1341, 1985.
33. Wilcken D.E.L., Hickey A.J.: Lifetime risk for patients with mitral valve prolapse of developing severe valve regurgitation requiring surgery. *Circulation* 78:10, 1988.
34. Lachman A.S., Bramwell-Jones D.M., Lahier T.B., et al.: Infective endocarditis in the billowing mitral leaflet syndrome. *Br. Heart J.* 37:326, 1975.
35. MacMahon S.W., Hickey A.J., Wilcken D.E.L., et al.: The risk of infective endocarditis in persons with mitral valve prolapse with and without precordial systolic murmurs. *Am. J. Cardiol.* 59:105, 1987.
36. Barnett H.J.M., Boughner D.R., Taylor W., et al.: Further evidence relating mitral-valve prolapse to cerebral ischemic events. *N. Engl. J. Med.* 302:139, 1980.
37. Nichol P., Kertesz A.: Two dimensional echocardiographic (2DE) detection of left atrial thrombus in patients with mitral valve prolapse and strokes. Circulation 59, 60(suppl. 2):11–18, 1979.
38. Duren D.R., Becker A.E., Dunninig A.J.: Long-term follow-up of idiopathic mitral valve prolapse in 300 patients: A prospective study. *J. Am. Coll. Cardiol.* 11:42, 1988.
39. Savage D.D., Devereux R.B., Garrison R.J., et al.: Mitral valve prolapse in the general population: II. Clinical features: The Framingham Study. *Am. Heart J.* 106:577, 1983.
40. Retchin S.M., Fletcher R.H., Earp J., et al.: Mitral Valve Prolapse. Disease or Illness? *Arch. Intern. Med.* 146:1081, 1986.
41. Braunwald E.: Valvular heart disease, in Braunwald E. (ed.): *Heart Disease.* Philadelphia, W.B. Saunders Co., 1980, pp. 1112–1141.
42. Carabello B.A.: Hemodynamic predictors of outcome in valve replacement. *Cardiology Board Review* 4:92, 1987.
43. Iturbe-Alessio I., Del Carmen Fonseca M., Mutchinik O., et al.: Risks of anticoagulant therapy in pregnant women with artificial heart valves. *N. Engl. J. Med.* 315:1390, 1986.
44. Hall J.G., Pauli R.M., Wilson K.M.: Maternal and fetal sequelae of anticoagulation during pregnancy. *Am. J. Med.* 68:122, 1980.
45. Bortolotti U., Milano A., Mazzucco A., et al.: Results of reoperation for primary tissue failure of porcine bioprostheses. *J. Thorac. Cardiovasc. Surg.* 90:564, 1985.
46. Antman E.M., Angoff G.H., Sloss J.J.: Demonstration of the mechanisms by which mitral regurgitation mimics aortic stenosis. *Am. J. Cardiol.* 42:1044, 1978.
47. Merendino K.A., Hessel E.A.: The murmur on top of the head in acquired mitral insufficiency. *J.A.M.A.* 199:392, 1967.
48. Carley J.E., Wong B.Y.S., Pugh D.M., et al.: Clinical significance of the V wave in the main pulmonary artery. *Am. J. Cardiol.* 39:982, 1977.
49. Burch G.E., Giles T.D., Colcolough H.L.: Pathogenesis of "rheumatic" heart disease: Critique and theory. *Am. Heart J.* 80:556, 1970.
50. Luisada A.A., MacCanon D.M., Kumar S., et al.: Changing views on the mechanism of the first and second sounds. *Am. Heart J.* 88:503, 1974.
51. Criley J.M., Chambers R.D., Blaufuss A.H., et al.: Mitral stenosis: mechanicoacoustical events, in Leon D.F., Shaver J.A. (eds.): *Physiological Principles of Heart Sounds and Murmurs.* New York, American Heart Association Monograph No. 46, 1975, pp. 149–159.
52. Thompson M.E., Shaver J.A., Heidenreich F.P., et al.: Sound, pressure, and motion correlates in mitral stenosis. *Am. J. Med.* 49:437, 1970.
53. Hatle L., Angelsen B.: *Doppler Ultrasound in Cardiology: Physical Principles and Clinical Application.* 2nd ed., Philadelphia, Lea & Febiger, 1985.
54. Cohen M.V., Gorlin R.: Modified orifice equation for the calculation of mitral valve area. *Am. Heart J.* 84:839, 1972.
55. Hugenholtz P.G., Ryan T.J., Stein S.W., et al.: The spectrum of pure mitral stenosis: Hemodynamic studies in relation to clinical disability. *Am. J. Cardiol.* 10:773, 1962.
56. Braunwald E.: Valvular heart disease, in Braunwald E. (ed.): Heart Disease. Philadelphia, W.B. Saunders Co., 1988, p. 1032.
57. Braunwald E., Braunwald N.S., Ross J., Jr., et al.: Effects of mitral-valve replacement on the

pulmonary vascular dynamics of patients with pulmonary hypertension. *N. Engl. J. Med.* 273:509, 1965.

58. Inoue K., Owaki T., Nakamura T., et al.: Clinical application of transverse mitral commissurotomy by a new balloon catheter. *J. Thorac. Cardiovasc. Surg.* 87:394, 1984.

59. McKay R.G., Grossman W.: Balloon valvuloplasty for treating pulmonic, mitral, aortic and prosthetic valve stenosis. In *Heart Disease Update I*. Braunwald, E. ed. Philadelphia, W.B. Saunders Co., 1988, pp. 3–7.

60. Olson L.S., Subramanian R., Edwards W.D.: Surgical pathology of pure aortic insufficiency: A study of 225 cases. *Mayo Clin. Proc.* 59:835, 1984.

61. Fortuin N.J., Craig E.: On the mechanism of the Austin-Flint murmur. *Circulation* 45:558, 1972.

62. Grayburn P.A., Handshoe R, Smith M.D., et al.: Quantitative assessment of the hemodynamic consequences of aortic regurgitation by means of continuous wave Doppler recordings. *JACC* 10:135, 1987.

63. Teague S.M., Heinsimer J.A., Anderson J.L., et al.: Quantification of aortic regurgitation utilizing continuous wave Doppler ultrasound. *JACC* 8:592, 1986.

64. Perry G.J., Helmcke F., Nanda N.C., et al.: Evaluation of aortic insufficiency by Doppler color flow mapping. *JACC* 9:952, 1987.

65. Greenberg B., Massie B., Bristow J.D., et al.: Long-term vasodilator therapy of chronic aortic insufficiency. A randomized double-blinded, placebo-controlled clinical trial. *Circulation* 78:92, 1988.

66. Gaasch W.H., Andrias C.W., Levine H.J.: Chronic aortic regurgitation: The effect of aortic valve replacement on left ventricular volume, mass and function. *Circulation* 58:825, 1978.

67. Henry W.L., Bonow R.O., Rosing D.R., et al.: Observations on the optimum time for operative intervention for aortic regurgitation: II. Serial echocardiographic evaluation of asymptomatic patients. *Circulation* 61:484, 1980.

68. Dehmer G.J., Firth B.G., Hillis L.D., et al.: Alterations in left ventricular volume and ejection fraction at rest and during exercise in patients with aortic regurgitation. *Am. J. Cardiol.* 48:17, 1981.

68a. Carabello B.A., Usher B.W., Hendrix G.H., et al.: Predictors of outcome for aortic valve replacement in patients with aortic regurgitation and left ventricular dysfunction: A change in the measuring stick. *JACC* 10:991, 1987.

69. Spring D.A., Folts J.D., Young W.P., et al.: Premature closure of the mitral and tricuspid valves. *Circulation* 45:663, 1972.

70. Teirstein P., Yeager M., Yock P.G., et al.: Doppler echocardiographic measurement of aortic valve area in aortic stenosis: A noninvasive application of the gorlin formula. *JACC* 8:1059, 1986.

71. Ross J., Jr., Braunwald E.: The influence of corrective operations on the natural history of aortic stenosis. *Circulation* 37(suppl. 5):61, 1968.

72. Frank S., Johnson A., Ross R., Jr.: Natural history of valvular aortic stenosis. *Br. Heart J.* 35:41, 1973.

73. Safian R.D., Berman A.D., Diver D.J., et al.: Balloon aortic valvuloplasty in 170 consecutive patients. *New Engl. J. Med.* 319:125, 1988.

74. Roberts W.C., Perloff J.K., Costantino T.: Severe valvular aortic stenosis in patients over 65 years of age. *Am. J. Cardiol.* 27:497, 1971.

75. Davison E.T., Friedman S.A.: Significance of systolic murmurs in the aged. *N. Engl. J. Med.* 279:225, 1968.

76. Caird F.I.: Heart disease in old age. *Postgrad. Med. J.* 39:408, 1963.

77. Lieppe W., Behar V.S., Scallion R., et al.: Detection of tricuspid regurgitation with two-dimensional echocardiography and peripheral vein injections. *Circulation* 57:128, 1978.

78. Grossman W.: *Cardiac Catheterization and Angiography*. Philadelphia, Lea & Febiger, 1980, p. 322.

Chapter 7

CONGENITAL HEART DISEASE

Approximately one infant in every 100 births has congenital heart disease, with one third of these dying in the first year if unattended. Thus, early diagnosis is mandatory for infants with heart disease. In this section only the most common lesions will be discussed. The registry of the Medical University of South Carolina (MUSC) revealed 1508 congenital cardiac defects from the 2496 patients in the pediatric cardiology registry over a two-year period. Table 7–1 indicates the congenital defects with their incidence. These lesions will be discussed under the following categories: left-to-right shunts, right-to-left shunts, pulmonary hypertension, obstructive defects, lesions that produce continuous murmurs, less common defects, and congenital heart defects in the adult.

LEFT-TO-RIGHT SHUNTS

Ventricular Septal Defect

Ventricular septal defects vary greatly in size and location. They can be in the membranous (beneath the aortic valve) portion of the septum or in the muscular portion which is further divided into the inlet (inflow portion of the right ventricle), trabecular, and outlet (infundibular) parts. The majority of the defects are in the membranous septum and are called perimembranous because they may extend into the adjacent portions of the muscular septum. The next most common defects occur in the trabecular portion of the muscular septum. Isolated defects in the inlet portion and in the outlet portion (beneath the aortic and pulmonic valve are often called infundibular defects) are not as common. Ventricular septal defects are seldom seen in adulthood because they either have closed off spontaneously or have had surgical repair. Hoffman and Rudolph[1] reported a 30% incidence of spontaneous closure of ventricular septal defects within the first 2 years of life and as high as 50% closure within 10 years. Perimembranous and trabecular muscular defects tend to close more frequently than the inlet and outlet types. Generally the smaller defects are the ones that close spontaneously, although there have been reports of larger ones with significant left-to-right shunts that have closed. Small ventricular septal aneurysms have developed with closure (especially the perimembranous type) and protrude into the right ventricle. At times such aneurysms retain a small opening, producing a left-to-right shunt with a holosystolic murmur or just in late systole. Tensing of the aneurysm can produce a systolic "clicking sound" along the left sternal border.

Table 7–1. 1508 Congenital Cardiac Defects from the 2496 Patients in the Pediatric Cardiology Registry of the Medical University of South Carolina Over a 2-Year Period*

Manifestation	Defect	Frequency, %	
Common left-right shunts	Ventricular septal	34	
	Atrial septal	15	
	Patent ductus	9	
			58
Common right-left shunts	Tetralogy of Fallot	7	
	Transposition of great vessels	3	
	Hypoplastic left ventricle	1	
	Tricuspid atresia	1	
			12
Common obstructive defects	Pulmonary stenosis	9	
	Aortic stenosis	5	
	Coarctation	4	
			18
Less common defects			4.6
Unlisted and complex defects			7
Total			99.6

*Courtesy of Arno Hohn.

The clinical picture and functional impairment depend primarily on the size of the defect and the status of the pulmonary vasculature and less on the location. The location may determine involvement of adjacent structures, such as the aortic valve or AV cushion. Small ventricular septal defects are referred to as Roger's disease. A small opening can produce a short, high-frequency systolic murmur. The murmur can become longer, harsher, and louder with larger defects, and often there may be an associated thrill. The murmur is heard best along the left sternal border, usually louder at the third and fourth intercostal spaces, and does not radiate well to the left axilla like that noted with mitral insufficiency. Those defects in the outlet septum may produce murmurs and thrills more prominent in the first or second left intercostal space with radiation upward. Large defects, with appreciable left-to-right shunts, have wide splitting of the second sound which varies with respiration, and the pulmonic component is accentuated. A flow diastolic, rumbling, low-pitched apical murmur may be present because of the increased flow across the mitral valve and may be preceded by a third heart sound. Hyperdynamic right and left ventricular lifts are present with such large shunts. Because of lack of support of the aortic root, aortic insufficiency may develop in 5 to 8% of patients with ventricular septal defects.[2] The defects in such cases (about 50%) are of the perimembranous or infundibular types. If pulmonary hypertension develops, the murmur can become faint or even disappear and is associated with a loud (often palpable) second sound at the pulmonic area with narrow splitting. A pulmonary ejection sound may be noted. The murmur of pulmonary insufficiency can develop (Graham Steell Murmur). Depending upon the size of the defect and the pulmonary vascular resistance, the ECG may be normal or show evidence of left and right ventricular hypertrophy or predominant right ventricular hypertrophy. Often with biventricular hypertrophy the midprecordial leads have large equidiphasic RS complexes (Katz-Waachtel sign). Likewise, the x ray of the chest may be normal or show biventricular and left atrial enlargement and prominence of the main pulmonary artery with increased pulmonary blood flow or predominant right ventricular enlargement and oligemic lung fields, depending on the size of the left-to-right shunt and

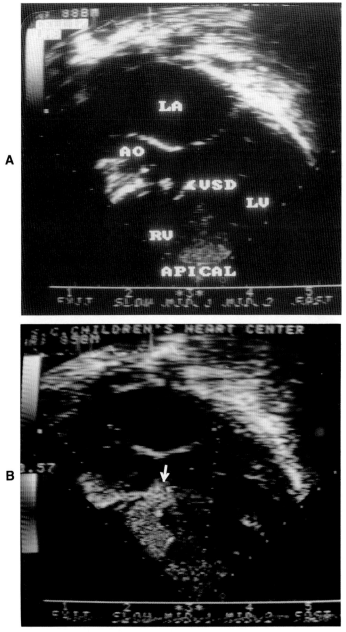

Fig 7–1. Membranous ventricular septal defect. A, Two-dimensional echocardiogram, apical view. Arrow points to ventricular septal defect (VSD). LA = left atrium, AO = aorta, LV = left ventricle, RV = right ventricle. B, Color flow Doppler shows VSD. The abnormal flow can be seen as a mosaic color high velocity shift from left to right ventricle (arrow) at the level of the VSD. (Courtesy of Dr. Derek A. Fyfe.)

VENTRICULAR SEPTAL DEFECT

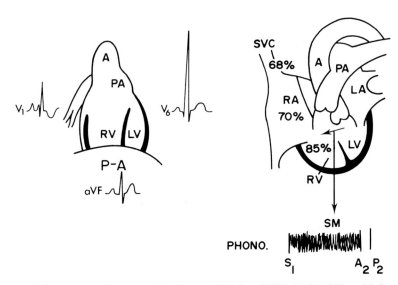

Fig 7–2. Main features of large ventricular septal defect (VSD). Right (RV) and left ventricular (LV) lifts. Splitting of the second sound in the pulmonic area. Pansystolic murmur (SM) maximum along lower left sternal border with thrill. At times mid-diastolic flow murmur at the apex. Electrocardiogram shows biventricular enlargement. Posteroanterior (P-A) view of chest shows biventricular and left atrial enlargement and prominence of the main pulmonary artery (PA) with pulmonary vascular engorgement. Cardiac catheterization shows a step-up in O_2 saturation from 70% in the right atrium (RA) to 85% in the right ventricle (RV). Arterial O_2 saturation is 95%. Shunt Q_p/Q_s is 2.5:1. Q_p = pulmonary blood flow; Q_s = systemic blood flow.

the pulmonary vascular resistance. Echocardiogram, especially two-dimensional, color and Doppler studies can show the defect and can exclude other congenital defects (Fig 7–1A,B). Heart catheterization studies demonstrate an oxygen step up in the right ventricle. Figure 7–2 depicts the main features of a large ventricular septal defect with a significant left-to-right shunt. The pulmonary artery pressure may be up slightly due to an increase in pulmonary blood flow or may be markedly elevated if pulmonary vascular changes occur with resulting pulmonary hypertension and even reversal of the shunt (Eisenmenger's syndrome).

A ventricular septal defect can communicate with the right atrium, either directly or from the right ventricle through deficiencies in the septal tricuspid leaflet. This type of communication can resemble the usual ventricular septal defect with some differences; for instance, the murmur is more rightward, the electrocardiogram shows right atrial enlargement and left ventricular volume overload. Atrial arrhythmias are common. X ray shows a large right atrium, and two-dimensional echocardiography and conventional and color flow Doppler can localize the defect.

Patients with small ventricular septal defects do not require treatment. Surgery is not indicated in asymptomatic patients with normal x ray of chest, normal ECG, and a left-to-right shunt of less than 1.5:1.0 pulmonary-systemic flow ratio. Symptomatic infants with large shunts who cannot be managed medically should have direct closure of the defect. Rarely pulmonary artery banding as a palliative procedure is recommended. Criteria for surgery in the school-aged child are a significant left-to-right shunt (>2.0:1.00) with a large heart or elevated pulmonary artery pressure. In adults, surgery is usually recommended if the flow ratio is above 1.5:1.00. At any age, surgery is contraindicated if the pulmonary vascular disease is so severe that the pulmonary to systemic vascular resistance is greater than 0.9. Between 0.75 and 0.9 and bidirectional shunting with small net left-to-right shunting, operation may be advised in a few institutions, although the long-term results are unpredictable. Pulmonary hypertension is not a contraindication to surgery as long as the pulmonary to systemic vascular resistance is less than 0.75.

ATRIAL SEPTAL DEFECT

Children with an atrial septal defect often have a frail or gracile habitus. One should be suspicious of an atrial septal defect if there are extremity abnormalities, such as hypoplastic thumb resembling a finger and in the same plane with the fingers (Holt-Oram syndrome).[3] Beside congenital bicuspid aortic valve, it is one of the most common congenital heart defects found in adults.

There are three types of atrial septal defects: ostium secundum, sinus venosus, and ostium primum. The secundum type is in the midatrial septum (region of fossa ovalis) and is the most common. The sinus venosus type of defect occurs high in the septum near the entrance of the superior vena cava in the right atrium. This type of defect is usually associated with anomalous pulmonary venous drainage. The ostium primum (partial atrioventricular canal) type of defect is located low in the anterior portion of the septum and may involve the membranous ventricular septum and have associated defects such as clefts or abnormal attachments of the septal leaflets of the mitral or tricuspid valve. These three types of defects have many common physical signs.

Atrial septal defect produces an ejection systolic murmur in the pulmonic area which is due to increased flow across the pulmonary outflow tract. The murmur characteristically radiates over both lung fields due to rapid blood flow in the peripheral pulmonary arteries. A thrill in the pulmonic area is unusual and, if present, usually indicates associated pulmonary stenosis. An important feature of an atrial septal defect is the wide fixed splitting of the second sound. The fixed splitting (not varying with respiration) is due to the usual normal increase in systemic venous return with inspiration and decrease during expiration associated with the shunt flow through the atrial septum undergoing the reverse. The shunt flow diminishes during inspiration and increases during expiration. These factors produce a constant right ventricular stroke volume overload during inspiration and expiration, which causes delay in pulmonic valve closure and thus accounts for the fixed degree of splitting. In some patients the fixed splitting persists after surgical correction, and this may be ascribed to right bundle-branch block or to right ventricular changes. The pulmonic component of the second sound is accentuated and the valve closure is palpable in the pulmonic area. A hyperdynamic, usually brief right ventricular lift is present. If the shunt is large, the increased flow across the tricuspid valve can produce a low-pitched, rumbling mid-diastolic flow type of murmur just along the left sternal border, at about the fourth intercostal space. This murmur can be confused with mitral stenosis, but it is best heard during inspiration and does not have the other associated characteristics. Patients may have at the apex a midsystolic click or late systolic murmur, indicating mitral valve prolapse. Up to 30% of patients with secundum atrial septal defects have mitral valve prolapse. The ECG usually reveals outflow tract right ventricular hypertrophy, resembling an incomplete right bundle-branch block. However, the QRS width can be normal. In adults, right bundle-branch block may be present. In the secundum and venosus types of defects right axis is usually present and in the primum type left axis is often noted. The left axis is probably due to a congenital variation in the conduction pathway. Atrial fibrillation or other supraventricular arrhythmias often occur in adults. Chest x rays demonstrate large pulmonary arteries with prominent tertiary branches due to the increased pulmonary blood flow. The right ventricle is enlarged, the aorta appears to be small, and the left atrium and left ventricle are normal. An M-mode echocardiogram reveals paradoxical systolic motion of the septum. The right ventricle is enlarged (Fig 7–3). These findings are not specific, for other lesions resulting in right ventricular volume load as tricuspid insufficiency may give similar findings. Two-dimensional echocardiography and conventional and color flow Doppler can confirm the diagnosis (Fig 7–4A,B). Heart catheterization studies demonstrate a step up in oxygen saturation in the right atrium.

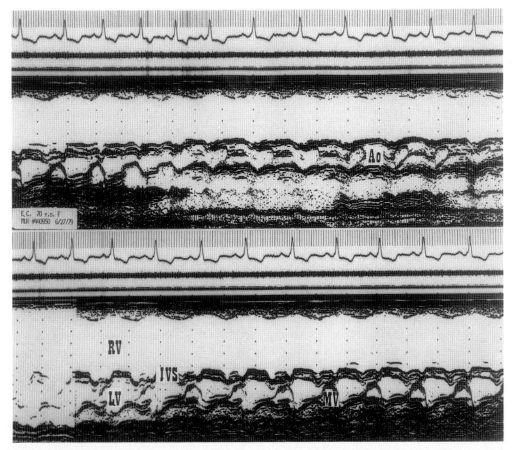

Fig 7–3. M-mode echocardiogram in a patient with a large atrial septal defect. Note the very large right ventricle (RV) and the paradoxical septal (IVS) motion. AO = aorta; RV = right ventricle; IVS = interventricular septum; LV = left ventricle; MV = mitral valve. (Courtesy of Dr. Bruce W. Usher.)

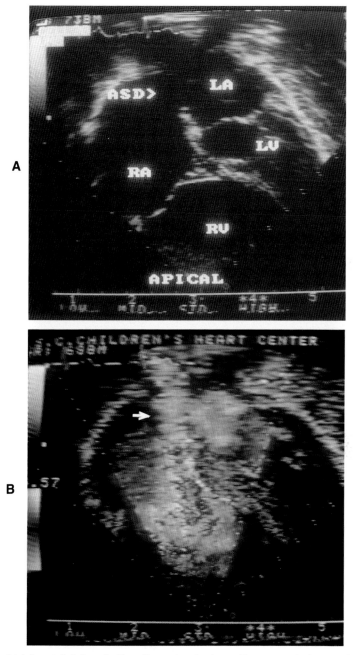

Fig 7–4. Atrial septal defect. A, Two-dimensional echocardiogram, apical view. Arrow points to atrial septal defect (ASD). LA = left atrium, RA = right atrium, RV = right ventricle, LV = left ventricle. B, Color flow Doppler shows ASD. Abnormal flow can be seen as orange-colored high-velocity shift at the level of the ASD (arrow). (Courtesy of Dr. Derek A. Fyfe.)

Figure 7–5 shows the main features of an atrial septal defect with a significant left-to-right shunt. An atrial septal defect with shunt of 1.5 to 1 (pulmonary to systemic flow ratio) or greater should be directly closed or patched, preferably after age 3. Many of these children can escape to adulthood before their lesions are detected because they are so well tolerated. However, with

ATRIAL SEPTAL DEFECT

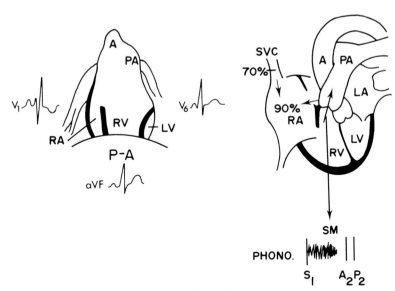

Fig 7–5. Main features of atrial septal defect (ASD). Hyperdynamic right ventricular lift. Second sound loud with fixed splitting in pulmonic area (A_2, P_2). Short ejection systolic murmur (SM) in pulmonic area. Mid-diastolic flow murmur at lower left sternal border. Electrocardiographic features of right ventricular outflow tract hypertrophy (resembling incomplete right bundle-branch block). Posteroanterior (P-A) view of chest reveals prominence of the main pulmonary artery (PA) with increased pulmonary blood flow. Right ventricular enlargement. Normal or even small-appearing aorta (A). Cardiac catheterization shows a step up in O_2 saturation from 70% in superior vena cava (SVC) to 90% in right atrium (RA). Arterial O_2 saturation is 95%. Shunt Q_p/Q_s is 4.7:1.00. Q_p = pulmonary blood flow; Q_s = systemic blood flow.

significant shunts, eventually atrial arrhythmias, heart failure, and, rarely, pulmonary hypertension can develop. Adults over age 60 have had surgery successfully.[4] Pulmonary hypertension is not a gauge of operability, since it is related to volume of pulmonary blood flow and pulmonary vascular resistance. However, pulmonary vascular resistance[5] is significant, for if it is over 640 dyne/sec/cm[5] or if the pulmonary to systemic vascular resistance ratio is equal to or greater than 0.7:1.0 (without a significant left-to-right shunt), surgery should not be advised.

Atrial septal defects can be associated with other anomalies such as anomalous pulmonary veins, endocardial cushion defects, and mitral valve disease.

As mentioned before, partial anomalous pulmonary venous drainage is most often noted with the sinus venosus defect and less so with the other types. One or more poulmonary veins drain into the the right atrium or systemic vein rather than into the left atrium. Clinically, the picture is simply that of an uncomplicated atrial septal defect. The chest x ray at times may show a shadow near the right side of the heart (venous drainage of right lung into inferior vena cava—scimitar sign).

Endocardial cushion defects with atrial septal defects can be complete with a defect in the ventricular septum and clefts in the mitral and tricuspid leaflets. The incomplete type is usually the ostium primum type with a cleft mitral valve. There can be variations between the incomplete and complete types.

Endocardial cushion defects are found often in mongolism (Down's syndrome). The complete type presents with biventricular lifts, findings of an atrial septal defect and murmurs of a ventricular septal defect, mitral insufficiency, and tricuspid insufficiency. One has to listen carefully, for each of the defects produces findings. In the incomplete type, the findings are those of an atrial septal defect with mitral insufficiency. Generally, if the ECG shows findings of an atrial septal defect with left-axis deviation or findings of an atrial and ventricular septal defect with left-axis, one should suspect an endocardial cushion defect. A long P-R interval may also be present. Chest x ray reveals the findings of an atrial septal defect and enlargement of the left atrium and ventricle in view of the endocardial cushion defect. At times the abnormal attachment of the mitral valve produces on left ventriculogram a "gooseneck" left ventricular outflow tract deformity.

The combination of an atrial septal defect and mitral stenosis is known as Lutembacher's syndrome.[6] It is still not clear whether the mitral stenosis is rheumatic or congenital in origin, although the majority consider it to be rheumatic. I suspect that some of these patients reported in the past probably did not have mitral stenosis; rather, the diastolic rumbling murmur was that of the tricuspid flow type associated with a large left-to-right atrial shunt. Echocardiography is helpful in distinguishing these two. Mitral stenosis increases the left-to-right shunt depending on the degree of the stenosis and the size of the atrial septal defect. The auscultatory findings of mitral stenosis may not be clear because of the decreased mitral flow caused by the shunt. The ECG can be that of an atrial septal defect with P wave changes indicating right and left atrial enlargement. The x ray of the chest will not show the pulmonary vein congestion of mitral stenosis and the left atrium may not be enlarged. The main pulmonary artery will be very prominent with increase in pulmonary arterial blood flow, and there will be right atrial and ventricular enlargement.

Patent Ductus Arteriosus

A patent ductus arteriosus is a connection between the pulmonary artery and the aorta which is present in the fetus but does not close off as it usually does 2 to 3 weeks after birth. It usually extends from the origin of the left pulmonary artery to just distal to the origin of the left subclavian artery. It may coexist with other anomalies such as ventricular septal defect, coarctation of the aorta, and pulmonary stenosis.

This defect is the most common cause of a continuous murmur (Gibson murmur). The murmur has a machinery quality, is usually heard louder during systole, and gradually reduces in intensity with diastole. It may be associated with crackling sounds called eddy sounds. The murmur is best heard in the pulmonic area, and frequently there is an associated systolic or continuous thrill. This thrill also may be felt in the suprasternal notch. A systolic thrill in the suprasternal notch should suggest a ductus, aortic stenosis, pulmonary stenosus, or, rarely, coarctation of the aorta. If the shunt is large, a distolic flow murmur may be audible at the apex. A left ventricular lift is usually present. The peripheral pulses are bounding, and there is a wide pulse pressure. If pulmonary hypertension occurs, the continuous murmur may disappear, with only a systolic component being audible. Patent ductus may be associated with the rubella syndrome (maternal rubella during the first 2 months of gestation). The ECG reveals left atrial and ventricular hypertrophy if the shunt is large, and the x ray shows a prominent aortic knob, left ventricular and left atrial enlargement, and a prominent main pulmonary artery with increase in pulmonary blood flow. Echocardiogram shows left atrial enlargement, and on M-mode this can be compared with aortic size. The ratio of the left atrial dimension to the aortic dimension is used to assess the size of the shunt. The ratio normally is between 0.7 and 0.85, and with large shunts it can be 1.2.[7] Left ventricular dilatation and excessive septal and posterior left ventricular wall motion can be noted. Two-dimensional echocardiography (Fig 7–6) and conventional and color flow Doppler can visualize the ductus. Heart catheterization studies demonstrate an oxygen step-up in the pulmonary artery, and the cineangiogram reveals a shunt from the aorta to the pulmonary artery. Figure 7–7 depicts the usual findings noted with a patent ductus arteriosus with a significant left-to-right shunt. Surgery should be recommended, and the ductus should be divided or ligated after 1 year of age or earlier if there is congestive heart failure. If a ductus is found in late life and there is a small shunt, surgery is usually not recommended. Surgery in the adult can present problems because the ductus can be calcified, brittle, and aneurysmal. Some symptomatic premature infants can be managed by using drugs that will inhibit prostaglandin synthesis, such as aspirin and indomethacin, and produce constriction of the ductus arteriosus, but side effects can occur.[8,9] Catheter closure has been done in children and in the future may be used in the older patient.

The aorticopulmonary septal defect (window) is a communication between the pulmonary trunk and ascending aorta and essentially has the same findings as those noted with a large patent ductus arteriosus.

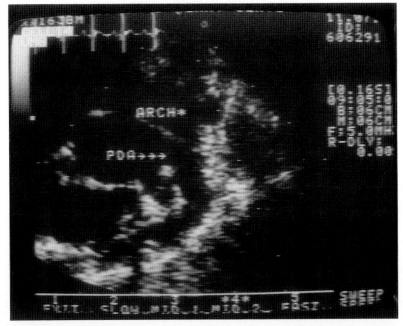

Fig 7–6. Patent ductus arteriosus (PDA). Two-dimensional echocardiogram (Suprasternal view) shows PDA (arrows). (Courtesy of Dr. Derek A. Fyfe.)

PATENT DUCTUS ARTERIOSUS

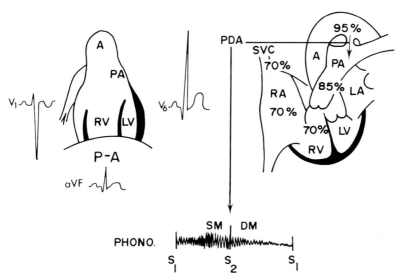

Fig 7–7. Main findings in patent ductus arteriosus (PDA). Left ventricular (LV) lift and late right ventricular (RV) lift. Continuous machinery-like murmur with systolic (SM) and diastolic (DM) components loudest in pulmonic area often associated with thrill. At times apical mid-diastolic flow murmur. Wide pulse pressure. Electrocardiogram shows left ventricular enlargement. Posteroanterior (P-A) view of chest shows left ventricular and left atrial enlargement and enlargement of main pulmonary artery (PA), with increased pulmonary blood flow and prominent aortic knob (A). Cardiac catheterization reveals a step-up in O_2 saturation from 70% in the right ventricle (RV) to 85% in the pulmonary artery (PA). Arterial O_2 saturation is 95%. Shunt Q_p/Q_s is 2.5:1. Q_p = pulmonary blood flow; Q_s = systemic blood flow.

RIGHT-TO-LEFT SHUNTS

These lesions usually are associated with cyanosis with the blood containing 5 g/dl or more of reduced hemoglobin. Secondary polycythemia will occur, and the arterial oxygen saturation is usually 85% or below. These right-to-left shunts may be associated with a decreased or increased pulmonary blood flow. In addition, any of the left-to-right shunts can develop pulmonary hypertension with reversal of the shunt from right to left (Eisenmenger reaction or hypertensive pulmonary vascular disease).

LESIONS WITH DECREASED PULMONARY BLOOD FLOW

Tetralogy of Fallot, pulmonary atresia, and tricuspid atresia are most commonly associated with a decreased pulmonary blood flow.

Tetralogy of Fallot

This is the most common cyanotic lesion after 1 year of age and consists of a ventricular septal defect (due to malalignment of the infundibular septum anteriorly), infundibular or pulmonary valve stenosis, right ventricular hypertrophy, and an aorta that overrides the ventricular septal defect. These patients often give a history of squatting after exercise and are subject to hypoxic spells. Squatting relieves the symptoms of dyspnea and faintness that can occur after exertion. The majority agree that with squatting there is an increase in systemic vascular resistance and a rise in the common ventricular pressure, producing an increase in pulmonary arterial blood flow, and thus more oxygenated blood reaches the left side of the heart. Guntheroth et al.[10] concluded from their studies that squatting produces a sustained reduction in venous return from the legs. After exercise the venous blood in the legs has a low oxygen saturation; consequently, the saturation of the mixed systemic venous return rises with squatting, and the mixture shunted from the right ventricle into the aorta has a higher oxygen content. Paroxysmal hypoxic spells (hyperpnea, severe cyanosis, and syncope) were thought to be due to infundibular spasm. Catecholamines were considered to be a factor, since some spells could be relieved by the use of β-adrenergic blocking agents. However, Guntheroth et al.[11] concluded that the respiratory center plays a part. Feeding and crying may produce a sudden increase in cardiac output with an increase in the right-to-left shunt, resulting in a fall in PaO_2 and pH and a rise in $PaCO_2$, which stimulate the sensitive respiratory center to produce hyperpnea. Hyperpnea further increases the cardiac output and thus perpetuates the problem. In addition, supraventricular tachycardias can precipitate attacks.

The clinical findings can vary depending on the size of the ventricular septal defect and the degree of right ventricular outflow obstruction. Severe outflow obstruction usually produces clubbing and cyanosis. However, the patient may be acyanotic (so-called pink tetralogy) if the right ventricular outflow obstruction is mild and the left-to-right shunt is dominant, even if the ventricular pressures are equal. A prominent A wave usually is not in the neck, as is seen with pulmonary stenosis with an intact ventricular septum, since the right and left ventricular pressures are equal. A harsh ejection systolic murmur is produced by the right ventricular outflow obstruction and is heard best at the second and third intercostal spaces to the left of the sternum and at times is associated with a thrill. This murmur may be faint if the obstruction is severe. The ventricular septal defect usually does not produce a murmur. The aortic component of the second sound is loud and pure and may be heard at the right or left base of the heart. An aortic ejection sound may be audible. At times there may be a continuous murmur if there is an associated ductus or if the pulmonary stenosis is severe in the form of atresia (pseudotruncus) and there is increased bronchial and nonbronchial systemic arterial collateral blood flow. A right ventricular lift is present, and the ECG reveals right ventricular hypertrophy. However, the hypertrophy seen with the tetralogy is not as severe as that seen with severe pulmonary stenosis and an intact ventricular septum.

X ray demonstrates right ventricular enlargement which in the PA view causes the apex to sit up and have the appearance of a sheep nose or be boot-shaped (coeur en sabot). The aorta is large. In about 25% of the cases there is a right aortic arch.[12] The lung fields appear oligemic. If the pulmonary stenosis is severe (pulmonary atresia) and the collateral circulation is prominent, the lungs have a lace-like appearance. M-mode and two-dimensional echocardiography will show the septal defect and overriding aorta. Right ventricular hypertrophy and aortic dilatation may be detected. Two-dimensional echocardiography can depict the ventricular septal defect and the overriding aorta (Fig 7–8) and evaluate the right ventricular outflow tract. Doppler (conventional and color flow) studies are also useful for assessing blood flow

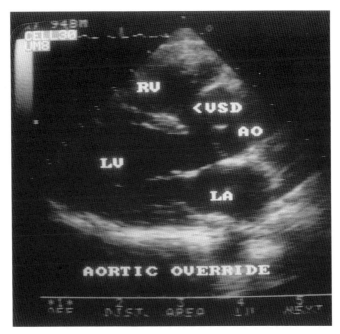

Fig 7-8. Tetralogy of Fallot. Two-dimensional echocardiograms (parasternal long axis) shows the ventricular septal defect (arrow) and the overriding aorta (AO). RV = Right ventricle, LV = left ventricle, LA = left atrium. (Courtesy of Dr. Derek A. Fyfe.)

through the ventricular septal defect and across the right ventricular outflow tract. Heart catheterization will reveal a low right ventricular outflow tract pressure (infundibular chamber) and elevation of pressure in the right ventricle to systemic levels. A right-to-left shunt can be demonstrated. Cineangiograms show the ventricular septal defect with the overriding of the aorta along with infundibular and valvular pulmonic stenosis and the size of the pulmonary annulus and the pulmonary arteries. Figure 7-9 shows the main features in tetralogy of Fallot.

Tetralogy patients can have many problems, such as hypoxic spells, infective endocarditis, polycythemia and blood-clotting problems, cerebral infarction or embolism, cerebral abscess, and, rarely, right ventricular failure. Hyperuricemia can occur because of the increased turnover of erythrocyte nucleic acid, which can precipitate acute gouty arthritis. Therefore, early total surgical correction should be done for all cases to avoid these complications. Previously a shunt procedure (creation of a surgical anastomosis between the aorta or subclavian artery and the pulmonary artery) was performed early in most cases, but presently this is advised only if there is severe hypoplasia of the pulmonary arteries, and then later in childhood total repair can be done. The Blalock-Taussig shunt is between the subclavian artery and the aorta, the Pott's shunt is between the descending aorta and pulmonary artery, and the Waterston shunt is between the ascending aorta and the pulmonary artery.

Tricuspid Atresia

This defect is characterized by absence of the tricuspid valve and orifice, atrial and ventricular septal defects, and underdevelopment of the right ven-

TETRALOGY OF FALLOT

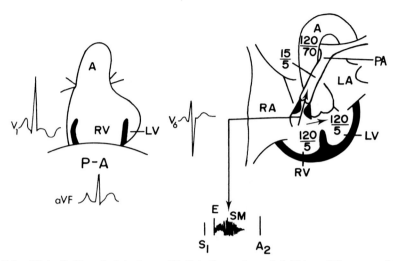

Fig 7–9.   Main findings in tetralogy of Fallot. Cyanosis and clubbing of fingers and toes. Right ventricular lift. Harsh ejection systolic murmur (SM) heard best at second and third left inter- costal spaces. The second sound is loud due to the aortic component (A_2). Aortic ejection sound (E) along left sternal border. Electrocardiogram shows right ventricular hypertrophy. Posteroanterior (P-A) view of chest reveals clear oligemic lung fields, an elevated apex (coeur en sabot), and a large aorta (A). Cardiac catheterization shows equal pressures in both ventricles and low pulmonary artery (PA) pressure. Right-sided angiocardiogram reveals the pulmonary stenosis, ventricular septal defect, and early opacification of the large aorta (A).

tricle. This defect can be subdivided into those with normally related great vessels or those with transposition of the great vessels.[13] In addition, associ- ated with each of these there may be other defects such as pulmonary hyperpla- sia, stenosis, or atresia, a patent ductus, or coarctation of the aorta. The ven- tricular septum can be intact, or there may be a variable-sized ventricular septal defect. The most common type of tricuspid atresia is that with normally related great vessels, a small ventricular septal defect and right ventricle, and pulmonic stenosis. The circulation from the venae cavae passes across the atrial septal defect, mixes with the pulmonary vein blood and then passes to the left ventricle where some goes out to the pulmonary arteries via the ven- tricular septal defect and the rest goes out the aorta. If the ventricular septum is intact, the ductus and the bronchial arteries may provide blood to the pul- monary bed.

Cyanosis appears early, and death may occur early. Rarely, patients may survive to the second decade, usually those with transposition and pulmonary stenosis. In some cases, pulmonary blood flow is increased (large ventricular septal defect and right ventricle and no pulmonary stenosis, or transposition without pulmonary stenosis), and the cyanosis may not be severe, and conges- tive failure can be present.

The most common type has a prominent A wave in the jugular pulse. A left ventricular lift may be palpable. The murmurs depend upon the defects, such as the ventricular septal defect, pulmonary obstruction, or ductus. The combination of cyanosis and ECG evidence of left axis and left ventricular hypertrophy are diagnostic. The ECG also may show right atrial enlargement. X ray of the chest usually demonstrates oligemic lung fields and left ventricular prominence. The lungs may be plethoric if a large ventricular septal defect is present without pulmonary stenosis or if there is transposition of the great vessels without pulmonary stenosis. M-mode and two-dimensional echocardiography can demonstrate the hypoplastic right ventricle, large left ventricular cavity, and no identifiable tricuspid valve. Conventional and color flow Doppler also are useful. Heart catheterization studies and angiocardiograms confirm the diagnosis.

Angiographic studies of the commonest type reveal the opaque medium going from the right atrium through an atrial septal defect into the left atrium and then into the left ventricle and from there to the right ventricle through a small ventricular septal defect with poor opacification of the right ventricle and pulmonary hypoplasia or stenosis. Figure 7–10 depicts the main features of the commonest type of tricuspid atresia. With pulmonary oligemia a surgical shunt procedure is usually recommended. Shunt procedures recommended have been vena caval to right pulmonary artery anastomosis (Glenn procedure) and systemic artery to pulmonary artery anastomosis (Blalock-Taussig procedure, Potts', or Waterson procedure). Other palliative procedures that can be done are balloon atrial septostomy in patients with an inadequate atrial communication, and pulmonary arterial banding in those with excessive pulmonary blood flow. Later, in some instances in children 5 years or older, a corrective procedure (Fontan operation) can be performed that completely separates the two circulations and physiologically corrects the anomaly. In this

TRICUSPID ATRESIA

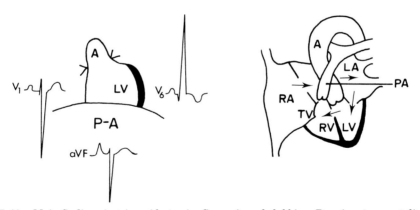

Fig 7–10. Main findings in tricuspid atresia. Cyanosis and clubbing. Prominent presystolic pulsation in the jugular veins. Left ventricular (LV) apical impulse palpable. Murmurs depend on associated defects. Electrocardiogram reveals left axis and left ventricular hypertrophy and right atrial enlargement. Posteroanterior (P-A) view of chest reveals straight right heart border, left ventricular prominence, and oligemic lung fields. Angiocardiogram reveals the opaque material going from the right atrium (RA) through an atrial septal defect into the left atrium (LA) and then into the left ventricle (LV) and from there to the right ventricle through a ventricular septal defect with very poor opacification of the right ventricle.

procedure, the right atrium is connected to the pulmonary artery by using a conduit with a valve, and another valve is inserted in the orifice of the inferior vena cava.[14] Subsequently, various modifications have been done, depending on the associated lesions such as pulmonary valvular or infundibular stenosis or a ventricular septal defect. Problems have been minimized by using direct wide atrioventricular or atriopulmonary anastomoses and avoiding the use of valved or nonvalved conduits and homograft valves.[15]

LESIONS WITH INCREASED PULMONARY BLOOD FLOW

The transpositions and truncus arteriosus are lesions that produce right-to-left shunts and usually increase pulmonary blood flow. However, the pulmonary blood flow can vary depending on the degree of pulmonary stenosis or pulmonary vascular resistance (hypertensive pulmonary vascular disease can occur within the first year of life). In this section emphasis will be placed on those lesions with increased pulmonary blood flow.

THE TRANSPOSITIONS

Many terms are used to designate the different positions of the atria, the ventricles, and the great vessels.[16] These terms should be understood to appreciate a segmental approach to the diagnosis of complex congenital heart disease. The normal position of viscera and atria is referred to as situs solitus and a mirror image as situs inversus. Situs ambiguus is said to be present when either situs solitus or inversus cannot be identified. Such cases have asplenia or polysplenia. Levocardia indicates that the apex is to the left, dextrocardia that it is to the right, and mesocardia that it is in the midline. A D-loop designates that the ventricles are in the proper position, and an L-loop that they are reversed. When the aortic origin is to the right of the pulmonary origin, the term D-normal is used, and for the reverse, L-normal is used. Malposition is the term used if the spatial relationship of the great arteries is abnormal in either the lateral or anteroposterior plane and the arteries are not transposed. In summary, the symbols used for this segmental approach are arranged in order as follows: relationship of viscera and atria; ventricular loop; and the relationship of the great arteries. For example, transposition of the great vessels (TGA) with situs solitus (S), D-ventricular loop (D), and with the aorta to the right (D) of the pulmonary artery arising from the right ventricle and the pulmonary artery from the left ventricle would be designated as TGA(SDD). If other abnormalities are present, these are abbreviated as ventricular septal defect (VSD) and then the designation is TGA(SDD) VSD.

The transpositions can exist as complete transposition of the great vessels, partial, as a double outlet right ventricle, or only a corrected transposition. In addition, there may be associated defects, such as pulmonary stenosis or tricuspid atresia, and shunts such as ventricular septal defect, patent ductus, or interatrial communications.

Complete Transposition of the Great Vessels (Situs Solitus, D-Loop, D Transposition or SDD)

In this most common form of transposition, the aorta originates from the right ventricle and the pulmonary artery from the left ventricle. Segmental analysis shows situs solitus (S) dextroventricular loop (D) and a rightward (D) and anterior aorta. There must be a shunt between the systemic and pulmonary circuits present for such patients to survive. This shunt may be at the atrial, ventricular, or pulmonary artery level. Cyanosis and dyspnea are usually present from birth and may be followed by congestive failure. Murmurs depend on the associated findings. At times mixing may be poor, and a murmur may be absent. The ECG can vary depending on the associated defects from pure right ventricular hypertrophy to biventricular hypertrophy. X rays of the chest reveal a narrow pedicle with cardiomegaly (egg-on-side or apple-hanging-from-a-string appearance) and pulmonary plethora. Cardiomegaly develops rapidly. Echocardiography has been helpful in establishing the diagnosis. It can identify the great vessels and their reversed origin and also may identify the associated defects. Doppler (conventionl and color flow) is also helpful in detecting the various defects. Heart catheterization and angiographic studies confirm the diagnosis. The aorta is seen arising anteriorly from the right ventricle with its valve more superior than normal and the pulmonary artery arising from the left ventricle. Figure 7–11 shows the main features of complete transposition of the great vessels.

A balloon atrioseptostomy should be done during heart catheterization. Rashkind and Miller[17] described this procedure, in which a small interatrial communication is enlarged by pulling a balloon catheter through the defect. A direct surgical creation of a large atrial septal defect is seldom necessary. After 3 to 9 months of age, total repair should be considered (Mustard[18] procedure). This procedure redirects the venous blood within the atria by excision of the septum and creates a new septum with a pericardial baffle or prosthetic material so positioned that the pulmonary vein blood flows across the tricuspid valve to the right ventricle and then out the aorta, and the caval blood flows across the mitral valve to the left ventricle and then into the pulmonary

COMPLETE TRANSPOSITION
OF GREAT VESSELS

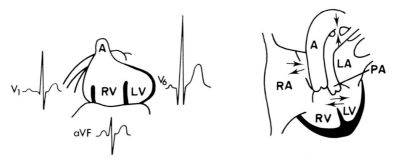

Fig 7–11. Main findings of complete transposition of great vessels. Cyanosis and clubbing. Murmur absent or depends on associated defects. Electrocardiogram depends on associated defects. Usually right ventricular or biventricular hypertrophy. Posteroanterior view of chest shows a narrow pedicle (egg-on-side appearance) and plethoric lung fields. Cardiac catheterization will reveal the associated defects and bidirectional shunting. Angiocardiogram shows the aorta (A) arising anteriorly from the right ventricle (RV) with the aortic valve more superior than normal and the pulmonary artery (PA) arising from the left ventricle (LV).

artery. The Senning[19] procedure is similar but is used less often. Instead of prosthetic material, it utilizes the atrial septum and right atrial wall for the creation of the intra-atrial baffle. Jatene et al.[20] performed anatomic correction by relocating the aorta and pulmonary artery to the proper chamber and reimplanting the coronary arteries. If a large ventricular septal defect is present, the pulmonary artery should be banded and surgical repair considered at 1 to 2 years of age. A shunt procedure (Rastelli) should be performed for those with a ventricular septal defect and severe pulmonary stenosis. A conduit is placed to connect the right ventricle and pulmonary trunk and a patch to close the ventricular septal defect that includes the aortic valve on the left ventricular side of the patch. If pulmonary vascular obstructive disease has developed, the prognosis is poor; however, a Mustard or Senning procedure, without closure of the ventricular septal defect, may give symptomatic improvement.

Double Outlet Right Ventricle (Situs Solitus, D-Loop, D-Malposition, or SDD)

The aorta and pulmonary artery arise from the right ventricle, and the only outlet from the left ventricle is through a ventricular septal defect. Segmental analysis in most cases identifies situs solitus (S) and dextroventricular loop (D), and the aortic origin is to the right of the pulmonary arterial origin (D-malposition). There are several variations of this defect depending on the location of the great vessels, location of the ventricular septal defect, and whether other associated defects are present, such as pulmonary stenosis (usually subpulmonary valve), patent ductus, coarctation of the aorta, and mitral valve obstruction. The Taussig-Bing type of defect is a condition in which the ventricular septal defect is subpulmonic, and the pulmonary artery may or may not straddle it.

The size and location of the ventricular septal defect and the presence or absence of pulmonary stenosis determine the findings. In most cases the ventricular septal defect is in the subaortic location, and the blood from the left ventricle goes preferably into the aorta. The clinical picture is that of an isolated large ventricular septal defect with pulmonary hypertension. Such patients can develop congestive failure. The Taussig-Bing type resembles clinically complete transposition of the great vessels with a ventricular septal defect and pulmonary hypertension. The clinical findings can resemble tetralogy of Fallot if there is associated pulmonary stenosis. Two-dimensional echocardiography may show the location of the great vessels and the discontinuity between the mitral and aortic valves. Conventional and color flow Doppler are also helpful. Angiocardiographic and catheterization studies will clarify the types of abnormality and allow corrective surgery. In some patients palliative procedures such as pulmonary artery banding or shunts (depending on the lesions) are done, and corrective surgery is deferred until an older age.

Corrected Transposition (Situs Solitus, L-Loop, L-Transposition or SLL)

Corrected transposition of the great arteries[21] as an isolated entity is rare. More than 95% have associated abnormalities such as a ventricular septal defect, AV valve abnormalities, pulmonary stenosis, and, at times, heart block. In corrected transposition the aorta lies anterior to the pulmonary artery and to the left, forming the upper left border of the heart. Anatomically, the coronary arteries are reversed in position: the right-sided ventricle has the structure of the left ventricle, and the left-sided ventricle has that of the right ventricle (ventricular inversion). Segmental analysis identifies situs solitus (S), ventricles inverted—L-loop (L) and the L-transposed aorta (L) arises from the left-sided right ventricle. Therefore, blood flows from the venae cavae to the right atrium through the mitral valve to the anatomic left ventricle to the pulmonary arteries and from the pulmonary veins through the tricuspid valve to the anatomic right ventricle and then into the aorta. The ECG reveals a small Q wave in the right precordial leads and an absence of a septal Q wave in V_6. First-degree atrioventricular block occurs in about 50% of these patients and complete AV block in about 10%. X ray of the chest may reveal the aorta forming the middle segment of the left border instead of the main pulmonary artery. The right pulmonary hilus is elevated. M-mode echocardiography reveals absence of continuity between the left AV valve and a semilunar valve and will show continuity between the right AV valve and the posterior semilunar valve. Two-dimensional echocardiography will show the inverted ventricles and other associated defects. Conventional and color flow Doppler are also useful. Heart catheterization and angiography will verify the diagnosis.

The isolated anomaly presents no symptoms or findings, whereas the nonisolated type depends on the associated abnormalities. There may be findings of a ventricular septal defect, pulmonary stenosis, or a systolic regurgitant murmur from the left AV valve.

Surgery may be required for the associated defects. The pathway of the conducting system and the coronary artery distribution can present surgical problems.

TRUNCUS ARTERIOSUS

This defect is characterized by having a single artery arising from both ventricles. The pulmonary arteries usually arise from one of several positions from a truncal vessel.[22] In type 1 the pulmonary arteries arise at the base of the truncal vessel from a single main pulmonary trunk; in type 2 the pulmonary arteries arise posteriorly from the ascending truncal vessel; in type 3 the pulmonary arteries arise laterally from the ascending truncus; and in type 4 there is no true pulmonary arterial system, and the lungs are supplied by way of the bronchial arteries. Type 4 is theoretically possible, but should be classified as pulmonary atresia with a ventricular septal defect rather than a truncus type. Patients with a truncus must have a ventricular septal defect to survive. Cyanosis is usually noted. If the pulmonary blood flow is good, cyanosis is less severe. Pulmonary blood flow is decreased if there is stenosis of the pulmonary arteries or severe pulmonary vascular obstructive disease.

Most patients with truncus arteriosus have increased pulmonary blood flow in early life (pulmonary vascular disease usually does not restrict flow until age 2). A parasternal life and a prominent apical impulse are present. A systolic ejection sound and a loud, single second sound can be present. A harsh systolic murmur is present over the precordium. A diastolic murmur due to truncal vessel insufficiency may occur. If pulmonary blood flow is restricted by either pulmonary stenosis or pulmonary vascular disease, the physical findings can be different. Cyanosis is more severe, and rarely the narrowed pulmonary arteries can produce continuous murmurs. The ECG may reveal left ventricular hypertrophy, biventricular hypertrophy, or right ventricular hypertrophy depending on the shunt and pulmonary blood flow. Right ventricular hypertrophy is predominant if the pulmonary blood flow is restricted. Likewise, chest x ray will depend on the hemodynamics. The chest x ray shows a wide pedicle with cardiomegaly and pulmonary vascular plethora, with the pulmonary arteries being higher than usual. If pulmonary blood flow is diminished, the pulmonary vasculature will be less prominent and cardiomegaly reduced. A right aortic arch can be noted in many patients. Echocardiography reveals the large truncal vessel overriding the ventricular septum, only one semilunar valve, and the left atrium enlarged. Conventional and color flow Dopper are also helpful. The diagnosis can be established by heart catheterization and angiocardiograms. Angiocardiography reveals a truncal vessel with the pulmonary arteries arising in one of several positions. Figure 7–12 reveals the main features of truncus arteriosus. All of these patients should be considered for surgery unless there is severe pulmonary vascular disease. Early in life, total correction should be attempted by the conduit procedure. In this operation the pulmonary arteries are disconnected from the aorta, and the resultant defect in the aorta is repaired. The right ventricle is opened, and the ventricular septal defect is patched. A valve-containing prosthetic conduit is used from the right ventricle to the pulmonary arteries. Surgery should be performed soon after birth, since pulmonary vascular obstructive disease can develop and cause early fatality. Truncal valve regurgitation may require valvular replacement.

PULMONARY HYPERTENSION

The Eisenmenger Complex

This condition was first described in patients who presented at birth with a large ventricular septal defect, pulmonary hypertension, overriding aorta, and reverse shunt, producing cyanosis.

TRUNCUS ARTERIOSUS

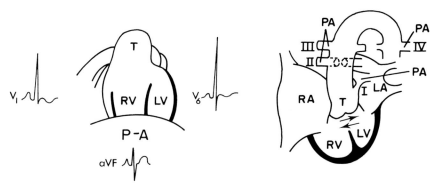

Fig 7–12.   Main findings of truncus arteriosus. Cyanosis usually noted. Systolic murmur and a continuous or diastolic murmur. Electrocardiogram may reveal right, left, or biventricular hypertrophy. Posteroanterior (P-A) view of the chest shows a large truncal (T) vessel, biventricular enlargement and pulmonary plethora. Angiocardiogram reveals a truncal vessel with the pulmonary arteries arising in one of several positions and frequently truncal valve insufficiency. Type IV is best classified as pulmonary atresia with a ventricular septal defect.

Eisenmenger's Syndrome

This term has been subsequently used to identify any shunt between the two circulations when the pulmonary vascular resistance (vascular resistance is calculated by dividing the mean arterial pressure by the flow through the artery) is equal to or greater than the systemic, producing a reversal of the shunt. This is caused by arteriolar lumen obstruction by intimal proliferation. Most often the shunt site is at the atrial, ventricular, or ductal level. Clinically, all of these patients present with essentially the same picture of pulmonary hypertension. Clubbing, polycythemia, and cyanosis are present, and a prominent A wave can be noted in the jugular venous pulse. The chest often appears emphysematous in shape (thorax of Davies), and a right ventricular lift is present. A right atrial sound may be heard. The second sound is narrowly split (may appear single) with a loud, palpable pulmonic component, and often there is some pulmonary insufficiency. This diastolic murmur (Graham Steell) simulates that of aortic insufficiency, except that it is heard best in inspiration and is associated with right heart enlargement and not left heart enlargement. In addition, it is not associated with the peripheral arterial findings seen with aortic insufficiency.

Frequently a pulmonic ejection sound is audible. With right ventricular dilatation secondary tricuspid insufficiency may develop, which produces a high-pitched systolic murmur along the left sternal border. The second sound may be of some aid in determining the site of the reversed shunt. Wide splitting of the second sound suggests that it is at the atrial level, physiologic splitting at the ductal level, and a single sound that it is at the ventricular level.[23] If the cyanosis is greater in the toes than in the upper extremities, the shunt could be at the ductal level. The ECG reveals right atrial and right ventricular hypertrophy. X rays demonstrate prominent central pulmonary arteries, which taper off peripherally, and right ventricular enlargement. M-mode echocardiography may show an absent or diminished posterior pulmonic valve leaflet A wave in pulmonary hypertension and midsystolic notching. Two-dimensional echocardiography can show the right atrial and ventricular enlargement and Doppler can give an estimate of the right ventricular systolic pressure by using the velocity of the tricuspid regurgitation jet and the Bernovilli equation. Color Flow Doppler is also useful. Cardiac catheterization, dye dilution studies, and angiocardiography establish the diagnosis of pulmonary hypertension and the site of the shunt. Figure 7–13 shows the main features of pulmonary hypertension secondary to Eisenmenger's syndrome. These patients are invariably inoperable and progressively worsen, but may attain middle age. However, survival is unusual beyond 50 years of age.[24] They can develop arrhythmias, hemoptysis, right heart failure, syncopal attacks, chest pain, and brain abscesses, and experience sudden death. Combined heart-lung transplantation has been performed.[25]

Primary Pulmonary Hypertension

Primary pulmonary hypertension may be difficult to differentiate clinically from Eisenmenger's syndrome. For this reason, we are discussing it in this section even though it is not known to be a congenital abnormality. Primary pulmonary hypertension is common in females and is usually seen between the

PULMONARY HYPERTENSION

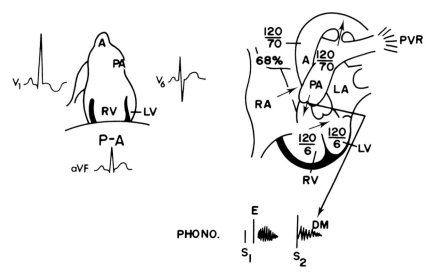

Fig 7–13. Main findings of pulmonary hypertension, Eisenmenger's syndrome. Cyanosis and clubbing. Right ventricular (RV) lift and palpable second (S_2) sound at pulmonic area, with second sound loud (at times split) and a pulmonic ejection sound (E), short systolic ejection murmur, and often a diastolic murmur (DM). Electrocardiogram shows right atrial and right ventricular hypertrophy. Posteroanterior (P-A) view of chest shows enlarged central pulmonary arteries that taper off peripherally. Cardiac catheterization reveals elevated right ventricular and pulmonary artery (PA) pressures and increased pulmonary vascular resistance (PVR). Angiocardiogram and dye dilution curves show the site of the central right-to-left shunt. Primary pulmonary hypertension: less cyanosis than in Eisenmenger's syndrome; otherwise, same findings. No shunt detected.

ages of 20 and 40. The exact etiology is not known, although there is much speculation. Raynaud's phenomenon,[26] anorexigenic agent (aminorex),[27] familial cases, oral contraceptives,[28] and thromboembolism[29] have all been associated with primary pulmonary hypertension and considered as possible factors in the cause or as aggravating mechanisms. Often primary pulmonary hypertension is compared with essential systemic hypertension and considered to be due to an increase in pulmonary vascular reactivity. Pathologically, thickening and fibrosis of the intima of small pulmonary arteries and arterioles, increased medial thickness, fibrinoid necrosis, necrotizing arteritis in the walls of muscular pulmonary arteries, and plexiform lesions (dilated, vein-like branches of hypertrophied muscular pulmonary arteries) have been described.[29] However, these are nonspecific and have been also found in Eisenmenger's syndrome. If there is no evidence of pulmonary emboli and venoocclusive disease pathologically and no evidence of cardiac shunts, the preceding lesions can be considered to be due to primary pulmonary hypertension.

These patients usually have decreased exercise tolerance, weakness, fatigue, at times have syncope on effort, and occasionally have angina. Dyspnea occurs progressively, and congestive heart failure develops. Initially, cyanosis may be absent, but later it can develop because of a right-to-left shunt through a patent foramen ovale. In addition, there is peripheral cyanosis due to the markedly reduced cardiac output. The physical findings are generally those seen with Eisenmenger's syndrome (see Fig 7–13). At present there is no effective therapy. Anticoagulant therapy is indicated if there is a possibility of multiple pulmonary emboli. Birth control pills are to be avoided because they may incite thromboembolic disorders. Drugs such as acetylcholine, tolazoline, isoproterenol, diazoxide, and hydralazine have been used with questionable results. Other agents being studied are prostacyclin, angiotension-converting enzyme inhibitors, and calcium channel blockers. Hydralazine and nifedipine can show favorable acute hemodynamic changes; however, the long-term use of these drugs does not appear to affect the overall outcome.[30] There have been few case reports of the long-term beneficial effect of nifedipine.[31,32] It appears at this time that calcium channel blockers should be used in patients with primary pulmonary hypertension. Perhaps it is best to begin at an early stage when pulmonary vasoconstriction is still reversible. Preliminary results with combined heart-lung transplantation indicate that it appears to be a realistic approach for patients with end-stage pulmonary hypertension.[33]

OBSTRUCTIVE DEFECTS

Pulmonary Stenosis

This lesion can be valvular, infundibular, or in the peripheral pulmonary arteries. An intact ventricular septum is rare in the infundibular or subvalvular type. Peripheral pulmonary artery stenosis is usually associated with other anomalies such as pulmonary valvular stenosis, supravalvular aortic stenosis, coarctation of the aorta, ventricular septal defect, or tetralogy of Fallot.

There are no unusual body characteristics except in individuals with a dysplastic valve who may have short stature, low-set ears, hypertelorism, ptosis, and mental retardation (Noonan's syndrome).[34] In the valvular type with intact ventricular septum, cyanosis is unusual unless there is an atrial communication. If the obstruction is moderate or greater, a prominent A wave is noted in the jugular pulse. The valvular lesion produces a murmur with features similar to those of aortic stenosis, that is, a harsh systolic crescendo-descrescendo murmur. It is maximum in the pulmonic area, radiates to the neck, especially on the left side, and is often associated with a thrill that may also be noted in the suprasternal notch. As in aortic stenosis, the greater the obstruction, the longer the murmur and the later its peak. An ejection sound is often present in the pulmonic area, louder with expiration, and splitting of the second sound is often heard, although the pulmonic component may be of reduced intensity. A right ventricular S_4 gallop may be present. The murmur will be lower along the left sternal border with the infundibular type of stenosis, and there will be no associated ejection sound. Patients with severe pulmonary stenosis develop tricuspid regurgitation and right heart failure. Both types present with a slow right ventricular lift. Electrocardiogram reveals different degrees of right ventricular hypertrophy, depending on the severity of the stenosis. X rays of the chest will show prominent central pulmonary arteries (unless it is the infundibular type) with normal or ischemic peripheral lung fields. M-mode echocardiography shows a prominent A wave depth and presystolic opening of the valve if both leaflets can be recorded. The severity and location of the stenosis can be assessed by two-dimensional echocardiography (Fig 7–14) and Doppler. Color flow Doppler is useful to detect other lesions.

Heart catheterization demonstrates a valvular or subvalvular gradient. Angiocardiograms show the stenotic area. Figure 7–15 demonstrates the main features of valvular pulmonary stenosis. In patients with normal cardiac output, if the peak systolic gradient across the pulmonic valve is up to 25 to 49 mm Hg, the stenosis is considered mild; if its 50 to 70 mm Hg, moderate; and if greater than 80 mm Hg, severe. Mild and moderate stenosis generally have a good prognosis with slow progression of the disease. Surgery or percutaneous balloon valvuloplasty[35,36] is indicated if the patient is symptomatic. However, in asymptomatic patients with moderate or severe stenosis there is no full agreement as to when to intervene. Balloon valvuloplasty appears to be effective and may produce long-term improvement. Therefore, it should be considered for those with moderate or severe stenosis even if they are asymptomatic. Those with significant subvalvular stenosis require surgical resection.

Peripheral pulmonary arterial stenosis rarely occurs without associated defects such as pulmonic valvular stenosis, ventricular septal defect, tetralogy of Fallot, and supravalvular aortic stenosis. These can produce ejection systolic murmurs away from the precordium over the lungs, and at times these murmurs may be continuous. Valvuloplasty or surgical repair depends on the location of the obstruction. The closer to the main pulmonary artery, the more likely intervention can be done.

Aortic Stenosis (Valvular, Subvalvular, Supravalvular)

Aortic valvular stenosis has been discussed in Chapter 6. Congenital bicuspid aortic valve has been reported in up to 2% of the population.[37] It is prev-

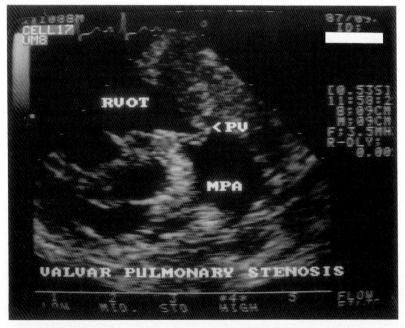

Fig 7–14. Pulmonary valvular stenosis. Two-dimensional echocardiogram (short axis) shows pulmonary valve (PV) stenosis (arrow). RVOT = Right ventricular outflow tract. MPA = Main pulmonary artery. (Courtesy of Dr. Derek A. Fyfe.)

PULMONARY VALVE STENOSIS

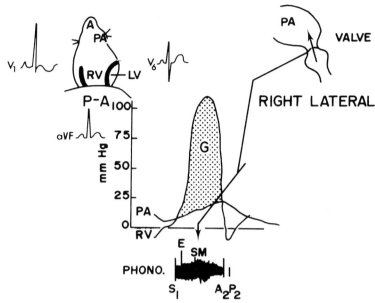

Fig 7–15. Main findings in pulmonary valvular stenosis. Prominent jugular venous a wave. Slow sustained right ventricular (RV) lift. Harsh ejection diamond-shaped systolic murmur (SM) at pulmonic area with thrill. Early systolic ejection (E) sound may be present at pulmonic area. P_2 often is faint, and there is splitting of the second sound (A_2, P_2). Electrocardiogram reveals right ventricular hypertrophy. Posteroanterior (P-A) view of chest shows poststenotic dilatation of main pulmonary artery (PA) and normal or oligemic lung fields. Cardiac catheterization shows systolic gradient (hatched area G) of 95 mm Hg across the pulmonic valve due to increased systolic right ventricular pressure over that in pulmonary artery (PA). Lateral angiocardiogram reveals small valve opening with jet of opaque material into the dilated pulmonary artery.

alent in Turner's syndrome (ovarian dysgenesis). Early on, these patients may have a short ejection systolic murmur with an aortic ejection sound best heard at the apex and, rarely, faint aortic insufficiency. The ECG and chest x ray are usually normal at this stage. M-mode echocardiography can reveal eccentric closure of the aortic valve leaflets (Fig 7–16). The thickened bicuspid valve can be noted best by two-dimensional echocardiography. Conventional and color flow Doppler flow studies can confirm and quantitate the degree of stenosis (gradient and valve area as discussed in Chap. 6). Most of these patients develop progressive calcification, usually after age 30, and in later life demonstrate significant aortic stenosis as was described in Chapter 6.

Subvalvular aortic stenosis may be just a membranous type located below the aortic valve. This is a localized fibrous ring in the left ventricular outflow tract. Another type is a long, tunnel-like, narrow fibromuscular channel. Subaortic stenosis can occur in Noonan's syndrome. Idiopathic hypertrophic subaortic stenosis is a muscular type of obstruction and will be considered in Chapter 12. The discrete subvalvular type does not produce an ejection sound; otherwise, its presentation is the same as that of the valvular type. Mild aortic regurgitation is often present. Two-dimensional echocardiography may localize the obstruction below the valve. M-mode shows the aortic valve opening in early systole, and immediately after opening, the valve partially closes with a

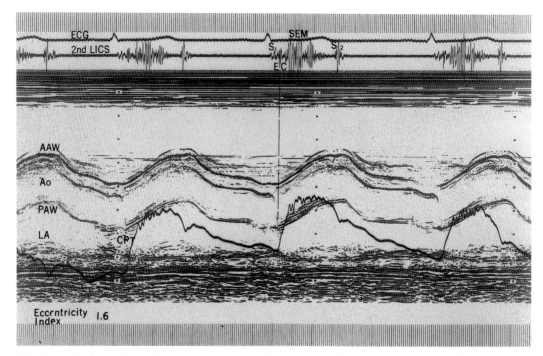

Fig 7–16. M-mode echocardiogram of a patient with aortic stenosis secondary to a bicuspid aortic valve. Note the eccentric anterior closure of the aortic valve. Aortic ejection click (EC) occurs (arrow) at full opening of the aortic valve. Phonocardiogram at the second left intercostal space (LICS) shows the aortic ejection click followed by an ejection systolic murmur (SEM). There is also shuddering in the carotid pulse tracing (CP). Eccentricity index is abnormal. ECG = electrocardiogram; SEM = systolic ejection murmur; EC = ejection click; AAW = anterior aortic wall; Ao = aorta; PAW = posterior aortic wall; LA = left atrium; CP = carotid pulse. (Courtesy of Dr. Bruce W. Usher.)

marked downward dip of the anterior leaflet, but this can also occur with IHSS.

Supravalvular aortic stenosis occurs just above the origin of the coronary vessels. There are several anatomic types. The commonest is a localized hourglass narrowing just above the valve. This lesion is often associated with other disorders and is referred to as Williams' syndrome.[38] Such patients may have an "elfin facies." They often have a high forehead, pointed chin, epicanthal folds, underdeveloped bridge of the nose and mandible, patulous lips, teeth malformation, strabismus, and are mentally retarded. This syndrome has been associated with idiopathic hypercalcemia of infancy; however, those beyond infancy have not had hypercalcemia.[39] The cardiovascular physical findings can resemble those of aortic valvular stenosis, except that the right carotid pulsation is more prominent than on the left (jet stream into the innominate artery), the right arm BP is higher, and the systolic murmur is louder in the first right intercostal space and transmitted well into the suprasternal notch and carotids and often may be associated with a thrill. Supravalvular aortic stenosis may be associated with peripheral pulmonary artery stenosis. Echocardiography, especially two-dimensional, shows the supravalvular narrowing. Doppler studies allow quantitation of the degree of the stenosis.

All of these types of aortic stenosis should have heart catheterization, left ventricular angiography, and supravalvular aortography prior to surgery.

Coarctation of the Aorta

Coarctation is a discrete narrowing, usually distal to the left subclavian artery or just distal to the ligamentum arteriosum. In infants and children who are symptomatic, the construction can be at the ductal or preductal connection. In older children, who are often asymptomatic, the legs may be small compared with the well-developed upper body. Arterial neck and suprasternal notch pulsations are prominent. A late systolic ejection murmur can be heard over the precordium, but is louder over the left side of the dorsal spine posteriorly. An ejection sound may be heard in the primary aortic area or at the apex. Often a congenital bicuspid valve with aortic stenosis or insufficiency may be present. Mitral insufficiency, patent ductus arteriosus, and a ventricular septal defect have also been noted. Berry aneurysms of the circle of Willis are often noted in patients with coarctation. A left ventricular lift is present, with systemic hypertension in the upper extremities and absent or weak delayed pulses in the femoral vessels. If the left subclavian artery comes off at or below the obstruction, there will be a BP difference between the two arms. Prominent collateral vessels can be noted coming off of the subclavian arteries anteriorly to the internal mammary arteries, epigastric arteries, and the lower extremities. Posteriorly, the parascapular arteries and intercostal arteries eventually supply the abdominal viscera. The dilated intercostal arteries can cause rib notching. The intercostal vessels and collateral vessels posteriorly about the scapula may produce visible and palpable pulsations and continuous murmurs. Coarctation of the aorta is often present in Turner's syndrome (ovarian dysgenesis). The ECG may show left ventricular hypertrophy but often is normal. Symptomatic infants may also show right ventricular hypertrophy. X ray of the chest reveals left ventricular enlargement and at times notching of the ribs. The dilated aorta above the coarctation, the indentation of the narrow segment, and the lower poststenotic dilatation can produce a "figure 3" configuration. Barium swallow will often show this as a reversed "3." Two-dimensional echocardiography may show the obstructed segment. Conventional and color flow Doppler can localize the level of the coarctation and estimate the pressure gradient across the narrowed segment. Heart catheterization and aortography should be done to demonstrate the exact site and length of the coarctation and to evaluate or detect the associated lesions. Elective operation is usually recommended between 4 and 6 years of age because, if it is done earlier, obstruction may recur. Figure 7–17 shows the main features of coarctation of the aorta. Surgery is usually indicated in all, especially if there is hypertension, rib notching, left ventricular enlargement, or heart failure. The coarctated segment should be resected. However, in infants and young children, subclavian patch angioplasty is often performed. Balloon dilation angioplasty may lead to aneurysm formation in the area of the coarctation. It has been effective for recurrent stenosis that can occur after surgery in infancy.[40] Surgery should be performed prior to development of major complications such as heart failure, dissection of the aorta, or bacterial endocarditis at the site of the jet lesion. Rupture of an aneurysm of the circle of Willis, rupture of the aorta without dissection, and later development of calcific aortic stenosis are other complications. It is interesting that after surgery the resting or exercise hypertension may remain in a few cases, indicating that, although

COARCTATION OF THE AORTA

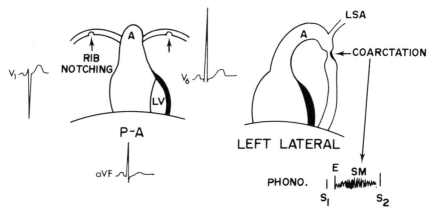

Fig 7–17. Main findings in coarctation of the aorta. Upper extremities may be better developed than lower. Left ventricular (LV) lift. The intercostal and collateral vessels posteriorly about the scapula may produce visible and palpable pulsations. Systolic ejection murmur (SM) often maximum over the left middorsal spine but can be heard over the precordium. Ejection (E) sound at primary aortic area or at the apex. Aortic systolic or diastolic murmur due to a bicuspid aortic valve. At times, a ductus murmur. Blood pressure in arms higher than in legs. Femoral pulses absent or weak and delayed. Electrocardiogram may be normal or show left ventricular hypertrophy. Posteroanterior (P-A) view of chest shows left ventricular enlargement and notching of the ribs. Left lateral angiocardiogram reveals the coarctation site usually distal to the left subclavian artery (LSA) with poststenotic dilatation. Cardiac catheterization can reveal the gradient across the narrow segment.

the mechanical factor has been removed, other nonunderstood factors come into play, maintaining the BP elevation. It is not uncommon during the first postoperative week to have significant hypertension. This could be a factor in those who develop the postcoarctation syndrome that is characterized by ileus, mesenteric vasculitis, and at times visceral infarction.

Hypoplastic Left Heart Syndrome

This is a common cause of congestive heart failure in newborns. There may be underdevelopment of the left ventricle, aortic valve atresia, mitral atresia, atresia or hypoplasia of the aortic arch, or a combination of these lesions. In addition, there may be endocardial fibroelastosis of the left atrium and ventricle. These infants are in respiratory distress with cyanosis and heart failure. Echocardiography shows the lesions and is diagnostic. Conventional and color flow Doppler are useful. There is no corrective operative procedure, and the defect almost always is fatal in the first year of life. Palliation has been reported by creating an atrial septal defect, pulmonary artery banding, aortic arch reconstruction and other staged procedures for the severely symptomatic infants. Few have survived these procedures. Human cardiac transplantation has been done and cardiac xenotransplantation has been attempted.

LESIONS THAT PRODUCE CONTINUOUS MURMURS

Patent ductus arteriosus, peripheral pulmonary artery stenosis, and persistent truncus have already been mentioned. Other causes of a continuous murmur are rupture of a congenital aneurysm of the sinus of Valsalva, coronary arteriovenous fistula, anomalous origin of coronary arteries, systemic arteriovenous fistula, and pulmonary arteriovenous fistula.

Rupture of a Sinus of Valsalva Aneurysm

The posterior (noncoronary) sinus aneurysms rupture into the right atrium, and those of the right sinus rupture into the right ventricle. Congenital aneurysms of the left aortic sinus are rare. The rupture can occur spontaneously or be secondary to bacterial endocarditis, and can present acutely with symptoms or with just a murmur and no symptoms. Patients with sudden rupture and symptoms usually have severe substernal chest pain, a continuous murmur, and heart failure. The murmur is loudest along the lower left sternal border and over the xiphoid area and often is associated with a thrill. The apical impulse is hyperdynamic, and a wide pulse pressure is present. The chest x ray usually resembles that of a patent ductus, and the ECG can show biventricular enlargement. Others can have a slow rupture, beginning with a small opening and continuous murmur, and later becoming symptomatic if the shunt increases. Most often one has to differentiate these from a patent ductus or a ventricular septal defect with aortic regurgitation. Two-dimensional echocardiography and Doppler (conventional and color flow) can establish the diagnosis. Heart catheterization and aortography confirm the diagnosis.

Ruptured aortic sinus aneurysms should be surgically repaired. Patients with bacterial endocarditis should have appropriate therapy and surgery later, unless uncontrolled heart failure or hemodynamic instability demands earlier repair.

Coronary Arteriovenous Communication

This coronary vessel defect most commonly communicates with the right ventricle or the coronary sinus. The right coronary artery is more frequently involved. The continuous murmur is usually located maximally at the site of communication on the venous side. It is maximum at the right sternal border if the coronary vessel enters the right atrium or coronary sinus and along the left sternal border if it enters the right ventricle. The patient may be asymptomatic unless the shunt is large and congestive failure occurs. Two-dimensional echocardiography and pulsed Doppler (including color flow) can detect the fistulas. Cardiac catheterization demonstrates a left-to-right shunt, and coronary arteriography or aortography shows the fistula. The coronary artery can be ligated near its entrance into the cardiac chamber or vessel.

Anomalous Origin of Coronary Arteries

The most common form of this anomaly is the left coronary artery originating from the pulmonary artery (Bland-White-Garland syndrome). Infants may have episodes of pallor, dyspnea, or cyanosis usually associated with any exertion such as feeding. Congestive heart failure can develop. Rarely, a patient will survive to adulthood because of good collateral circulation; such patients often have a continuous murmur. Frequently an apical systolic murmur is audible. The ECG may show an anterolateral infarction pattern. Two-dimensional echocardiography and conventional and color flow Doppler may be diagnostic, especially in infants. Thallium stress test may show perfusion defects. The diagnosis is established by cardiac catheterization, aortography, and right coronary arteriography. If there is good collateral circulation, the anomalous coronary artery can be ligated at its origin from the pulmonary artery. The anomalous coronary artery has been anastomosed to the aorta directly or bypassed with a vein graft in older children, followed by ligation of the artery near its pulmonary origin.

Systemic Arteriovenous Fistula

This is usually acquired and most often involves the peripheral vessels, as with gunshot wounds. It may be congenital. In the presence of undiagnosed heart failure, one should listen over every scar, no matter how small, for a continuous murmur of arteriovenous fistula, since this is a surgically correctable lesion. A wide pulse pressure can be noted and if one compresses the fistula, the heart rate will slow (Branham's sign). If an extremity is involved, it becomes warm and large, and dermatitis and edema can develop. The congenital types are often multiple and nonlocalized and do not respond to repair or excision as well as the acquired types.

Pulmonary Arteriovenous Fistula

This lesion will usually produce cyanosis due to the right-to-left shunt, and the continuous murmur will be heard over the lung area involved. This may be present with or without Osler-Weber-Rendu disease (hereditary hemorrhagic telangiectasia). Chest x ray may show one or more masses. The diagnosis can be made with pulmonary arteriography. Resection of the involved lung area can be performed or, if possible, through dissection the pulmonary artery and vein can be ligated and the aneurysm excised. Catheter embolization has been used in selected cases.

LESS COMMON DEFECTS

There are many rare and at times complex congenital heart defects. Some of them have been discussed, and a few more will be briefly mentioned.

Ebstein's Anomaly

In this anomaly the septal and posterior leaflets of the tricuspid valve are attached downward from the anulus to the right ventricular wall. Thus, the right atrium and the upper part of the right ventricle above the displaced leaflets form a common chamber. Most cases have a patent foramen ovale or atrial septal defect. The functional right ventricle is small, and, rarely, there may be associated pulmonary stenosis or a ventricular septal defect. Clinically, there may be slight cyanosis, tricuspid insufficiency, and a quiet precordium. Multiple heart sounds are audible (the tricuspid component of the first soon can be loud and clicking, the so-called "sail sound"), and supraventricular arrhythmias are common. The ECG shows prominent P waves and right bundle branch block with low voltage. Deep Q waves can be present in the inferior and precordial leads. The type B Wolff-Parkinson-White syndrome may be present in about 10% of cases. X ray of the chest shows marked cardiomegaly with reasonably clear lung fields. The right atrium forms a prominent right heart border. The M-mode echocardiogram will reveal delayed tricuspid valve closure compared with the mitral valve. The diagnosis can be made by two-dimensional echocardiography and conventional and color flow Doppler. Cardiac catheterization and angiography can confirm the diagnosis. Many surgical procedures have been performed for symptomatic patients. The atrial septal defect can be repaired, atrial portions of the right ventricle can be obliterated by plication of the line of attachment of the displaced tricuspid leaflets to the anulus fibrosus, and the tricuspid valve can be replaced. This procedure has been performed with some success.[41]

Total Anomalous Pulmonary Venous Drainage

In this anomaly, the pulmonary venous (usually as a common trunk) and systemic venous drainages are into the right atrium. The total anomalous pulmonary venous connection may be in several other areas, such as below the diaphragm to the portal system or inferior vena cava, to a persistent left superior vena cava, or to the coronary sinus. The supradiaphragmatic connections are the most common and may have obstruction. The infradiaphragmatic types occur less often and are always obstructed. An atrial septal defect is always present. Cyanosis and congestive failure appear early in life, and chest x ray may show a widened superior mediastinum giving a "snowman" or "figure 8" appearance if the return is to an anomalous left vertical vein, a left innominate vein, and a right superior vena cava. The diagnosis should be confirmed with cardiac catheterization and angiography. Operation is indicated in symptomatic infants and can be delayed in asymptomatic ones for several months. Balloon atrial septotomy can be life-saving in the sick infant with a small atrial septal defect.

Dextrocardia and Other Cardiac Malpositions

Levocardia indicates that the apex is to the left, dextrocardia that it is to the right, and mesocardia that it is in the midline. Dextrocardia actually means right-sided position of the heart due to the inherent cardiac malposition and not to displacement of the heart (dextroposition as due to pulmonary pathology). As mentioned before, situs solitus describes the normal position of the atria and viscera—namely, the right atrium and liver are on the right side and the stomach and left atrium are on the left—whereas situs inversus is the reverse. Situs ambiguus indicates that situs solitus or inversus cannot be identified (usually in cases of asplenia or polysplenia). Dextrocardia with situs inversus is referred to as situs inversus totalis, and dextrocardia with situs solitus is referred to as isolated dextrocardia. "Isolated levocardia" is used if there is levocardia with situs inversus. Patients with isolated dextrocardia or isolated levocardia have almost 100% incidence of cardiac anomalies, whereas patients with situs inversus totalis have a 3 to 10% incidence.[42]

It is important in the approach to diagnosis of dextrocardia that the location of the atria be determined as well as their relationship to the viscera. In most cases the right atrium will retain its position with relation to the liver; e.g., if the liver is on the left, the right atrium will also be on the left side. The P wave is positive in lead I in normal patients. If there is atrial inversion, the P wave will be negative in lead I and aVl and upright in aVr situs inversus with either dextrocardia or levocardia). Situs solitus with either a normally positioned heart or dextrocardia has an upright P wave in lead 1 and aVl and inverted in aVr. However, ectopic left atrial pacemakers and reversal of right and left arm leads can cause confusion. Atrial inversion is associated with a left-sided liver and right-sided stomach. The most reliable method for atrial location is the position of the inferior vena cava. This position may be identified by two-dimensional echocardiography or nuclear or venous angiography. If the atrial positions are not clear, one should suspect the asplenia or polysplenia syndrome. The asplenia patients frequently have dextrocardia and complex cardiac anomalies and severe cyanosis and pulmonary stenosis, whereas the polysplenia patients have frequent but less complex cardiac anomalies, levocardia is more common in polysplenia patients, who frequently have interruption of the inferior vena cava with azygous continuation. Howell-Jolly bodies, Heinz bodies, and abnormally shaped red blood cells are noted in patients with asplenia, but are nonspecific. Following determination of the atrial locations, the ventricles should be located and their relationship to the atria established. The QRS complex of the ECG can be of some help. If there are no other cardiac anomalies, a qRs pattern in a particular precordial position can indicate that the left ventricle is in the underlying area, and an rS pattern that the right ventricle is in the underlying area. Two-dimensional echocardiography can be used to detect the ventricular morphology. Angiographic studies will show the location of the ventricles by their trabeculations and shape and by location of the valves. If the ventricles are in normal relationship, then the patient has a d-loop, and for the reverse, an l-loop. If the atria are connected to the proper ventricle, the AV connection is said to be concordant; if not, discordant. In addition, the relationship of the great vessels to the ventricles should be established. If the spatial relationships of the great arteries are normal, this is called D-normal. It is L-normal if this relationship is reversed. Malposition refers to an abnormal spatial relationship. Echocardiography has been helpful in establishing this relationship, which can be confirmed by aortography and selective coronary arteriography. Finally, the type of conus (subpulmonic, subaortic, bilateral, or absent) should be determined by echocardiography or angiography. The subpulmonic conus is noted with normally related great vessels. Conventional and color flow Doppler are also helpful.

Kartagener's syndrome is a combination of situs inversus totalis, sinusitis, and bronchiectasis.

In summary, dextrocardia can be evaluated by this segmental approach of VanPraagh and Vlad[43] by detecting the site of the atria, ventricles, and great vessels.[44] This can be done by a combination of the physical examination, chest x ray, ECG, and echocardiographic findings, and, if other associated anomalies are suspected, by cardiac catheterization with selective cineangiography. Many today use only the term dextrocardia for all hearts on the right side and do not use such terms as dextroversion, mirror image or isolated dextrocardia, or dextroposition. Various terms, abbreviations, and symbols are used to designate the visceroatrial situs, location of ventricles, and location of great vessels and their various connections as mentioned earlier in this chapter.

CONGENITAL HEART DEFECTS IN THE ADULT (UNCORRECTED AND CORRECTED)

Surgery has corrected many of the congenital heart lesions in infants and children (Table 7–2). However, many patients who are inoperable or have had palliative procedures may live to adulthood. In addition, many cases have been overlooked and not considered to have a congenital lesion until they were

Table 7–2. Indications for Surgery for the Common Types of Congenital Cardiac Defects*

Manifestation	Defect	Indications for Surgery	Optimal Age and Procedure
Left-right shunt	Ventricular septal defect	Left to right shunt above 2.0:1.00 or elevated pulmonary artery pressure or enlarged heart. In adult, shunt above 1.5:1.00	Direct closure or patch: 3 years and older or earlier if in failure or with pulmonary hypertension
	Atrial septal defect	Shunts 1.5:1.00 or greater	Direct closure or patch: 3 years and older or earlier if in failure
	Patent ductus	All, unless found late in life with small shunt	Divided or ligated; over 6 months of age or earlier if in failure
Right-left shunt	Tetralogy	All	Total correction in the first several years of life or earlier if symptomatic. At times shunt before total repair
	Transposition of great vessels	All, except those with severe pulmonary hypertension	Balloon atrioseptostomy: total repair after age 3 months (Mustard or Senning) with pulmonary stenosis (Rastelli)
	Tricuspid atresia	Small pulmonary blood flow	Shunt, after age 4 possible corrective procedure (Fontan)
	Truncus arteriosus	All, unless there is severe pulmonary vascular disease	Before age 3–6 months, total correction
Obstructive defects	Pulmonary stenosis	Gradient of 50 mm Hg or greater	Balloon valvuloplasty or surgery; 3 years and older or earlier if in failure
	Aortic stenosis	Symptomatic, asymptomatic if gradient 75 mm Hg or greater or the valve area is 0.5 cm^2/m^2 or less	Valvotomy; any age in childhood; later valve replacement if necessary
	Coarctation of aorta	All	Segment resected; 4–6 years or earlier if symptomatic

*Generally, unless the patient is symptomatic, surgery should be deferred until after 1 year of age, but preferably should be done before the patient enters school.

adults. Frequently congenital lesions simulate acquired heart disease, especially valvular types or cardiomyopathy. Bicuspid aortic valve and atrial septal defect are the most frequent congenital lesions noted in adults. Less common lesions encountered are pulmonary stenosis, patent ductus, coarctation of the aorta, Ebstein's anomaly, tetralogy of Fallot, and the Eisenmenger syndrome. Attention may be drawn to these because of such complications as arrhythmia, heart failure, or endocarditis. The clinical features are essentially those described for children with some minor differences. Often the first clue has been the appearance of the heart and pulmonary vasculature in the chest x ray. Atrial septal defect is a common congenital cardiac lesion seen in adults and frequently has been overlooked as mitral stenosis because of the flow-type diastolic tricuspid murmur produced by the large left-to-right shunt. Coarctation of the aorta may be followed for years for systemic hypertension, because the blood pressure was not checked in the legs. Cyanotic lesions are at times mistaken as a form of chronic lung disease. Total correction of many of these lesions can be performed even in adulthood when indicated at a relatively low risk. Some are inoperable such as the Eisenmenger syndrome.

Since patients operated on for congenital heart disease now live longer, there is a new group of cardiac patients available for study. Many with complete repair have residual abnormalities. However, regardless of whether residual abnormalities are present or not, patients may be asymptomatic or symptomatic. Although the mechanical defect has been corrected, myocardial changes may be present and become progressively worse, leading to arrhythmias and heart failure. Atrial septal defects can be closed, yet the patient may continue to have atrial arrhythmias, or they can develop for the first time. Chronic congestive heart failure, tricuspid and mitral insufficiency, or pulmonary vascular obstructive disease can be present. Patients with repaired ventricular septal defects can develop progressive pulmonary hypertension, especially if they had moderate preoperative elevation of the pulmonary vascular resistance. Patients with repaired tetralogy of Fallot may have pulmonary valve insufficiency, and if the right ventricular outflow tract was patched, an aneurysm can develop at that site. Ventricular arrhythmias and conduction defects have been noted. Patients having had surgery for coarctation can continue to have some obstruction or hypertension at rest or especially with exercise. Porcine valves can deteriorate and calcify, and patients who have had an aortic valve commissurotomy may have restenosis or develop aortic insufficiency. The aortic anulus may fail to enlarge to meet body growth, and a second operation may be necessary.

Many patients with repaired congenital lesions can develop tachyarrhythmias or bradyarrhythmias or complete heart block. Sudden death is more common following repair of tetralogy of Fallot or transposition of the great vessels. Patients with uncomplicated secundum atrial septal defect repaired by direct suture without a prosthetic patch and those who have had ligation and division of a patent ductus arteriosus do not require endocarditis prophylaxis. Except for these two conditions, others who have had cardiovascular surgery, especially those with prosthetic valves, should have prophylaxis as was required for the patient without surgery undergoing dental, genitourinary, or gastrointestinal studies and other procedures.

Besides the usual routine examinations and tests, patients with repaired congenital heart defects should have echocardiographic and Holter monitoring annually, and promptly if symptoms occur. In addition, many should have exercise stress tests, for cardiac performance may be below normal with exercise, even though it is normal at rest.

Table 7–2 summarizes the indications for surgery for the common types of congenital cardiac defects.

REFERENCES

1. Hoffman J.I.E., Rudolph A.M.: The natural history of ventricular septal defects in infancy. *Am. J. Cardiol.* 16:634, 1965.
2. Tatsuno K., Konno S., Sakakibara S.: Ventricular septal defect with aortic insufficiency. *Am. Heart J.* 85:13, 1973.
3. Smith A.T., Lack G.H., Jr., Taylor G.J.: Holt-Oram syndrome. *J. Pediatr.* 95:538, 1979.
4. Nasrallah A.T., Hall R.J., Garcia E., et al.: Surgical repair of atrial septal defect in patients over 60 years of age. *Circulation* 53:329, 1976.
5. Reed W.A., Dunn M.I.: Long-term results of repair of atrial septal defects. *Am. J. Surg.* 121:724, 1971.
6. Steinbrunn W., Cohn K.E., Selzer A.: Atrial septal defect associated with mitral stenosis: The Lutembacher syndrome revisited. *Am. J. Med.* 48:295, 1970.
7. Feigenbaum H.: *Echocardiography.* 4th Ed., Philadelphia, Lea & Febiger, 1985, p. 417.
8. Friedman W.F., Hirschklau M.J., Printz M.F., et al.: Pharmacologic closure of patent ductus arteriosus in the premature infant. *N. Engl. J. Med.* 295:526, 1976.
9. Nadas A.S.: Patent ductus revisited. *N. Engl. J. Med.* 295:563, 1976.
10. Guntheroth W.G., Morgan B.C., Mullins G.L., et al.: Venous return with knee-chest position and squatting in tetralogy of Fallot. *Am. Heart J.* 75:313, 1968.
11. Guntheroth W.G., Morgan B.C., Mullins G.L.: Physiologic studies of paroxysmal hyperpnea in cyanotic congenital heart disease. *Circulation* 31:70, 1965.
12. Knight L., Edwards J.E.: Right aortic arch: Types and associated cardiac anomalies. *Circulation* 50:1947, 1974.
13. Tandon R., Edwards J.E.: Tricuspid atresia: A reevaluation and classification. *J. Thorac. Cardiovasc. Surg.* 67:530, 1974.
14. Fontan F., Baudet E.: Surgical repair of tricuspid atresia. *Thorax* 26:240, 1971.
15. Girod D.A., Fontan F., Deville C., et al.: Long-term results after the Fontan operation for tricuspid atresia. *Circulation* 75:605, 1987.
16. VanPraagh R.: Terminology of congenital heart disease: Glossary and commentary. *Circulation* 56:139, 1977.
17. Rashkind W.J., Miller W.W.: Creation of an atrial defect without thoracotomy: A palliative approach to complete transposition of the great arteries. *J.A.M.A.* 196:991, 1966.
18. Mustard W.T.: Successful two-stage correction of transposition of the great vessels. *Surgery* 55:469, 1964.
19. Senning A.: Surgical correction of transposition of the great vessels. *Surgery* 45:966, 1959.
20. Jatene A.D., Fontes V.F., Paulista P.P., et al.: Anatomic correction of transposition of the great vessels. *J. Thorac. Cardiovasc. Surg.* 72:364, 1976.
21. Schiebler G.L., Edwards J.E., Burchell H.B., et al.: Congenital corrected transposition of the great vessels: A study of 33 cases. *Pediatrics* 27(part 2):851, 1961.
22. Collett R.W., Edwards J.E.: Persistent truncus arteriosus: A classification according to anatomic types. *Surg. Clin. North Am.* 29:1245, 1949.
23. Wood P.: The Eisenmenger syndrome or pulmonary hypertension with reversed central shunt. *Br. Med. J.* 2:701, 1958.
24. Young D., Mark H.: Fate of the patient with Eisenmenger syndrome. *Am. J. Cardiol.* 28:658, 1971.
25. McGregor C.G.A., Jamieson S.W., Baldwin J.C., et al.: Combined heart-lung transplantation for end-stage Eisenmenger's syndrome. *J. Thorac. Cardiovasc. Surg.* 91:443, 1986.
26. Winters W.L., Jr., Joseph R.R., Learner N.: "Primary" pulmonary hypertension and Raynaud's phenomenon: Case report and review of the literature. *Arch. Intern. Med.* 114:821, 1964.
27. Gurtner H.P.: Pulmonary hypertension; "plexogenic pulmonary arteriopathy" and the appetite depressant drug aminorex: Post or propter? *Bull. Eur. Physiopathol. Respir.* 15:897, 1979.
28. Kleiger R.E., Boxer M., Ingham R.E., et al.: Pulmonary hypertension in patients using oral contraceptives: A report of six cases. *Chest* 69:143, 1976.
29. Wagenvoort C.A., Wagenvoort N.: Primary pulmonary hypertension: A pathologic study of the lung vessels in 156 clinically diagnosed cases. *Circulation* 42:1163, 1970.

30. Rich S., Brundage B.H., Levy P.S.: The effect of vasodilator therapy on the clinical outcome of patients with primary pulmonary hypertension. *Circulation* 71:1191, 1985.
31. Fisher J., Borer J.S., Moses J.W., et al.: Hemodynamic effects of nifedipine versus hydralazine in primary pulmonary hypertension. *Am. J. Cardiol.* 54:646, 1984.
32. Lunde P., Rasmussen K: Long-term beneficial effect of nifedipine in primary pulmonary hypertension. *Am. Heart J.* (Brief Communications) 108:415, 1984.
33. Jamieson S.W., Stinson E.B., Oyer P.E., et al.: Heart and lung transplantation for pulmonary hypertension. *Am. J. Surg.* 147:740, 1984.
34. Noonan J.A.: Hypertelorism with Turner phenotype: A new syndrome with associated congenital heart disease. *Am. J. Dis. Child.* 116:373, 1968.
35. Kan J.S., White R.I., Mitchell S.E., et al.: Percutaneous transluminal balloon valvuloplasty for pulmonary valve stenosis. *Circulation* 69:554, 1984.
36. Gibbs J.L., Stanley C.P., Dickenson D.F.: Pulmonary balloon valvuloplasty in late adult life. *Int. J. Cardiol.* 11:237, 1986.
37. Roberts W.C.: The congenital bicuspid aortic valve: A study of 85 autopsy cases. *Am. J. Cardiol.* 26:72, 1970.
38. Williams J.C.P., Barratt-Boyes B.G., Lowe J.B.: Supravalvular aortic stenosis. *Circulation* 24:1311, 1961.
39. Folger G.M., Jr.: Further observations on the syndrome of idiopathic infantile hypercalcemia associated with supravalvular aortic stenosis. *Am. Heart J.* 93:455, 1977.
40. Allen H.D., Marx G.R., Ovitt T.W., et al.: Balloon dilation angioplasty for coarctation of the aorta. *Am. J. Cardiol.* 57:828, 1986.
41. Hardy K.L., Roe B.B.: Ebstein's anomaly: Further experience with definitive repair. *J. Thorac. Cardiovasc. Surg.* 58:553, 1969.
42. Hanson J.S., Tabakin B.S.: Primary and secondary dextrocardia: Their differentiation and the role of cineangiocardiography in diagnosing associated congenital cardiac defects. *Am. J. Cardiol.* 8:275, 1961.
43. VanPraagh R., Vlad P.: Dextrocardia, mesocardia and levocardia: The segmental approach to diagnosis in congenital heart disease, in Keith J.D., Rowe R.D., Vlad P. (eds.): *Heart Disease in Infancy and Childhood,* New York, Macmillan Publishing Co., 1978.
44. Rao R.S.: Dextrocardia: Systemic approach to differential diagnosis. *Am. Heart J.* 102:389, 1981.

Chapter 8

INNOCENT HEART MURMURS

The interpretation of heart murmurs is based on their timing, intensity, location, radiation, duration, quality, and pitch. In addition, the features of the first and second sounds and extra sounds (such as ejection sounds, clicks, and opening snaps) are important in evaluating the significance of heart murmurs.

The following classification of Freeman and Levine[1] is used most commonly by observers to describe the intensity of murmurs:

Grade I—Murmur difficult to hear and not immediately apparent.
    II—Faintest murmur immediately heard.
    III—Intermediate intensity.
    IV—Intermediate intensity with thrill.
    V—Loudest murmur heard with rim of stethoscope touching skin.
    VI—Murmur audible with stethoscope removed from chest wall.

Innocent murmurs are usually grade I to a maximum of grade III intensity and not associated with significant heart disease. It is often difficult to assess the significance of a murmur, especially in a child. In addition, the generalist finds it difficult to know when to refer a child to a cardiologist for evaluation of a murmur, especially when the x ray and ECG are normal. About 50 to 75% of all children have an innocent heart murmur heard at one time or another, and we should not make them and their families psychologic cripples. The murmur should be explained to the patient (depending on his age) and to the parents. The parents should not be told that the child will outgrow the murmur, even though frequently innocent murmurs disappear by adolescence. Detection of a heart murmur also brings up many other questions pertaining to restriction from sports or other activities, life insurance eligibility, type of occupation, risk of pregnancy and noncardiac surgery, and endocarditis prophylaxis. Such problems are important to the patient's future, and the answers depend on whether the murmur is innocent or organic, and, if organic, the degree of impairment. Rarely are elaborate hemodynamic studies necessary for evaluation.

Innocent murmurs are referred to as systolic ejection type, cardiorespiratory, venous hum, mammary souffle, and innocent carotid and supraclavicular bruit.

THE INNOCENT SYSTOLIC EJECTION MURMUR

The innocent systolic ejection murmur is the most common type of innocent murmur and is noted more often in adolescents and young adults. However, at times it may be heard in the newborn. The murmur may be due to the small normal pressure gradient which exists early in systole between each ventricle

295

and its respective great vessel. It is more intense in early systole because, during this time, the peak blood flow and velocity of flow are maximal even if the basal cardiac output is normal.[2] Any condition that increases the cardiac output and blood flow can increase this normal gradient and produce or accentuate such a murmur—anemia, fever, hyperthyroidisim, exercise, and pregnancy. It arises in the ventricular outflow tracts, near the aortic or pulmonic valve, or at the level of the great vessels. The murmur is typically diamond-shaped (crescendo-decrescendo), peaks in early or midsystole, and has a harsh or blowing quality of medium frequency. The vibratory Still's murmur is a variant of the innocent ejection murmur and has a musical, buzzing, groaning, or twanging quality. It was previously thought to originate from the pulmonic valve, but now the source is thought to be the subaortic area or the aortic valve.[3] It can be confused with a small muscular ventricular septal defect, and, if it is heard at the apex, with mitral insufficiency.

The intensity of the innocent systolic ejection murmur depends on the stroke volume and velocity of blood flow, width of chest (frequently noted in the straight back syndrome), and proximity of the great vessels to the chest wall. Turbulent flow in the pulmonary artery[4] or aorta[5] can produce the murmur, probably more so in the pulmonic area, which is close to the anterior chest. Also, the right ventricular outflow tract narrows with systole due to bulging of the membranous septum. It is most often heard in the pulmonic area, downward along the left sternal border and occasionally at the apex, and becomes louder on lying down and with exercise. It may be heard in all these areas in the same patient.

The innocent systolic ejection murmur must be differentiated from mild aortic stenosis, mild valvular pulmonary stenosis, or an atrial septal defect. Table 8–1 gives the differentiating clinical features. The ejection sounds and splitting of the second sound are the determining factors, since the murmur can be the same in all four situations. The pulmonic ejection sound occurring with pulmonary valvular stenosis may be mistaken for the first sound. During inspiration, this ejection sound decreases in intensity or disappears because the right ventricular end-diastolic pressure exceeds the pulmonary artery pressure and the stenotic pulmonic valve moves to the open position, therefore having less systolic motion.[6] A systolic thrill may be present even with mild pulmonary stenosis. The ECG can be normal in the four situations in Table 8–1. However, the ECG may show right ventricular outflow hypertrophy (rSR' in V_1), and the x ray may show an enlarged pulmonary artery segment with increased pulmonary vascular markings in patients with atrial septal defects. The pulmonary artery segment may also be enlarged with valvular pulmonary stenosis. Echocardiography and Doppler have been of great help in ruling out organic disease.

In the presence of a normal-sized heart, if there is normal splitting of the second sound, no ejection sound or diastolic murmur, the systolic ejection murmur is probably innocent.

CARDIORESPIRATORY MURMUR

This murmur probably is due to compression of the lung during inspiration with movement of air in the bronchial tree as the heart contracts.[7] Often it is heard in patients with pectus excavatum or with some other chest deformity or in the presence of atelectasis, pulmonary consolidation, or pleural or pericar-

Table 8–1. Differential Diagnosis of Basal Systolic Ejection Murmur

	Systolic Ejection Murmur	Radiation of Murmur	Early Ejection Sound	Second Sound	Lift
Innocent murmur	Usually heard best at pulmonic area	Insignificant	No	Normal	No
Mild pulmonary valvular stenosis	Usually heard best at pulmonic area	Infraclavicular	Yes; best heard at the pulmonic area with expiration	Split but not fixed	Possible right ventricular
Mild aortic stenosis	Usually heard best at aortic area	To neck and apex	Yes; at the aortic area, but usually heard best at the apex and does not vary with respiration	Normal	No
Atrial septal defect	Usually heard best at pulmonic area	To lungs	Yes and no	Wide, fixed, splitting	Right ventricular

dial adhesions. The murmur is high-pitched, squeaky, or swishing in systole and is heard best along the left sternal border and apex with inspiration; it may not be heard if breathing is held at expiration.

VENOUS HUM

This murmur is often heard in children and is due to venous flow in the neck veins. The murmur is continuous with early diastolic accentuation and is often musical. It may be heard over either side of the neck (supraclavicular areas) or chest, but most often is on the right. It is loudest in the sitting position and varies with head position (brought out by turning the head to the side opposite the murmur) or can be obliterated by compression of the neck veins. Rarely, it can be confused with a patent ductus arteriosus. The ductal murmur is loudest in late systole, has a harsher quality, is heard well in the recumbent position, and cannot be obliterated with pressure of the jugular veins. The venous hums can be heard not only in children but also in patients with thyrotoxicosis, anemia, pregnancy, or in any hyperkinetic state.

THE MAMMARY SOUFFLE

This continuous or, rarely, systolic murmur occurs in late pregnancy, after the third month, and early postpartum; it is especially common in the mother who is nursing her child. It is most frequently heard in the second right or left intercostal spaces and down along either sternal border. Firm pressure with the stethoscope directly or with the finger in the relevant intercostal space lateral to the stethoscope bell can obliterate the murmur. The exact mechanism for this murmur is not clear; however, Tabatznik et al.[8] suggest that the murmur arises at the site of anastomosis between branches of the aortic intercostal arteries and branches of the internal mammary artery. They considered the phonocardiographic features of the murmur as being of arterial origin rather than venous, which is still thought by some to be the cause. This murmur can be mistaken for a patent ductus arteriosus, systemic or pulmonary arteriovenous fistulas, or combined aortic stenosis and insufficiency. Obliteration of the mammary souffle by compression should differentiate it from these.

CAROTID AND SUPRACLAVICULAR BRUIT

These early systolic murmurs (bruit) are frequently heard in adolescents and young adults and are associated with hyperkinetic states, such as anxiety, or with anemia. They are often heard in the supraclavicular areas, especially on the right, and are rarely associated with a thrill. They radiate poorly to the upper chest and therefore should not be confused with aortic or pulmonic valve murmurs. Such murmurs may be eliminated by deep pressure in the supraclavicular area, compressing the subclavian artery against the first rib,[9] or by hyperextension of the shoulders. In young children and infants, similar murmurs may be heard over the cranium. If they are the only findings, they are benign cranial bruit.

IMPORTANT FACTS ABOUT MURMURS

1. Innocent murmurs are most often short, early to mid-systolic ejection types beginning after the first sound and ending well before the second

sound. However, it should be recognized that the systolic ejection murmur, even though it is most commonly innocent, can indicate an abnormality of the semilunar valves, cardiac chambers, or the great vessels. Pansystolic murmurs, beginning with the first sound and extending to the second sound, and late systolic murmurs, beginning after the first sound at about mid-systole and extending to the second sound, are organic murmurs.

2. It is a fallacy to think that innocent murmurs decrease or disappear after exercise. An increase in cardiac output due to any cause will increase the intensity of all murmurs.

3. Intensity is less indicative of the severity of the murmur than is the length of the murmur. A loud murmur may be due to a small lesion, and a faint murmur may be associated with a severe lesion.

4. Diastolic murmurs usually are abnormal. These are most often due to direct structural changes, but they can also be secondary to other cardiovascular abnormalities.

5. If a thrill is present, the murmur is practically always organic, although the lesion may be small.

6. A murmur noted in a cyanotic patient is usually organic.

7. If the ECG and chest x ray are normal, the murmur may not be hemodynamically significant but could well be organic.

8. Judge murmurs by the company they keep. Other evidences of heart disease, such as cardiomegaly, ECG abnormalities, ejection sounds, mid or late systolic clicks, or an opening snap suggest that the murmur is organic.

9. One should consider an atrial septal defect as the most likely congenital lesion or mitral valve disease as the most likely acquired lesion in a woman age 40 or older who is not cyanotic and has a history of a heart murmur, even prior to auscultation.

10. When in doubt, the patient should be referred to a cardiologist.

11. Echocardiography and conventional and color Doppler are useful in the diagnosis of murmurs and for obtaining hemodynamic information. These studies have reduced the need for cardiac catheterization studies to clarify the etiology of a murmur.

REFERENCES

1. Freeman A.R., Levine S.A.: The clinical significance of the systolic murmur: A study of 1,000 consecutive "noncardiac" cases. *Ann. Intern. Med.* 6:1371, 1933.
2. Abrams J.: Auscultation of heart murmurs. *Primary Cardiol.* 7:21, 1981.
3. Wennevold A.: The origin of the innocent "vibratory" murmur studied with intracardiac phonocardiography. *Acta Med. Scand.* 181:1, 1967.
4. deLeon A.C., Perloff J.K., Twigg H., et al.: The straight back syndrome. *Circulation* 32:193, 1965.
5. Stein P.D., Sabbah H.N.: Aortic origin of innocent murmurs. *Am. J. Cardiol.* 39:665, 1977.
6. Hultgren H.N., Reeve R., Cohn K., et al.: The ejection click of valvular pulmonic stenosis. *Circulation* 40:631, 1969.
7. Harvey W.P.: Innocent versus significant murmurs. *Curr. Probl. Cardiol.* 1:7, 1976.
8. Tabatznik B., Randall T.W., Hersch C.: The mammary souffle of pregnancy and lactation. *Circulation* 22:1069, 1960.
9. Fowler N.O., Marshall W.J.: The supreclavicular arterial bruit. *Am. Heart J.* 69:410, 1965.

Chapter 9

PULMONARY HEART DISEASE

CHRONIC COR PULMONALE

Chronic cor pulmonale is a condition in which hypertrophy and dilatation of the right ventricle, with or without failure, result from certain disease states affecting the function or structure of the lungs. This does not include pulmonary changes occurring in diseases primarily affecting the left side of the heart or associated with congenital heart disease. The common factor preceding right ventricular hypertrophy is always pulmonary hypertension secondary to changes in the pulmonary vascular bed.

The incidence of cor pulmonale is difficult to estimate, since its frequency varies considerably in different areas, and the death certificates are reported differently. A review of 801 consecutive autopsied cases of heart disease of all types from the files of the Medical University Hospital of South Carolina reveals 77 (9.2%) cases of cor pulmonale. It is impossible at present to give a realistic figure, but the incidence of cor pulmonale probably ranges from 5 to 10% of all cases of organic heart disease. Cor pulmonale is at least five times more common in men than in women, and about 75% of the patients are over 50 years of age.[1]

PATHOGENESIS AND PATHOLOGY

Increased pulmonary vascular resistance and pulmonary hypertension are the major factors always present in cor pulmonale. In addition, abnormal blood gases (acidosis and hypoxia) may directly affect the myocardium. The following four mechanisms may be important primary or secondary contributors to the pulmonary hypertension and myocardial depression: (1) alveolar hypoventilation (net and general), (2) reduction of pulmonary vascular bed, (3) intrapulmonary vascular shunts, and (4) myocardial factors.

Alveolar Hypoventilation

Net alveolar hypoventilation is characterized by a normal or increased minute volume, but a decrease in effective alveolar ventilation results from mismatching of ventilation and perfusion within the lung. Alveolar hypoventilation produces hypoxia and hypercapnia, and the net form of alveolar hypoventilation is often encountered in chronic airway obstruction (emphysema, bronchitis, or combinations). Alveolar hypoxia, by its local effect on vessels and by stimulation of neurohumoral mechanisms, increases pulmonary vascular resistance by pulmonary arteriolar vasoconstriction. Harvey et al.[2] have shown that an increase in the hydrogen ion concentration of the circulating blood is also associated with vasoconstriction in the pulmonary vascular tree in patients with chronic obstructive pulmonary disease (COPD) and that it can potentiate the response to hypoxia. Hypoxia also produces polycythemia with hypervolemia, increased venous return with an increased cardiac output, increased viscosity with increased pulmonary vascular resistance, and resultant pulmonary hypertension. Pulmonary hypertension eventually leads to right ventricular hypertrophy and failure.

General alveolar hypoventilation is characterized by a decrease in minute volume. This is often due to a CNS lesion, depression of respiration by drugs, extreme obesity, or dysfunction and deformity of the thoracic musculoskeletal system. After prolonged periods of pulmonary hypertension, chronic cor pulmonale ensues and right heart failure. In general alveolar hypoventilation, the ventilatory driving mechanism is decreased, which probably accounts for the development of pulmonary hypertension. Therefore hypoxia and hypercapnia can initiate and sustain pulmonary hypertension, which leads to cor pulmonale.

Reduction in Pulmonary Vascular Bed

If reduction in the pulmonary vascular bed were the only factor involved, more than 50% of the pulmonary vascular bed would have to be eliminated, since pneumonectomy does not produce cor pulmonale. Destruction usually occurs in extensive fibrotic diseases of the lung. Alveolar hypoxia is the most important cause of pulmonary hypertension in COPD, and compromise of the total capillary bed is of secondary importance. The mean intra-alveolar pressure is elevated because of the great degree of air trapping that occurs with a prolonged expiratory phase and a shortened inspiratory phase. Therefore the pulmonary capillary bed, already damaged through alveolar wall fenestration, is further compromised by the transmitted extramural pressure. Microthromboembolic complications in the lungs may cause further loss of function. Regardless of the type of lung disease, intraluminal or extraluminal obstruction of the pulmonary vascular bed may be an important factor, in association with hypoxia, in the production of pulmonary hypertension. In addition, chronic hypoxia alone can produce structural changes (muscularization) in the pulmonary arterioles, further increasing pulmonary resistance and hypertension.[3]

Intrapulmonary Vascular Shunts

Precapillary shunts may develop between the bronchial and pulmonary arteries in chronic lung disease[4] (especially in bronchiectasis) and anastomoses between the bronchopulmonary veins and pulmonary veins may appear.[5] The importance of these may be negligible, although in the presence of a restricted vascular bed they may add to the pulmonary hypertension.

Myocardial Factors

There is much debate as to whether cor pulmonale produces left heart dysfunction. Studies have shown both normal and abnormal left ventricular function.[6,7] However, often such patients with left ventricular dysfunction may have independent underlying left ventricular disease (often coronary artery disease or systemic hypertension). Low myocardial oxygen tension, high CO_2 tension, polycythemia, and intrapulmonary vascular shunts may precipitate left ventricular dysfunction even in a mildly diseased left ventricle. Autopsy studies have shown biventricular hypertrophy in the absence of abnormalities of the left ventricle. Michelson[8] found biventricular hypertrophy in 32 autopsies of patients who had chronic lung disease with no evidence of congenital defects, valvular incompetence, coronary disease, nephrosclerosis, sytemic hypertension, or any other entity known to cause left ventricular hypertrophy. On a percentage basis, the hypertrophy was greater in the right ventricle. The author has reviewed 97 autopsied cases of cor pulmonale and has found that 83 had biventricular hypertrophy. Thirty-six of these had a significant degree of coronary atherosclerosis but no other cause for left ventricular enlargement. Degenerative changes of myocardial fibers and replacement by fibrous tissue have been found in cor pulmonale. Currently it can be stated that it is uncommon for cor pulmonale to impair left ventricular function and that usually, when left ventricular dysfunction is present with cor pulmonale, it is due to associated coronary disease or hypertension.

Regardless of the cause, if left ventricular failure occurs, it can aggravate cor pulmonale by increasing lung water, so pulmonary compliance is reduced, airway resistance is increased, the work of breathing is increased, and there is interference with gas exchange.[9]

FUNCTIONAL CLASSIFICATION

Functional classification is of practical importance in terms of instituting appropriate therapy. It is based on whether alveolar hypoventilation or the reduction in pulmonary vascular bed is the more prominent feature. However, it should be emphasized that there is some overlapping and that alveolar hypoxia producing arteriolar constriction is the most important factor in the production of pulmonary hypertension. This classification is illustrated in Table 9–1.

Pulmonary diseases, according to the conditions that produce the chronic alveolar hypoventilation, may be subdivided into anatomical changes in the lung (chronic airway obstruction), defective function of chest bellows (chronic neuromuscular disorders, pleural thickening, kyphoscoliosis, and obesity), diminished ventilatory drive (CNS lesions), or high altitudes.

In certain obese persons a cardiopulmonary syndrome may develop referred to as the Pickwickian syndrome.[10] Patients with this syndrome may manifest cyanosis, polycythemia, somnolence, and edema. The mechanism for the hypoventilation initially was thought to be the exogenous obesity, especially since such patients improved with weight loss. However, this does not appear to be the sole factor. These individuals may also have underactive chemore-

Table 9–1. Functional Classification of Causes of Cor Pulmonale*

Alveolar Hypoventilation	Cor Pulmonale	Reduction in Pulmonary Vascular Bed
Chronic airway obstruction	Silicosis	Restrictive lung disease
Defective chest bellows		Pulmonary emboli
Diminished ventilatory drive		

*Modified from Gazes P.C.: Chronic cor pulmonale, in Hurst J.W., Logue R.B. (eds.): *The Heart*, (ed. 2. New York, McGraw-Hill Book Co., 1970).

ceptors or oxygen sensors, and may improve with progesterone (respiratory stimulant).[11]

Since the advent of study of sleep patterns, it has been found that sleep apnea syndromes can cause apneic periods during sleep with hypoxemia, hypercapnia, and pulmonary hypertension. Brady- and tachyarrhythmias can occur.[12] These patients often have morning headaches, daytime somnolence, personality changes, and apneic periods during sleep, with periods of loud snoring. The apnea can be of the central, obstructive, or mixed types.[13] Abnormalities of the brainstem can cause respiratory center depression. Upper airway obstruction can be due to enlarged tonsils, the tongue, or collapse of pharyngeal walls.

Pectus excavatum (funnel chest) is a congenital anomaly characterized by depression of the lower end of the sternum which rarely produces any cardiopulmonary problems. Ejection-type systolic murmurs are heard over the pulmonic area or along the left sternal border. The cause of these murmurs has been thought to be due to compression of the great vessels or compression of the outflow tract of the right ventricle. Displacement of the heart to the left causes the apical impulse to appear prominent. The second heart sound is often split, or a third heart sound may be detected. Electrocardiographic changes also are common, including right axis deviation, persistence of the juvenile pattern with T wave inversion in the right precordial leads, and incomplete right bundle-branch block. In the PA chest x ray, the heart may appear enlarged and displaced to the left. Lateral view reveals the sternal depression and AP narrowing. Angiocardiography has shown compression of the right ventricle with imprint on the outflow tract and infundibulum. Cardiac catheterization may show a postsystolic dip with an elevated end-diastolic pressure in the right ventricle and a slight gradient across the pulmonary valve. These findings may be misinterpreted as indicating organic heart disease. This malformation rarely has been found to cause cardiac or pulmonary dysfunction necessitating corrective surgery. Even though it usually causes no organic disease, surgery may be indicated for the cosmetic effect and relief or prevention of psychologic problems.

Pectus carinatum (pigeon chest) usually causes no cardiac problems. Pectus excavatum and carinatum do not produce cor pulmonale. However, these can be associated with kyphoscoliosis, which leads to abnormal function of the respiratory muscles, compression of the lung, interference with gas exchange, and possible interference with growth and development of alveoli and pulmonary arteries.

Pulmonary diseases that produce significant destruction of functioning pulmonary parenchyma and reduction of the pulmonary vascular bed, in contrast to those seen with primarily alveolar hypoventilation, are characterized by the development of cor pulmonale in the late stages of the disease secondary to pulmonary hypertension which is usually irreversible. Intraluminal obstruction is usually due to pulmonary emboli. Extraluminal obstruction due to restrictive lung diseases is characterized by impaired pulmonary oxygen diffusion and abnormal ventilation-perfusion ratios. Restrictive lung diseases are associated with diffuse interstitial fibrosis with development of pulmonary hypertension. Most of the interstitial diseases are idiopathic. Granulomatous disease, interstitial fibrosis, or occupational pneumoconiosis should be considered. Interstitial fibrosis may have a chronic or an acute course (Hamman-Rich syndrome).

Neither alveolar hypoventilation nor reduction in pulmonary vascular bed diseases appears in pure form, but there are often combinations, such as those seen with silicosis.

DIAGNOSIS

It is essential to determine the type of pulmonary disease and to determine if cor pulmonale is present to institute proper therapy.

Clinical Features of Pulmonary Disease

Diseases that produce alveolar hypoventilation (primarily chronic airway obstruction) must be differentiated from those that produce alveolar capillary diffusion defects (primarily restrictive lung disease).

Clinically, patients with chronic airway obstruction (namely, bronchitis with or without emphysema) have a chronic cough, bouts of bronchitis, and exertional dyspnea for a period of 5 to 10 years prior to development of cardiac disability. Examination shows them to be dyspneic, orthopneic, and cyanotic; they cough ineffectually, and their eyes are protuberant, injected, and chemotic. Cough syncope can occur. The neck veins of these patients, even when heart failure is not present, are frequently distended as a consequence of the marked changes in intrapleural pressure. The distended veins collapse briskly during inspiration under these circumstances. The lack of inspiratory collapse of the neck veins may aid in identifying those patients with a venous abnormality due to heart failure. The chest may resemble a rectangle, with manubrium upward and forward, and the back has a rounded buffalo appearance. In the presence of CO_2 retention, Cheyne-Stokes breathing is rarely encountered. Papilledema may appear, probably the result of a combination of right-sided failure, hypercapnia, and hypoxemia, associated with a secondary elevation in cerebral spinal fluid (CSF) pressure.[14] There is no convincing evidence that polycythemia is a factor in producing the papilledema. There is wheezing in the lungs, and rhonchi are present. Clubbing of the digits and pulmonary hypertrophic osteoarthropathy occur rarely unless the bronchitis is complicated by another disease such as bronchiectasis or carcinoma of the lung.

Patients with obstructive emphysema, a normal hematocrit, and a Pco_2 near normal have been identified as "pink puffers." In contrast, patients with mild obstructive emphysema and predominantly chronic bronchitis, raised hematocrit, and a high Pco_2 are known as "blue bloaters" and more frequently develop cor pulmonale.[15] The "blue bloaters" have a much greater ventilation perfusion inequality than the "pink puffers."

In contrast, the patient with restrictive lung disease has dyspnea with tachypnea and symptoms of hyperventilation (paresthesias and light-headedness) and may be cyanotic, especially after exercise. The configuration of the chest may be normal. Fine end-inspiratory rales are present at the lung bases, and there is no evidence of bronchial obstruction.

Pulmonary Function Tests

Pulmonary diseases also may be differentiated by tests of pulmonary function. Ventilation, diffusion, and perfusion (blood flow) are involved in delivering oxygen and removing CO_2 from the pulmonary capillary bed. Mechanics of breathing should be evaluated to define the type of abnormality and are primarily studied by spirometric measurements that include the total and timed vital capacity and maximum voluntary ventilation (maximum breathing capacity). Lung volumes can be determined noninvasively by specialized techniques. Diffusion is determined by the uptake of carbon monoxide, and pulmonary blood flow is determined by perfusion lung scans or by heart catheterization. Alveolar ventilation measurements are included in the determination of the diffusing capacity. These tests of diffusion and blood flow are fairly inexpensive, only take 10 minutes, and require specialized equipment and technical aid. They are usually performed in medical centers that have special cardiopulmonary laboratories. In actual clinic practice, after careful history taking and physical and x-ray examinations of the chest, sufficient knowledge of pulmonary function may be obtained by performing the basic spirometric tests and measuring the arterial blood gases with very simple apparatus (Table 9–2).

Arterial gas measurements are significant not only as aids in diagnosis, but also at intervals as a guide to therapy. Pulse oximeters offer reliable, inexpensive, and noninvasive determinations of arterial oxygen saturation (SaO_2).

Clinical Features of Cor Pulmonale

The primary problem is first to recognize the type of pulmonary disease and then to determine if cor pulmonale is present. It is difficult to make a clinical

Table 9–2.   **Pulmonary Function Studies**

Spirometric Tests	Chronic Airway Obstruction	Restrictive Lung Disease
Vital capacity, L (FVC)	N or D	D
Functional residual capacity (FRC)	I	D
Total lung capacity (TLC)	I	D
Forced expiratory volume in 1 sec, L (FEV_1)	D	N or D
FEV_1/FVC %	D	N or I
Maximum mid-expiratory flow, L/sec (MMEF)	D	N or D
Peak flow, L/min	D	N or D
Maximum voluntary ventilation, L/min (MVV)	D	N or D

Arterial Blood Gases	At Rest	100% O_2	After Exercise	At Rest	100% O_2	After Exercise
pH	N or D	May D	D	N	N	I
Pco_2	N or I	N or I	I	N or D	N	D
Po_2	D	I	D	N or D	I	D
Sao_2	D	I	D	N or D	I	D

N = normal; D = decreased; I = increased.

diagnosis of cor pulmonale prior to the development of heart failure, since right ventricular hypertrophy and dilatation are difficult to detect early. It is also difficult to decide whether failure of the right side of the heart is present or symptoms and findings are due entirely to the chronic airway obstruction. Heart failure may be insidious and appear as further impairment of pulmonary function, as though the chronic airway obstruction were becoming more severe. The usual findings of early congestive failure often are masked by those of chronic airway obstruction. Cough, dyspnea, orthopnea, peripheral edema due to inactivity and venous stasis, and a palpable liver because of a low diaphragm may be present in chronic airway obstruction without heart failure. Hepatic congestion may be present, or hypoxic liver damage may exist before clinical cardiac failure is recognized in severe obstructive airway disease.[16] The neck veins may be distended without congestive failure, but usually are more congested on expiration and collapse on inspiration.

In early cor pulmonale, due to chronic airway obstruction, the pulse is usually bounding, and the extremities, ears, and nose are warm. The BP may be elevated with a wide pulse pressure, and the cardiac output can be increased. However, in the early stages the cardiac output may also be normal or low.[17] The level of cardiac output depends on many factors, including changes in arterial blood gases, acid-base balance, myocardial reserve, hypervolemia, and the state of the pulmonary vascular bed.[18] In the more advanced stages, the cardiac output is low; the patient is cold and may be cyanotic, confused, somnolent, or even comatose.

The apex beat is difficult to localize because of distention of the overlying lung. A systolic thrust of the right ventricle rarely may lift the sternum, and the hypertrophied right ventricle often can be felt protruding beneath the xiphosternum on palpation in the epigastric area. A right ventricular S_3 gallop with inspiratory accentuation may be audible near the sternum or in the epigastrium, and the pulmonic second sound is accentuated and there may be a systolic ejection sound suggesting pulmonary hypertension. When heart failure is present, the jugular venous pressure is usually elevated, as noted when the patient is lying at an angle of 45 degrees from the horizontal. Its level may be difficult to determine because of fluctuations produced by the great variations in intrapleural pressure due to respiratory effort.

Retrograde filling will aid in recognizing true elevation of venous pressure. Cheyne-Stokes respiration is rarely seen with CO_2 retention, and hydrothorax from heart failure due to chronic airway obstruction is rare.[19] The liver will be enlarged (not just displaced downward) and tender. Dependent edema is a common feature, and ascites may occur. If treatment is not effective, increasing respiratory depression and worsening of cardiac failure will ensue, with deepening coma and cyanosis, a rising pulse rate, falling BP, and increasing peripheral vasoconstriction, recognizable by the development of cold extremities. These findings indicate a falling cardiac output and are grave prognostic features. Pulmonary emboli and acute coronary thrombosis are complications which may produce a similar terminal picture. These, rather than terminal cor pulmonale, should be suspected in a patient with chronic obstructive airway disease and cyanosis when there is no significant CO_2 retention.

In addition to masking right ventricular failure, chronic airway obstruction often presents findings suggestive of left ventricular failure. The problem is further accentuated when aging changes in the thoracic cage (senile emphysema) and failure of the left side of the heart must be differentiated from chronic airway obstruction. Differentiation is important, especially with regard to therapeutic considerations. The history is often rewarding. Orthopnea, paroxysmal nocturnal dyspnea, pulsus alternans, and frothy sputum, especially with little wheezing, are features that suggest left ventricular failure, whereas repeated bouts of bronchitis and progressive dyspnea for many years suggest pulmonary disease. A palpable apical impulse, S_3 gallop (at the apex and louder with expiration), and pulsus alternans favor the diagnosis of left ventricular failure. Chest x rays and ECGs may be of aid, especially if they clearly demonstrate either right or left ventricular hypertrophy. Arterial gas studies point to chronic airway obstruction if there is CO_2 retention and a low arterial pH, unless there is pulmonary edema, when CO_2 retention may occur without primary lung disease. Therapeutic tests may be dangerous; however, when in doubt it is usually safe to administer aminophylline, which is of therapeutic value in both cases. A Swan-Ganz catheter may be inserted for proper differentiation. In pure cor pulmonale, the pulmonary artery diastolic pressure is elevated and the pulmonary wedge pressure is normal. The diastolic-wedge pressure gradient is smaller in left ventricular failure. Both pressures can be elevated if cor pulmonale is complicated by left ventricular failure.

Since bronchial obstruction produces greater than normal increase in intrathoracic negative pressure during inspiration, patients with chronic airway obstruction may have a paradoxical pulse. This introduces the problem of differentiation from pericardial effusion with tamponade or constrictive pericarditis, since both conditions may cause distended neck veins, hepatomegaly, diminished heart sounds, and low ECG voltage. The patient with known chronic airway obstruction also may develop pericardial effusion or constriction from another associated condition, thus causing further confusion. Other studies, such as pericardial scan, echocardiogram, or even heart catheterization, may be necessary to clear the picture.

In patients with restrictive lung disease, the cardiac output may be normal or low; therefore, these patients are not warm and do not have bounding pulses. A right ventricular lift is easier to detect than in chronic airway obstruction, since there is usually less increase in the PA diameter of the chest. At times the high pulmonary artery pressure may produce a diastolic murmur of pulmonary valve insufficiency, a systolic murmur of tricuspid insufficiency (both louder with inspiration), a pulmonary systolic ejection sound, and a prominent venous jugular A wave. Heart failure occurs when there is severe hypoxia and is usually terminal and seldom reversible, as it sometimes is with chronic airway obstruction.

Roentgenographic Studies

These aid in determining the underlying type of pulmonary disease. The heart may be large or may appear normal. The enlargement that occurs is confined to the pulmonary arteries, right ventricle, and right atrium and is best seen in the lateral projections. In chronic airway obstruction, the small vertical heart may be dilated but without apparent increase in size, and only by comparison with previous films can this dilatation be detected. If other films are not available, after recovery from failure, cardiomegaly can be suspected if the heart returns to its previous smaller size. The marked changes in the heart size as a patient goes in and out of failure suggest that dilatation may be more important than hypertrophy (Fig 9–1).

Electrocardiographic Findings

These findings in chronic cor pulmonale have been well described.[20] The main positive ECG signs are right-axis deviation of greater than 110 degrees, conduction defects producing an rSR' complex in the right precordial leads, and classic right ventricular hypertrophy in V_1 or V_3R with dominant R waves (Rs, R, QR, qRs and qR). Tall R waves in the right precordial leads are unusual in chronic airway obstructive disease and are seen more often in the restrictive lung diseases, which produce a greater degree of right ventricular hypertrophy. In fact, Fishman,[21] in an autopsy study, showed that the right ventricular enlargement criteria were absent in two thirds of patients with chronic obstructive pulmonary disease who had right ventricular hypertrophy. The tall peaked P waves in leads II, III, and aV_F (axis greater than +60 degrees) are often present. There is debate as to whether these P waves actually indicate right atrial hypertrophy or are due to positional changes because of the chronic airway obstruction. Often with the "P pulmonale" there is right axis and clockwise rotation (rS in V_5 to V_6).[22] Arrhythmias are not frequent, but acute hypoxic periods, even in the absence of heart failure, produce paroxysmal arrhythmias, primarily atrial in origin, such as atrial tachycardia, multifocal atrial tachycardia, atrial flutter, atrial fibrillation, and atrial tachycardia with block. These arrhythmias may disappear with improvement of the hypoxic state. A normal tracing may be noted in well-advanced cases of cor pulmonale; therefore, the absence of ECG evidence of right ventricular disease does not exclude this lesion. Many factors are responsible for the ECG

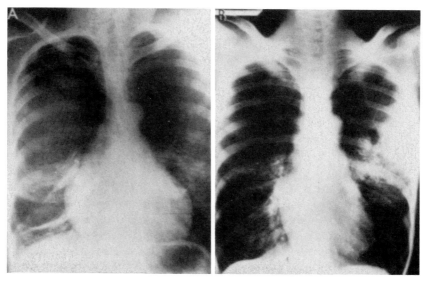

Fig 9–1. Chest x rays of a 38-year-old woman with chronic obstructive airway disease and cor pulmonale. **A,** patient in right heart failure. **B,** after therapy note the decrease in heart size.

changes, such as elevated pulmonary artery pressures and resistances, myocardial ischemia due to relatively insufficient coronary blood flow, metabolic disorders, and positional changes.

Echocardiographic and Radionuclide Studies

Many individuals with pulmonary artery hypertension and right ventricular enlargement do not have clinical, ECG, or chest x ray findings of right ventricular enlargement. Noninvasive techniques, such as thallium 201 myocardial imaging,[23,24] gated equilibrium bloodpool imaging,[25] first-pass radionuclide angiocardiography,[26] and echocardiography,[27] are useful in detecting right ventricular enlargement and dysfunction in patients with chronic lung disease. Doppler echocardiography can assess tricuspid regurgitation and, using the Bernoulli equation, can estimate the right ventricular systolic pressure. If there is no obstruction to right ventricular outflow, the pulmonary artery pressure will also be known (see Fig 6–4).

TREATMENT

Initially, the pulmonary hypertension should be vigorously treated before the cardiac failure. Pulmonary hypertension, hypoxia, and hypercapnia may be aggravated by associated heart failure. First controlling the pulmonary hypertension by effective ventilation, increased oxygenation, and lowering of CO_2 reduces the load on the heart and allows a better therapeutic response.

Pulmonary Hypertension

Early treatment has been stressed by many, since rapidly ensuing death in patients with acute and chronic lung disease is often due to cor pulmonale superimposed on acute respiratory failure, regardless of whether infection is present. The following is an outline of therapy for alveolar hypoventilation, particularly that associated with chronic airway obstruction (namely, bronchitis with or without emphysema).

Smoking

The patient with chronic bronchitis and emphysema should stop smoking permanently. The avoidance of air pollution is more difficult, since this depends on the efforts of industry in each locale.

Oxygen

Oxygen is essential in relieving pulmonary hypertension but has to be administered properly. Carbon dioxide, oxygen, and hydrogen concentrations (pH) are important factors in the control of respiration. Although CO_2 is the primary stimulant, hypoxemia may stimulate the respiratory center reflexly through the chemoreceptors located in the carotid and aortic bodies. In advanced chronic airway obstruction, a patient is unable to eliminate CO_2, and increased arterial P_{CO_2} and respiratory acidosis develop. As a result of CO_2 retention, the pH is increased, depressing the respiratory center and leaving hypoxemia via the peripheral chemoreceptors as the major stimulus. Removing this hypoxemic stimulus by giving oxygen improperly may result in apnea, further CO_2 retention, coma, and death unless the problem is anticipated and ventilatory control with a respirator is instituted. Many patients with such a condition can tolerate oxygen without adverse effects if it is given in lower concentrations, especially with a mechanical respirator. During oxygen administration the patient should be observed carefully, and frequent measurements of arterial blood gases should be performed. Levine et al.[28] showed that long-term continuous oxygen administration improves clinical status, increases exercise tolerance, reverses secondary polycythemia, and causes a decrease in pulmonary arteriolar resistance. Continuous or nocturnal oxygen therapy at home for patients with COPD has been shown to be effective in the prevention and treatment of cor pulmonale.[29] The U.S. (NIH-sponsored) trial and the English (MRC) trial showed that survival is best for those who received oxygen for the longest portion of the day.[30,31]

Bronchodilators, β_2 Agonists, and Vasodilators

Vaporized bronchodilators used with or without a positive pressure apparatus may be effective in alleviating bronchospasm and mucosal edema and improving net alveolar ventilation. The removal of tracheobronchial secretions by tracheobronchial aspiration is of utmost importance. The patient should be taught the technique of postural drainage. Terbutaline, a selective β_2 agonist, has been shown to decrease biventricular afterload and to improve both right and left ventricular ejection fractions while decreasing pulmonary and systemic vascular resistances and improving airway flow in obstructive pulmonary diseases.[32,33] Klugman et al.[34] showed that sublingual nifedipine (a calcium antagonist) decreased pulmonary and systemic vascular resistances and increased cardiac index without changing the oxygen saturation. Future studies will determine the actual value of such vasodilators.

Aminophylline administered by suppository or carefully by slow infusion is often effective in relieving extreme bronchospasm. It also produces pulmonary arteriolar dilation, with reduction in pulmonary artery pressure and pulmonary vascular resistance, and reduction in right and left ventricular end diastolic pressures.[35] Long-acting theophylline (Theo-dur) orally has produced moderate improvement in biventricular performance immediately and this improvement has been sustained during long-term follow-up.[36] Serum theophylline levels should be checked because theophylline may aggravate or precipitate arrhythmias such as multifocal atrial tachycardia, which occurs often with chronic lung disease.

Antibiotics

The patient with an acute exacerbation of chronic lung disease often has pulmonary infection, at times without a febrile or leukocytic response. This complication is so common, in fact, that it should be a major target for the therapeutic attack. It is difficult to isolate the responsible bacteria, so treatment must be empirical. Penicillin or a broad-spectrum antibiotic can be used unless cultures reveal an organism that is more sensitive to a specific antibiotic.

Sedation

It is obvious that the use of morphine and other narcotics is contraindicated because of the further respiratory depression that may be produced. Barbiturates and tranquilizers also may be harmful. If sedation is absolutely necessary, chloral hydrate may be administered by mouth or rectum. As a general rule, it is unwise to use sedation except for facilitating ventilatory control by respirators.

Steroids

A trial of adrenal corticosteroids is indicated at times with careful evaluation of the results and continuation in those who show a satisfactory response.[37] Long-term steroid therapy is much more controversial and cannot be recommended generally in patients with chronic airway obstruction because of the lack of efficacy and the potential complications. Results of most studies have shown that prolonged use of steroids produces only minor changes in pulmonary function, although some patients obtain a certain degree of symptomatic relief.

Acid-Base Regulation

Hypokalemia and systemic alkalosis may develop because of diuretics, steroids, and removal of large volumes of carbon dioxide from the lung with respirators without concomitant removal of bicarbonate by the kidneys.[38] It is obvious that, in addition to frequent determination of the concentration of blood gases, there also should be electrolyte evaluations.

Surgery

Beside tracheostomy in certain cases, surgical removal or obliteration of large bullae may be of value. Intensive studies are being made of the immunology and use of lung transplantation; however, it is still being performed in only a few centers.

The necessity of a balanced approach in the treatment of chronic obstructive lung disease should be emphasized, especially when respiratory acidosis ensues. Overtreatment or attempts to correct any individual chemical factor may result in a more serious problem that may be potentially fatal.

Many of the therapeutic measures mentioned in chronic obstructive lung disease should be tried for restrictive lung defects, especially use of oxygen and antibiotics. There is no known direct therapy for the primary pulmonary disease. In the granulomas (proved by biopsy), the use of adrenal corticosteroids has offered some hope of limiting the cellular proliferation that causes the alveolar capillary diffusion defect. However, it is not always possible to control the degree of pulmonary fibrosis, and there are many side effects from the steroids.

CARDIAC FAILURE

Once the pulmonary hypertension is being treated, attention should be given to the cardiac failure.

Digitalis

The use of digitalis in patients with cor pulmonale is still controversial, unless left heart failure or a supraventricular tachyarrhythmia is present.[39] Studies have shown that it does improve right ventricular function in cor pulmonale.[40] Currently, most favor digitalis if there is associated left heart failure, a supraventricular arrhythmia, or overt right heart failure that fails to respond to other therapy for pulmonary hypertension.[41] Hypoxia and acidosis increase the sensitivity to digitalis; therefore, it should be given after these have been controlled.

Diuretics

As in other forms of congestive failure, diuretics may be employed. If hypervolemia is present, pulmonary function may be improved by the use of diuretics. Pulmonary gas exchange can be compromised by excess flow in the lung which increases pulmonary vascular resistance. Diuretics can decrease the total blood volume and lower the pulmonary artery pressure.[42] However, these should be given cautiously because excessive volume depletion can decrease cardiac output and diuretics can produce hypokalemic metabolic alkalosis and so reduce the CO_2 ventilatory drive on the respiratory centers.

Phlebotomy

The role of phlebotomy is still not clear, but since blood viscosity increases abruptly between a hematocrit value of 60% and 70%, most physicians recommend phlebotomy when the hematocrit exceeds 60%. The increased viscosity could impede blood flow, decrease the delivery of oxygen to tissue, and increase the danger of thromboembolism. Phlebotomy may improve right ventricular function by reducing pulmonary arterial pressure and pulmonary vascular resistance.[43]

Vasodilators

Vasodilation has been used to reduce pulmonary artery pressure (afterload), which can lead to right ventricular failure. Hydralazine and nifedipine have been found to reduce pulmonary vascular resistance and increase cardiac output over short periods of time.[44,45] Further studies are needed to evaluate their chronic use.

With present therapy, cor pulmonale can be better treated and prevented, although the prognosis for the underlying lung disease has not improved greatly. Home-care programs may reduce the need for repeated hospitalizations. Oxygen therapy can be given at home. It is imperative to prevent episodes of prolonged severe dyspnea by limiting activities and treating asthmatic episodes and pulmonary infections with the use of bronchodilators, expectorants, and antibiotics, and in some cases administering steroids for continuous wheezing to reduce allergic edema and bronchospasm. Patients should be strongly urged to discontinue cigarette smoking. Arterial gases should be determined to detect impending pulmonary failure. Unilateral and bilateral lung transplantation, and combined heart-lung transplantation have become feasible in selected patients with end-stage lung disease because there have been improvements in immunosuppression and surgical techniques.[46]

PULMONARY EMBOLISM

Acute Cor Pulmonale

Pulmonary embolism is the most frequent acute illness detected in a general hospital. It is found in up to 25% of all autopsies and is even more frequent in patients dying of congestive failure. Fatal pulmonary embolism has been estimated to occur in about 150,000 patients and nonfatal embolism in about 600,000 per year, and the incidence continues to rise.[47,48]

Pulmonary embolism is the most common cause of acute cor pulmonale. Obstruction to the pulmonary arteries occurs with associated reflex vasoconstriction, bronchoconstriction, pulmonary hypertension, and acute right heart failure. The broncho- and vasoconstriction can be mediated by serotonin and thromboxane A_2. In addition, the coronary circulation may be impaired, and left ventricular failure also develops. The emboli usually arise from a thrombus in the proximal deep venous system in the leg or pelvic veins in over 90% of instances. The risk is lower if the thrombosis is only in the calf veins.[49] Superficial thrombophlebitis and thrombosis in the arms are seldom associated with pulmonary emboli.[50] These also can originate from the right atrium, usually when associated with heart failure or atrial fibrillation. Emboli of fat, air, tumor, bone marrow, myxoma, or amniotic fluid are rare. Pulmonary emboli may or may not produce pulmonary infarction. Most often, when infarction occurs, the occlusion is in the medium-sized pulmonary vessels in the distal branches,[51] and the collateral circulation from the bronchial arteries are impaired. Usually either pulmonary venous hypertension or systemic hypotension is noted when the bronchial collateral circulation is impaired. In addition, initially pulmonary emboli with or without infarction can occur without the development of acute or chronic cor pulmonale. It is therefore essential to recognize the clinical features of pulmonary emboli occurring alone or with pulmonary infarction prior to the development of pulmonary hypertension.

Clinical Findings

Unfortunately, many do not suspect pulmonary emboli (PE) unless there is evidence of thrombophlebitis and the pulmonary findings of infarction. Failure to make the diagnosis clinically is well documented by postmortem studies. One should have a high index of suspicion if the setting is proper or there are predisposing factors, such as with surgical procedures, fractures, periods of prolonged bed rest, debilitating diseases (such as carcinoma), oral contraceptives, congestive heart failure, and childbirth. The elderly and obese are more prone to pulmonary emboli. Findings of thrombophlebitis such as swelling in the legs and pain in the calves often are absent. Positive signs such as inflating the BP cuff over the calf producing pain at pressures below the patient's systolic pressure (Lowenberg's sign) or with dorsiflexion of the foot (Homan's sign) are rather rare.

Pulmonary embolism can appear as three different clinical syndromes: (1) Nonspecific findings in patients with submassive pulmonary emboli: These patients do not have evidence of pulmonary infarction or acute cor pulmonale, but in the proper setting they should be suspected of having pulmonary emboli if they have sudden episodes of undiagnosed dyspnea. Other clues are tachycardia, arrhythmias, fever, and episodes of hypotension and apprehension. Often these patients are overlooked as having the hyperventilation syndrome. They probably represent a significant group with pulmonary emboli, and because of the nonspecific findings the diagnosis is difficult. (2) Pulmonary infarction: Even though this is the most familiar manifestation, it does not occur in all patients. These patients will have chest pain, signs of pleurisy, at times hemoptysis, dyspnea, and often an infiltrate demonstrated in the chest x ray. A pulmonary infarction may appear as an infiltrate, plate-like atelectasis, wedge-shaped density, or as a pleural effusion. (3) Acute cor pulmonale: Acute cor pulmonale can occur with or without shock. If the embolism occludes more than 60% of the pulmonary circulation, the right ventricle will dilate, and right heart failure develops. Shock, cyanosis, and cardiac arrest can occur. A large A wave may be noted in the jugular venous pulse if sinus rhythm is present. A right ventricular lift often is noted. On auscultation, S_3 and S_4 gallops, louder during inspiration, may be heard. The pulmonic second sound is loud, and there can be splitting. Rarely, a systolic murmur is heard, and a thrill is palpable in the pulmonic area due to partial stenosis produced by the pulmonary clot. This murmur may be a scratchy sound associated with pulmonary artery dilatation and often is mistaken for a pericardial friction rub. Tricuspid insufficiency may develop with a prominent V wave and a pulsating liver. With massive emboli, rarely inspiratory filling of the neck veins (Kussmaul's sign) can appear.

The ECG may reveal right axis with an S_1, Q_3 pattern and clockwise rotation, right atrial enlargement, T wave inversion in the precordial leads V_1 to V_3, or right bundle-branch block. Such findings are noted when the embolism has produced acute cor pulmonale. However, they occur in less than 25% of such cases and are more diagnostic if the changes are transient. Nonspecific ST-T changes occur in most patients with pulmonary emboli. In addition, arrhythmias may be noted. The chest film is frequently normal. The x ray may reveal dilatation of the central pulmonary arteries and right ventricular enlargement. Rarely, an era of radiolucency is detected in an area distal to the pulmonary vessel obstruction as compared to other areas of the lung. There may be evidences of a pulmonary infarction.

Laboratory Studies

The triad of Wacker et al.[52] of an elevated LDH, a normal serum glutamic oxaloacetic transaminase (SGOT), and an elevated serum bilirubin to differentiate pulmonary embolism and infarction from other clinical entities has been found to be of little value. The arterial Po_2 is decreased below 75 mm Hg while breathing room air. However, it can be normal in those with submassive pulmonary embolism. Bronchitis, emphysema, cardiac failure, and the age of the patient should be taken into consideration in evaluating the arterial Po_2. Radioisotope lung scanning has become readily available to evaluate abnormalities of pulmonary perfusion. An abnormal lung scan, especially in the presence of a normal chest x ray, favors pulmonary embolism. Many other lesions, such as pneumonia, atelectasis, neoplasms, or effusions, can produce abnormal lung scans. Ventilation scanning with xenon may suggest pulmonary embolism if segmental perfusion defects have normal ventilation. A negative lung scan and a normal arterial Po_2 constitute good evidence against a pulmonary embolism. It has become customary to report ventilation-perfusion (V/P) scans as low, moderate, high, or indeterminate probability as compared to pulmonary angiography.[53] Studies have shown that those with high probability have a greater than 85% incidence of pulmonary embolism.[54] In the other categories, the results have been variable, probably because of the populations studied. However, patients with low probability appear to have an incidence of pulmonary embolism of less than 15%. Selective pulmonary angiography is the only definitive method of detecting pulmonary emboli (Fig 9–2). Whenever, after blood gases and ventilation-perfusion scans, the diagnosis is in doubt, rather than embarking on long-term therapy, angiography should be done. Venous thrombosis is detected clinically in about 30% of pa-

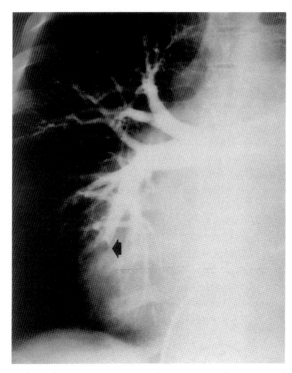

Fig 9–2. Selective right pulmonary arteriogram in a patient who sustained a pulmonary embolism, showing abrupt cut-off of the right descending pulmonary artery (arrow).

tients with pulmonary emboli. Radioactive fibrinogen, Doppler ultrasound, impedance plethysmography, and venography have been used to assess the deep veins. In one series of patients, 95% had an abnormal impedance plethysmography of those who had documented angiographic emboli.[48] In the cases with suspected embolism, if the impedance test was abnormal, 90% had a positive pulmonary angiogram, and if the test was normal, only 10% had a positive pulmonary angiogram. Two recent trials showed that serial impedance plethysmography used alone is an effective diagnostic tool for clinically suspected deep-vein thrombosis (DVT).[55,56]

Treatment

An important question often asked is "Which studies are necessary for diagnosis before therapy is begun?" The answer can vary depending on the availability of studies. Assuming that the hospital has the facilities for all studies and the patient might have a pulmonary embolism and is not in shock, then one can give 5000 units I.V. of heparin unless there is a contraindication. If the ventilation-perfusion scan is negative, another diagnosis should be sought. If it indicates high probability and the clinical suspicion is high, heparin therapy should be continued. If it indicates low probability, pulmonary angiogram should be done to confirm or exclude the diagnosis only if the clinical suspicion is high. Pulmonary angiography should be done if the probability is moderate or indeterminate and if thrombolytic therapy or vena caval interruption is contemplated.

If angiography is not available and the ventilation-perfusion scan is positive or even suspicious, then, according to clinical judgment, whether the patient is in shock or not, therapy should be started.

Supportive therapy and heparin (unless there is a contraindication) are begun, and once diagnosis is confirmed the heparin is continued. A loading dose of 5000 to 10,000 units is given I.V., followed by 1500 units per hour by pump infusion. After 4 hours of therapy, the partial thromboplastin time (PTT) should be checked and the heparin adjusted to control the PTT at two to three times the control level. The PTT should be checked ever 4 hours until the rate of the infusion has been established. Duration of heparin therapy depends on response, but usually is continued for 7 to 10 days, which allows time for thrombi in the deep veins to become firmly attached to the vein or undergo lysis. Warfarin is started about 2 to 3 days before discontinuing heparin. The warfarin is continued for at least 6 months, and longer if the predisposing factors are still present.

Acute cor pulmonale is usually caused by a massive pulmonary embolism and requires supportive therapy. Oxygen should be administered, and morphine for severe pain. Isoproterenol drip (2 to 4 mg per 500 ml of 5% glucose in water) should be started for hypotension. After pulmonary angiography, thrombolytic therapy should be started in an attempt to lyse the clot (unless there is a contraindication as brain lesion, recent surgery, or trauma). If thrombolytic therapy is not successful, pulmonary embolectomy should be considered. The thrombolytic agents streptokinase and urokinase have been evaluated by NIH-sponsored studies.[57,58] The usual dosage for streptokinase for pulmonary embolism is 250,000 IU over 30 minutes, followed by 100,000 IU per hour for 24 hours; for urokinase it is 4400 IU/kg over 10 minutes followed by 4400 IU/kg per hour for 12 to 24 hours. Thrombin time, plasma fibrinogen, fibrin split products, prothrombin time, and partial thromboplastin time should be monitored to confirm that adequate fibrinolysis has been achieved. Tissue plasminogen activator (t-PA) has been used effectively for pulmonary embolism and may in the future be considered the thrombolytic agent of choice because it is relative fibrin-selective and may cause less bleeding.[59]

Interruption of the inferior vena cava is considered for the following situations: recurrence of emboli in the face of adequate anticoagulation therapy, contraindication to anticoagulant therapy, septic pelvic thrombophlebitis with emboli, pulmonary embolectomy, and multiple recurrent pulmonary emboli. Transvenous devices (umbrella or filters) can be inserted under angiographic control. The Mobin-Uddin[60] and Kimray Greenfield filters have been used, with the latter being preferred by some surgeons. Ligation or external clip of the inferior vena cava can be used for septic embolization if the patient does not respond to antibiotics and heparin and for patients that have an intracaval device that has migrated to an incorrect position.

Every attempt should be made to prevent pulmonary emboli. Fortunately, most patients survive the first episode but one should not wait for this to occur. If deep vein thrombosis is detected clinically or if suspected and detected by impedance plethysmography or other methods as mentioned earlier, it should be treated the same as if acute pulmonary embolism has occurred with heparin followed by warfarin. Deep vein thrombosis should be prevented. Therefore, it is important to use preventive measures in individuals with the proper setting and predisposing factors for pulmonary emboli. Prolonged bed rest should be avoided and leg motion should be encouraged. The NIH consensus conference has made recommendations for prophylactic treatment to prevent DVT and PE.[61] In general, this can be summarized as follows: High-risk groups (40 years or older, obese, or with a history of prior DVT or PE) undergoing major general surgery, urologic surgery, or gynecologic surgery should receive low-dose heparin, 5000 units subcutaneously every 8 to 12 hours at least until the patient is ambulatory. The panel recommended that orthopedic patients undergoing elective hip surgery or knee reconstruction should receive, for at least 7 days or longer, one of the following regimens: low-dose warfarin, dextran, or adjusted-dose heparin. They did not recommend low-dose heparin for orthopedic surgery. Recently an overview of the results of all randomized trials in general, orthopedic, and urologic surgery was published.[62] The overview of all the orthopedic trial results showed that low-dose heparin does greatly reduce the incidence of fibrinogen-detected DVT and PE and mortality just as it did in the general surgery and urologic trials. Individual orthopedic studies were not large enough to have a chance of detecting even a halving in the thrombosis rate.

From these reviews, I would recommend low-dose heparin (starting a few hours before surgery) for high-risk patients (40 years or older, obese, or with a prior history of DVT or PE) undergoing major general, urologic, orthopedic, or gynecologic surgery and continuing it at least until the patient is ambulatory. External pneumatic compression should be used for those who are undergoing neurosurgery. Pregnant patients with a prior history of DVT or PE may be treated antenatally with low-dose heparin (time of onset of therapy is arbitrary) and continued postpartum.

Other regimens that have been recommended for prevention of DVT and PE include external pneumatic compression and gradient stockings, alone or in combination with heparin or heparin/dihydroergotamine. These can be tailored according to the patient's disease and risks. Aspirin has not been shown to be effective.

REFERENCES

1. Spain D.M., Handler B.J.: Chronic cor pulmonale: Sixty cases studied at necropsy. *Arch. Intern. Med.* 77:37, 1946.
2. Harvey R.M., Enson Y., Betti R., et al.: Further observation on the effect of hydrogen ion on the pulmonary circulation. *Circulation* 35:1019, 1967.
3. Fried R., Meyrick B., Rabinovetch M., Reid L.: Polycythemia and the acute hypoxic response in awake rats following chronic hypoxia. *J. Appl. Physiol.* 55:1167, 1983.
4. Liebow A.A., Hales M.R., Lindskog G.E.: Enlargement of the bronchial arteries and their anastomoses with the pulmonary arteries in bronchiectasis. *Am. J. Pathol.* 25:211, 1949.
5. Liebow A.A.: The bronchopulmonary venous collateral circulation, with special reference to emphysema. *Am. J. Pathol.* 29:251, 1953.
6. Krayenbuehl H.P., Turina J., Hess O.: Left ventricular function in chronic pulmonary hypertension. *Am. J. Cardiol.* 41:1150, 1978.
7. Baum G.L., Schwartz A., Llamas R., et al.: Left ventricular function in chronic obstructive lung disease. *N. Engl. J. Med.* 285:361, 1971.
8. Michelson N.: Bilateral ventricular hypertrophy due to chronic pulmonary disease. *Dis. Chest* 38:435, 1960.
9. Fishman A.P.: Chronic cor pulmonale. *Am. Rev. Respir. Dis.* 114:775, 1976.
10. Burwell C.S., Robin E.D., Whaley R.D., et al.: Extreme obesity associated with alveolar hypoventilation—a Pickwickian syndrome. *Am. J. Med.* 21:811, 1956.
11. Lyons H.A., Huang C.T.: Therapeutic use of progesterone in alveolar hypoventilation associated with obesity. *Am. J. Med.* 44:881, 1968.

12. Burrek B.: The hypersomnia-sleep apnea syndrome: Its recognition in clinical cardiology. *Am. Heart J.* 107:543, 1984.

13. Guilleminault C., Tilkian A., Dement W.C.: The sleep apnea syndrome. *Ann. Res. Med.* 27:465, 1976.

14. Stevens P.M., Austen K.E., Knowles J.H.: Prognostic significance of papilledema in the course of respiratory insufficiency. *JAMA* 183:161, 1963.

15. Cherniak R.M., Naimark A.: The management of chronic respiratory insufficiency, in Safar P. (ed.): *Respiratory Therapy.* Philadelphia, F.A. Davis Co., 1965.

16. Thomas A.J., Rees H.A., Saunders R.A.: Liver function in pulmonary heart disease. *Br. Heart J.* 27:791, 1965.

17. Burrows B., Kettel L.S., Niden A.H., et al.: Patterns of cardiovascular dysfunction in chronic obstructive lung disease. *N. Engl. J. Med.* 286:912, 1972.

18. Lim T.P.K., Brownlee W.E.: Pulmonary hemodynamics in obstructive lung disease. *Dis. Chest* 53:113, 1968.

19. Harvey R.M., Ferrer M.I.: A clinical consideration of cor pulmonale. *Circulation* 21:236, 1960.

20. Scott R.C.: The electrocardiogram in pulmonary emphysema and chronic cor pulmonale. *Am. Heart J.* 61:843, 1961.

21. Fishman A.P.: State of the art: Chronic cor pulmonale. *Am. Rev. Respir. Dis.* 114:775, 1976.

22. Padmavati S., Raizada V.: Electrocardiogram in chronic cor pulmonale. *Br. Heart J.* 34:658, 1975.

23. Berger H., Wackers F., Mahler D., et al.: Right ventricular visualization on thallium-201 myocardial images in chronic obstructive pulmonary disease: Relationship to right ventricular function and hypertrophy. *Circulation* 62(suppl. 3):103, 1980.

24. Ohsuze F., Handa S., Kondo M., et al.: Thallium-201 myocardial imaging to evaluate right ventricular overloading. *Circulation* 61:620, 1980.

25. Strauss H.W., Pitt B.: Evaluation of cardiac function and structure with radioactive tracer techniques. *Circulation* 57:645, 1978.

26. Berger H.J., Matthay R.A., Loke J., et al.: Assessment of cardiac performance with quantitative radionuclide angiocardiography: Right ventricular ejection fraction with reference to findings in chronic obstructive pulmonary disease. *Am. J. Cardiol.* 41:897, 1978.

27. Hirschfeld S., Meyer R., Schwartz D.C., et al.: The echocardiographic assessment of pulmonary artery pressure and pulmonary vascular resistance. *Circulation* 52:643, 1975.

28. Levine B.E., Bigelow D.B., Hamstra R.D., et al.: The role of long-term continuous oxygen administration in patients with chronic airway obstruction with hypoxemia. *Ann. Intern. Med.* 66:639, 1967.

29. Petty T.L., Neff T.A., Creagh C.E., et al.: Outpatient therapy in chronic obstructive pulmonary disease. *Arch. Intern. Med.* 139:28, 1979.

30. Nocturnal oxygen therapy trial group. Continuous or nocturnal oxygen therapy in hypoxemic chronic obstructive lung disease. A clinical trial. *Ann. Intern. Med.* 93:391, 1980.

31. MRC Working Party: Long-term ancillary oxygen therapy in chronic hypoxic corpulmonale complicating chronic bronchitis and emphysema. A clinical trial. *Lancet* 1:681, 1981.

32. Matthay R.A., Berger H.J.: Cardiovascular performance in chronic obstructive pulmonary disease. *Med. Clin. North Am.* 65:489, 1981.

33. Teule G.J.J., Majid P.A.: Hemodynamic effects of terbutaline in chronic obstructive airways disease. *Thorax* 35:536, 1980.

34. Klugman S., Fioretti P., Carnerini F.: Acute hemodynamic effects of nifedipine in pulmonary hypertension. *Circulation* 62:III–134, 1980.

35. Parker J.O., Ashekian P.B., DiGiorgi S., et al.: Hemodynamic effects of aminophylline in chronic obstructive pulmonary disease. *Circulation* 35:365, 1967.

36. Matthay R.A., Berger H.J., Davis R., et al.: Prolonged improvement in cardiac performance by oral long-acting theophylline in chronic obstructive pulmonary disease. *Circulation* 60:107, 1979.

37. Beerel F., Hershel J., Tyler J.M.: Controlled study of the effort of prednisone on airflow obstruction in severe pulmonary emphysema. *N. Engl. J. Med.* 268:226, 1963.

38. Refsum H.E.: Hypokalemic alkalosis with paradoxical aciduria during artificial ventilation of patients with pulmonary insufficiency and high plasma bicarbonate concentration. *Scand. J. Clin. Lab. Invest.* 13:481, 1961.

39. Green L.H., Smith T.W.: The use of digitalis in patients with pulmonary disease. *Ann. Intern. Med.* 87:459, 1977.

40. Smith D.E., Bissett J.K., Phillips J.R., et al.: Improved right ventricular systolic time intervals after digitalis in patients with cor pulmonale and chronic obstructive pulmonary disease. *Am. J. Cardiol.* 41:1299, 1978.

41. Moritz E.D., Matthay R.A.: Cor pulmonale: Diagnosis and management. *J. Respir. Dis.* 1:34, 1980.

42. Gertz I., Hedensteirna G., Wester P.O.: Improvement in pulmonary function with diuretic

therapy in the hypervolemic and polycythemic patient with chronic obstructive pulmonary disease. *Chest* 75:146, 1979.

43. Weisse A.B., Moschos C.B., Frank M.J., et al.: Hemodynamic effects of staged hematocrit reduction in patients with stable cor pulmonale and severely elevated hematocrit levels. *Am. J. Med.* 58:92, 1975.

44. Rubin L.J., Handel F., Peter R.H.: The effects of oral hydralazine on right ventricular end-diastolic pressure in patients with right ventricular failure. *Circulation* 65:1369, 1982.

45. Simonneau G., Escourrou P, Duroux P., et al.: Inhibition of hypoxic pulmonary vasoconstriction by nifedipine. *N. Engl. J. Med.* 304:1582, 1981.

46. Toronto lung transplant group: Unilateral lung transplantation for pulmonary fibrosis. *N. Engl. J. Med.* 314:1140, 1986.

47. Dalen J.E., Alpert J.S.: Natural history of pulmonary embolism. *Prog. Cardiovasc. Dis.* 17:259, 1975.

48. Sharma G.V.R.K., Sasahara A.A.: Diagnosis and treatment of pulmonary embolism. *Med. Clin. North Am.* 63:239, 1979.

49. Moser K.M., Lemoine J.R.: Is embolic risk conditioned by location of deep venous thrombosis? *Ann. Intern. Med.* 94:439, 1981.

50. Husni E.A., Williams W.A.: Superficial thrombophlebitis of lower limbs. *Surgery* 91:70, 1982.

51. Dalen J.E., Haffajee C.I., Alpert J.S., et al.: Pulmonary embolism, hemorrhage, and pulmonary infarction. *N. Engl. J. Med.* 296:1431, 1977.

52. Wacker W.E., Rosenthal M., Snodgrass P.J., et al.: A triad for the diagnosis of pulmonary embolism and infarction. *JAMA* 178:8, 1961.

53. Biello D.R., Mattar A.G., Osei-Wusu A., et al.: Interpretation of indeterminate lung scintigrams. *Radiology* 133:189, 1979.

54. Hull A.D., Hirsh J., Carter C.J., et al.: Diagnostic value of ventilation-perfusion lung scanning in patients with suspected pulmonary embolism. *Chest* 88:819, 1985.

55. Hull, R.D., Hirsh J., Carter C.J., et al.: Diagnostic efficacy of impedance plethysmography for clinically suspected deep-vein thrombosis. A randomized trial. *Ann. Intern. Med.* 102:21, 1985.

56. Huisman M.V., Büller H.R., Ten Cate J.W., et al.: Serial impedance plethysmography for suspected deep venous thrombosis in outpatients. The Amsterdam general practitioner study. *N. Engl. J. Med.* 314:823, 1986.

57. Urokinase pulmonary embolism trial: Phase I results. *JAMA* 214:2163, 1974.

58. Urokinase-streptokinase embolism trial: Phase II results. *JAMA* 229:1606, 1974.

59. Goldhaber S.Z., Vaughan D.E., Markis J.E., et al.: Acute pulmonary embolism treated with tissue plasminogen activator. *Lancet* 2:886, 1986.

60. Mobin-Uddin K., Utley J.R., Bryant L.R.: The inferior vena cava umbrella filter. *Prog. Cardiovasc. Dis.* 17:391, 1975.

61. Consensus Conference: Prevention of venous thrombosis and pulmonary embolism. *JAMA* 256:744, 1986.

62. Collins R., Scrimgeour A., Yusuf S., et al.: Reduction in fatal pulmonary embolism and venous thrombosis by perioperative administration of subcutaneous heparin. Overview of results of randomized trials in general, orthopedic, and urologic surgery. *N. Engl. J. Med.* 318:1162, 1988.

Chapter 10

DISEASES OF THE AORTA

CARDIOVASCULAR SYPHILIS

Syphilis has become uncommon, and therefore fewer of its cardiovascular complications are seen. The incidence has been reduced because of public health measures, drugs, and better public education. The organism responsible *(Treponema pallidum)* is almost always acquired sexually, and there is often a latent period of 10 to 30 years prior to the development of cardiovascular syphilis. Usually the ascending aorta is involved via the lymphatics of the adventitia, leading to medial destruction and loss of elastic tissue and weakening of the aortic wall with formation of an aneurysm. The intima becomes scarred (tree bark appearance), and atheroma and calcification can be superimposed. Calcification is not specific for syphilis, but when present it is more often seen in the first part of the ascending aorta, whereas with atherosclerosis it is noted usually in the aortic knob. The coronary ostia may be narrowed because of the syphilitic aortitis. The aortic valve leaflets become separated at their commissures because of dilatation and weakening of the annulus with resultant aortic insufficiency. Myocardial involvement by gumma is rare.

Often a history of past treatment for syphilis is elicited. Before development of aortic insufficiency or an aneurysm, a loud tambour second sound in the aortic area can suggest aortitis in the presence of positive serologic tests for syphilis. Aortic insufficiency demonstrates essentially the same findings as noted with rheumatic aortic insufficiency (see Chap. 6). Because of the large stroke volume, calcification in the annulus, and stiffness of the aortic leaflets at the base, a systolic murmur is often heard in the primary aortic area, and a systolic thrill is palpable in the suprasternal notch even though there is no aortic stenosis. The marked dilatation of the aortic root may cause the aortic insufficiency murmur to be louder to the right of the sternum. It is often well heard along the left sternal border down to the apex and is high-pitched and crescendo-decrescendo. The sudden distention of the dilated aorta in early systole can produce an ejection sound. An apical mid-diastolic low-pitched, rumbling murmur (Austin Flint) may occur with severe aortic insufficiency and be mistaken for mitral stenosis. However, this murmur is not associated with a loud first heart sound and an opening snap, as is often the case with organic mitral stenosis. Most likely this murmur is due to the aortic regurgitant jet of blood during diastole pushing the aortic leaflet of the mitral valve toward closure and to the rapidly rising left ventricular diastolic pressure, which also impedes opening of the mitral valve and interferes with flow from the left atrium.[1]

An echocardiogram is useful in differentiating organic mitral stenosis from the Austin Flint murmur. Rarely, secondary to syphilis an aortic cusp may rupture or evert, producing a dove-coo type of diastolic murmur. Such a murmur may produce a thrill, which usually is not common with aortic insufficiency. A wide pulse pressure is often present, depending on the degree of aortic insufficiency. Many peripheral vascular signs have been noted, such as a bifid carotid (pulsus bisferiens), pistol-shot sounds over the peripheral arteries (Traube's sign), diastolic murmur proximal to constriction of an artery (Duroziez's sign), nodding of the head (de Musset's sign), water-hammer or collapsing pulse (Corrigan's pulse), alternate flushing and blanching of the capillary bed (Quincke's pulse), and a marked increase in leg BP over that in the arms (Hill's sign).

Patients may have angina which is often prolonged and can occur at night. The angina can be due to coronary ostial narrowing, aortic insufficiency, associated coronary artery disease, or a combination of these. Eventually heart failure can develop.

Infection with *T. pallidum* stimulates the host's defense mechanisms and produces a complex antibody response. Serologic testing detects these antibodies. There are two categories of serologic tests, nontreponemal and treponemal antigens. The VDRL test is the most commonly used nontreponemal test, and the fluorescent treponemal antibody absorption test (FTA-ABS) is the most commonly used treponemal antigen test. The *Treponema pallidum* immobilization (TPI) test and the Reiter protein complement-fixation test (RPCF) are also used. False-positive VDRL tests can occur with collagen and autoimmune types of diseases. In such cases the FTA-ABS or other treponemal antigen tests should be performed, as well as CSF examination.

Treatment should be started if syphilis is proved or highly suspected. Penicillin is the treatment of choice. Herxheimer's reaction has been suspected in a few cases when the patient has fever a few hours after treatment. Many penicillin schedules have been recommended. For cardiovascular syphilis, procaine penicillin, 600,000 units I.M. daily for 15 days, or benzathine penicillin-G (Bicillin), 2.4 million units I.M. weekly for 3 weeks, is recommended. If the patient is allergic to penicillin, tetracycline, 500 mg orally four times per day for 30 days, is given. If the patient cannot take tetracycline, erythromycin, 500 mg orally four times daily should be taken for 30 days. The VDRL and FTA-ABS may remain positive for many years after adequate therapy.

Luetic aneurysms producing symptoms may have to be excised and the aortic valve replaced for significant aortic insufficiency (see Chap. 6).

THORACIC AORTIC DISEASE

Aneurysms

Aneurysms of the thoracic aorta are most commonly due to arteriosclerosis rather than syphilis. Medial degeneration and weakness of the aorta produce the dilatation, which is often accelerated by hypertension. The arteriosclerotic types are more common in the arch and descending aorta. The luetic types, though rare today, are noted more often in the ascending aorta. An aneurysm may be fusiform or spindle-shaped or saccular with a narrow pedicle. Aneurysm of the ascending aorta is often referred to as the aneurysm of signs, since compression of neighboring structures produces obstruction to the superior vena cava with resultant suffusion of the face, edema, cyanosis, and swelling of the neck and upper arms. The aortic leaflets can become distorted, producing aortic regurgitation. Erosion into the sternum on either side may produce a pulsating mass. Aneurysm of the arch of the aorta is known as the aneurysm of symptoms, since compression on neighboring structures can produce respiratory symptoms, hoarseness, or dysphagia. A tracheal tug also may be present. In addition, there may be inequality of the pulses and BP in the upper extremities. Rupture can occur into the surrounding structures. Aneurysm of the descending aorta is usually found on a routine film, since it may be large prior to producing any symptoms.

Thoracic aneurysms are usually detected by chest x ray and confirmed by cardiac fluoroscopy and aortography. Aneurysms can contain clots which, on aortography, can obscure the actual size and extent of the aneurysm. CT scanning with contrast medium and MRI can identify the aneurysms and in some instances obviates the need for aortography. Two-dimensional echocardiography can define the aneurysm, but not as clearly as it defines abdominal aneurysms.

Surgical treatment is recommended for thoracic aneurysms if they are 7 cm or more in diameter or if they are producing symptoms, provided the patient is otherwise in good health.

Marfan's Syndrome

Marfan's syndrome[2] is a heritable disorder of connective tissue fibers. The changes in the aorta resemble those of medical cystic necrosis described by Erdheim years ago. Aneurysmal dilatation of the sinuses of Valsalva and pulmonary arteries can occur. Dilatation of the ascending aorta and valve ring may result in aortic insufficiency (Figs 10–1 and 10–2). Dissecting aneurysm frequently occurs. In fact, Marfan's syndrome is the leading cause of dissecting aneurysm under age 40. The aorta can rupture without a dissection. Myxomatous changes of the mitral valve leaflets with redundant chordae can produce multiple systolic clicks and mitral insufficiency. Myxomatous changes can also occur in the aortic valve leaflets without aortic dilatation. Such valves are noted at surgery without the patient's having other criteria for the diagnosis of Marfan's syndrome, and are classified as forme fruste of this syndrome. The diagnosis of Marfan's syndrome is suspected because of other features, such as skeletal, muscle, and eye abnormalities. Among these are a slender body with sparsity of subcutaneous fat, high arched palate, disproportionate long bones, arachnodactyly, loose ligaments and loose-jointedness, hypotonic muscles, pectus carinatum or pectus excavatum. Other stigmata are dislocation of the lens, retinal detachment, iridodonesis (tremor of the iris), and myopia. The aortic sinuses and valvular changes can be evaluated by the use of echocardiography and Doppler. Magnetic resonance imaging (MRI) and digital subtraction angiography (DSA) are also useful for following patients. A thin aorta found at surgery suggests a forme fruste of Marfan's in the absence of other diagnostic features. The connective tissue defect makes surgery, although required for symptomatic aneurysms or aortic insufficiency or mitral insufficiency, technically very difficult with recurrent complications. At times

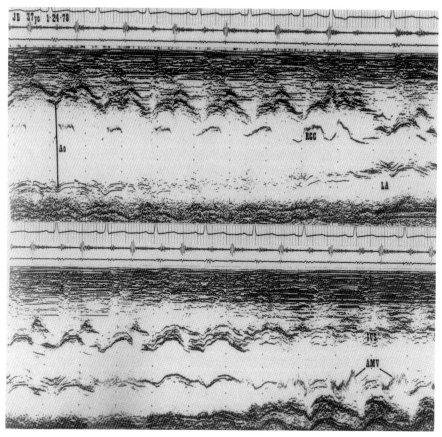

Fig 10–1. M-mode echocardiogram of a patient with Marfan's syndrome. Note dilated aorta *(arrow)* at level of the aortic sinuses. Marked diastolic fluttering of the anterior mitral valve leaflet (AMV) is present due to aortic insufficiency. AO = aorta; RCC = right coronary cusp; LA = left atrium; IVS = intraventricular septum; AMV = anterior mitral valve leaflet. (Courtesy of Dr. Bruce W. Usher.)

the surgery may be successful, yet the patient worsens because of underlying cardiomyopathy that may occur with Marfan's syndrome.

Annuloaortic Ectasia

Medial degenerative changes can cause dilatation of the annulus and proximal aorta with development of aortic regurgitation or dissection. This can occur to some degree in all patients with Marfan's syndrome. Chest x ray shows marked dilation of the aortic root and ascending aorta. This can be detected easily with echocardiography (Fig 10–3), CT scan, MRI, and aortography. When the aortic regurgitation becomes severe and symptomatic, surgery is required but can be difficult because of the weak tissues, and the coronary arteries may have to be reimplanted or bypassed with saphenous vein grafts.

Aortic Arch Syndrome

Aortic arch syndrome (Takayasu's, pulseless disease, or brachiocephalic syndrome) is a term used for stenosis and occlusion of the aortic arch and its great

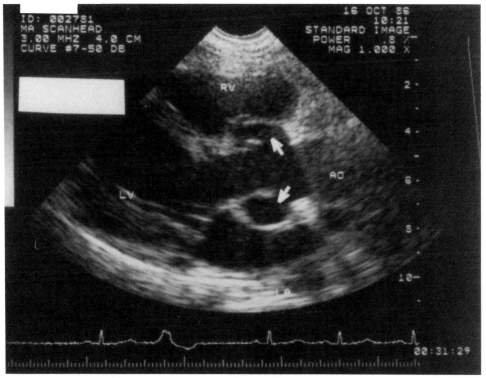

Fig 10–2. Two-dimensional echocardiogram of a patient with Marfan's syndrome. Note aneurysmal dilatation *(arrows)* of the sinuses of Valsalva. RV = Right ventricle; AO = aorta; LV = left ventricle. (Courtesy of Dr. Bruce W. Usher.)

vessels and in certain types may be associated with constitutional symptoms such as fever, malaise, anemia, or an elevated sedimentation rate. Atherosclerosis, syphilis, congenital aortic arch anomaly, and arteritis are some of the causes.

Takayasu's disease[3] is found most often in Orientals, but occurs worldwide and is noted particularly in women. It is an arteritis involving the aorta and its branches (aortic arch, brachiocephalic and thoracoabdominal vessels). Other vessels such as the pulmonary arteries may also be involved. A specific etiology for this arteritis is not known, although there is some evidence that it may be an autoimmune disease. Many patients have systemic symptoms such as fever, malaise, weight loss, arthralgias, night sweats, and pleuritic pain. Leukocytosis, anemia, and elevated sedimentation rate are noted. This acute phase subsides and these patients show symptoms and signs due to the obstructed vessels as noted with other conditions that involve the aorta. Involvement of the renal arteries can produce systemic hypertension, and, rarely, this arteritis may be responsible for primary pulmonary hypertension.

Giant cell arteritis may involve the aorta and its branches and occurs more commonly in the elderly. It may give symptoms similar to those of Takayasu's arteritis. Granulomatous inflammation more often involves the small and medium arteries such as the temporal. Patients can have constitutional symptoms such as fever and malaise. Involvement of the temporal vessels produces

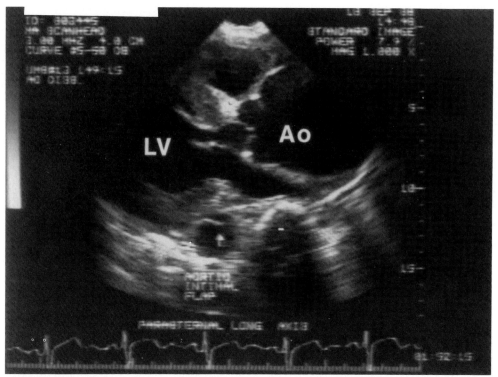

Fig 10–3. Two-dimensional echocardiogram of a patient with annuloaortic ectasia. Note the dilated pear-shaped aortic root (Ao). Arrow points to intimal flap in descending aorta consistent with dissection. LV = left ventricle. (Courtesy of Dr. Bruce W. Usher.)

headaches and tenderness over the vessel. If the ophthalmic artery is involved, blindness may occur. Activity of the arteritis can be followed by the sedimentation rate, which in most cases is high. The diagnosis is confirmed by biopsy, usually of the temporal artery.

Dizziness, syncope, ocular manifestations, claudication of the arms and jaws, paresthesia, and coldness of the extremities and the subclavian steal (retrograde flow from the vertebral artery to the arm distal to a stenotic subclavian artery producing vertebral-basilar system ischemic symptoms) are some of the features that may be associated with all types of the aortic arch syndrome. Radial and carotid pulses may be unequal or absent, and bruits are audible over the narrow sites. The term reversed coarctation describes the state in which the upper body pulses are diminished and the BP is higher in the legs. Aortic regurgitation can occur with all of these syndromes and with other conditions that may include arteritis such as psoriatic arthritis, relapsing polychondritis, Reiter's syndrome, ankylosing spondylitis, and arthritis with ulcerative colitis.

Although the aortic arch syndrome is discussed as an isolated entity, conditions producing it frequently involve other aortic branches and can produce signs and symptoms depending on the vessels involved: e.g., abdominal angina can occur if the mesenteric vessels are involved, and claudication can occur if the leg vessels are involved.

The diagnosis of the vessels involved is confirmed by aortography. Depending on the etiology, calcification, irregular intimal surface, saccular aneurysm, and even completely occluded vessels may be seen. Lande and Rossi[4] described a "rat-tail" appearance of the descending thoracic aorta in Takayasu's arteritis.

Treatment depends on the conditions. Surgery is indicated depending on the symptoms and location of the obstructed vessels. Rarely, the aortic valve may need replacement. Adrenal corticosteroids are recommended for the arteritis conditions (Takayasu's and giant cell). Anticoagulation and immunosuppressive therapy have also been given in Takayasu's disease.

ABDOMINAL AORTIC DISEASE

Aneurysms

An aneurysm is a dilatation of an artery, and it may be fusiform or saccular. At times a false aneurysm can occur in which the walls of the vessel are destroyed and the aneurysmal sac is composed of perivascular clot and connective tissue. Abdominal aortic aneurysms usually are due to arteriosclerosis and less often to infections (mycotic) or trauma. Often these are found during a routine examination. Symptoms are sudden pain in the abdomen, back, loin, or testicular area. These symptoms usually indicate leakage, dissection, or perforation. Sudden collapse and shock indicate rupture. Rarely, microemboli from the aneurysm can shower the small vessels of the feet, producing areas of ischemia or gangrene. Some aneurysms may rupture and close off spontaneously. These are sealed by forming a hematoma or false blood vessel. Ecchymosis of the flank or perineum indicates retroperitoneal bleeding. Gastrointestinal bleeding may occur due to an aortoenteric fistula. Abdominal aneurysms usually are noted between 50 and 80 years of age and are more common in males. The most characteristic feature is a pulsatile mass which the patient may be aware of. It may be mistaken for a mass overlying the aorta, but the expansile pulsation laterally usually indicates an aneurysm. A tortuous aorta may cause confusion. For this reason it is important to palpate from the lateral aspects of the abdomen medially until the aortic pulsations are felt. The distance between these pulsations is the width of the aorta. If one routinely does this, it is less likely that an aneurysm would be missed. A tortuous aorta may give a prominent pulsation near the lateral aspect of the abdomen suggesting an aneurysm, yet its other medial pulsation will be felt as an aorta of normal width, about 2 cm. The aneurysm may be tender, indicating sudden enlargement or leakage. Bruit may be present over the aneurysm and iliac and femoral vessels because frequently there is associated peripheral arterial insufficiency. Anteroposterior and lateral views of the abdomen may show linear calcification outlining the aneurysm. However, calcification may not be noted in 25% of patients.[5] Abdominal ultrasound has become an excellent method of detecting and sizing an aneurysm; it also can detect an intraluminal thrombus. In fact, it may be better than aortography, for on aortography a thrombus may give a reduced width of the aneurysm. However, in most hospitals aortography is still performed because it will outline associated vascular lesions as renal and peripheral artery stenosis. Fortunately, 95% of abdominal aneurysms are below the renal arteries. This information is important to the surgeon. MRI and CT scan can also define the aneurysm.

Surgery is indicated immediately if there is rupture or impending rupture as suggested by pain, increase in size of the aneurysm, or tenderness; otherwise, mortality is 100%. If the patient is otherwise in good health, surgery should be performed when an aneurysm is first noted even if the patient is asymptomatic, especially if the aneurysm is 6 cm or larger. One study[6] showed that 59% of patients survived for 1 year after the aneurysm was detected, and 19% for 5 years. If the aneurysm was greater than 6 cm in size, then the survival rate for 1 year was 47.5% and for 5 years 6%. Unfortunately, some 50% of patients have other associated diseases. These must be taken into consideration prior to elective surgery. Absolute contraindications to surgery are intractable congestive failure, metastatic cancer, uremia, and chronic lung disease with CO_2 retention. The majority agree that if an aneurysm is producing symptoms or is 6 cm in diameter or greater, surgery should be performed. There is not full agreement as to the indication for surgery if the aneurysm is 4 cm to less than 6 cm. One study[7] showed that aneurysms between 4 cm and 7 cm had a 25% incidence of rupture, suggesting that surgery should be performed for aneurysms as small as 4 cm. Surgery is recommended for such small aneurysms unless the patients are poor surgical risks, in which case they should be followed up closely for symptoms and increasing size of the aneurysm, which demand surgery. An aneurysm can expand on an average of 0.4 to 0.52 cm in diameter per year.[8,9] If the patients have evidence of associated carotid or coronary artery disease,[10] they should be evaluated and surgery performed if indicated for these lesions prior to resection of the aneurysm.

Leriche's Syndrome

This syndrome is caused by atherosclerotic occlusion of the terminal aorta and iliac vessels. Patients have several months of symptoms of ischemia characterized by pain in the buttocks or thighs occurring with exertion and relieved by rest. Calf claudication may also be present. Such patients often complain of impotence. Femoral pulses are reduced or absent and bruits are common over the lower abdomen and femoral vessels. Surgery is usually indicated for those who have severe intermittent claudication.

Saddle Embolus

The majority of such emboli to the aortic bifurcation come from the left side of the heart (myocardial infarction, ventricular aneurysm, atrial fibrillation, prosthetic valves, atrial myxoma, fungal endocarditis). A paradoxical systemic embolism from the venous side can occur through an atrial septal defect or patent foramen ovale. Chronically ill patients (usually with malignancies) develop intracardiac thrombi that can embolize (marantic endocarditis). Such patients have sudden, severe pain in the legs. Pain can also be noted in the lower abdomen, lumbosacral area, and perineum. Numbness, paresthesias, absent leg pulses, and cold, pale legs can be noted. The embolic material can be removed by a Fogarty balloon-tipped catheter, and if not successful, surgery can be performed. Heparin and later warfarin anticoagulation is used postoperatively.

Atheromatous Emboli

Microcholesterol emboli can occur to small vessels. These emboli originate from atherosclerotic material in the aorta and its major branches. They can occur spontaneously, after surgery or after cardiac catheterization. The clinical findings depend on the vessels involved. Emboli to peripheral vessels can produce skin necrosis, ischemic toes, livedo reticularis, and purpuric spots. Even renal failure can occur if the kidneys are showered with small emboli. There is no specific therapy for the emboli; however, at times surgery can be performed on the source.

TRAUMA TO THE AORTA

Nonpenetrating injury can cause rupture of the aorta, usually sudden acceleration-deceleration forces such as those associated with automobile accidents. The aorta may rupture just above the aortic valve or just distal to the left subclavian artery. Penetrating injuries, such as stab wounds, can also enter the aorta. The diagnosis is often obscured because of other injuries and lack of specific findings. Increased BP in the upper extremities, reduced lower extremity pulses, and x-ray evidence of a widened mediastinum should suggest aortic rupture. Once aortic rupture is suspected, it should be confirmed, if the patient's condition allows, with CT scanning with contrast or aortography and surgery performed immediately.

CONGENITAL ANOMALIES OF THE AORTA

Many of these, such as coarctation, are discussed in Chapter 7 on congenital heart lesions.

During embryonic development there are six pairs of aortic arches that connect the truncus arteriosus to the dorsal aorta. The truncus partitions into the aorta and pulmonary artery and portions of the six aortic arches disappear. The first, second, and fifth sets of arches completely disappear; the proximal portions of the sixth arch became the pulmonary arteries, and the distal portion becomes the ductus arteriosus. The third arch connects the internal carotid with the external to the common carotid artery, the left fourth arch becomes the connection between the left carotid and subclavian arteries, and the right fourth arch forms the proximal portion of the right subclavian artery.[11] A variety of anomalies is possible if these regressions do not occur properly. A right aortic arch occurs in only 0.1 to 0.14% of the population and is frequently associated with other congenital anomalies, such as tetralogy of Fallot, pulmonary atresia, ventricular septal defects, truncus arteriosus, and tricuspid atresia. A double aortic arch (persistence of right and left fourth embryonic aortic arches) can encircle the esophagus and trachea and result in symptoms of dyspnea, stridor, cough, and dysphagia. The barium-filled esophagus can show compression on the esophagus. Aortography confirms the diagnosis, and surgery is indicated if symptoms are present. Other combinations of abnormal regression of the arches can produce different types of vascular rings. Persistent cervical aortic arch is usually benign (persistence of the third aortic arch, with regression of the fourth) and may be on the right or left and present as a supraclavicular pulsating mass. Fluoroscopy, x rays, and an esophagram can often indicate the diagnosis, which can be confirmed with aortography. Surgery is seldom required. Congenital kinking of the aorta (pseudocoarctation) may produce a mediastinal mass and reduction in the femoral pulses. Aortography can confirm the diagnosis and exclude true coarctation. The abnormality is produced by a sharp angulation of the aorta at the ligamentum arteriosum attachment. It is often associated with the anomalies noted with true coarctation, such as a bicuspid aortic valve, ventricular septal defect, corrected transposition, and aneurysm of the sinus of Valsalva. Usually surgery is required only for the associated anomalies or complications such as associated aneurysm of the left subclavian artery or aneurysm proximal or distal to the kink.

AORTIC DISSECTION

The incidence of dissecting aneurysm of the aorta is approximately 1 per 10,000 hospital admissions and noted in 1 per 360 autopsies. It varies from one locality to another depending on the age and racial distribution; e.g., Pate et al.[12] estimated an incidence as high as 20 patients per million in the Memphis area. Most of these aneurysms occur between the ages of 40 and 70 years and are about three times more frequent in men. Seventeen percent of patients in one series were over 70 years of age.[13] When it is present in a patient under age 40, one must consider Marfan's syndrome or a congenital aortic anomaly. Hypertension and degeneration of the aortic media (cystic necrosis) are predisposing factors. Schlatmann and Becker[14] looked at apparently normal aortas and concluded that the changes of medial degeneration are essentially the same as those of medionecrosis and are more frequent and extensive in older persons, especially if hypertension is present. However, these same changes occur to a lesser degree in older patients (normal aging) and hypertensive patients without dissection. Rarely the changes are primarily those of atherosclerosis or syphilis. It appears that medial degeneration, motion of the aorta and hydrodynamic forces related to the pulse wave produced by each cardiac beat, and systolic BP act upon the proximal aorta, resulting in intimal tear with dissection.[15] There is no definite relationship to activity or trauma. A proximal tear is present in 90% of instances, through which the longitudinal cleavage of the aortic media communicates with the true lumen. A distal intimal tear may also be present, thus producing a double-barreled aorta. The dissection can lead to aortic wall rupture, cardiac tamponade, exsanguination, major vessel occlusion, or aortic regurgitation. DeBakey and co-workers[16] classify dissections as to their anatomic pattern (Fig 10–4). The more common type I begins in the ascending aorta, and the intimal tear is just above the aortic valve. Type II is rare and is limited to the ascending aorta. Type III

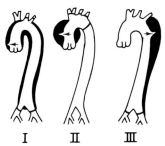

I   II   III

Fig 10–4.   Classification of dissecting aneurysm of the aorta. Type I involves the ascending aorta and extends distally. Type II is limited to the ascending aorta. Type III originates near or below the left subclavian artery and extends distally. (Modified from DeBakey M.E., et al.: Surgical management of dissecting aneurysm of the aorta. *J. Thorac. Cardiovasc. Surg.* 49:130, 1965.)

begins at or just distal to the origin of the left subclavian artery. It may be limited to the descending thoracic aorta (type IIIa). Types I and III (type IIIb) may extend to the abdominal aortic bifurcation and into its major terminal branches.[17] This classification has been modified into type A and B, depending on the presence or absence of involvement of the ascending aorta.[18] Type A dissections have the intimal tear in the ascending aorta in three positions: ascending aorta, transverse arch, or the descending aorta. (Type A includes the DeBakey types I and II.) Type B dissections occur distal to the origin of the left subclavian (type III of DeBakey) and do not include the ascending aorta. Type A dissections occur in 66% of all cases and type B in 33%.

Sudden, excruciating pain is the most common complaint. It reaches its greatest intensity immediately and does not increase in onset, as frequently occurs with acute myocardial infarction. It may begin in the chest or abdomen, anterior or posterior, and may radiate upward or downward according to the direction of the dissection. Rarely, the pain may not be severe, especially when there is shock and the patient is confused. The physical findings depend on the area involved. Absent or diminished pulses, aortic insufficiency, sternoclavicular joint pulsation, shock, cyanosis, fever, and tachycardia may occur. Partial occlusion of the branches of the aorta, such as the carotid and subclavian, can produce murmurs over these vessels and a difference in the BP between the upper extremities. The BP may be high, even though the patient appears to be in shock. At times neurologic deficits occur. Rupture into the pericardial cavity can produce cardiac tamponade and may produce syncope.[19] Most often when the pain is in the chest, the diagnosis of acute myocardial infarction is entertained. However, the lack of Q waves in the ECG and serum enzyme elevation and the persistence of pain, especially with hypertension in the presence of a shock-like state, should make one suspicious of a dissection. Chest films may reveal progressive widening of the aorta and at times intimal calcification separated from the outer edge of the aortic shadow. The aortic knob can be obliterated and the trachea displaced to the right. Pleural effusions, namely, on the left, can develop. These findings are of greater significance if prior films are available for comparison. Echocardiography can detect proximal dissection by outlining the aortic root. However, CT scanning with contrast is even better because it can detect proximal and distal dissections. MRI has also been used in diagnosis and has the advantage of not requiring contrast injection. The diagnosis should be confirmed by aortography, especially since the patient may need surgery. It also gives some idea of the prognosis. Up to 40% of deaths due to dissection occur in the first 48 hours, and fewer than 10% of patients are alive after 1 year. Medical therapy has improved the survival rate up to 80%.

Wheat[15] introduced pharmacologic treatment to reduce the propulsive stress on the aortic wall and prevent spread of the dissection. Because the pulsatile flow is considered more important than the absolute BP levels, agents are used to reduce the velocity of left ventricular ejection (dV/dt) and systolic blood pressure.

Drug therapy is the initial treatment of choice for all patients with dissection. However, serious complications such as severe aortic regurgitation, aortic rupture, cardiac tamponade, or compromise to a vital organ may require immediate surgery. Wheat recommends reducing the systolic BP to 100 to 120 mm Hg by use of trimethaphan camsylate (Arfonad) IV in a solution of 1 to 2 mg/ml (500 mg in 500 ml of 5% dextrose in water) at a flow rate to reduce the BP to the desired level. Sodium nitroprusside is often given initially because the patient may become tachyphylactic to trimethaphan or develop side effects such as urinary retention, constipation, or hypotension. Prior to use of sodium nitroprusside, the patient should receive propranolol, methyldopa, or reserpine to reduce the adrenergic-stimulating effect that occurs because of relaxation of the peripheral vascular bed. Sodium nitroprusside is begun at a rate of 0.5 to 2.0 μg/kg/minute IV and increased as necessary. The BP level must be adequate to maintain urinary output and cerebral and coronary perfusion.

Propranolol (80 to 160 mg orally daily, or 1 mg I.V. every 4 hours or sooner to produce adequate β blockade) has replaced reserpine, and sometimes, especially if the patient is normotensive, may be the only drug administered. Calcium channel blockers have been used with some success but need more study. In some cases, blood volume may have to be restored because of loss into the dissecting hematoma.

Once the patient is stable (BP controlled and pain relieved if possible), aortography should be performed to confirm the diagnosis and the location of the dissection. Community hospitals without the facilities for aortography and surgery should send such patients (once reasonably stable) to a center that is prepared for more definitive management. If the dissection involves the ascending aorta (type A—includes DeBakey types I and II), surgery should be performed. The mortality today with surgery is 15% to 30%.[15] This improvement is due to the initial drug therapy stabilizing the patient and to the development of better surgical skills. Type B (includes DeBakey type III) dissections are distal to the left subclavian artery, but for therapeutic purposes, dissections that originate in the transverse arch are also included if the dissection has not involved the ascending aorta. Such dissections are initially treated with drugs. If the patient's pain is relieved and the condition is stable, drug therapy is continued on a long-term basis. Surgical intervention is indicated for type B dissections if, in spite of maximum therapy, there is evidence of progression of the dissection, impending rupture, or an inability to control the BP or pain or both within four hours. Progression of the dissection is indicated by evidence of compromise or occlusion of the carotid, renal, or other major vessels, or by the development of aortic insufficiency. Acute saccular aneurysm, blood in the pleural or pericardial cavities, and continuous pain in spite of therapy may be evidence of impending rupture of the dissecting hematoma.

Stable chronic dissections presenting 2 weeks or later after onset, regardless of the type, respond better to their respective medical or surgical therapies.

In summary, we feel that the various classifications of dissecting aneurysms do not need many descriptive details. However, it is important to recognize that drug therapy is the initial course in all cases, and if the ascending aorta is involved, surgery should be performed (at times immediately if a life-threatening complication occurs); for other locations, drug therapy should be continued unless there is evidence of spread of the dissection or other complications.

After the acute phase, all patients should have a continuation of drug therapy, even if surgery was performed. The BP should be maintained with oral preparations of β-blockers, diuretics, and other drug combinations as discussed in Chapter 5. The patients should be closely observed because a sacular aneurysm can develop in 14 to 20% of patients or aortic insufficiency in 10% of patients.[4] Such complications require surgery.

REFERENCES

1. Fortuin N.J., Craige E.: On the mechanism of the Austin Flint murmur. *Circulation* 45:558, 1972.
2. McKusick V.A.: *Heritable Disorders of Connective Tissue.* ed. 4. St. Louis, C.V. Mosby Co., 1972.
3. Lupi-Herrera E., Sanchez-Torres G., Marcushamer J., et al.: Takayasu's arteritis: Clinical study of 107 cases. *Am Heart J.* 93:94, 1977.
4. Lande A., Rossi P.: The value of total aortography in the diagnosis of Takayasu's arteritis. *Radiology* 114:287, 1975.
5. Retief P.J., Loubser J.S.: Diagnosis and treatment of abdominal aortic aneurysm: A report of 82 cases. *S. Afr. Med. J.* 56:67, 1979.
6. Szilagyi D.E., Smith R.F., DeRusso F.J., et al.: Contribution of abdominal aortic aneurysmectomy to prolongation of life. *Ann. Surg.* 164:678, 1966.
7. Darling R.C., Messina C.R., Brewster D.C., et al.: Autopsy study of unoperated abdominal aortic aneurysms: The case for early resection. *Circulation* 56(suppl 2):161, 1977.
8. Bernstein E.F., Chan E.L.: Abdominal aortic aneurysm in high-risk patients. Outcome of selective management based on size and expansion rate. *Ann. Surg.* 200:255, 1984.
9. Delin A., Ohlsen H., Swedenborg J.: Growth rate of abdominal aortic aneurysms as measured by computed tomography. *Br. J. Surg.* 72:530, 1985.
10. Young A.E., Couch N.P.: Coronary artery disease and aortic aneurysm surgery. *Lancet* 1:1005, 1977.
11. Langman J., van Mierop L.H.S.: Development of the cardiovascular system, in Moss A.J., Adams F.H. (eds.): *Heart Disease in Infants, Children and Adolescents.* Baltimore, Williams & Wilkins Co., 1968.
12. Pate J.W., Richardson R.L., Eastridge C.E.: Acute aortic dissections. *Am. Surg.* 42:395, 1976.
13. Wheat M.W., Jr., Harris P.D., Malm J.R., et al.: Acute dissecting aneurysms of the aorta: Treatment and results of 64 patients. *J. Thorac. Cardiovasc. Surg.* 58:344, 1969.
14. Schlatmann T.J.M., Becker A.E.: Histologic changes in the normal aging aorta: Implications for dissecting aortic aneurysm. *Am. J. Cardiol.* 39:13, 1977.
15. Wheat M.W., Jr.: Acute dissecting aneurysms of the aorta: Diagnosis and treatment—1979. *Am. Heart J.* 99:373, 1980.
16. DeBakey M.E., Henly W.S., Cooley D.A., et al.: Surgical management of dissecting aneurysm of the aorta. *J. Thorac. Cardiovasc. Surg.* 49:130, 1965.
17. DeBakey M.E., McCollum C.H., Crawford E.S., et al.: Dissection and dissecting aneurysms of the aorta: Twenty-year follow-up of five hundred twenty-seven patients treated surgically. *Surgery* 92:1118, 1982.
18. Dailey P.O., Trueblood H.W., Stinson E.B., et al.: Management of acute aortic dissection. *Ann. Thorac. Surg.* 10:237, 1970.
19. Slater E.E., DeSanctis R.W.: The clinical recognition of dissecting aortic aneurysm. *Am. J. Med.* 60:625, 1976.

Chapter 11

INFECTIVE ENDOCARDITIS

For many years bacterial endocarditis has been divided into acute and subacute types. Acute endocarditis usually is due to a virulent organism, with rapid progression of the disease if untreated. Subacute bacterial endocarditis (SBE) is more insidious and is usually due to *Streptococcus viridans*. However, today this classification is not used as often because certain organisms can produce an acute or a chronic course. The so-called most benign microorganisms can produce devastating complications, such as valvular perforation and cerebral embolization. In view of the extensive use of antibiotics, the distinction is not as clear-cut today as it was formerly. Actually, since many nonbacterial organisms can produce endocarditis, the term infective endocarditis is probably most accurate.

Endocarditis usually occurred in the past in patients with known rheumatic valvular disease, congenital heart lesions, or after cardiac surgical procedures. Recently this has changed. Only 50% of patients have had known heart disease, although 90% have murmurs on admission.[1] An increased frequency has been noted on normal heart valves, especially in the drug addicts. Mitral valve prolapse has now been detected with increasing frequency as an underlying lesion susceptible to endocarditis. About 2 to 4% of patients with prosthetic heart valves develop endocarditis. Elderly patients with atherosclerosis in the ascending aorta and valve have an aortic systolic murmur which is due to sclerosis rather than stenosis and predisposes to infective endocarditis. This has also been noted in patients with calcification of the mitral valve annulus[2] and in patients with idiopathic hypertrophic subaortic stenosis (IHSS).[3] In IHSS the aortic or mitral valve can be involved.

With the decreased incidence of acute rheumatic fever, the incidence of underlying rheumatic heart disease in endocarditis has declined from 90% of all cases to about 40 to 60%. The aortic and mitral valves are most commonly affected and rarely the tricuspid and pulmonic valves. Endocarditis most frequently occurs on mild lesions such as mild mitral or aortic insufficiency rather than on a severely damaged valve. However, it can occur on the more severe lesions, on mitral stenosis, and in the presence of atrial fibrillation and congestive heart failure.

The most common underlying congenital lesions are ventricular septal defect, patent ductus arteriosus, bicuspid aortic valve, and pulmonic stenosis. Endocarditis rarely occurs in a patient with atrial septal defect. Tetralogy of Fallot is the most common cyanotic lesion involved. Persistent bacteremia with no obvious focus of infection may suggest endothelial surface involvement. In one instance we saw such a case following heart catheterization.

Rodbard[4] showed how high pressure can drive an infected fluid into a low-pressure sink and deposit bacterial colonies in this low-pressure area. This study explained the distribution of lesions occurring in endocarditis; e.g., in aortic insufficiency the lesions occur on the ventricular surface of the aortic valve, in mitral insufficiency on the atrial surface of the mitral valve, and in ventricular septal defect on the right ventricular side of the defect. In a review, Arnett and Roberts[5] reported on 137 autopsy cases of endocarditis. They classified these cases in the following groups depending on the sites of the vegetations: involvement of right-sided valves, left-sided valves, prosthetic valves, aortic and mitral valves after valvulotomy or valvuloplasty, congenital cardiac disease with shunt, and the mural endocardium. They described the gross and histologic abnormalities in the various stages of endocarditis. The organisms deposit at the site of the diseased valves, endocardium, or the endothelium of a blood vessel and form friable vegetations consisting of platelets, thrombi, fibrin, red and white blood cells, and bacteria. These vegetations can cause necrosis of the tissue and may break off easily, producing peripheral embolization. Abscesses can occur in the valve rings and in the myocardium. There may be leaflet destruction or ruptured chordae. Pericarditis can occur from a ruptured valve ring abscess, from transmural acute myocardial infarction, and from rupture of a myocardial abscess into the pericardium. Myocardial inflammation as foci of nonsuppurating interstitial and perivascular inflammation (Bracht-Wächter bodies) can occur. Emboli can be noted in the coronary arteries. The most common feature of endocarditis on a prosthetic valve is infection at the site of attachment of the valve prosthesis with a valve ring abscess.

ETIOLOGY

The incidence of the various causative organisms is difficult to assess today because the organism flora has changed since the widespread use of antibiotics. Endocarditis is usually due to the α-hemolytic streptococcus (viridans), the *Streptococcus faecalis* (enterococcus), or to the staphylococcus. *Streptococcus bovis* is a nonenterococcal group D streptococcus that is being found more frequently and is commonly associated with cancer of the colon.[6] Since the advent of cardiac surgery and the indiscriminate use of opiates by addicts, other organisms have become a part of the endocarditis picture, such as *Staphylococcus aureus* and *albus,* hemolytic streptococcus, *Pseudomonas aeruginosa,* and other gram-negative infections, fungi, and nonpathogenic bacteria such as *Serratia marcescens.* Whereas previously pneumococcal and gonococcal endocarditis were frequent, these are rather unusual today. In addition, there still remain typical clinical cases of endocarditis with negative blood cultures. Such cases may range up to about 15%. Anaerobes, *Hemophilus influenzae,* fungi, and brucellae may be the infecting organism in such cases with persistently sterile blood cultures. The portal of entry may give a clue to the type of organism involved. *Streptococcus viridans* infection occurs frequently after dental procedures. Enterococcal infections can occur after genitourinary and GI tract procedures or in women after abortion or giving birth. Staphylococcal, gram-negative bacterial, and fungal infections occur in drug addicts and after open heart surgery.

DIAGNOSIS

Clinical Findings

In the presence of cardiac disease, a history of significant fever (rarely is fever absent) demands careful evaluation for endocarditis. Unexplained fever for more than 7 days' duration in a patient with congenital or rheumatic heart disease or with a heart murmur from any cause should be considered to be due to bacterial endocarditis until proved otherwise. In addition, multisystem involvement should direct attention to the possibility of this disease. Besides fever, the patient's complaints are variable, but usually include tiredness, weight loss, vague abdominal or flank pain, arthralgias, and at times severe musculoskeletal backache. The physical findings may be limited to the presence of fever and abnormal cardiovascular findings. Changing heart murmurs or the development of new murmurs can indicate valvular damage because of the vegetations or perforation of the valve or of the chordae tendineae. Heart murmurs may be absent initially. This is especially true when the right side of the heart is involved. In fact, a murmur may not appear with vegetations on the tricuspid valve.[7] However, it is important to listen carefully, for the murmur may be heard only with inspiration along the left lower sternal border. Prominent C-V jugular venous pulses may be the first clue to the presence of tricuspid insufficiency. In addition, a bicuspid aortic valve may be present without a murmur and only an aortic ejection sound, or there may be only a midsystolic click without mitral insufficiency. Arrhythmias, including heart block (abscess in septum), can occur. Pericarditis is rare and may be due to rupture of a mycotic aneurysm, a coronary embolism with myocardial infarction, rupture of a mural or valve ring abscess, or uremia. Cardiac failure may occur even when the infection appears to have been eradicated. Embolization can cause many other organ systems to be involved. Petechiae can appear on the skin or mucous membranes. Splinter hemorrhages may occur under the nail beds but are nonspecific.

The significance of petechiae and splinter hemorrhages is greater if these are noted to appear during repeated examinations. Osler's nodes are small, red, tender lesions occurring on the tips of the fingers or the toes, along the palms of the hands, or on the plantar surface of the feet. Janeway's lesions are painless and appear as ecchymotic or macular spots on the palms or soles. Splenomegaly can occur and may be painful due to metastatic abscesses and infarcts. The patient may present with a vascular lesion of the CNS. Mycotic aneurysms can result in intracerebral or subarachnoid hemorrhage and even meningitis. Hemorrhages can appear in the retina, at times with white spots in their center (Roth's spots). Retinal vessel embolism can cause visual loss, and metastatic septic endophthalmitis can occur. Embolism to the GI tract may produce symptoms. At times a ruptured mycotic aneurysm of the vessels of the GI tract may produce GI hemorrhage. Pulmonary embolism can occur when the infective endocarditis is localized to the right side of the heart. The underlying lesion in such cases is usually a congenital heart lesion or right-sided valvular lesion. These patients can have episodes of hemoptysis, cough, chest pain, and pulmonary infiltrates. Clubbing of the fingers and toes is rare and is usually a late manifestation in untreated cases. Microemboli frequently occur in the kidneys. In the proper setting microscopic hematuria is an important diagnostic clue. Multiple emboli or proliferative glomerulonephritis can eventually produce renal insufficiency. Circulating immune complexes are partly responsible for the peripheral signs of vasculitis (Osler's nodes, Janeway's lesions, Roth's spots, splinter hemorrhages, glomerulonephritis, and synovial joint inflammation). Peripheral lesions were much more common in the pre-antibiotic era, when the active disease had a long course. An organism with high virulence, such as coagulase-positive staphylococci and pneumococci, may produce a dramatic picture with sudden onset of high fever, extreme toxic signs, and cardiac failure.

Prosthetic valve endocarditis (PVE) can be classified as early-onset if it develops within 2 months after operation and late-onset if it develops more than 2 months after operation.[8] The most frequent causes in the early-onset group were *Staphylococcus aureus* (44%) and gram-negative bacilli (38%), and associated mortality was 86% and 83%, respectively. Viridans streptococci (41%) and gram-negative bacilli (31%) were the most frequent agents in the late-onset group, and the mortality was 25% and 22%, respectively. Early-onset PVE has become less common since surgical techniques have improved and prophylactic antibiotics are administered in the perioperative period. However, late-onset PVE has become more frequent as this constantly enlarging population ages. Yet, the overall incidence has decreased. The aortic valve is most often involved. Late-onset PVE is usually caused by the same microorganisms that cause native valve endocarditis and is easier to cure than early-onset PVE. The case fatality rate has not decreased over the past two decades. One report of 14 large studies showed 78% case fatality for early PVE and 46% for late PVE.[9,10] The portal of entry for the early-onset group was I.V. catheters, pneumonitis, urinary catheters, contamination of blood by the oxygenator, and wound infections, and for the late-onset, antecedent trauma, surgical operations, or dental work. Clinically there may be diminished intensity of the opening or closing sound of the prosthesis. A new murmur can indicate perivalvular peak or improper closure or opening of the valve. However, such findings can occur in the absence of endocarditis.

Endocarditis is being seen more frequently on the tricuspid valve in parenteral drug abusers. *Staphylococcus aureus, Streptococci viridans* and gram-negative organisms are the most common causes. The injection apparatus and drugs used by addicts are often not the source of the staphylococcal infection, but such patients often have staphylococci in the nasopharynx and on the skin.[11] Endocarditis involving the tricuspid valve can be manifested by pneumonitis, pulmonary emboli, evidence of tricuspid insufficiency (murmur and right-sided gallops may be present or absent or present only with inspiration). Peripheral manifestations such as splinter hemorrhage are not common. Hepatomegaly and splenomegaly can occur.

Echocardiography

Echocardiography has become useful for detecting vegetations on heart valves and suspecting the presence of endocarditis (Figs 11–1 and 11–2). Traditional physical findings in acute situations, as with severe aortic insufficiency due to endocarditis, are often absent. In addition, echocardiography can detect vegetations in patients with negative blood cultures who have received inadequate therapy. However, the presence of vegetations does not in-

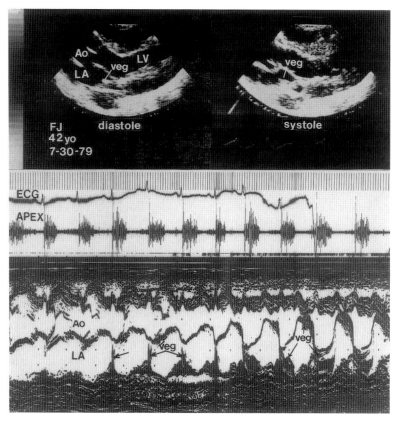

Fig 11-1. Echocardiogram (two-dimensional, *top*) and M-mode (*bottom*) showing vegetations on the mitral valve due to infective endocarditis. Note that vegetations protrude in the left atrium. Phonocardiogram at the apex reveals a systolic murmur of mitral insufficiency. Ao = aorta; LA = left atrium; Veg = vegetation; LV = left ventricle; ECG = electrocardiogram. (Courtesy of Dr. Bruce W. Usher.)

dicate active lesions, and the absence of vegetations does not exclude endocarditis. Vegetations usually must be greater than 3 mm to be detected. False-positive results can be due to calcified or thickened valves, flail valvular leaflets, rupture of the chordae tendineae, or prosthetic valves. Amsterdam[12] reported that two-dimensional echocardiography detects 50 to 80% of cases of infective endocarditis. The sensitivity of M-mode for detection of vegetations is 40 to 50%.[13] Echocardiography in combination with phonocardiography can aid in detecting the severity of the valvular lesions and is useful for following such patients. For example, premature closure of the mitral valve (see Fig 6-16) can help in determining the time for aortic valve replacement for acute aortic insufficiency.[14,15] Doppler echocardiography (including color flow) is of value in following changes in murmurs and assessing their severity.

Gallium Scanning

Gallium 67 scanning has not proven to be diagnostic of infective endocarditis because of the high incidence of false-negative results. One report detected a myocardial abscess.[16]

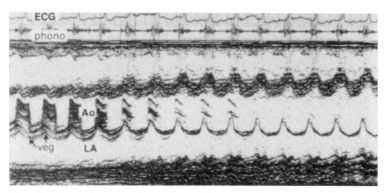

Fig 11–2. M-mode echocardiogram of a patient with severe acute aortic regurgitation due to bacterial endocarditis. Vegetations (*arrows*) on aortic valve that can be noted to prolapse into the left ventricular outflow area. AO = aorta; LA = left atrium; Phono = phonocardiogram; Veg = vegetations. (From Usher B.W., Hendrix G: Severe acute aortic regurgitation: Early recognition and management of life-threatening syndrome. *J. Cardiovasc. Med.* 5:169–181, 1980. Used by permission.)

Laboratory Findings

Anemia and leukocytosis are common and the sedimentation rate is usually elevated. Red blood cells may be found in the urine. Proteinuria, RBC casts, and hematuria are noted with acute proliferative glomerulonephritis. Intravascular infection can give rise to antibodies, hypocomplementemia, rheumatoid factor, and immune complexes, but none is specific for infective endocarditis. Circulating immune complexes are much higher with infective endocarditis than with septicemia not due to infective endocarditis.[17]

Blood Culture

All of the preceding clinical and other studies can strongly suggest endocarditis, which can be confirmed by positive blood cultures. The blood should be cultured both aerobically and anaerobically. There is often discussion pertaining to the optimal time that blood cultures should be drawn and the number of cultures obtained. When bacteremia is present, it is usually persistent, and at least five to six blood cultures should be obtained at 10-minute intervals. Approximately 5 ml of blood should be used for each 30 to 50 ml of medium. After the cultures are drawn, antibiotic therapy should be started based on clinical judgment especially in those who have an acute onset, until the culture results are known. In the subacute forms of infection, therapy can be delayed for a few days until definitive microbiologic results are known. Approximately 5 to 20% of patients thought to have infective endocarditis have persistently negative blood cultures, depending on the population studied. Negative blood cultures may occur because of the absence of endocarditis, prior administration of antibiotics, and the presence of unusual microorganisms which do not grow in the routine media. At times it is best in patients with negative cultures to stop the antibiotic therapy and reculture. There is no specific period of time after the antibiotics are stopped at which the cultures may become positive. However, the longer the period during which the patient received antibiotics, the longer it may take for cultures to become positive. A single positive blood culture when the others of the series are negative can represent contamination. Bacterial sensitivity to antibiotics is best determined by their minimal inhibitory concentration (MIC) and minimal bactericidal concentration (MBC), and the serum bactericidal titers (SBTs) are used to adjust the antibiotic dosage.

DIFFERENTIAL DIAGNOSIS

The clinical picture of infective endocarditis can be confused with many other disease states that give somewhat similar findings, such as nonendocardic septicemias or disseminated lupus erythematosus. Other causes of fever such as influenza, pneumonia, sickle cell anemia, postcardiotomy syndrome, rheumatoid arthritis, meningitis, brain abscess, stroke, acute pericarditis, vasculitis, or lymphomas have to be excluded. Left atrial myxoma should always be considered, since this can produce changing murmurs and emboli. Frequently, in addition to blood cultures, extensive studies must be performed to establish a diagnosis. Among these are urine and stool cultures, serologic studies, and even biopsies. The problem is solved if blood cultures are positive, but when they are negative and the clinical picture is suggestive of endocarditis, one must use clinical judgment if other studies do not yield a diagnosis. A patient with known rheumatic heart disease may develop fever, and in such a case one has to differentiate infective endocarditis from a recurrent attack of acute rheumatic fever. Often in acute rheumatic fever, features such as polyarthritis, erythema marginatum or subcutaneous nodules may not be present. The sedimentation rate and antistreptolysin titers may be high in both conditions. Hematuria, proteinuria, splenomegaly, and bland emboli also can occur in acute rheumatic fever. The presence of acute pericarditis would be more in favor of acute rheumatic fever, although it can occur in acute cases of endocarditis. At times, when the blood cultures are negative, the differential may depend on a therapeutic trial. If the patient fails to respond to antibiotic therapy and promptly responds to salicylates, acute rheumatic fever may be present. After open heart surgery, if fever persists beyond 10 days, it is imperative to undertake investigation for bacterial endocarditis.

TREATMENT

Medical Therapy

The choice of antibiotics is determined on the basis of the causative organism and its sensitivity. Tube dilution sensitivity studies are superior to routine disk sensitivity studies. Disk sensitivity studies do not distinguish bactericidal from bacteriostatic activity and do not separate the most sensitive from more resistant organisms. Bactericidal agents (penicillin, streptomycin, cephalosporin, or vancomycin) should be used if possible instead of bacteriostatic agents (erythromycin, tetracycline, lincomycin, or chloramphenicol). Most cures of endocarditis have been with the penicillins and cephalosporins. Traditionally, serum bactericidal titers (SBTs) have been monitored periodically and the dosage adjusted to produce titers of 1:8. However, a multi-center study using a standardized protocol recommended for optimal medical therapy peak (30 minutes after I.V. or 1 hour after I.M. injection) SBTs of 1:64 or more and trough (less than 30 minutes before next dose) SBTs of 1:32 or more. These titers were associated with bacteriologic cure in all patients. The SBTs of 1:8 had statistically significant predictive accuracy at trough antibiotic levels only. The SBT was a poor predictor of bacteriologic failure or clinical outcome.[18] The sensitivity test and the serum bactericidal tests are in vitro assessments of antibiotic therapy and should be considered along with the clinical course.

Penicillin remains the drug of choice for most infections. The patient often gives a history of penicillin allergy. It is important to dwell upon this history because frequently it is not a true allergy. In some instances desensitization has been accomplished, and the patient was able to tolerate full therapy. Some investigators suggest that antihistamines and steroids be given if there is a question of allergy, or they recommend other antibiotics. Table 11–1 lists many of the causative agents with the preferable initial therapy. Naturally, these regimens may have to be varied, depending on the response. Oral penicillin treatment has been recommended for *streptococcus viridans* but is rather unreliable, since absorption is variable and gastrointestinal symptoms can occur, superinfections are not eliminated and the patient may omit doses. It is seldom advised unless for some reason I.V. therapy cannot be given. In such instances, oral penicillin V plus probenecid can be tried. A combination of penicillin and streptomycin parenterally for 2 weeks has been sucessful in patients who have highly penicillin-susceptible viridans streptococci and no complications such as shock, extracardiac foci of infection, or intracardiac abscess. This short-course regimen is not recommended in patients whose infection involves prosthetic valves or other prosthetic materials. If the patient

TABLE 11–1.   Usual Therapy for Infectious Endocarditis*

Causative Agent	Antibiotics		Duration of Treatment
Streptococcus viridans	Penicillin G, 12 million units/day I.V.	→	4 wk
	plus streptomycin, 0.5 g every (q) 12 hr I.M.	→	2 wk
Enterococcus	Penicillin G, 20 million units/day IV	→	6 wk
	plus gentamicin, 3 mg/kg/day in two divided doses		
Staphylococcus aureus	Nafcillin, 12–16 g/day I.V., or oxacillin,	→	6 wk
	12–16 g/day I.V., or if the infecting strain is pencillin-sensitive (nonpenicillinase-producing), then	→	6 wk
	penicillin G, 40 million units/day I.V., or if	→	6 wk
	penicillin-allergic, cephalothin, 12 g/day	→	6 wk
	I.V., or vancomycin, 1 g q 12 h I.V.	→	6 wk
Gram-negative bacilli	Depending on susceptibility tests, ampicillin, 12–16 g/day I.V. or ticarcillin or piperacillin 18 g/day I.V. or ceftriaxone 2 g/day I.V. or other third-generation cephalosporin 6 g/day I.V.	→	6 wk
	plus gentamicin or tobramycin, 5 mg/kg/day or amikacin, 15 mg/kg/day in divided doses	→	6 wk
Fungal	Amphotericin B, 1.2 mg/kg/day I.V. or every other day if nephrotoxicity develops, plus usually surgery	→	3–6 mo

*Source: Courtesy of W. Edmund Farrar.
MIC = minimual inhibitory concentration.

with *Streptococcus viridan* endocarditis does not respond to penicillin and streptomycin, then cephalothin (Keflin) or vancomycin can be given. Vancomycin is the drug of choice in patients with immediate-type hypersensitivity to penicillin. Cephalosporins should not be used in patients with this immediate type reaction. Other antibiotics used in enterococcal endocarditis are ampicillin and vancomycin. Endocarditis can be caused by staphylococci that are coagulase-positive (*Staphylococcus aureus*) or coagulase-negative (*Staphylococcus epidermidis* and various other species). Both types can infect either native or prosthetic valves. However, most cases of endocarditis due to coagulase-negative organisms occur in patients with valvular prostheses. The treatment of *S. aureus* endocarditis is outlined in Table 11–1. Coagulase-negative staphylococci are usually methicillin-resistant and respond to vancomycin in combination with rifampin and gentamicin. Prosthetic valve endocarditis caused by methicillin-susceptible coagulase-negative staphylococci responds to a semisynthetic penicillinase-resistant penicillin in combination with rifampin and gentamicin. If the patient is allergic to penicillin, a first-generation cephalosporin or vancomycin can be substituted for the penicillinase-resistant penicillin.[18a] Gram-negative endocarditis may respond to a combination of an antigram-negative penicillin or third-generation cephalosporin plus an aminoglycoside (gentamicin, tobramycin, or amikacin); choice of agents must be guided by the results of susceptibility tests.

Many antibiotics can produce toxic reactions; e.g., streptomycin can produce eighth nerve toxicity, and nephrotoxicity can occur with gentamicin. Streptomycin should not be given to patients with renal involvement. The duration and dosage of therapy with such antibiotics should be observed carefully and kidney function monitored.

Fungal endocarditis is becoming more frequent because of prolonged antibiotic therapy, intravascular portal of entry, and cardiac valve abnormalities requiring prosthetic valves. Most endocarditis in drug addicts is bacterial, but there is an increased incidence of fungal endocarditis in such patients. The aortic valve is most often involved, and many cases are due to *Candida albicans*. During I.V. therapy for bacterial endocarditis, there is an increased incidence of superimposed infections with *Candida*. Blood cultures are often positive for *Candida* but not in endocarditis due to other fungi. Because of the bulk of the vegetative mass on the valve, changing heart murmurs and large vessel emboli should suggest fungal endocarditis. Fungal involvement of valves usually requires operation; however, rates of cure with or without adjunctive surgical intervention are low. Amphotericin B (fungizone) is the most useful drug for fungal endocarditis and is continued for 6 to 8 weeks after surgical removal of the infected valve. Nausea, vomiting, and nephrotoxicity may prevent adequate therapy. 5-Fluorocytosine (dosage is 50 to 150 mg/kg at 6-hour intervals) may provide in vivo synergism with amphotericin therapy.

When endocarditis is strongly suspected and blood cultures are negative, therapy should be begun with penicillin G (20 to 40 million units daily I.V.) plus gentamicin (1.7 mg/kg I.V. every 8 hr) for 4 to 6 weeks. If the patient has a prosthetic valve, vancomycin (7.5 mg/kg I.V. every 6 hr) plus gentamicin (1.7 mg/kg I.V. every 8 hr) should be given for 4 to 6 weeks. If there is no response after a few days, the penicillin should be increased, or if the course is fulminant and acute, drugs used for resistant staphylococcus infections should be added.

The recurrence of fever during treatment may indicate drug fever, phlebitis, or embolism and not an unsatisfactory choice of antibiotic.

Surgical Therapy

Surgical therapy is indicated if the patient is deteriorating (because of intractable failure, emboli, or organisms resistant to therapy) and has a correctable lesion. Other indications are septal abscess, recurrence of endocarditis, involvement of AV junctional area, or aneurysms of the sinuses of valsalva. It probably should be performed after a few weeks of therapy but, if necessary, prior to this. This is particularly so for patients with infective endocarditis and acute aortic insufficiency who often need early surgery because of congestive heart failure, or if early mitral valve closure (steep rise in left ventricular diastolic pressure exceeding the elevated left atrial pressure in late diastole) is demonstrated by echocardiography. In fact, Richardson et al.[19] recommended that patients with staphylococcal endocarditis should have surgery regardless of the hemodynamic status. However, most agree that patients with native valve endocarditis due to *Staphylococcus aureus* should be treated medically unless moderate or severe heart failure is present. Appropriate antibiotic therapy even for a few days is better than none. Surgical removal of the tricuspid or pulmonic valve without immediate valve replacement may be necessary for right-sided cases of endocarditis when the infection cannot be eradicated.[20]

Fungal endocarditis is usually an indication for early valve replacement because of the resistance of fungus to medical therapy and the high incidence of emboli.[21]

As mentioned earlier, mortality rates are greater in patients who develop endocarditis early (within 2 months) after prosthetic valve insertion.[8] Often such patients require reoperation along with appropriate antibiotic therapy, especially if during therapy the infection continues, heart failure develops, emboli occur, prosthesis is unstable or obstructed, heart block occurs, or the cause is fungal. Again, Richardson et al.[19] advised early surgery in this group, even without hemodynamic deterioration, if the staphylococcus was the isolate. Prognosis is better for the prosthetic valve endocarditis that occurs late after surgery (after 2 months), and such patients are treated medically unless hemodynamic deterioration occurs, in which case reoperation is performed.

After treatment is completed, patients should be followed up closely, with temperature recordings and repeated cultures at least up to 4 weeks.

PROGNOSIS

Up to 6 months following completion of antibiotic therapy bacterial relapse may occur. Usually, if there is a recurrence after this time, a new infection should be considered.

Before the advent of effective antibiotics, mortality was high. In the pre-antibiotic era, infection was the most common cause of death in patients with bacterial endocarditis, but now congestive heart failure is the most common cause. At times a bacterial cure may be achieved, yet the patient has irreparable cardiac damage with congestive heart failure or develops many sterile emboli or rupture of mycotic aneurysms. Mortality is higher in patients who develop aortic or mitral insufficiency during the endocarditis, whereas preexisting aortic or mitral insufficiency is better tolerated with superimposed endocarditis, unless the insufficiency worsens. The cause of the endocarditis often determines the prognosis. The prognosis is better for *Streptococcus viridans* and worse for infections due to the staphylococcus, enterococcus gram-negative bacteria and fungi.

PROPHYLAXIS

All patients with valvular lesions, congenital heart lesions, or prosthetic valves should have antibiotic prophylaxis against bacterial endocarditis prior to dental procedures or surgery of the GI, urinary, respiratory, or genital tracts, as outlined in Chapter 17. This includes, besides the usual valvular and congenital lesions, mitral valve prolapse, calcified mitral anulus, hypertrophic subaortic stenosis, intracardiac prosthesis, and patches, and excludes uncomplicated secundum atrial septal defect repaired by direct suture without a prosthetic patch and ligated or divided patent ductus arteriosus.

REFERENCES

1. Garvey G.J., Neu H.C.: Infective endocarditis—an evolving disease. *Medicine* 57:105, 1978.
2. Burnside J.W., Desanctis R.W.: Bacterial endocarditis on calcification of the mitral annulus fibrosis. *Ann. Intern. Med.* 76:615, 1972.
3. Wang K., Gobel F.L., Gleason D.F.: Bacterial endocarditis in idiopathic hypertrophic subaortic stenosis. *Am. Heart J.* 89:359, 1975.
4. Rodbard S.: Blood velocity in endocarditis. *Circulation* 27:18, 1963.
5. Arnett E.N., Roberts W.C.: Active infective endocarditis: A clinicopathologic analysis of 137 necropsy patients. *Curr. Probl. Cardiol.* 1:7, 1976.
6. Kein R.S., Recco R.A., Catalano M.T., et al.: Association of streptococcus bovis with carcinoma of the colon. *N. Engl. J. Med.* 297:800, 1977.
7. Banks T., Fletcher R., Ali N.: Infective endocarditis in heroin addicts. *Am. J. Med.* 55:444, 1973.
8. Wilson W.R., Jaumin P.M., Danielson G.K., et al.: Prosthetic valve endocarditis. *Ann. Intern. Med.* 82:751, 1975.
9. Cowgill L.D., Addonizio V.P., Hopeman A.R., et al.: Prosthetic valve endocarditis. *Curr. Probl. Cardiol.* 11:623, 1986.
10. Mayer K.H., Shoenbaum, S.C.: Evaluation and management of prosthetic valve endocarditis. *Proc. Cardiovasc. Dis.* 25:43, 1982.
11. Tuazon C.U., Hill R., Sheagren J.N.: The microbiologic study of street heroin and infection paraphernalia. *J. Infect. Dis.* 129:327, 1974.
12. Amsterdam E.A.: Valve and limitations of echocardiography in endocarditis. *Cardiology* 71:229, 1984.
13. Mintz G.S., Morris M.D., Kotler N.: Clinical value and limitations of echocardiography. *Arch. Intern. Med.* 140:1022, 1980.
14. DeMaria A.N., King J.F., Salel A.F., et al.: Echocardiography and phonography of acute aortic regurgitation in bacterial endocarditis. *Ann. Intern. Med.* 82:329, 1975.
15. Assey M.E., Usher B.W.: Echocardiography in diagnosing and managing aortic valve endocarditis. *South. Med. J.* 74:558, 1981.
16. Spies S.M., Meyers S.M., Barresi A., et al.: A case of myocardial abscess evaluated by radionuclide techniques: A case report. *J. Nucl. Med.* 18:1089, 1977.
17. Bayer A.S., Theofilopoulos A.N., Tillman D., et al.: Use of circulating immune complex levels in the serodifferentiation of endocarditis and nonendocarditic septicemias. *Am. J. Med.* 65:58, 1979.
18. Weinstein M.P., Stratton C.W., Ackley A., et al.: Multicenter collaborative evaluation of a standardized serum bactericidal test as a prognostic indicator of infective endocarditis. *Am. J. Med.* 78:262, 1985.
18a. Bisno A.L., Dismukes W.E., Durack D.T., et al.: Antimicrobial treatment of infective endocarditis due to viridans streptococci, enterococci, and staphylococci. *JAMA* 261:1471, 1989.
20. Arbulu A., Thomas N.W., Wilson R.F.: Valvulectomy without prosthetic replacement. A lifesaving operation for tricuspid pseudomonas endocarditis. *J. Thorac. Cardiovasc. Surg.* 64:103, 1972.
21. Utley J.R., Mills J., Roe B.B.: The role of valve replacement in the treatment of fungal endocarditis. *J. Thorac. Cardiovasc. Surg.* 69:255, 1975.

Chapter 12

MYOCARDIAL DISEASE

Advances in cardiac investigative studies have unveiled a large group of patients primarily with disease of the heart muscle, excluding changes due to hypertension or valvular or coronary artery disease. The cause of many of these conditions remains obscure. The terminology and classification of these myocardial diseases have caused considerable confusion. Various terms, such as primary and secondary myocardial disease, cardiomyopathy, myocardiopathy, myocardosis, myocardial hypertrophy, and others have been used. It is preferable to use the terms "primary" (heart muscle disease of unknown cause) and "secondary" (heart muscle disease of known or suspected cause, often associated with or due to a systemic disease) cardiomyopathies and to further classify these by using Goodwin's[1] functional pathologic classification: congestive, hypertrophic, and restrictive. The congestive type is now called dilated cardiomyopathy and has primary dilated ventricles and impaired systolic function. The hypertrophic type has an increase in myocardial mass, often with asymmetric septal involvement, good contractility and without dilatation, and the restrictive type has a small cavity and can resemble hemodynamically constrictive pericarditis. The latter two types have impaired ventricular filling (diastolic dysfunction). However, there may be overlapping between these three types. Myocarditis will be discussed as a separate entity.

CARDIOMYOPATHIES

The various primary and secondary types (Table 12–1) will be discussed according to Goodwin's functional pathologic classification. Regardless of which classification is used, there will be overlapping.

Dilated Cardiomyopathy

This is the most common type and can occur with both primary (idiopathic) and secondary cardiomyopathies. The ventricles are dilated, and there is impaired systolic ventricular function. Yet the patient may be asymptomatic for several years. Often no cause is found and the final diagnosis is listed as idiopathic dilated cardiomyopathy.

Patients, when symptomatic, often complain of fatigue, weakness, and exertional dyspnea. At times pulmonary edema can occur. Eventually there are symptoms of right-sided failure, such as abdominal swelling and peripheral edema. On physical examination, congestive heart failure is a common feature. The internal jugular pulsations are high into the neck, and there is a narrow pulse pressure and at times pulsus alternans. Cardiomegaly (right and

Table 12–1. Cardiomyopathies

Primary (Idiopathic)	Secondary
Peripartum	Alcoholic
Familial	Granulomatous (sarcoidosis)
Hypertrophic	Connective tissue disease
Endomyocardial fibrosis	Infiltrative
	Neuromuscular diseases
	Metabolic diseases
	Nutritional diseases
	Physical agents
	Toxic agents
	Hematologic diseases

left lifts but not sustained) is usually present, with S_3 and S_4 gallops. Due to the altered architecture of the ventricles, the murmurs of mitral and tricuspid insufficiency can develop. Later, hepatomegaly and peripheral edema are noted. Any type of arrhythmia can occur, but most common are sinus tachycardia, PVBs, and atrial fibrillation. Thrombi can originate in the peripheral veins or in the atria and ventricles, with resulting pulmonary and systemic emboli. Besides the arrhythmias, other ECG features may be biatrial enlargement, biventricular enlargement, conduction disturbances, ST-T changes, and at times Q waves due to myocardial destruction simulating myocardial infarction. The QRS complexes may show low voltage. X rays of the chest (Fig 12–1) will reveal cardiomegaly, predominantly of the left ventricle, and pulmonary congestion. Eventually gross generalized cardiomegaly can occur. Echocardiography (M-mode and two-dimensional and Doppler, Fig 12–2) reveals a dilated heart with poor function, with the mitral valve on M-mode seen clearly in the dilated left ventricle, well separated from the septum. These studies are helpful in excluding primary valvular and pericardial disease and in evaluating ventricular function. Radionuclide studies also show the dilated ventricles and a reduced left ventricular ejection fraction. Cardiac catheterization usually reveals elevated pulmonary capillary wedge, left atrial, and left ventricular end-diastolic pressures. The coronary vessels are usually normal and appear large.

Often no cause for the congestive cardiomyopathy can be found, and it is referred to as idiopathic congestive cardiomyopathy. Usually other types of cardiac disease, such as coronary artery disease, hypertension, and valvular and congenital disease, must be excluded. Alcoholic and peripartum cardiomyopathy present with the picture of dilated cardiomyopathy.

Alcoholic cardiomyopathy. The interest in this entity has been revived because of studies that have shown a decrease in left ventricular performance in normal subjects as well as in those with cardiac disease associated with ethanol intake.[2,3] The mechanism by which alcohol produces dilated cardiomyopathy is not known. Histochemical and ultrastructural studies have not identified specific diagnostic changes due to alcohol. Among the biochemical effects reported are alteration of ionic permeability of cardiac cells, reduced intracellular calcium transfer, reduced myofibrillar ATPase, increased triglyceride extraction, and decreased protein synthesis.[4] Ethanol and its metabolite may be responsible for these biochemical effects. One study[4a] concluded that my-

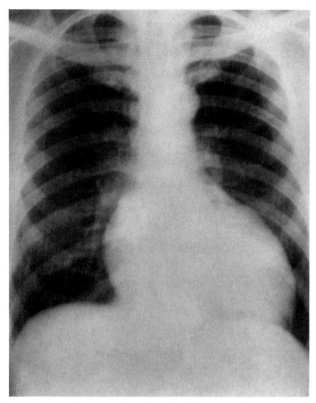

Fig 12–1. Cardiomegaly in a 62-year-old male with dilated cardiomyopathy.

opathy of skeletal muscle and cardiomyopathy are common among persons with chronic alcoholism. Alexander[5] has described myocardial changes in heavy beer drinkers. The cobalt additive, used in the past to prevent excessive foaming, has been implicated as one factor in this disease. Alcoholic cardiomyopathy most often is noted in men who have been drinking beer, wine, or whiskey for several years. Even though it is noted mostly in alcoholics, often in indigent patients, it can also be found in patients with higher economic and social status. Such patients might be successful salesmen who drink heavily at night while entertaining their customers, yet abstain during the daytime while working. Unexplained persistent sinus tachycardia may be the only early sign of the development of cardiomyopathy. Patients may present for the first time with congestive failure, or the disease can be insidious in onset, and the first symptoms are due to arrhythmias, namely, premature beats of various types and atrial fibrillation. Some weekend drinkers and those who drink during the holiday season have developed arrhythmias, and this has been referred to as the "holiday heart syndrome."[6] Subsequently, chronic drinkers develop exertional dyspnea, which becomes progressive. Cardiomegaly often occurs, and the ECG reveals T wave changes or conduction defects. These and other findings are similar to those already described for dilated cardiomyopathy in general. These patients may not have cirrhosis of the liver or beriberi, suggesting that the alcohol may have a direct toxic effect on the heart. They

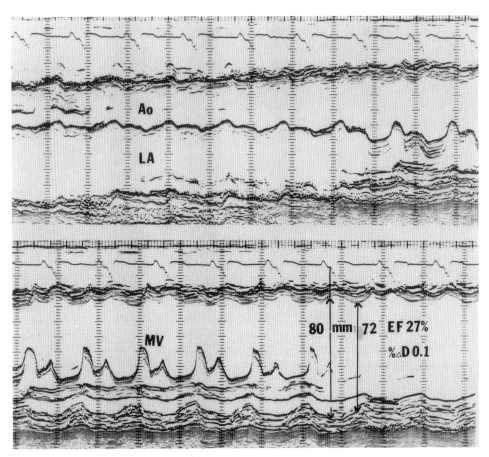

Fig 12–2. M-mode echocardiogram in a patient with dilated cardiomyopathy. Note the dilated hypokinetic left ventricle and left atrium (LA). The ejection fraction (EF) and left ventricular fractional shortening (%ΔD) are markedly reduced. Ao = aorta; LA = left atrium; MV = mitral valve; EF = ejection fraction, %ΔD = left ventricular fractional shortening. (From Usher B.W.: Role of echocardiography in evaluating patients with congestive heart failure. Reprinted by permission of *Medical Times,* 1982, vol. 110, no. 6.)

should be persuaded to stop drinking alcoholic beverages, because the condition, if detected early, may be reversible—otherwise, permanent damage will eventually occur.

Peripartum heart disease. This condition formerly was referred to as postpartum, but peripartum is more appropriate because it also can occur during the last month of pregnancy. Usually this diagnosis is considered if cardiac failure develops in the last month of pregnancy or within 6 months postpartum in a patient with absence of prior heart disease or a cause of the heart failure. It is more common in older, multiparous women and is more frequently associated with toxemia and with twins.[7] The cause and exact relationship to pregnancy are not known, but some studies suggest immunologic factors.[8] The picture is that of a congestive cardiomyopathy. The condition may be reversible, but with subsequent pregnancies recurs, and eventually the changes become permanent, with a downhill course characterized by heart failure and pulmonary and systemic emboli.

Hypertrophic Cardiomyopathy

This has been given a variety of names, but most prefer hypertrophic cardiomyopathy (HCM). There is an increase in ventricular mass, the ventricular cavity is small, and there is impedance to diastolic filling (diastolic dysfunction). The ventricular septum is often thicker than the free left ventricular wall. Because of this latter finding, the term asymmetric septal hypertrophy (ASH) has been used, and if this is associated with left ventricular outflow obstruction, the term idiopathic hypertrophic subaortic stenosis (IHSS) is used. The obstruction to left ventricular ejection is due to narrowing of the outflow tract by the hypertrophied ventricular septum and the anterior leaflet of the mitral valve.[9] It is now recognized that there are a variety of forms of HCM and not just the asymmetric type with or without obstruction. These vary in terms of the patterns and extent of their left ventricular hypertrophy. Other forms that have been noted are concentric left ventricular hypertrophy (symmetric thickening of the left ventricle free wall and septum), hypertrophy confined to the anterior or posterior septum or to the anterolateral free wall and an unusual form confined to the apex (described by the Japanese).[10] The pattern is diffuse in most patients, involving the septum and large portions of the anterolateral free wall with less involvement of the posterior segment of the free wall. Rarely, the right ventricle is involved. Histologic features are bizarrely arranged and shaped muscle cells,[11,12] myocardial scarring, and abnormalities of the small intramural coronary arteries. Hypertrophic cardiomyopathy is genetically transmitted as an autosomal dominant trait. Screening all asymptomatic relatives by echocardiography has been suggested, especially if there has been sudden death in the family. Because the morphologic expression of HCM may not be complete until adulthood, children with a genetic predisposition but normal echocardiographic study should undergo repeat studies at 3-year intervals until adulthood.[13]

The clinical picture varies depending on the presence or absence of left ventricular outflow obstruction. Patients can complain of dyspnea, angina, palpitation, dizziness, and syncope, or be asymptomatic. The first clinical manifestation can be sudden death. On physical examination, those without obstruction may have only a left ventricular lift and an audible and palpable S_4. Those with obstruction (IHSS) have certain additional classic findings. The carotid pulse is brisk and can be bifid due to prominent percussion and tidal waves. This is in contrast to the pulse of aortic valvular stenosis, in which the carotid pulse upstroke is slow and of low amplitude. The apical impulse can be bifid or triple. These are due to the left ventricular lift, interruption of systolic ejection due to the obstruction, and to atrial contraction. A variable intensity, late harsh ejection systolic murmur, simulating to some degree valvular aortic stenosis, is audible but is usually best heard along the left sternal border and at the apex. It radiates to the base of the heart but not into the neck. A systolic thrill may be present. The murmur decreases in intensity with an increase in left ventricular volume, which decreases the obstruction as can occur with sudden lying down, squatting, or the use of phenylephrine (Neo-Synephrine). Amyl nitrite, the Valsalva maneuver, or standing will intensify the murmur due to a decrease in left ventricular volume, which increases the obstruction. A murmur of mitral insufficiency may also be present due to changes in the mitral valve or its apparatus. Rarely a low-pitched mitral diastolic murmur can be heard due to left ventricular inflow obstruction by the thick septum or abnormal filling or to transmitral flow because at times the mitral regurgitation can be severe.

The chest x ray may show a normal-sized heart, but eventually left ventricular enlargement due to hypertrophy can be noted. If significant mitral regurgitation is present, the left atrium is enlarged. The ECG reveals left ventricular hypertrophy and, in addition, may simulate an infarction pattern, with deep Q waves in the inferior and left precordial leads (Fig 12–3). The Q waves can be due to septal hypertrophy and fibrosis. However, Cosio et al.[14] found that myopathic septal muscle has different electrophysiologic properties from those of the remainder of the myocardium that may account for the septal Q waves. The apex form of HCM has giant T wave inversion in the midprecordial leads.[10] Left atrial enlargement and ventricular arrhythmias may be present. Atrial fibrillation can be a late finding. The echocardiogram has certain features that are helpful in the diagnosis. The septal hypertrophy should give a septal to free wall ratio of 1.3 to 1.0 or more at the end of diastole for the diagnosis of ASH. Two-dimensional echo will rule out the false positives that may be noted on M-mode. The anterior leaflet of the mitral valve during systole can be displaced toward the septum (SAM), and midsystolic closure of the aortic valve is noted if there is a gradient. SAM can be found in other conditions as left ventricular hypertrophy, conditions that have increased in contractility and in transposition of the great arteries. The decrease in left ventricular compliance can produce a decreased rate of closure of the mitral

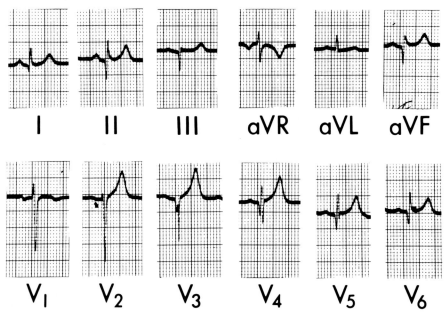

Fig 12–3. Electrocardiogram of a patient with idiopathic hypertrophic subaortic stenosis (IHSS). Note deep Q waves in the inferior and anterior leads that simulate an infarction. (From Gazes P.C.: Recognition of acute myocardial infarction, in *Chest Pain: Problems in Differential Diagnosis*, vol. 3, No. 1. By permission of Biomedical Information Corp., New York. Copyright 1977 by Marion Laboratories, Inc., Kansas City, Mo.)

valve. Figure 12–4 shows the features of IHSS. Two-dimensional echocardiography can demonstrate clearly the septal hypertrophy, mitral valve motion, and small left ventricular cavity. In addition, it can show the segmental hypertrophy in other locations as at the apex and free wall. Doppler studies confirm the presence of mitral regurgitation. Radionuclide scanning can also detect HCM. Cardiac catheterization and angiocardiograms can outline the obstruction and show a subvalvular gradient which may be labile. Amyl nitrite, a Valsalva maneuver, or isoproterenol can produce or increase the gradient. The left atrial and left ventricular end-diastolic pressures are often

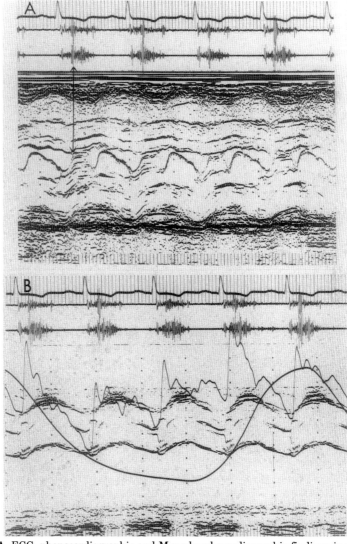

Fig 12–4. **A**, ECG, phonocardiographic and M-mode echocardiographic findings in patient with idiopathic hypertrophic subaortic stenosis (IHSS). Note typical murmur with "septal slap" (*arrow*), asymmetric septal hypertrophy and systolic anterior motion of the mitral valve (*arrow*). **B**, further features of this patient. Note bifid carotid pulse (spike and dome) and midsystolic aortic valve closure. (Courtesy of Dr. Bruce W. Usher.)

elevated. The arterial pressure tracing may have a "spike and dome" configuration (Fig 12–4, B). After a spontaneous or provoked premature ventricular contraction, the increased contractility with the next beat will produce a decrease in pulse pressure in the arterial tracing. Figure 12–5 summarizes the main features seen in IHSS.

Patients who have symptoms of dyspnea, syncope, angina, or documented arrhythmias should be treated with a β-adrenergic blocking agent. Most experience to date has been with propranolol. One study indicated that for relief of symptoms, doses greater than 320 mg per day may be necessary.[15] β-blockers decrease the determinants of myocardial oxygen consumption, prevent increase in outflow obstruction that can occur with exercise, and improve diastolic ventricular filling. It is still not known whether asymptomatic patients should be treated, for it has not been shown that sudden death can be prevented. One study showed that asymptomatic ventricular arrhythmia is common in patients with hypertrophic cardiomyopathy and its frequency was not reduced with β-adrenergic blocking therapy.[16] Patients should have a 24-hour Holter monitoring. If patients have arrhythmias or a family history of sudden death, even though they have no other symptoms, they should be treated with propranolol and an antiarrhythmic drug if necessary. Amiodarone can be effective for the treatment of supraventricular or ventricular tachyarrhythmias that do not respond to conventional antiarrhythmic agents.[17] However, disopyramide (Norpace) in some patients relieved symptoms by decreasing the pressure gradient because of its negative inotropic effect, which could be due to the effect on calcium kinetics.[18] Sudden death can occur in those with or

IDIOPATHIC HYPERTROPHIC SUBAORTIC STENOSIS (IHSS)

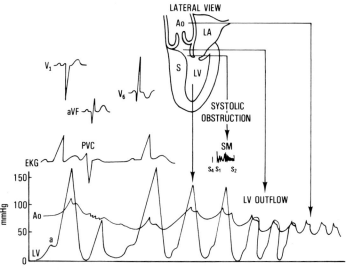

Fig 12–5. Main findings in IHSS. Left ventricular lift and double or triple apical impulse. Ejection systolic murmur (SM) loudest along the left sternal border and at the apex. S_4 sound prominent. Carotid pulse and aortic pressure (Ao) have a brisk upstroke and are bifid (spike and dome). ECG shows left ventricular hypertrophy and deep Q waves. The aortic pulse pressure is diminished following a premature ventricular contraction (PVC). Left ventricular (LV) pressure drops in the outflow tract and remains at this level into the aorta (Ao). Lateral view ventriculogram reveals systolic left ventricular outflow obstruction.

without obstruction.[19] It also can occur with strenuous exercise. In one study[20] of sudden death in 29 patients, 14 had hypertrophic cardiomyopathy. Such patients should be advised to avoid strenuous exercise. Sudden death is more common in younger patients and is rare after age 40. Some families have a malignant form of the disease and a propensity to sudden death.[21] One study concluded that the natural history of hypertrophic cardiomyopathy may be more benign than can be inferred from published reports from referral institutions that include highly symptomatic patients. Twenty-four outpatients who were asymptomatic or had mild symptoms were followed for a mean period of 4.4 years and none died or had clinical deterioration.[21a] Recently verapamil has been used with some success in symptomatic patients with IHSS not responding to a β-adrenergic blocker.[22] However, one must be careful, for calcium blockers can decrease afterload (especially nifedipine) due to arteriolar vasodilation, and thus they may increase the obstruction and the gradient. Verpamil should not be used in patients with high left ventricular filling pressure for pulmonary edema or sudden death can occur. If the hypertrophic cardiomyopathy is without obstruction, calcium blockers may increase exercise tolerance by improving diastolic function, i.e., increasing the compliance of the left ventricle, probably because isovolumic expansion is calcium-dependent. Atrial fibrillation can be catastrophic, and if the response is not immediate with administration of I.V. propranolol, then dc shock should be carried out. Digitalis can increase contractility and the obstruction, so generally it should not be used. However, if the atrial fibrillation cannot be reverted or is recurrent, the ventricular rate can be controlled with digitalis alone or with propranolol. Digitalis can also be used if there is heart failure without evidence of left ventricular outflow obstruction. Some patients may be transformed from the typical HCM to a dilated form of cardiomyopathy. This may be due to left ventricular scarring, myocardial infarction, or after surgical resection of the septum. Long-term oral anticoagulants should be given if the atrial fibrillation is established.[23] Drugs that can reduce preload, such as nitrates and diuretics, should be avoided because they may increase the obstruction. Prophylactic therapy for bacterial endocarditis should be given, especially for the obstructive type. A portion of the thickened septum can be resected (myotomy-myectomy) in patients who do not respond to medical therapy and have a resting systolic gradient of over 50 mm Hg. Occasionally the mitral valve is replaced to relieve the subaortic obstruction.

Restrictive Cardiomyopathy

Restrictive cardiomyopathy is not as common as the congestive and hypertrophic types. Patients have good systolic function, but ventricular filling is impeded (diastolic dysfunction) because the endocardial or myocardial disease produces rigid walls that do not stretch well. Endomyocardial fibrosis is the most common cause; however, in the Western world, amyloid is more common. Other causes are hemochromatosis, glycogen storage, fibroelastosis, neoplastic infiltration and collagen-vascular diseases.

Such patients complain of weakness and dyspnea. The jugular venous pulsations can be elevated and the pulse pressure narrow. Mitral and tricuspid murmurs may be present because of papillary muscle involvement or distortion of the ventricular cavities. S_4 and S_3 gallops may be audible. Kussmaul's sign (inspiratory increase in venous pressure) can be noted. This latter finding and findings of systemic visceral congestion can make it difficult to differentiate this condition from constrictive pericarditis. The ECG may show nonspecific ST-T changes, conduction disturbances, left ventricular hypertrophy, or diminished QRS voltage. Echocardiography may reveal a thickened left ventricle. Hemodynamic studies may resemble constrictive pericarditis. Pressures in all chambers are elevated, but in restrictive conditions the left-sided pressures are usually higher and the systolic pulmonary artery pressure is often greater than that in constrictive pericarditis. The ventricular pressure curves can show the early diastolic dip with rapid rise to a plateau as noted with constrictive pericarditis (see Chap. 13). Endomyocardial biopsy, CT scanning and MR imaging are helpful in differentiating these two conditions.

Amyloidosis. Amyloidosis is an infiltrative form of cardiomyopathy that can produce a restrictive picture. It can present with or without other organ involvement. It is usually associated with a monoclonal gammopathy or plasma cell myeloma.[24] The diagnosis is easier if there are extracardiac features. Patients may have a beefy appearance of the face and macroglossia. Pupura, peripheral neuropathy, autonomic nerve involvement (which can produce postural hypotension), and polyarthropathy may be present. The cardiac manifestations can be those described previously for restrictive cardiomyopathies. However, with extensive involvement, systolic dysfunction can occur, and the picture of congestive cardiomyopathy can develop. The ECG can resemble an old anteroseptal infarction with low QRS voltage and infrequently an old inferior infarction. Arrhythmias and conduction defects can be present. Cardiomegaly is noted on chest x ray. Echocardiography may show increased ventricular wall, septum, atrial wall, and valvular thickening, with a normal or small ventricular cavity. Two-dimensional echocardiography shows a granular sparkling appearance of the thickened myocardium. The diagnosis can be made by rectal biopsy, although it has also been demonstrated in biopsy of other tissues, such as the gingiva. Satisfactory treatment for amyloidosis is not available. Patients are sensitive to digitalis. Conduction abnormalities may occur that require insertion of a pacemaker.

Endomyocardial fibrosis. Tropical endomyocardial fibrosis and Löffler's disease (hypereosinophilic syndrome) are now considered as the same entity,[25] although that seen in the tropics has less eosinophilia and the two diseases have some different clinical presentations. Eosinophils are present in multiple organs. Eosinophilic infiltration of the heart produces focal necrosis, mural thrombi, and endomyocardial fibrotic thickening. Both ventricles can be involved, as well as the mitral and tricuspid valves. Heart failure can develop, and embolic phenomenon can occur. Tropical endomyocardial fibrosis has a right ventricular form, a left ventricular form, or a mixed form with both ventricles affected. Cardiac involvement in Löffler's disease is often biventricular. The symptoms and findings of these two variants of the same disease depend on the ventricle involved. Predominant right-sided disease may present with the cardiac findings of a restrictive cardiomyopathy. Endomyocardial biopsy may establish the diagnosis. Corticosteroids are of questionable value. Heart failure is treated in the usual manner, and anticoagulants should be considered to prevent embolism. Surgical resection of the thickened endocardium with repair or replacement of the mitral or tricuspid valves (if there is significant regurgitation) has given some short-term improvement.[26]

Myocardial Involvement in Systemic Diseases

Many systemic diseases can produce cardiac involvement. Usually the cardiac picture, if the myocardium is diffusely involved, is that of the congestive type, although combinations of the restrictive and congestive types can occur. Several of these entities will be briefly discussed, since there are no specific cardiac findings and the diagnosis is made by recognizing the systemic disease or agent that involved many organ systems.

Sarcoidosis. Approximately 25% of patients with sarcoidosis have cardiac involvement at autopsy.[27] Granulomas can be noted in the myocardium, conduction system, ventricular septum, papillary muscle, pericardium, and in the aorta. Findings of systemic sarcoidosis can be present as fever, dyspnea, skin nodules, and keratoconjunctivitis sicca. However, only the cardiac manifestations may be present. The patient can present with arrhythmias—namely, ventricular—or heart block. In fact, one should suspect sarcoidosis in a young person with complete AV heart block. Mitral regurgitation can occur because of infiltration into the papillary muscle or left ventricular enlargement. Sudden death is common in patients with cardiac involvement. Pulmonary sarcoid is more prevalent in the black population. Chest x ray may reveal hilar adenopathy and pulmonary infiltrates. Extensive pulmonary involvement can produce cor pulmonale. Hyperglobulinemia of the gamma fraction, hypercalcemia, and a negative tuberculin test should make one suspect sarcoid. Thallium 201 imaging may show cold spots in the myocardium. Definite diagnosis depends on biopsy of nodes or skin lesions if these are present. Endomyocardial biopsy may reveal the diagnosis. Corticosteroids may be beneficial. Arrhythmias are difficult to control, but with addition of corticosteroids, results have been better. A permanent pacing is necessary for complete heart block.

Connective tissue diseases. Lupus erythematosus, progressive systemic sclerosis (scleroderma), polyarteritis nodosa, dermatomyositis, rheumatoid arthritis, ankylosing spondylitis, and Reiter's syndrome can directly or indirectly involve the myocardium. The diagnosis is generally made because of the extracardiac manifestations. Most of these conditions are autoimmune disorders.

Lupus erythematosus (LE) is a fairly common disease noted more often in women. It can involve the skin, joints, kidneys, heart, and brain. It frequently involves the pericardium, but can also involve the endocardium and myocardium. Nonbacterial verrucae are nonspecific vegetations involving primarily the mitral valve, although the other valves may be involved. This endocardial involvement is referred to as Libman-Sacks disease. Fibrinoid necrosis can involve the interstitial tissues and blood vessels in the myocardium. Arteritis of the coronary vessels can produce myocardial infarction. The diagnosis is suspected because of the other systemic findings and the ANA findings. The finding of blood LE cell is specific if rheumatoid arthritis, drug reactions, or lupoid hepatitis can be excluded. Corticosteroids and at times immunosuppressive agents are given along with the cardiac medications necessary if arrhythmias or heart failure are present.

Scleroderma produces changes in the skin, esophagus, intestines, kidneys, lungs, and heart. Pericarditis and myocardial fibrosis can occur, but no valvular involvement has been noted. The picture may be that of a restrictive cardiomyopathy, but if the involvement is extensive, a congestive cardiomyopathy picture develops. Kidney involvement can produce hypertension with further strain on the heart. Rarely, cor pulmonale can occur because of pulmonary parenchymal or pulmonary vascular lesions. Raynaud's phenomenon is commonly present. Cutaneous lesions and GI tract symptoms, especially esophageal, suggest the diagnosis. The term crest syndrome has been used when there are calcinosis, Raynaud's phenomena, esophageal abnormality, sclerodactyly, and telangiectasia. The cardiac lesions have been detected by the use of radionuclide studies and echocardiography. Indomethacin can be given for pericarditis. Steroids have been used for the pericardial and myocardial changes, although the benefits are uncertain. The interrelationship between structural and functional (vasospastic) small-vessel disease is not clear. If Raynaud's phenomenon of the heart occurs, as has been hypothesized to account for the myocardial pathology,[28] vasodilators (nitrates and calcium-blockers) may be of value. Since angiotensin can cause direct vascular injury, captopril (angiotension-converting enzyme inhibitor) has been used, especially for renal involvement.[29] White blood cell and differential counts should be made, for neutropenia has rarely (0.3% of patients) been observed in patients taking captopril, especially in those with SLE and renal impairment. The counts should be performed before starting treatment, at approximately 2-week intervals for the first 3 months of therapy, and periodically thereafter.

Polyarteritis nodosa is a necrotizing vascular disease that can involve the coronary arteries and even produce a myocardial infarction. The skin and many organ systems can be involved. The renal involvement can cause systemic hypertension, which is noted in most cases. Biopsy of active inflammatory sites, such as the skin, muscles, or testicles, may prove the diagnosis. The prognosis is grave, but treatment with steroids may give some improvement.

Mucocutaneous lymph node syndrome can have periarteritis lesions. This has been referred to as "Kawasaki disease," which can involve the coronary arteries in infants and produce aneurysms of the coronary arteries, myocardial infarction, and sudden death.[30]

Polymyositis and dermatomyositis (skin involvement) are diffuse inflammatory diseases affecting the striated muscles, skin, and joints. The cardiac muscle, pericardium, and conducting system can be involved. Arrhythmias of all types may be frequent. Corticosteroids and immunosuppressive drugs have been of some benefit.

Rheumatoid arthritis is recognized by the characteristic joint deformities. Nodular granulomas can involve the heart, and arteritis of the small vessels can occur. Pericarditis has been noted frequently by echocardiography, even though it may not produce symptoms. There may also be myocardial and valvular involvement. Conduction disorders can occur. Anti-inflammatory drugs and corticosteroids are usually prescribed.

Ankylosing spondylitis is now considered separate from rheumatoid arthritis, even though they are related. This involves the dorsal spine and eventually produces kyphosis and immobilization of the spine. This inflammatory lesion can affect the aortic root and the basal portion of the aortic cusps and produce aortic insufficiency.[31] Reiter's syndrome[32] can produce similar aortic root involvement. Conjunctivitis, iritis, urethritis, keratotic skin lesions, and arthritis complete this picture of Reiter's syndrome.

Infiltrative diseases. Amyloid has already been discussed. Hemochromatosis and glycogen storage disease also are in this category. Hemochromatosis is due to excessive deposits of iron in the connective tissue, liver, heart, and many other organs of the body. It can be idiopathic or secondary to increased dietary iron, drugs, increased absorption in pancreatic insufficiency, chronic anemias, or chronic liver disease, or to transfusions. Iron is deposited in the myocardium and conducting system with resultant fibrosis, cardiomegaly, and heart failure. A restrictive or dilated cardiomyopathy can develop. Skin pigmentation (bronze appearance), diabetes, hepatomegaly, and cardiac failure should alert one to the diagnosis. Liver biopsy can establish the diagnosis. Phlebotomies, reducing iron intake, and iron-chelating agents (such as desferrioxamine) may help. Heart failure is treated in the usual way.

Glycogen storage disease is an abnormality of carbohydrate metabolism due to a deficiency of acid maltase (Pompe's disease). As a result, there is excessive glycogen in cardiac and skeletal muscles and other tissues. Heart failure occurs early in life, and massive cardiomegaly with thickened ventricles can be present. Muscle weakness, neurologic abnormalities, and a large tongue are other features. Skeletal muscle biopsy can confirm the diagnosis by demonstrating increased glycogen. Death usually occurs within the first year of life and is the result of heart failure or lung complications.

Neuromuscular diseases. Progressive muscular dystrophies, especially the Duchenne type, are hereditary and characterized by progressive muscular weakness. The myocardium may be involved, and often characteristic ECG features can appear. The changes simulate an anterolateral infarction in that the R waves are prominent in the V_1 position, and there are deep Q waves in the left precordial leads. Becker's muscular dystrophy has a late onset and survival to middle age is not uncommon. All four cardiac chambers can be involved. Limb-girdle dystrophy of ERB presents with progressive weakness of the hips and shoulders and cardiac involvement is infrequent. Landouzy-Dejerine (facioscapulohumeral) dystrophy begins with facial involvement and then progresses to the arms and shoulders. Cardiac involvement may be atrial standstill (absence of P waves in the electrocardiogram and of A waves in the jugular venous pulse). Friedreich's disease, due to degeneration of the spino-cerebellar tracts, corticospinal tract, medulla, and cerebellum, may have myocardial involvement (hypokinesis or hypertrophy of left ventricle) in addition to progressive ataxia. Myotonic dystrophy (Streinert disease) characterized by muscle weakness and atrophy may develop cardiomegaly and AV and bundle-branch block. The His-Purkinje system is involved more than the myocardium.

Metabolic diseases. Endocrine diseases associated with cardiomyopathy will be discussed in Chapter 14. Electrolyte disturbances such as deficiencies of potassium, phosphate, or magnesium can produce cardiomyopathy. Hypokalemia can be suspected from the ECG ST-T changes, U waves, and prolonged Q-T interval. Individuals consuming large quantities of aluminum hydroxide gel, which binds phosphate, can develop cardiomegaly and failure, which can clear with phosphorus replacement.[33] Hypomagnesemia can occur with excessive alcohol intake.

Mucopolysaccharidosis is associated with mucopolysaccharide deposits in the tissues. One type, Hunter-Hurler syndrome, has deposits in the myocardium, thickening and fibrous nodules in the valves, and intimal proliferation of the coronary and pulmonary arteries. Cardiomegaly and murmurs of mitral and aortic insufficiency may develop. Other features are skeletal abnormalities, hepatosplenomegaly, corneal clouding, and mental retardation. Excessive amounts of mucopolysaccharides are excreted in the urine.

Nutritional diseases. Beriberi cardiomyopathy can be due to thiamine (vitamin B_1) deficiency and is most likely to occur in alcoholics. The peripheral vascular resistance is decreased. The cardiac picture is that of high-output failure similar to thyrotoxicosis. The skin is warm, pulse pressure is widened, and the cardiac apical impulse is prominent. Other findings such as peripheral neuritis, glossitis, dermatitis, and anemia may be present.

Selenium (a trace element) deficiency in China has been shown to produce a dilated cardiomyopathy, and a case was reported in this country in an occidental patient.[34]

Physical agents. Radiation to the thorax during radiotherapy may produce pericardial, coronary artery, and myocardial damage. Chronic pericarditis with or without effusion or constriction and myocardial fibrosis can occur. Such events usually appear several months to years after the exposure, seldom immediately.

Extreme cold or heat, by producing changes in the peripheral circulation, can be detrimental to patients with heart disease. They can directly damage the myocardium. Myocardial hemorrhage and infarction can occur. The electrocardiogram in hypothermia may develop a "J type" deflection between the QRS and the ST segment (Osborne wave).

Electricity and lightning can produce cardiac damage. Annually there are over 1200 deaths from electric current accidents and lightning injuries.[35] Amperage (amperes = volts/ohms) is the measure of current flow per unit of time and is the most important single factor in human electrocution. The following approximations as to various effects of current flow in humans for 60 Hz alternating currents are generally recognized:[36]

> 0.001 amperes—barely perceptible tingle
> 0.016 amperes—"let go" current
> 0.020 amperes—muscular paralysis
> 0.100 amperes—ventricular fibrillation
> 2.000 amperes—ventricular standstill

Dry skin resistance can be up to 100,000 ohms. Therefore, one in contact with 120 volts (common household current) would get 0.001 amperes (120 volts/100,000 ohms), which gives a tingle. However, water or sweat-soaked skin resistance often drops to 1000 ohms and, in this case, the amperes would be 0.120 (120 volts/1,000 ohms), which can produce ventricular fibrillation. The electrical injuries that require intensive care are often caused by high tension trauma (over 350 volts). Almost all electrical injuries are caused by alternating current. Low-tension injuries (less than 350 volts) commonly lock a person to the contact, whereas above this usually throws the subject from the site of contact. Lightning injury is the most common form of direct current trauma. Lightning bolts usually contain 12,000 to 20,000 amperes and may reach energies of a hundred million volts and over 200,000 amperes peak current.[37] This degree of energy is seldom reached in high-voltage injuries. The lightning current passes through the body and is dissipated in the ground. Depending on the amount of electrical energy, duration of the current, resistance of skin, and course of the current, a variety of systemic findings can occur. Electricity and lightning can cause burns and neurologic or cardiac injuries. Vascular injuries are common if the current follows the path of blood vessels. Many arrhythmias and ST-T changes can occur which may be transient or permanent. Lightning can produce myocardial contusion or necrosis with ECG changes resembling an infarct.[38] Late findings can occur as myoglobinuria. Lightning more often induces ventricular standstill and electrical injuries induce ventricular fibrillation. Respiratory arrest produced by lightning often lasts longer than asystole. One must be prepared to give basic and advanced cardiac life support to victims with such injuries.

Toxic agents. Many drugs and chemicals can affect the myocardium and cause cardiac toxicity, hypersensitive reactions, or cardiomyopathy. Among these are psychotherapeutic agents and sedatives, such as phenothiazine and antidepressant drugs; antibiotics and chemotherapeutic agents, such as penicillin, streptomycin, antimalarials, and emetine; antineoplastic agents, such as adriamycin; and metallic compounds, such as arsenic, antimony, and cobalt. Even drugs used to treat cardiac problems can be toxic.

Not all drug reactions will be discussed, for there are many excellent reviews[39] on this subject; only those recently encountered more frequently will be mentioned. Many of these produce only arrhythmias, not the full picture of a cardiomyopathy.

Tricyclic antidepressant drugs may produce toxicity by their myocardial depression, anticholinergic, or adrenergic neuron effects.[40] However, toxicity is usually noted in patients who have received high doses or have severe impairment of myocardial performance. Toxic doses can produce arrhythmia, myocardial infarction, heart failure, and sudden death. Imipramine (Tofranil), Nortriptyline (Aventyl, Pamelor) and amitriptyline (Elavil) can delay conduction velocity and resemble a type I antiarrhythmic drug such as quinidine. Amitriptyline (Elavil) has the greatest anticholinergic effect, and desipramine (Pertofrane, Norpramin), trazodone (Desyrel) and maprotiline (Ludiomil) the least anticholinergic effect. Doxepin and amitriptyline have the greatest α-adrenergic blocking effect. The tricyclic antidepressant drugs can produce postural hypotension. It is important to select an antidepressant drug with consideration of the patient's cardiac problem. Such drugs may be given safely to many patients with cardiovascular disease. Newer preparations with fewer cardiac effects will soon be available.

Doxorubicin (Adriamycin), an antineoplastic agent, can produce cardiac toxicity. Early evidence of cardiac changes may be arrhythmias, ST-T changes, and decrease in QRS voltage. Heart failure is unusual in dosages below 550 mg/m^2.[41] However, cardiotoxicity can occur with lower doses. Sequential radionuclide studies (MUGA) can detect early changes. Endomyocardial biopsy detects toxicity more often than noninvasive studies.

Lithium is a popular drug used for manic-depressive disease. It can produce ST-T changes, arrhythmias, and, rarely, heart failure.

Certain drugs can produce hypersensitive reactions, such as penicillin, phenylbutazone, methyldopa, and others. Anaphylaxis, serum sickness, and vaccines may produce myocardial reactions. Direct myocardial changes are noted by ECG abnormalities, myocarditis, and arrhythmias.

Hematologic diseases. Leukemia, polycythemia vera, and sickle cell anemia may affect the heart. Myocardial infiltration can occur in 50% of patients with leukemia and rarely in Hodgkin's disease. The cardiac and other manifestations of sickle cell anemia can mimic those of acute rheumatic fever. Mitral systolic and diastolic murmurs may appear. The chronic anemia and thrombosis of small intracardiac vessels produce myocardial changes. Thrombosis of the small pulmonary arteries and pulmonary endarteritis may lead to cor pulmonale.

MYOCARDITIS

Myocarditis is an inflammation of the myocardium and can be due to bacterial, viral, fungal, or parasitic infections. It is often idiopathic (Fiedler's). Bacterial infections with streptococcus, staphylococcus, and others can produce myocardial involvement. Such changes can occur directly by microorganisms or indirectly by bacterial toxins, such as those from diphtheria, pneumonia, or streptococcal infections, or may occur as an autoimmune reaction as noted with acute rheumatic fever. Myocarditis may be encountered during systemic infections such as those with typhoid fever, meningococcemia, and acute rheumatic fever. Coxsackievirus B is the most common viral cause of myocarditis. Measles, mumps, influenza, infectious mononucleosis, chickenpox, and generalized vaccinia are other causes. Actinomycosis, histoplasmosis, coccidioidomycosis, and moniliasis and other fungal infections can invade the myocardium. Parasites such as malaria, trypanosomiasis, trichinosis, or schistosomiasis also may involve the myocardium. One study[42] reported that 50% of 60 patients with human immunodeficiency virus (HIV) infection had unsuspected cardiac abnormalities (left ventricular dilatation and hypokinesis, pericardial effusion, repolarization ECG changes, and ventricular tachycardia) as detected by echo and Holter monitoring. The abnormalities were higher in patients with more advanced disease (AIDS) than those who were asymptomatic.

The clinical features of myocarditis are nonspecific. Fever, weakness, sinus tachycardia, arrhythmias, gallops, cardiomegaly, heart failure, and leukocytosis are some of the common features in severe cases. Pericarditis may be present. The tachycardia is often persistent and is out of proportion to the fever. Most patients do not have findings so overt or so severe. Many have only transient ECG changes that indicate subclinical or focal myocardial involvement. At times the symptoms and findings of the systemic illness (rash, arthralgias, pulmonary symptoms) may mask the cardiac features.

Electrocardiographic, echocardiographic, and radioisotope studies, x ray of the chest, and cardiac catheterization do not give any specific findings that can indicate the etiology of the myocarditis. These procedures can detect cardiomegaly and pericardial effusion and also help to exclude other types of cardiac conditions. Special viral studies (antibody titer during acute phase and at 2 and 6 weeks), cultures (blood, throat washing, feces, urine), monospot test, tests for cold agglutinins and surface antigens (hepatitis), and other tests depending on the clinical features should be done. Gallium scintigraphy has shown myocardial uptake in some studies but lacks sensitivity and specificity.

At times right ventricular endomyocardial biopsy may detect inflammatory changes. Biopsy material should be cultured and examined by electron microscopy and immunofluorescent techniques.

Treatment is directed at the specific cause, if one is identified. However, often supportive therapy and the usual therapy for heart failure, arrhythmias, and other cardiac complications are all that can be done. Immunosuppressive agents (prednisone and azathioprine) may be beneficial to patients with acute inflammatory myocarditis, but the evidence is circumstantial.[43,44]

Patients can have a fulminating course with myocarditis, with death; they may recover but continue to have different degrees of cardiac damage; or they may recover completely.

ENDOMYOCARDIAL BIOPSY

Cardiac biopsy has been performed more extensively during the past several years since specific indications have evolved and the procedure is safe.[45,46] It has led to a significant increase in our understanding of the etiology and pathogenesis of dilated cardiomyopathy. Myocarditis, infiltrative diseases such as amyloidosis, heart transplant rejection, and doxorubicin (adriamycin) cardiotoxicity can now be detected by biopsy. Myocarditis may be detected in 10 to 15% of patients with cardiomyopathy who have unexplained ventricular arrhythmias, syncope, new-onset congestive failure, and extreme fatigue.[46] Such cases at times can respond to immunosuppressive drugs.[43,44] Table 12–2 lists the indications for myocardial biopsy. The right and left ventricles can be biopsied. However, because most myocardial diseases are diffuse, the right ventricle is most often the sampling site. Currently the left ventricle is usually biopsied for research purposes.

APPROACH TO UNDIAGNOSED CARDIOMEGALY

It is best to approach the patient with cardiomegaly with a set classification of conditions to avoid misdiagnosis. The following classification has been of help to me when faced with this problem:

1. Usual types of heart disease. Rheumatic, valvular, hypertensive, syphilitic, coronary, and congenital heart disease are the commonest.
2. High-output syndromes. These conditions have altered O_2 tension, metabolic defects or shunts decreasing the peripheral vascular resistance, as occurs in hyperthyroidism, beriberi, anemia, systemic arteriovenous fistula, cor pulmonale, hepatic disease, Paget's disease of bone, or polycythemia vera.
3. Specific hypertensive conditions. Hypertension associated with renal arterial or parenchymal diseases, pheochromocytoma, primary aldosteron-

Table 12–2. **Indications For Endomyocardial Biopsy**

1. Detecting myocarditis
2. Detecting infiltrative myocardial disease
3. Differentiating restrictive from constrictive heart disease
4. Detecting and grading cardiac transplant rejection
5. Detecting and grading adriamycin cardiotoxicity

ism, Cushing's syndrome, and coarctation of the aorta are included in this category.

4. Endocardial lesions other than rheumatic. Infective endocarditis, carcinoid, Marfan's syndrome, lupus, and rheumatoid should be considered.

5. Myocardial diseases. Primary and secondary cardiomyopathies or myocarditis must be excluded.

6. Pericardial diseases. Pericardial effusion can mimic a large heart.

REFERENCES

1. Goodwin J.F.: Prospects and predictions for the cardiomyopathies. *Circulation* 50:210, 1974.
2. Friedman H.S., Lieber C.S.: Cardiotoxicity of alcohol. *Cardiovasc. Med.* 2:111, 1977.
3. Regan T.J., Levinson G.E., Oldewurtel H.A., et al.: Ventricular function in noncardiacs with alcoholic fatty liver: Role of ethanol in the production of cardiomyopathy. *J. Clin. Invest.* 48:397, 1969.
4. Regan T.J.: Alcoholic cardiomyopathy. *Prog. Cardiovasc. Dis.* 27:141, 1984.
4a. Urbano-Marquez A., Estrugh R., Navarro-Lopez F., et al.: The effects of alcoholism on skeletal and cardiac muscle. *New Engl. J. Med.* 320:409, 1989.
5. Alexander C.S.: Cobalt-beer cardiomyopathy: A clinical and pathological study of twenty-eight cases. *Am. J. Med.* 53:395, 1972.
6. Ettinger P.O., Wu C.F., DeLaCruz C., et al.: Arrhythmias and the "holiday heart": Alcohol-associated cardiac rhythm disorders. *Am. Heart J.* 95:555, 1978.
7. Demakis J.G., Rahimtoola S.H., Sutton G.E., et al.: Natural course of peripartum cardiomyopathy. *Circulation* 44:1053, 1971.
8. Knobel B., Melamud E., Kishon Y.: Peripartum cardiomyopathy. *Israel J. Med. Sci.* 20:1061, 1984.
9. Braunwald E., Morrow A.G., Cornell W.P., et al.: Idiopathic hypertrophic subaortic stenosis: Clinical, hemodynamic and angiographic manifestations. *Am. J. Med.* 29:924, 1960.
10. Yamaguchi H., Ishimura T., Nishiyama S., et al.: Hypertrophic non-obstructive cardiomyopathy with giant T-waves (apical hypertrophy): Ventriculographic and echocardiographic features in 30 patients. *Am. J. Cardiol.* 44:401, 1979.
11. Maron B.J., Roberts W.C.: Quantitative analysis of cardiac muscle cell disorganization in the ventricular septum of patients with hypertrophic cardiomyopathy. *Circulation* 59:689, 1979.
12. Maron B.J., Epstein S.E.: Hypertrophic cardiomyopathy. Recent observations regarding the specificity of three hallmarks of the disease: Asymmetric septal hypertrophy, septal disorganization and systolic anterior motion of the anterior mitral leaflet. *Am. J. Cardiol.* 45:141, 1980.
13. Maron B.J.: Hypertrophic cardiomyopathy. *Cardiology* 2:(June)1, 1988.
14. Cosio F.G., Moro C., Alonso M.: The Q waves of hypertrophic cardiomyopathy, an electrophysiologic study. *N. Engl. J. Med.* 302:96, 1980.
15. Frank M.J., Abdulla A.M., Watkins L.O., et al.: Long-term medical management of hypertrophic cardiomyopathy: Usefulness of propranolol. *Eur. Heart J.* 4:155, 1983.
16. McKenna W.J., Chetty S., Oakley C.M., et al.: Arrhythmias in hypertrophic cardiomyopathy: Exercise and 48 hour ambulatory electrocardiographic assessment with and without beta adrenergic blocking therapy. *Am. J. Cardiol.* 45:1, 1980.
17. McKenna W., Harris L., Rowland E., et al.: Amiodarone for long-term management of patients with hypertrophic cardiomyopathy. *Am. J. Cardiol.* 54:802, 1984.
18. Pollick C.: Muscular subaortic stenosis. Hemodynamic and clinical improvement after disopyramide. *N. Engl. J. Med.* 307:997, 1982.
19. Frank S., Braunwald E.: Idiopathic hypertrophic subaortic stenosis: Clinical analysis of 126 patients with emphasis on the natural history. *Circulation* 37:759, 1968.
20. Maron B.J., Roberts W.C., McAllister H.A., et al.: Sudden death in young athletes. *Circulation* 62:218, 1980.
21. Shah P.M.: Controversies in hypertrophic cardiomyopathy. *Curr. Probl. Cardiol.* 11:567, 1986.
21a. Spirito P., Chiarella F., Carratino L., et al.: Clinical course and prognosis of hypertrophic cardiomyopathy in an outpatient population. *New Engl. J. Med.* 320:749, 1989.
22. Rosing D.R., Kent K.M., Borer J.S., et al.: Verapamil therapy: A new approach to the pharmacologic treatment of hypertrophic cardiomyopathy: 1. Hemodynamic effects. *Circulation* 60:1201, 1979.
23. Henry W.L., Morganroth J., Pearlman A.S.: Relation between echocardiographically determined left atrial size and atrial fibrillation. *Circulation* 53:273, 1976.
24. Glenner G.G.: Amyloid deposits and amyloidosis: The B-fibrilloses (second of two parts). *N. Engl. J. Med.* 302:1333, 1980.

25. Roberts W.C., Buja L.M., Ferrans V.J.: Löfflers's fibroplastic parietal endocarditis: Eosinophilic leukemia, and Davies' endomyocardial fibrosis: The same disease at different stages? *Pathol. Microbiol.* 35:90, 1970.
26. Cherian G., Vijayaraghavan G., Krishnaswami S., et al.: Endomyocardial fibrosis: Report on the hemodynamic data in 29 patients and review of the results of surgery. *Am. Heart J.* 105:659, 1983.
27. Silverman K.J., Hutchins G.M., Buckley B.H.: Cardiac sarcoid: A clinicopathologic study of 84 unselected patients with systemic sarcoidosis. *Circulation* 58:1204, 1978.
28. Buckley B.H., Ridolfi R.L., Salyer W.R.: Myocardial lesions of progressive systemic sclerosis: A cause of cardiac dysfunction. *Circulation* 53:483, 1976.
29. Lopez-Ovejero J.A., Saal S.D., D'Angelo W.A., et al.: Reversal of vascular and renal crisis of scleroderma by oral angiotensin-converting enzyme blockade. *N. Engl. J. Med.* 300:1417, 1979.
30. Landing B.H., Larson E.J.: Are infantile periarteritis nodosa with coronary artery involvement and fatal mucocutaneous lymph node syndrome the same? Comparison of 20 patients from North America with patients from Hawaii and Japan. *Pediatrics* 59:651, 1977.
31. Buckley B.H., Roberts W.C.: Ankylosing spondylitis and aortic regurgitation: Description of the characteristic cardiovascular lesion from study of eight necropsy patients. *Circulation* 48:1014, 1973.
32. Paulus H.E., Pearson C.M., Pitts W.: Aortic insufficiency in five patients with Reiter's syndrome. *Am. J. Med.* 53:464, 1972.
33. Darsee J.R., Nutter D.O.: Reversible severe congestive cardiomyopathy in three cases of hypophosphatemia. *Ann. Intern. Med.* 88:867, 1978.
34. Johnson R.A., Baker S.S., Fallon J.T., et al.: An occidental case of cardiomyopathy and selenium deficiency. *N. Engl. J. Med.* 20:1210, 1981.
35. Dixon G.F.: The evaluation and management of electrical injuries. *Crit. Care Med.* II:384, 1983.
36. Wright R.K., Davis J.H.: The investigation of electrical deaths: A report of 220 fatalities. *J. Forensic Sci.* 25:514, 1980.
37. Cooper M.I.: Lightning injuries: Prognostic signs for death. *Ann. Emerg. Med.* 9:134, 1980.
38. Hanson G.I., McIlwraith G.R.: Lightning injury: Two case histories and a review of management. *Br. Med. J.* 4:271, 1973.
39. Aviado D.M.: Drug action, reaction, and interaction: II. Iatrogenic cardiopathies. *J. Clin. Pharmacol.* 15:641, 1975.
40. Jefferson J.W.: A review of the cardiovascular effects and toxicity of tricyclic antidepressants. *Psychom. Med.* 37:160, 1975.
41. Lefrak E.A., Pitha J., Rosenheim S., et al.: A clinicopathologic analysis of adriamycin cardiotoxicity. *Cancer* 32:302, 1973.
42. Ross A.M., Levy W.S., Simon G.L., et al. Clinically silent cardiac abnormalities in patients with human immunodeficiency virus infection. Abstract: Association of University Cardiologists Meeting, Carmel, CA, Jan. 1989.
43. Mason J.W., Billingham M.E., Ricci D.R.: Treatment of acute inflammatory myocarditis assisted by endomyocardial biopsy. *Am. J. Cardiol.* 45:1037, 1980.
44. O'Connell J.B., Robinson J.A., Henkin R.E., et al.: Immunosuppressive therapy in patients with congestive cardiomyopathy and myocardial uptake of Gallium-67. *Circulation* 64:780, 1981.
45. O'Connell J.B., Costanzo-Nordin M.R., Subramanian R., Robinson J.A.: Dilated cardiomyopathy: Emerging role of endomyocardial biopsy. *CPC* XI:450, 1986.
46. Fowles R.E., Mason J.W.: Cardiac biopsy to diagnose and guide therapy in patients with myocardial disease. *Cardiac Impulse* 5:1, 1984.

Chapter 13

PERICARDIAL DISEASES

Inflammation of the pericardium can produce clinical and pathologic changes of acute pericarditis, pericarditis with effusion, chronic constrictive pericarditis, or calcific pericarditis without constriction. The pericardial reaction may be purulent, hemorrhagic, fibrinous, or serofibrinous. Table 13–1 lists some of the various causes of pericarditis.

ACUTE PERICARDITIS

Acute pericarditis can be seen with any of the causes listed in Table 13–1. The visceral pericardial membrane has no pain fibers and the parietal membrane carries pain fibers, from the phrenic nerve, only in the lower part. The afferent nerves of pain perception enter the spinal cord at the level of C_3-C_5 via the phrenic nerve. These factors may explain the absence of pain that may be noted in some types of pericarditis at times, such as uremic pericarditis. Involvement of adjacent structures (such as the mediastinum, diaphragm, and pleura) also may contribute to the pain. The pain distribution of pericarditis can be similar to that of an acute myocardial infarction. It can be precordial or substernal and radiate into the neck, jaw, arms, interscapular region, trapezius muscle at the back of the shoulder and neck, or upper abdomen. The pain may be dull, heavy, or achy as noted with infarction. However, it may have certain distinguishing features, such as being sharp, aggravated by deep inspiration and coughing, and less intense on sitting up and leaning forward. Some patients never have pain and seek attention only because of other symptoms. Dyspnea can occur because of splinting of the chest from pain or because of significant pericardial fluid. Immediate fever may be present, especially with the infectious types. A pericardial friction rub (produced by the friction of the fibrinous surfaces of the two pericardial membranes) is often present (but its absence does not exclude acute pericarditis) and is heard best along the left sternal border in the sitting-up and bending-forward positions. At times, rubs may be heard only with the patient positioned on his hands and knees. It may appear intermittently, and its intensity may vary. Up to three components may be audible (see Fig 13–6). These are associated with atrial systole, ventricular systole, and ventricular diastole. Most often, only a two-component rub is audible with sounds during atrial and ventricular systole. Occasionally there may only be a one-component rub, which is difficult to differentiate from a systolic murmur. Frequent auscultation will solve the problem, for a single-component rub can become a two- or three-component rub or can disappear. At times a rub can produce a palpable thrill. This is noted more often with uremic

Table 13–1.   Etiology of Pericarditis

1. Acute idiopathic (nonspecific)
2. Infectious
     Bacterial
     Viral
     Tuberculous
     Fungal
     Parasitic
3. Associated with a general disease
     Rheumatic fever
     Rheumatoid arthritis
     Lupus erythematosus
     Scleroderma
     Uremia
     Myxedema
4. Involvement of contiguous structures
     Acute myocardial infarction and postinfarction syndrome
     Postpericardiotomy syndrome
     Dissecting aneurysm
     Esophageal disease
     Pulmonary disease
5. Neoplastic
6. Trauma
7. Radiation
8. Drugs

pericarditis. One can simulate a pericardial rub by placing a hand over an ear and scratching its dorsal surface to and fro with the other hand. A pericardial rub may be audible even when there is significant pericardial fluid. Left pleural rubs may cause confusion. However, such rubs are heard best with inspiration and disappear when the breath is held, whereas a pericardial rub persists when the breath is held. The ECG may reveal diffuse ST segment elevation except in the leads that face the endocardial surface such as a V_R or at times some of the right precordial leads (Fig 13–1). Spodick[1] describes four stages in acute pericarditis. Stage 1 is characterized by ST segment elevation and is the

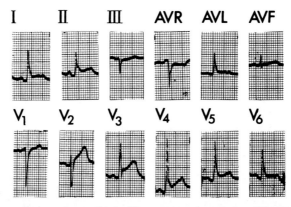

Fig 13–1.   Electrocardiogram in a patient with acute purulent pericarditis. Note the ST elevation in all the leads except aVR and V_1.

most diagnostic. In stage 2 the ST segment is isoelectric, and later in stage 2 there may be T wave flattening. In stage 3 the T waves become inverted, and they return to normal in stage 4. The PR segment may be depressed in the first two stages and represents subepicardial atrial injury. It should be emphasized, however, that the changes may not go through all four stages (only in approximately 50% of patients). Instead there may be only ST elevation and a return to normal without later T wave inversion. On the other hand, the T wave inversion may be the first sign, since the acute process was missed, and in such instances the ECG is nonspecific because there are so many other conditions that can produce T wave inversion. The T waves during evolution can become deeply inverted, simulating an evolving subendocardial (nontransmural) infarct, and can persist for several months, remain to some degree inverted permanently, or clear. Reciprocal ST depression and Q waves differentiate acute myocardial infarction from pericarditis. Likewise, normal early repolarization (Fig 13–2), which must be distinguished from acute pericarditis, does not produce reciprocal ST depression and it is often localized in just a few leads. This is most often noted in blacks. Spodick[2] reported that an ST-segment deviation in both limb and precordial leads, with a horizontal mean ST-vector orientation to left of the mean T vector and ST-segment depression in lead V_1 favors pericarditis. On the other hand, a vertical mean ST-vector and isoelectric ST segment in V_6 favor early repolarization. Another study[3] showed that an ST:T ratio <0.25 in V_6 suggests a normal variant. The patients represented in Figure 13–2 conform to this ratio. Since heart position, body habitus, and the time of the tracing vary, however, I believe that the description of the ST-segment elevation is more helpful than such ratios.[4] The ST-segment elevation of acute pericarditis most often comes straight off the QRS complex or is downwardly concave, whereas that of early repolarization is upwardly con-

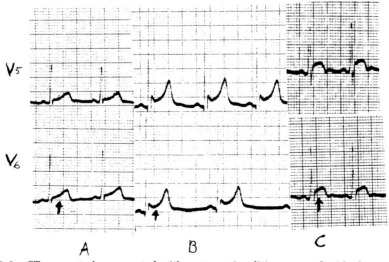

Fig 13–2. ST-segment changes noted with acute pericarditis compared with changes of early repolarization. Note that the ST segment of acute pericarditis (A) comes straight off of the QRS complex or can be downwardly concave (C). The ST-segment elevation of early repolarization is usually upwardly concave (B). The ST:T ratio in A and C in V_6 is >0.25 mV. (From Gazes, P.C.: Pericarditis. *Cardiovasc. Dis. Chest Pain* 1:3, 1985.)

cave. In addition, early repolarization is frequently associated with increased R-wave amplitude, especially in the left precordial leads. However, it should be recognized that at times, when the early repolarization is diffuse, it is almost impossible to differentiate it from acute pericarditis. Pericardial effusion can produce low QRS voltage and electrical alternans. Arrhythmias usually indicate additional heart disease, but can be associated with the inflamed pericardium being contiguous to the sinoatrial node or to atrial wall involvement. Supraventricular arrhythmia, such as atrial flutter and fibrillation, is most often noted with neoplastic or tubercular pericarditis. Unless pericardial fluid develops, the x ray may remain normal or there may be only the findings of an underlying cardiac problem. Cardiac isoenzymes may be elevated, indicating epicarditis or myocarditis (see Chapter 4).

PERICARDITIS WITH EFFUSION

This can occur with all the causes listed in Table 13–1. The patients may begin with the picture of acute or subacute pericarditis or with x-ray evidence of an enlarged heart shadow with or without clinical evidence of congestive failure. As a result, pain may or may not be present and abdominal swelling or pain in the right upper quadrant due to liver distension may be the presenting complaints. Exertional dyspnea is usually present, yet the lungs are often clear. Dyspnea can occur because of atelectasis associated with lung compression. Orthopnea may occur, and the patient often leans forward in order to breathe well. Dysphagia can develop from esophageal compression, hiccups from phrenic nerve compression, and hoarseness from recurrent laryngeal compression. A pericardial friction rub may be audible even when there is a large effusion. The apical impulse is often absent, and the precordium is quiet, but a palpable apical impulse does not exclude pericardial effusion. The heart sounds may be decreased in intensity but may be normal, and a third heart sound (pericardial knock) may be present. Dullness in the left base posteriorly below the angle of the left scapula with bronchial breathing (Ewart's sign) is not often elicited. The ECG usually shows low voltage and inverted T waves. The P, QRS, and T waves may show electric alternans due to the swinging motion of the heart. Chest x ray reveals an enlarged cardiac silhouette, often with clear lung fields (Figs 13–3,A and 13–4,A). However, the heart silhouette may be of normal size, yet significant pericardial effusion can be present. Cardiac fluoroscopy with the image intensifier may reveal diminished pulsations and the epicardial fat pad inside the cardiac silhouette. Echocardiography has become a very valuable and easy noninvasive method to detect pericardial effusion. An echo-free area will be noted between the myocardium and the pericardium (Figs 13–5 and 13–6). Two dimensional echo studies can even detect localized effusions, and with large effusions the swinging motion of the heart can be appreciated, which produces total electric alternans noted in the ECG. Echocardiography has reduced the need for other methods, such as CT or radionuclide scanning, CO_2 venous injection, angiography, MR imaging, and heart catheterization for detecting pericardial effusions.

Cardiac Tamponade

Cardiac tamponade may develop when pericardial fluid interferes with diastolic filling and is related to the rapidity of fluid accumulation and the

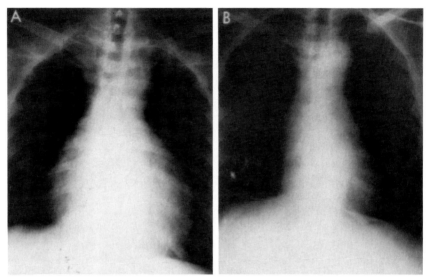

Fig 13–3. A, x-ray of cardiac tamponade postcoronary vein bypass graft surgery due to bleeding. Echocardiogram (see Fig 13–5) and pericardial scan indicated pericardial fluid. **B,** note reduction in the size of the cardiac silhouette after 400 ml of blood was aspirated from the pericardial sac.

distensibility of the pericardium and not the quantity of fluid (see Fig 13–3,A). Less than 100 ml accumulating suddenly, such as from hemopericardium due to trauma, can produce cardiac tamponade, yet with tuberculous pericarditis (see Fig 13–4,A), a large quantity of fluid can develop slowly before tamponade occurs. The most common causes of cardiac tamponade are hemopericardium secondary to trauma, infectious pericarditis, idiopathic or viral, uremic or neoplastic disease. In fact, it can occur with almost all types of pericarditis. In cardiac tamponade, diastolic filling of the ventricles is impaired, ventricular

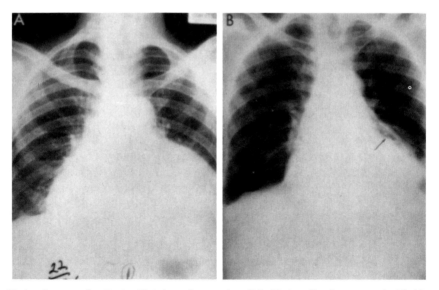

Fig 13–4. A, x ray of patient with tuberculous pericardial effusion. **B,** after removal of fluid, note air in pericardial sac *(arrow)* and thickened pericardium.

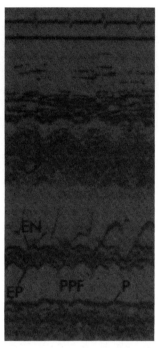

Fig 13–5. Echocardiogram of patient shown in Figure 13–3 demonstrating posterior pericardial effusion (PPF). Note echo-free space between epicardium (EP) and parietal pericardium (P). The myocardium is represented between the endocardium (EN) and the epicardium.

diastolic pressures are raised, and stroke volume is reduced. Tachycardia develops to maintain the cardiac output, and a narrow pulse pressure occurs. The jugular venous pulsations are often up to the angle of the jaw, and marked X descent can be seen in the acute types. Hepatomegaly is usually present. Pulsus paradoxus is an important finding and should be tested for by the use of the BP cuff. The systolic pressure is determined and lowered a few millimeters at a time. A paradoxical pulse is present when during inspiration sounds are not heard after lowering the BP 10 mm or more. It also may be noted in bronchial asthma, obstructive emphysema, pneumothorax, and massive pulmonary embolism. Marked negative intrathoracic pressure with inspiration in these conditions can produce a decrease in left heart filling. There are many theories explaining the mechanism of the paradoxical pulse in cardiac tamponade. The most logical explanation is that with inspiration there is a drop in the elevated intrapericardial pressure which results in an increased venous return to the right atrium and ventricle with an increase in right ventricular dimensions and a shift of the interventricular septum toward the left ventricle, reducing left ventricular volume, which results in a fall in aortic flow and systolic blood pressure.[5,6] Normally these changes occur with inspiration to a slight degree and become exaggerated with cardiac tamponade. Other factors of some importance are negative thoracic pressure transmitted to the aorta, inspiratory traction on the taut pericardium, and reflex changes due to lung distention.

    Low pressure cardiac tamponade can occur with tuberculosis, neoplastic

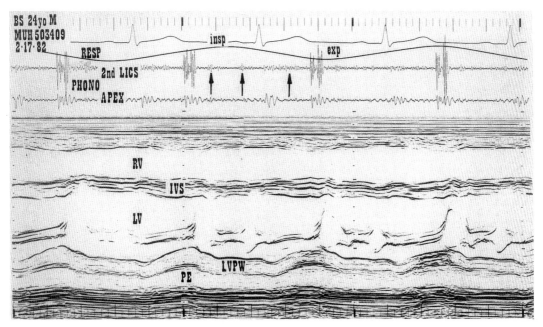

Fig 13–6. M-mode echocardiogram in a patient with pericardial effusion (PE). Note (*arrows*) the three component pericardial friction rub in the phonocardiogram. Resp = respiration; Insp = inspiration; Exp = expiration; LICS = left intercostal space; Phono = phonocardiogram; RV = right ventricle; IVS = interventricular system; LV = left ventricle; LVPW = left ventricular posterior wall; PE = pericardial effusion. (Courtesy of Dr. Bruce W. Usher.)

pericarditis concomitantly with dehydration as from excessive diuresis.[7] Such patients may not have the classic findings of cardiac tamponade, the neck veins may be normal or only slightly elevated, blood pressure normal and pulsus paradoxus may be absent. Recognizing that the patient has a condition that may involve the pericardium should lead to other studies. Echocardiography and right heart catheterization establish the diagnosis.

Echocardiography can confirm the diagnosis of pericardial fluid and may give clues that cardiac tamponade is present. During cardiac tamponade, diastolic right atrial and right ventricular collapse can be noted. Diastolic collapse of the left atrium can also occur if fluid is behind the left atrium. M-mode images can also show diastolic compression of the right ventricle. The heart may show a pendular swinging motion which is often associated with electrical alternans (Fig 13–7). There may be total alternans involving the P waves, QRS complex, and T waves, which is more common with tamponade than just QRS alternation.

Catheterization of the right heart and measurement of the intrapericardial pressure confirm the diagnosis. The right atrial, right ventricular diastolic and intrapericardial pressures are elevated to a similar degree. There also may be some elevation of the right ventricular and pulmonary artery systolic pressures. If the patient's condition is unstable, one should perform pericardiocentesis based on clinical judgment rather than consuming valuable time with studies.

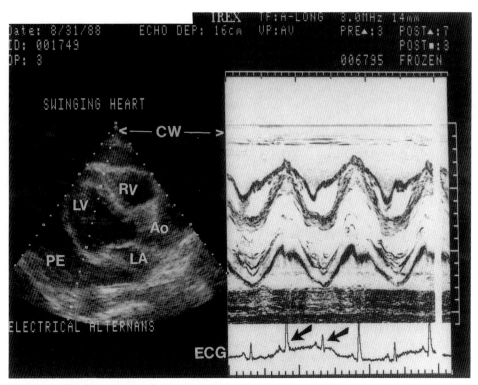

Fig 13–7. Cardiac tamponade in a patient with carcinoma of the lung. M-mode and two-dimensional echocardiogram reveal a large pericardial effusion (PE) with a swinging heart motion, diastolic collapse of the right ventricle and left atrium, and electrical alternans. Note in the M-mode tracing that when the cardiac wall swings anteriorly, the QRS voltage is high (*arrow*) and low (*arrow*) when it swings posteriorly. Ao = aorta, RV = right ventricle, LV = left ventricle, LA = left atrium.

Pericardiocentesis

Pericardial aspiration is performed (ideally in the cardiac catheterization laboratory with ECG and hemodynamic monitoring) to remove fluid for diagnostic purposes (see Fig 13–4,B) and therapeutically for the relief of cardiac tamponade (see Fig 13–3,B). Two-dimensional echocardiography may help choose the safest insertion sites. In a patient with acute cardiac tamponade, removal of only 100 ml of fluid may be lifesaving. The procedure is performed with the patient's chest elevated to a 45-degree position from the horizontal. I prefer the subxiphoid approach with the needle inserted in the angle between the left costal arch and the xiphoid and directed posteriorly toward the right shoulder while maintaining suction on the syringe. The precordial lead of the ECG is attached to the aspirating needle with a sterile connector. The myocardium has been reached if ST elevation is recorded (Fig 13–8) and the right atrium reached if the P-Q interval is elevated. Ventricular and atrial arrhythmias can appear. When the heart is touched, the needle should be withdrawn slightly. If bloody fluid is obtained, its hematocrit should be compared with that of the patient's peripheral blood to be certain that the cardiac cavity has not been entered. However, in trauma, the hematocrit of the blood fluid and that of venous blood may be the same. Failure of the bloody fluid to clot is

V₁

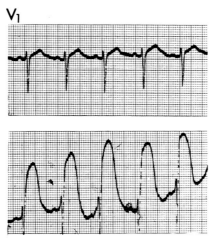

Fig 13–8. Top strip of ECG represents lead V_1. Note in bottom strip the marked ST elevation in V_1 when the aspirating needle touched the myocardium.

further evidence that it is not from within the heart. Injection of contrast medium with fluoroscopic observation can clarify the problem. Once the needle is in the pericardial space, a soft catheter is advanced over a guidewire and the guidewire is removed. Fluid can then be aspirated from the catheter. At times, pericardiotomy and evacuation of fluid and clots may be necessary, especially if pericardiocentesis is unsuccessful or accumulation of fluid recurs. Surgery is usually necessary if the cardiac tamponade is due to trauma. When cardiac tamponade has been relieved, the cause should be determined and treated appropriately. Expansion of the intravascular volume by I.V. crystalloids or plasma expanders may improve the venoatrial gradient and BP until pericardiocentesis or surgery can be performed. In hypotensive patients, in addition to fluid challenge, inotropic agents may be infused as an aid in maintaining the arterial pressure.

Diagnostic pericardiocentesis is controversial and is not performed as often today, since it does carry some risk and since more information can be obtained and better drainage accomplished with surgical intervention. By limited subxiphoid pericardiotomy, pericardial tissue can be obtained for study and multiple aspirations can be avoided. The fluid should be studied for cells, organisms, and fungi by smear and culture, tumor cells, proteins, enzymes, LE cells, sugar, amylase, cholesterol, latex fixation, and complement level. Grossly bloody fluid should suggest tuberculosis or neoplasm, whereas sanguinous fluid occurs primarily in lupus, tuberculosis, idiopathic pericarditis, and rheumatoid pericarditis.

CONSTRICTIVE PERICARDITIS

Often the etiology of constrictive pericarditis cannot be found. Tuberculosis at one time was the most common cause, but with improved therapy, fewer cases are now seen. Other causes are trauma, radiation therapy, collagen diseases, viral, uremic, neoplastic, pyogenic and cardiac surgery.

The clinical picture can vary depending on the rapidity of development of the constriction and whether it is diffuse or localized. One type has been referred to as effusive-constrictive pericarditis.[8] This type occurs more rapidly and presents as a combined picture of cardiac tamponade and constriction, with fluid between the visceral and parietal layers and thickening of the visceral pericardium. After the fluid is removed, the picture is that of constriction. This has been noted with radiation, tuberculosis, metastatic disease, and chronic renal failure.[9]

Often past symptoms of acute or subacute pericarditis may be overlooked, and the patient's complaints when initially seen are of abdominal swelling and peripheral edema with slight or no dyspnea. The jugular veins become distended, and because of the high venous pressure the external jugular veins may become thickened and overlooked as veins, and the internal jugular pulsations may be minimal and show diminished respiratory variation. Kussmaul's sign (inspiratory increase in the venous pressure) may be present, and the jugular venous pulse shows a deep trough of the Y wave. The precordium is usually quiet, but a diastolic knock coinciding with a sudden deceleration in filling of a restricted ventricle may be palpable and audible. Constriction in the AV groove can produce murmurs of mitral or tricuspid stenosis, and such patients often are misdiagnosed as having rheumatic heart disease.[9a,10] In addition, this is compounded by the fact that atrial fibrillation is often present, and the diastolic knock sound is mistaken for an opening snap. The lungs are usually clear, but pleural effusions can be present. There is marked hepatomegaly and frequently ascites. When the neck veins are overlooked, these patients are followed as having cirrhosis of the liver. Variable degrees of peripheral edema are present, but less so compared with the ascites. Pulsus paradoxus is rarely noted. Low QRS voltage with inverted T waves usually are seen in the ECG. The P waves are often notched and widened, and about 30% may have atrial flutter or fibrillation. Right axis and a pattern resembling right ventricular hypertrophy have been reported. This was found in 6 out of 122 cases. In only 1 with fibrotic annular subpulmonic constriction was there a plausible cause.[11] Flat mid and late diastolic motion of the posterior left ventricular wall, rapid early diastolic slope of the mitral valve (E to F), early diastolic notch in septal motion, atrial systolic notch in septal motion, and premature opening of the pulmonic valve have been described as M-mode echocardiographic signs of constrictive pericarditis. Two-dimensional echocardiography can suggest constriction by showing normal systolic function, abnormal diastolic function, abnormal septal motion, increased thickness of the pericardium, and dilatation of the inferior vena cava and hepatic veins. However, none of these findings is specific. The heart size may be normal or enlarged on chest film. Pleural effusions are common. A normal-sized heart on x ray with clear lung fields with a clinical picture of heart failure should suggest constrictive pericarditis. Calcification may be present in the pericardium. At times calcification can be seen even though the patient has no symptoms or other findings. Often this nonconstrictive,[12] adhesive form of pericarditis is found on a routine x ray. Liver function studies can be abnormal, which may be misinterpreted as due to cirrhosis. Severe venous hypertension can cause a protein-losing gastroenteropathy with hypoalbuminemia. Cardiac catheterization studies in constrictive pericarditis will reveal elevated mean right atrial, pulmonary arterial diastolic, pulmonary capillary wedge, or left atrial and right and left ventricular end-diastolic pressures to almost identical levels.

The elevated right and left atrial pressures may have "M" configurations. Rapid early right and left ventricular diastolic dips are followed by a plateau of elevated end-diastolic pressures (square root sign). Right ventricular and pulmonary systolic pressure may be moderately elevated. Figure 13–9 shows the main features of constrictive pericarditis. Similar hemodynamic findings can be noted in patients with restrictive cardiomyopathy (amyloidosis, scleroderma, idiopathic). The left ventricular end-diastolic pressure may be higher and the cardiac output lower than with constriction. Tyberg et al.[13] described different left ventricular filling patterns in restrictive amyloid cardiomyopathy and constrictive pericarditis with the use of digitized left ventriculograms. Patients with amyloid had no plateau in the diastolic left ventricular filling volume curve, and their left ventricular filling rate was slower than normal during the first half of diastole, whereas patients with constrictive pericarditis had a sudden premature plateau in the diastolic left ventricular volume filling curve and the left ventricular filling rate was faster than normal during the first half of diastole. In addition, restrictive cardiomyopathy may have findings of secondary tricuspid insufficiency, and the ECG may show left ventricular hypertrophy or bundle-branch block. Endomyocardial biopsy is helpful if the results are positive, but a negative finding does not rule out restrictive cardiomyopathy. Computed tomography and MRI may also aid in the differentiation. If, after the various studies, the diagnosis is still in question, an exploratory thoracotomy is warranted.

CONSTRICTIVE PERICARDITIS

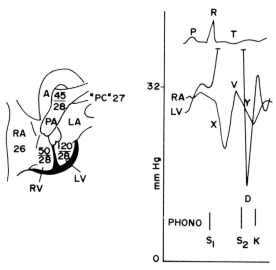

Fig 13–9. Main findings in constrictive pericarditis: Neck veins distended and Kussmaul's sign. Heart sounds normal or quiet. Diastolic pericardial knock (K) sound. Electrocardiogram shows low voltage and often atrial fibrillation. X ray reveals normal heart size or slight cardiomegaly. Calcification in pericardium at times. Cardiac catheterization studies show that the mean right atrial (RA), pulmonary arterial diastolic (PA), pulmonary capillary wedge (PC), and right (RV) and left ventricular (LV) end-diastolic pressures are elevated to identical levels (26–28 mm Hg). Right atrial pressure pulse and that of the capillary wedge have an "M" pattern. Early diastolic dips (D) of both ventricular pressures are present.

Once the diagnosis of constrictive pericarditis is established and the patient has symptoms of constriction, pericardiectomy should be performed. If tuberculous pericarditis is active or suspected, antituberculous therapy should be administered for at least 2 weeks prior to surgical resection.

Occult Constrictive Pericarditis

Occult constrictive pericarditis should be suspected if a patient has a history of pericarditis or trauma and chronic symptoms of fatigue, chest pain, and dyspnea without evidence of cardiac disease. The diagnosis can be made after rapid expansion of the intravascular volume with the rapid administration of 1 L of normal saline, if the monitored pressures show diastolic equilibration— namely, the pulmonary capillary wedge, pulmonary artery diastolic, right ventricular end-diastolic, and mean right atrial pressures—are identically elevated.[14] Pericardiectomy has relieved such patients of disabling symptoms.

Effusive-Constrictive Pericarditis

As mentioned earlier, Hancock[8] described this intermediate form of constriction as a combination of cardiac tamponade and constriction, and after fluid is removed the constriction prevails. Patients have fatigue, exertional dyspnea, and chest heaviness. The jugular venous pulse is elevated with a prominent X descent, and after the fluid is removed a prominent Y descent. Cardiomegaly is noted on x ray, and the echocardiogram reveals findings of pericardial fluid. Pericardial calcification is unusual. The underlying disease, if detected, should be treated and pericardiectomy performed.

SPECIFIC TYPES OF PERICARDITIS

Acute idiopathic or nonspecific. The cause of this type of pericarditis is unknown. Some cases are associated with such viruses as Coxsackie B, Echo, mumps, or influenza. Often such patients have a preceding upper respiratory illness and then suddenly develop chest pain and fever. Frequently a pericardial rub is heard and effusion develops. Cardiac tamponade can occur and later constriction. The pericardial effusion may be serous or hemorrhagic. A pleural effusion also may be present. Leukocytosis often is noted. The acute course usually lasts from 1 to 3 weeks. However, recurrent attacks can occur. In some cases such recurrences may be due to an autoimmune process. Treatment is symptomatic, and corticosteroids are given if the attack does not subside or is recurrent. The use of antibiotics should be discouraged, for they are of no value. The patient should have bed rest and chair rest with bathroom privileges for at least 2 weeks. Morphine or meperidine (Demerol) can be given for chest pain. Aspirin, 600 mg, or indomethacin (Indocin), 25 to 50 mg every 6 hours, will aid because of the analgesic and anti-inflammatory effects of these drugs. Ibuprofen (Motrin), 400 mg four times daily and other types of nonsteroidal anti-inflammatory agents are also effective. If corticosteroids become necessary, I would give 60 mg of prednisone (or its equivalent) daily in divided doses for 1 to 2 weeks or until clinical resolution, and then taper it at a rate of 5 to 10 mg every third day. Steroid dosages should not be reduced abruptly, because rebound can occur. Aspirin or indomethacin may be started as tapering is begun. Cardiac tamponade seldom develops, but should this happen, pericardiocentesis should be done. Rarely, pericardial resection may be necessary for patients who have recurrence of attacks when steroids are withdrawn if they have become steroid-dependent.

Bacterial. Microorganisms such as staphylococci, pneumococci, streptococci, or gram-negative aerobic bacilli may be associated with septicemia, post-thoracotomy, or spread from the lungs or pleura to involve the pericardium. The staphylococcus has become the most common causative organism. Since the introduction of antibiotics, pyogenic pericarditis has declined. Undiagnosed types of pericarditis may be partially treated pyogenic types, because physicians use antibiotics so early today for many infections before detecting the causative microorganism. Gram stain and cultures of the aspirated effusion should be performed. The antibiotic of choice depends on the organism isolated and the results of sensitivity studies. Surgical drainage often is necessary along with the antibiotic therapy. Cardiac tamponade or later constriction can occur, especially if the patient has had inadequate or insufficient prolonged therapy.

Tuberculous. This type of pericarditis is not common today and is primarily seen without pulmonary involvement, arising probably from infected peribronchial, peritracheal, or mediastinal nodes. A prior history of tuberculosis may be obtained. The onset may be abrupt, but is usually insidious. Malaise and fever may be present for several months before signs of pericarditis appear. A pericardial rub may be noted or pericardial fluid detected. The effusion can be large before signs and symptoms of compression occur. The fluid may be serous or hemorrhagic. Cardiac tamponade or effusive-constrictive pericarditis can occur and, later, constriction. The ECG may reveal only inverted T waves and not ST elevation, since these patients often are seen after the tuberculous process has been present for several weeks. Atrial fibrillation or flutter can occur. The patient may be considered to have congestive failure until pericardial effusion is suspected because of the chest x ray or echocardiogram. The tuberculin skin test is positive in up to 75% of cases. Tubercle bacilli in the pericardial fluid or by guinea pig inoculation and cultures are found only in about 50% of patients. It may take as long as 6 to 8 weeks for the results of cultures. Therefore, it is usually best to begin therapy if the skin test is positive, the patient has a reasonable history, pericardial effusion is present, and no other cause has been detected, rather than wait for the results of the cultures. After 2 to 3 weeks of therapy, if the patient is not improving, a pericardial biopsy should be performed, as well as pericardiectomy. The therapy can be altered accordingly if the biopsy shows some other condition. Otherwise, antituberculous therapy should be continued. If the clinical evidence strongly supports a tuberculous etiology, therapy should be started even if the cultures and animal inoculations are negative. Early therapy may prevent constrictive pericarditis. Sagrista-Sauleda et al.[15] suggested the following diagnostic procedures: three samples of sputum or gastric aspirate for turbercle bacilli investigation if the acute pericarditis lasts longer than 1 week or the clinical findings are severe; pleural or lymph node biopsy suggested by the clinical findings; measurement of adenosine deaminase activity in pleural fluid if pleural effusion is present (activity >45 μ/liter may justify invasive procedures as pericardiocentesis or pericardial biopsy); and pericardiocentesis when there is therapeutic need and pericardial biopsy when significant disease persists ≥3 weeks or when there is a strong suspicion of tuberculosis. Using this diagnostic approach, they diagnosed tuberculous pericarditis in 13 patients out of a group of 294 who were consecutively admitted for primary acute pericardial disease. Fifty percent of the 13 cases developed subacute constrictive pericarditis requiring pericardiectomy within 3.5 months of admission.

Many combinations of therapy including isoniazid, ethambutal (Myambutal), rifampin (Rimactine), streptomycin, and pyrazinamide have been used. At present, our group prefers isoniazid 300 mg per day and rifampin 600 mg per day for 9 months. Because both of these drugs can be hepatotoxic, liver function studies should be checked periodically. Isoniazid can produce disorders of the nervous system, especially peripheral neuritis. These can be prevented by the use of 50 to 100 mg of pyridoxine orally per day. The addition of corticosteroids has been advocated by some to minimize the possibility of adhesions and constriction, but its value has not been clearly shown. If, in spite of therapy, the cardiac silhouette is persistently enlarged, the venous pressure is persistently elevated, and dyspnea, hepatomegaly, or ascites remain, then pericardiectomy should be performed. The earlier it is recognized that medical therapy will fail, the easier pericardiectomy can be done. Extended chronic constriction with fibrosis and calcification can produce a major surgical problem. During the surgical procedure, the myocardium can be torn and the coronary arteries injured.

Fungal. Fungal diseases such as histoplasmosis, aspergillosis, nocardiosis, blastomycosis, candidiasis, and coccidioidomycosis, can produce pericarditis. Since the advent of antibiotics, fungi are found in 20% of the cases with suppurative pericarditis. In addition, those who are on immunosuppressive agents and drug addicts are at increased risk. Diagnosis is usually established by culture of the pericardial fluid or by pericardial biopsy. Rising complement fixations titers may aid. Amphotericin B therapy can be used as for systemic involvement, pericardiocentesis if acute cardiac tamponade develops, and pericardiectomy if constriction occurs.

Rheumatic pericarditis. Isolated pericarditis in acute rheumatic fever is rare. It is usually associated with pancarditis. At times the endocarditis may be overlooked because murmurs are obscured by the pericardial effusion. Constriction rarely occurs with rheumatic pericarditis (see Chap. 6).

Rheumatoid arthritis. Rheumatoid disease can involve all structures of the heart, especially the pericardium. Often the pericarditis is not detected clinically and only recognized at autopsy. Recently many of these have been uncovered by the use of the echocardiogram. Usually the other features of rheumatoid arthritis are apparent (see Chap. 12).

Lupus erythematosus. Pericarditis may be the first feature of SLE. It may be of the dry type, or an effusion can develop. Cardiac tamponade or constriction rarely occur. Other manifestations of lupus are usually present or will appear later. A positive test for antinuclear antibodies and for lupus cells usually indicates the diagnosis (see Chap. 12).

Scleroderma. Acute and chronic pericarditis are not uncommon in scleroderma and often do not produce symptoms. Effusion can develop but it rarely produces tamponade. Echocardiography has demonstrated the common occurrence of pericardial involvement in scleroderma. The pericardial fluid has no diagnostic features. The diagnosis of scleroderma depends on the other visceral and skin findings (see Chap. 12).

Uremia. Pericarditis is usually a late finding in uremia. A pericardial friction rub is often present, is loud, and may produce a thrill. Effusion can develop and even constriction since the advent of renal dialysis and transplantation. Significant pericardial effusion and tamponade can occur during dialysis. Because of dialysis and renal transplantation, pericarditis is no longer considered a terminal event. It is usually treated by augmenting dialysis and supportive care. Pericardiocentesis, pericardial window, or pericardiectomy may be necessary, especially if during the dialysis the patient's condition worsens. Steroids or indomethacin given orally have been effective in some cases, especially for those who are febrile and in much pain. The steroids also have been injected into the pericardial sac through an indwelling polyethylene catheter which has been inserted for drainage.

Myxedema. Large effusions develop with myxedema but do not produce tamponade or constriction. The other clinical features of myxedema are diagnostic along with the laboratory studies (see Chap. 14).

Acute myocardial infarction, postinfarction syndrome, and postpericardiotomy syndrome. Pericarditis can develop with a transmural myocardial infarction. Usually a pericardial rub is present, but not in all cases. Often when a rub is not heard it is tempting to consider return of pain due to the spread of the infarction. The pericarditis associated with infarction usually clears up in a few days. In some cases, 2 weeks after the onset of infarction, fever, pericarditis, pleuritis, and pneumonitis can occur. The initial attack may be 3 months later, and recurrent attacks can occur for months or even years. The features of this postmyocardial infarction syndrome (Dressler's syndrome[16]) are similar to those of the postpericardiotomy syndrome, which is a complication of surgery that can occur whenever the pericardium is entered. It also may occur after hemopericardium due to trauma. Engle et al.[17] noted high titer of heart-reactive antibody in the serum of patients in whom the postpericardiotomy syndrome developed after intrapericardial surgery. Usually the syndrome clears in 2 to 4 weeks with aspirin or indomethacin (use with caution in patients with severe coronary artery disease) treatment. One must be cautious, since salicylates may suppress platelets and cause intrapericardial bleeding. Corticosteroids are given for severe or recurrent attacks, and, rarely, pericardiectomy is necessary.

Dissecting aneurysm. Dissection may produce a leak into the pericardial sac. Usually when this occurs, the patient also develops aortic insufficiency, which, combined with the severe chest pain, makes diagnosis of the dissecting aneurysm most likely (see Chap. 10).

Neoplastic. The most common primary tumor of the heart is mesothelioma. Carcinoma of the lung or breast, melanoma, lymphomas, and leukemia are the most common neoplastic diseases that can invade the pericardium.[18,19] Appropriate therapy for the malignancy, such as radiotherapy or chemotherapy, should be given. Cardiac tamponade can occur as the presenting feature before one suspects malignancy. Pricardiocentesis and intrapericardial chemotherapy or pericardial surgery may be necessary. Nitrogen mustard, thiotepa, radioactive gold, and quinacrine (Atabrine) are some of the agents given by intrapericardial instillation. These agents cause severe pain, and bone marrow toxicity can be produced by the alkylating agents.[20] Tetracycline hydrochloride has been instilled because it is nontoxic and less irritating.[21] This procedure is repeated every 48 hours through an indwelling pericardial cannula until total sclerosis develops or no more fluid can be drained.

Trauma. Trauma can produce hemopericardium and cardiac tamponade. Removal of only 50 ml of fluid may be lifesaving until thoracotomy can be done and the lacerated myocardium or bleeding vessel is sutured. Later, recurrent pericarditis can occur as noted with the postpericardiotomy syndrome, or even constriction can develop. These complications can be managed in the same way as when they occur from other causes.

Radiation. After radiation therapy, acute pericarditis, chronic effusion, or even constriction can occur. Often such cases are overlooked because the history of radiation therapy was not noted, and the pericarditis can appear months or years later. Corticosteroids may reduce the effusion. Rarely, constrictive pericarditis can occur.

Drugs. Pericarditis can be induced by drugs or can present as a part of the lupus-like picture produced by certain drugs. Hydralazine and procainamide most often have been implicated. Cardiac tamponade and constriction are rare. Usually the pericarditis clears when the drug is stopped.

Unusual pericardial effusions. Cholesterol pericarditis may be of unknown etiology or noted with myxedema, rheumatoid disease, or tuberculosis. Rarely, constriction can occur. Chylopericardial effusion is even rarer. It can be related to trauma or chest surgery, or be idiopathic. The effusion is milky and clears when ether is added. Often patients have no symptoms and cardiac tamponade is rare.

Congenital Defects

Congenital pericardial defects usually occur on the left side; however, there may be total absence of the pericardium. These defects are important, for they may be confused with congenital heart defects or may be associated with other congenital heart anomalies. Most patients do not have symptoms or unusual physical findings. The apical impulse can be prominent if there is complete absence of the left pericardium or total absence of the pericardium. X-ray findings usually give the clue to the diagnosis. With partial absence of the left pericardium, the pulmonary artery segment or left atrial appendage is prominent, and with complete absence of the left pericardium, the heart is shifted to the left. In addition, with complete absence of the left pericardium, there may be lung tissue between the inferior border of the heart and the left hemidiaphragm, which can be demonstrated by radionuclide perfusion of the lung.[22] This latter procedure is less hazardous than the production of a pneumopericardium to demonstrate the defect. The ECG may show right-axis deviation and clockwise rotation of the precordial leads, with the transitional zone to the left. Surgery is usually not required, unless there is herniation of the heart with symptoms, as can rarely occur with partial defects.

REFERENCES

1. Spodick D.H.: Electrocardiogram in acute pericarditis: Distribution of morphologic and axial changes by stages. *Am. J. Cardiol.* 33:470, 1947.
2. Spodick D.H.: Differentiation characteristics of the electrocardiogram in early repolarization and acute pericarditis. *N. Engl. J. Med.* 295:523, 1976.
3. Ginzton L.E., Laks M.M.: The differential diagnosis of acute pericarditis. *Circulation* 65:1004, 1982.

4. Gazes P.C.: Pericarditis. *Cardiovasc. Dis. Chest Pain* 1(4):3, 1985.
5. Settle H.P., Adolph R.J., Fowler N.O.: Echocardiographic study of ventricular dimensions in cardiac tamponade: Effects of respiration and pericardiocentesis. *Circulation* 56:951, 1977.
6. Shabetai R., Fowler N.O., Fenton J.C., et al.: Pulsus paradoxus. *J. Clin. Invest.* 44:1882, 1965.
7. Shabetai R.: The pericardium and its disorders. *Baylor Cardiol. Series* 10(2):5, 1987.
8. Hancock E.W.: Subacute effusive constrictive pericarditis. *Circulation* 43:183, 1971.
9. Boltwood C.M., Shah P.M.: The pericardium in health and disease. *Curr. Probl. Cardiol.* 9(5):9, 1984.
9a. Bergh N.P., Krause F., Linder E.: Some aspects of diagnosis and treatment of chronic pericarditis. *Acta Chir. Scand.* 128:683, 1964.
10. McGuinn J.B., Zipes D.P.: Constrictive pericarditis producing tricuspid stenosis. *Arch. Intern. Med.* 129:487, 1977.
11. Chesler E., Mitha A.S., Matisonn R.E.: The ECG of constrictive pericarditis—Pattern resembling right ventricular hypertrophy. *Am. Heart J.* 91:420, 1976.
12. Harvey R.M., Ferrer M.I., Catheart R.T., et al.: Mechanical and myocardial factors in chronic constrictive pericarditis. *Circulation* 8:695, 1953.
13. Tyberg T.I., Goodyer A.V.N., Hurst V.W. III, et al.: Left ventricular filling in differentiating restrictive amyloid cardiomyopathy and constrictive pericarditis. *Am. J. Cardiol.* 47:791. 1981.
14. Kilman J.W., Bush C.A., Wooley C.F., et al.: The changing spectrum of pericardiectomy for chronic pericarditis: Occult constrictive pericarditis. *J. Thorac. Cardiovas. Surg.* 74:688, 1977.
15. Sagrista-Sauleda J., Permanyer-Miralda G., Soler-Soler J.: Tuberculosis pericarditis: Ten year experience with a prospective protocol for diagnosis and treatment. *J.A.C.C.* 11:724, 1988.
16. Dressler W.: The post-myocardial infarction syndrome: A report of forty-four cases. *Arch. Intern. Med.* 103:28, 1959.
17. Engle M.A., McCabe J.C., Ebert P.A., et al.: The postpericardiotomy syndrome and antiheart antibodies. *Circulation* 49:401, 1974.
18. Roberts W.C., Body G.P., Westlake P.T.: The heart in acute leukemia: A study of 420 autopsy cases. *Am. J. Cardiol.* 21:388, 1968.
19. Glancy D.L., Roberts W.C.: The heart in malignant melanoma: A study of 70 autopsy cases. *Am. J. Cardiol.* 21:555, 1968.
20. Fracchia A.A., Knapper W.H., Carey J.T., et al.: Intrapleural chemotherapy for effusion from metastatic breast carcinoma. *Cancer* 26:626, 1970.
21. Davis S., Sharma S.M., Blumberg E.D., et al.: Intrapericardial tetracycline for the management of cardiac tamponade secondary to malignant pericardial effusion. *N. Engl. J. Med.* 299:1113, 1978.
22. D'Altoria R.A., Caro J.Y.: Congenital absence of the left pericardium detected by imaging of the lung: Case report. *J. Nucl. Med.* 18:267, 1977.

Chapter 14

MISCELLANEOUS CARDIAC PROBLEMS

PREGNANCY AND THE HEART

Normal pregnancy can stimulate heart disease because symptoms of dyspnea, orthopnea, palpitation, and peripheral edema can occur as a result of the mechanical effects of the pregnancy and the hemodynamic adjustments. This is compounded by the fact that clinically the heart may appear enlarged and basal systolic murmurs are common. Extracardiac systolic and continuous murmurs may be present because of the increased blood flow to the breasts. The first heart sound may be increased and a loud second sound (may be persistently split with expiration) may be heard in the pulmonic area and a prominent third sound at the apex. At times it may be difficult to evaluate a murmur during pregnancy, and one must wait several weeks postpartum to complete the evaluation. In fact, murmurs of mitral and aortic insufficiency may decrease in intensity during pregnancy because of the associated decrease in peripheral vascular resistance. The heart may appear enlarged on x ray due to the high diaphragm. There is straightening of the left sternal border, increase in hilar vascular markings, and the left atrium appears enlarged. These findings may simulate mitral stenosis. The ECG may show nonspecific ST-T changes, and PABs and PVBs can be present.

The cardiac output begins to increase in the first trimester and reaches a peak by the 20th to 24th week (30 to 40% above the nonpregnant level). Previously it was thought that the cardiac output fell in late pregnancy (studies in supine position), but subsequent studies[1] in the lateral recumbent position show that it may be maintained until term. In the supine position the enlarged uterus compresses the inferior vena cava and decreases the venous return. Stroke volume is mainly responsible early in pregnancy for the increase in cardiac output, and later the increased heart rate plays a more significant part. The cardiac output intermittently rises with uterine contractions during labor, and postpartum it returns to normal in a few weeks. Peripheral vascular resistance decreases. Blood volume increases as the cardiac output increases, but reaches its peak (32 weeks) more gradually and remains at this level until term.[2] It increases at about 40% above the nonpregnant level. One of the major factors is sodium and water retention associated with activation of the renin-angiotensin system. The hemoglobin falls during pregnancy because the plasma volume increase is greater than that of the RBC volume. The majority of patients develop peripheral edema, with about 8.5 L of water accumulation during a normal pregnancy,[3] primarily due to salt retention. Raised venous pressure in the lower extremities also contributes to the edema. In view of these hemodynamic factors, heart failure may occur with increasing frequency as the pregnancy advances in the cardiac patient, with the majority of episodes occurring in the third trimester (almost 50% of these in the last 4 weeks). Mortality in the cardiac patient has declined over the years because of better treatment, both medical and surgical, prior to pregnancy.

The New York Heart Association functional classification has been revised (see Chap. 1) and is an excellent guide to the management of such patients. This category has been replaced by a new classification of the patient's overall cardiac status and prognosis (see Table 1–3). Patients with a cardiac status uncompromised or only slightly compromised tolerate pregnancy well, whereas patients with moderately compromised or severely compromised cardiac status tolerate pregnancy poorly. Therefore, patients in the latter two groups should be advised to avoid pregnancy until they have improved with medical or surgical therapy (if an operable lesion is present). The pregnant cardiac patient should be advised to reduce her activities and salt intake. If heart failure develops, she should have bed rest and be treated in the usual manner for heart failure. One study[4] showed that the serum digoxin concentration in the pregnant cardiac patient is only about half that noted 1 month post partum, even though the maintenance dose was the same. They postulated that this could be due to increased maternal blood volume and glomerular filtration rate (GFR). In view of this, it would be best to increase the maintenance dosage during pregnancy if the clinical response is not adequate while following serum levels. Digitalis does cross the placenta, and the same serum concentration as in the mother may be found in the newborn.[4] However, this has not been a problem. Diuretics and vasodilators can be used during pregnancy. There has been little experience with ACE inhibitors.

Termination of pregnancy is rarely indicated today. Vaginal delivery is preferable to cesarean section, unless there is an obstetric indication for the latter. In special instances, cardiac surgery (even open heart surgery) has been performed during the pregnancy. At the onset of labor, antibiotics for bacterial endocarditis prophylaxis (see Chap. 17) should be started, especially in patients with valvular abnormalities and in some cases of congenital heart defect. The American Heart Association does not recommend prophylaxis in routine vaginal delivery without urethral catheterization. However, such patients frequently require urethral catheterization. Labor, delivery, and the puerperium may present further problems.

As would be expected during the child-bearing age, valvular and congenital heart disease are the most common types of heart disease encountered with pregnancy. In addition, the spectrum of heart disease in pregnancy has changed because of the reduced incidence of rheumatic fever and because patients with congenital heart disease are now living longer owing to corrective surgery; they also tolerate pregnancy better. Tables 14–1 and 14–2 illustrate this changing spectrum by comparing more recent admissions of pregnant cardiac patients to the obstetric service at the Medical University of South Carolina (MUSC) with past data from other institutions.[5–9] Ten patients in

Table 14–1. Various Incidences of Heart Disease in Pregnancy

Study	Incidence (%)	Mortality (%)	Rheumatic (%)	Congenital (%)
Mendelson[6] (1940–1950)	2.3–3.7	0.8	91	4
Etheridge[7] (1960s)	0.5	1.0	84*	11
Adams[8] (1960)	1.2–3.7	0.1	75–95	—
Szekely[9] (1960–1970)	0.5–1.5	0	75	25
MUSC†[5] (1975–1979)	0.4–1.3	0	58	28

*Only 70% have a definite history of rheumatic fever.
†Medical University of South Carolina.
(From Leman R.B., Assey M.E.: Heart disease and pregnancy. *South. Med. J.* 74:944, 1981, used with permission.)

the MUSC group were thought to have organic heart disease; on further evaluation they were shown to have functional murmurs.

Rheumatic Heart Disease

Patients with mitral stenosis can develop pulmonary congestion and pulmonary edema because of the increase in cardiac output, heart rate, and sodium retention. In fact, pregnancy may be the first time the patient experiences symptoms. The increased flow across a fixed narrow valve orifice may result in high left atrial and pulmonary artery pressures to produce such symptoms. Atrial arrhythmias may be a precipitating factor for the development of failure

Table 14–2. Types of Heart Disease in the Study Population at MUSC* From 1975 to 1979 (180 Pregnancies, 67 Patients)

Disease	Incidence
Rheumatic heart disease (31/67)	
Mitral valve	17 (4 pure mitral stenosis)
Aortic valve	4
Both valves	2
Not specified	8
Congenital heart disease (15)	
Ventricular septal defect	8
Pulmonary stenosis	4
Atrial septal defect	1
Bicuspid aortic valve	1
Tetralogy of Fallot	1
Miscellaneous	
Barlow's (mitral prolapse)	2
IHSS†	2
Cardiomyopathy	4
Rhythm disturbances (5)	
Paroxysmal atrial tachycardia	3
Wolff-Parkinson-White syndrome	1
Second-degree AV block	1
Functional murmurs	10

*Medical University of South Carolina.
†Idiopathic hypertrophic subaortic stenosis.
(From Leman R.B., Assey M.E.: Heart disease and pregnancy. *South. Med. J.* 74:944, 1981, used with permission.)

or of an aggravating factor. Atrial fibrillation is the most common atrial arrhythmia, and the ventricular rate should be slowed immediately. Digitalis or
a combination of digitalis and a β-adrenergic blocking agent are usually effective. Beta-adrenergic blocking agents do cross the placenta and are present
in breast milk. There have been a few case reports of a small placenta, intra-
uterine growth retardation, fetal respiratory depression at birth, and fetal
postnatal hypoglycemia and bradycardia occurring when the mother had received continuous propranolol therapy during pregnancy.[10,11] Despite these
observations, the benefits of β-blockers in most cases outweigh the potential
disadvantages. The use of verapamil with digoxin to control the ventricular
rate of atrial fibrillation in pregnancy has not been evaluated, but appears
feasible. If the patient does not respond favorably to drug therapy, dc shock can
be performed, especially if the atrial fibrillation is associated with pulmonary
edema. Quinidine can be given safely[12] to prevent recurrences of atrial fibrillation. Atrial fibrillation can lead to atrial thrombi and systemic emboli. The
majority of patients can be managed medically and do not require surgery. The
surgical group is small, since the majority today have had surgery prior to
pregnancy. Surgery should be done only in a lifesaving situation. Closed mitral valvotomy for mitral stenosis can be done at any time, but if open heart
surgery is required, it is best delayed until after the first trimester, since
cardiopulmonary bypass in early pregnancy may affect the fetus. Balloon valvuloplasty is a possible alternative. However, it requires cardial fluoroscopy
(radiation exposure) and can produce hypotension which can affect fetal blood
flow. Patients who have had prior valve replacement present a problem regarding anticoagulant therapy, so that many physicians advise tissue valves
for women of child-bearing age. Oral anticoagulants cross the placenta and
may produce fetal hemorrhage or have a teratogenic effect if given early in
pregnancy.[13,14] For prosthetic valves, it has been recommended that heparin
be given during the first trimester (it does not cross the placenta), oral anticoagulants until the 37th week of gestation, and heparin again instead of the
oral anticoagulant until labor. The heparin is discontinued during labor, restarted 12 to 24 hours after delivery, and continued until oral anticoagulant
has an adequate effect.[14] Others advocate the use of self-administered heparin
subcutaneously throughout pregnancy except for the period prior to onset of
labor, when it should be given intravenously (see Chap. 6).

During the first few days, postpartum patients with mitral stenosis are
prone to develop pulmonary edema. Immediately postpartum, the contracting
uterus may deliver up to 1,000 ml of blood rapidly into the circulation.[15]

Mitral regurgitation is usually well tolerated. Atrial arrhythmias can be
managed as for mitral stenosis. Congestive heart failure usually can be controlled medically, and surgery is seldom necessary.

Aortic stenosis is not frequently noted in pregnancy. Hypovolemia should be
avoided in such cases. If the aortic stenosis is severe and symptoms cannot be
controlled, surgery may be required. If the patient has a prosthetic valve,
anticoagulant therapy should be managed as was recommended for the mitral
valve prosthesis. Aortic insufficiency is usually tolerated well, and seldom is
surgery required. The murmur of aortic or mitral insufficiency may decrease
or disappear during pregnancy due to the decrease in peripheral vascular
resistance. Postpartum, as the peripheral vascular resistance returns to nor-

mal, such murmurs may appear for the first time or become accentuated. This may lead to unnecessary studies for endocarditis, especially if the patient has fever.

Echocardiography and Doppler (including color flow) are safe procedures and allow appropriate assessment of the severity of valvular lesions. Chest x rays are not done often now, but if necessary after the first trimester, they can be done safely with shielding. No data are available as to the use of balloon valvuloplasty in pregnant patients with aortic or mitral stenosis.

Congenital Heart Disease

Fortunately, most of the patients have had surgery prior to the child-bearing age. Patients with left-to-right shunts (atrial and ventricular septal defect and patent ductus) who have not had surgery usually tolerate pregnancy well, and if heart failure develops, it can be controlled medically. Surgery is considered if medical treatment fails. Right-to-left shunts (Eisenmenger's complex and tetralogy of Fallot are the most common) present great problems with pregnancy. Pregnancy should be avoided, for there is a 50% abortion rate[16] in mothers with cyanotic heart disease, and if severe pulmonary hypertension is present the maternal mortality is over 50%.[17] Therapeutic terminaton of the pregnancy should be seriously considered, but has to be individualized. If patients refuse abortion, high right-sided filling pressures should be maintained; therefore, it is important to avoid blood loss and decreased venous return. At delivery, to control volume, A Swan-Ganz catheter should be inserted. However, cesarean section is preferable to spontaneous labor and delivery, although both have a high maternal risk.

Coarctation of the aorta is associated with an increase in mortality. One study[18] reported 13 maternal deaths in 147 patients who had 380 pregnancies. Six patients died from aortic rupture, 2 from cerebrovascular accidents, 3 from heart failure, 1 from aortic valve endocarditis, and 1 from undetermined causes. Aortic dissection is more common in such patients. Fetal mortality is also increased in coarctation. Uncomplicated cases should have vaginal delivery at term. Previously cesarean section was recommended, but it has been shown that the strain of labor is probably not an important factor in production of aortic rupture or dissection, since most of these occur before the onset of labor.[19] Surgical repair during pregnancy is only considered if symptoms or signs of aortic dissection develop or if there is excessive uncontrolled hypertension.

Congenital third-degree AV block is usually tolerated well during pregnancy. However, Stokes-Adams attacks can occur, and pacing may become necessary.

Infective Endocarditis

Diagnosis is more difficult in pregnant patients because changing murmurs of a normal pregnancy may cause one to overlook significant changes due to infection. Antibiotic treatment of endocarditis is the same as in nonpregnant patients. Although the American Heart Committee does not recommend antibiotic prophylaxis in the pregnant patient with valvular or congenital heart disease, I would recommend its use at the onset of labor and up to 24 hours postpartum or until the infection is cleared if there is a peripartum infection or septic abortion.

Hypertension

Essential hypertension predating the pregnancy or preeclampsia developing during the last trimester should be treated. Preeclampsia is more likely to develop in the patient with known essential hypertension. The decrease in systemic vascular resistance that occurs with pregnancy should be considered in the patient with essential hypertension. At times if the patient is receiving therapy, dosages may have to be reduced. Diuretics—namely, thiazides—may produce hypovolemia, hyponatremia, thrombocytopenia, neonatal jaundice, and may impair placental function.[17,20] Excessive reduction in plasma volume may be harmful to the fetus. Unless there is heart failure, these agents should not be used. Methyldopa and hydralazine are often recommended.[21] Hydralazine may also increase uterine blood flow. As mentioned previously, the use of β-adrenergic blockers in pregnancy has been questioned, since they may affect the fetus. However, Rubin,[22] in a review, concluded that β-blockers for hypertension seem to confer benefits on the fetus. He does state that these were not controlled studies. At present it is best to use other forms of therapy first, and if the response is not good, use the β-blockers. The treatment of hypertension related to toxemia of pregnancy is discussed in Chapter 5.

Coronary Artery Disease

Formerly it was unusual to find coronary disease in the pregnant patient. However, it is now being noted with increasing frequency, probably related to cigarette smoking and the use of oral contraceptives.[23] In addition, spasm has become an important factor. Recently, I encountered a pregnant patient with Prinzmetal's angina.

Treatment of the pregnant patient with coronary disease is also a problem. As mentioned before, there have been case reports of adverse effects of β-adrenergic blocking agents on the fetus.[10,11] In addition, nifedipine (Procardia) has been shown to be teratogenic and embryotoxic in rats when given in doses much greater than the maximum recommended human dose.[24] However, there are no adequate and well-controlled studies in pregnant women. Therefore, it is best that β-adrenergic blocking agents and calcium channel blockers be given to such patients only if the potential benefit justifies the potential risk to the fetus, and then only after discussion with the patient and her husband. Coronary arteriography should be avoided because of the dangers of fluoroscopic exposure, unless the patient does not respond to therapy and is at great risk from unstable angina.

Mitral Valve Prolapse

This is a common finding, especially in young females. The physical findings may vary with the hemodynamic changes of pregnancy. Unless the mitral insufficiency is severe, it presents no problems for the pregnant patient. Arrhythmias are managed in the usual manner as in the nonpregnant patient. During labor and delivery, endocarditis prophylaxis should be given.

Idiopathic Hypertrophic Subaortic Stenosis

This condition can be affected by the hemodynamic changes of pregnancy. Some of these can be beneficial and others undesirable. The increased blood volume may lessen the obstruction, but this can be offset by the decrease in peripheral vascular resistance. At the time of delivery, compression of the inferior vena cava by the uterus, especially in the supine position, decreases venous return, and, if there is also blood loss, the outflow obstruction can be increased. Hypovolemia should be avoided. If the patient develops angina, syncope, or tachyarrhythmias during pregnancy, a β-adrenergic blocker should be administered. During labor and delivery, endocarditis prophylaxis is recommended.

Marfan's Syndrome

The risk of death from dissection or aortic rupture is high in pregnant patients with Marfan's syndrome. Such patients should avoid pregnancy and, if pregnancy occurs, termination should be recommended, especially if the aortic root is widened significantly. Such patients often have mitral valve prolapse and aortic regurgitation, and if they go on to labor should have endocarditis prophylaxis. Cesarean section is preferable to labor and vaginal delivery.

Cardiac Arrhythmias

Arrhythmias can occur in the pregnant patient who has no evidence of cardiac disease. Usually no therapy is necessary for PABs and PVBs. Supraventricular tachycardia (reentrant type) usually can be stopped by carotid sinus pressure or drugs. Recently I.V. verapamil has become the drug of choice. As yet there have been no reports on adverse effects of this drug on the mother or fetus. In cases refractory to medical therapy, direct current shock therapy has been done without deleterious effect on the fetus.[25] The management of atrial fibrillation has already been discussed. Digitalis should be avoided if atrial fibrillation is present and the patient has the Wolff-Parkinson-White syndrome. Atrial flutter responds best to direct current shock. Ventricular tachycardia rarely has been noted during pregnancy and can be terminated by I.V. lidocaine. A pacemaker for complete heart block is inserted only if the patient is having heart failure or Stokes-Adams attacks.

Peripartum cardiomyopathy was discussed in Chapter 12. The reader is referred to a review of the heart and pregnancy that has been published by McAnulty et al.[25a]

THYROID AND THE HEART

There is still debate as to whether an abnormal thyroid state produces heart disease. Many suggest that the demands on the heart unveil subclinical heart disease such as coronary disease or hypertension. However, autopsy studies have revealed cardiac dilatation and hypertrophy in patients without evidence of other cardiac disease. Similar findings have been noted by echocardiography. Sandler and Wilson[26] reported reversible cardiac changes in young patients with thyrotoxic disease. Some of these cardiac changes could be potentially fatal. Another study of juvenile hyperthyroidism showed that patients with no known cardiac disease can develop mitral regurgitation, cardiomegaly, and congestive heart failure.[27]

Hyperthyroidism

Hyperthyroidism develops because of excessive thyroid hormone secretion (production of triiodothyronine, T_3, and/or thyroxine, T_4) that can occur with diffuse toxic goiter (Graves' disease), toxic multinodular goiter (Plummer's disease), toxic adenoma, at times with subacute thyroiditis if inflammation is sufficient to release stored hormone, or from excessive thyroid hormone intake. By increasing the activity of membrane-bound NA^+-K^+-ATPase, thyroid hormone increases cellular oxygen consumption.

The cardiac output is increased in hyperthyroidism by tachycardia and peripheral vasodilatation and decreased peripheral vascular resistance. The peripheral vasodilatation is due to the increased heat from the increased metabolic rate, oxygen consumption, and oxygen requirements of the tissues. The hyperdynamic state in thyrotoxic patients resembles that of increased adrenergic activity. Data do not clearly support the idea that this is due to excessive output of catecholamines, increased sensitivity to catecholamines, or decreased catecholamine uptake by nervous tissue. Buccino et al.[28] suggested that thyroxine has a direct effect on the heart independent of tissue catecholamine stores. The thyroid hormone effects on the heart are additive to those of the adrenergic system. However, another study suggests that part of the action of thyroid hormone is to sensitize myocardial cells in culture to added catecholamines.[29] This action can be treated with β-blockers.

Typical hyperthyroidism features may be present such as tachycardia, e.g., nervousness, sweaty palms, tremors, weight loss, and heat intolerance. Proptosis, lid-lag, and a diffusely enlarged thyroid gland may be noted. On the other hand, the hyperthyroidism may be masked (apathetic hyperthyroidism), and subtle findings such as rapid atrial fibrillation not responding to digitalis, unexplained tachycardia, frequent bowel movements in the presence of congestive heart failure (usually constipation exists), and warm feet (especially in a woman) suggest the diagnosis. Cardiac findings in hyperthyroidism are usually noted in patients over 40 years of age. The cardiac manifestations may be an overactive apical impulse, elevated systolic pressure with widened pulse pressure, systolic flow murmurs, atrial arrhythmias, and congestive failure. The increased blood flow across the mitral and tricuspid valves can produce diastolic murmurs that may simulate mitral and tricuspid stenosis. Third and fourth heart sounds may be present. At the second or third left intercostal space a systolic scratching sound (Means-Lerman scratch) may be heard which can be erroneously considered as a friction rub or crescendo murmur. It is probably due to a dilated hyperdynamic pulmonary artery contacting the chest wall. In toxic nodular goiter, the cardiac manifestations may be more prominent than the symptoms of thyrotoxicosis.

Besides sinus tachycardia or atrial arrhythmias, occasionally different degrees of AV heart block may be noted. The T waves may be prominent, the QRS complexes may be of increased amplitude, or there may be nonspecific ST-T changes. The roentgenogram of the chest may show normal appearance of the heart, prominence of the pulmonary artery, or generalized cardiomegaly (pear-like configuration). The diagnosis is usually made by demonstrating an elevated free serum T_4 level. Total serum T_4 is nonspecific and can be elevated because of increased thyroxine-binding globulin (TBG) associated with the intake of estrogens, pregnancy, hepatitis, and perphenazine.[30] T_3 thyrotoxicosis should be considered in some cases, especially with nodular goiter. In such cases the serum T_3 is elevated and the T_4 is normal. The thyrotropin-releasing hormone–thyroid-stimulating hormone (TRH–TSH) test may be useful in mild cases or when both T_3 and T_4 are normal. After intravenous TRH, the TSH rise is absent in hyperthyroidism. There is a recently developed TSH assay that measures small amounts of TSH and allows detection of suppressed TSH in the hyperthyroid state. Excessive intake of thyroid hormone (thyrotoxicosis factitia) gives a low radioactive iodine uptake test. This latter test is also helpful if ^{131}I therapy is planned.

There are three major therapeutic choices for patients with hyperthyroidism: radioactive iodine, antithyroid drugs (propylthiouracil or methimazole), and subtotal thyroidectomy. In addition, the β-adrenergic effects of hyperthyroidism may be controlled with propranolol (40 mg three times per day or more often) or other β-blockers as an adjunct to any of these three approaches, until euthyroidism is present. Most physicians now prefer the use of radioactive iodine as the therapy of choice in patients with hyperthyroid heart disease and in the older population. Occasionally, with a small goiter, recent hyperthyroidism, and minimal clinical findings, antithyroid drugs may be used (propylthiouracil, 100 mg, or methimazole, 10 mg every 8 hours). In the rare patient who is a candidate for subtotal thyroidectomy, preoperative preparation with antithyroid drugs and propranolol may be necessary for several months until the patient is euthyroid. In emergency situations, patients with hyperthyroidism may be prepared for surgery with large doses of propranolol alone. Iodides (SSKI, 5 drops three times per day) may be used to decrease release of thyroid hormone from the gland either as preoperative preparation or for several weeks after radioactive iodine treatment along with antithyroid agents, while awaiting maximal radiation effects. In the latter case, iodides should not be used until 1 week after radioactive iodine is given. Digitalis is given if atrial fibrillation or heart failure is present. However, its effect is limited until the hypermetabolic state is partially controlled. Beta-blockers can aid digoxin to slow the ventricular response. If atrial fibrillation does not revert to a normal sinus rhythm once the hyperthyroid state is under control, then quinidine is added and, if necessary, cardioversion is performed.

Myxedema

The heart in myxedema is affected by mucoid infiltration, myofibrillar swelling, muscle-cell necrosis, and interstitial fibrosis. It is still not clear if myxedema patients have an increased incidence of coronary artery disease, although some studies suggest this.[31] The patients complain about cold weather, sluggishness, fatigue, dyspnea, and orthopnea. They are often mentally dull. The hair is coarse, the skin is dry and puffy, and the voice is hoarse. There is a slow return of the reflex response. Bradycardia usually is present. In this clinical setting, myxedema should be suspected, especially if the patient had prior thyroidectomy. The ECG in addition to the slow rate will reveal low voltage and inverted T waves (Fig 14–1). Most of the cardiac enlargement noted on the x ray is due to pericardial effusion. Laboratory studies of elevated

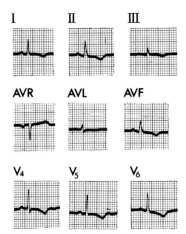

Fig 14–1. Electrocardiogram in myxedema. The heart rate was 55 beats per minute. Note the low voltage and diffusely inverted T waves.

cholesterol and reduced levels of serum T_4 and radioactive iodine uptake confirm the diagnosis. A serum thyroxine-stimulating hormone (TSH) analysis determines if primary hypothyroidism (elevated TSH) or pituitary hypothyroidism (low TSH) is present.

Thyroid hormones should be replaced slowly because angina, heart failure, and major arrhythmias, especially ventricular, can be precipitated. Thyroxine (Synthroid), 0.05 mg daily, is started and increased gradually every week to a maintenance level. It is now recognized that replacement levels of thyroxine are decreased with age. Most patients under age 65 tolerate replacement doses of 0.125 to 0.15 mg of thyroxine. Most older patients do well with a daily oral dose of 0.1 mg. The smallest dose that will reduce the TSH level to normal should be selected to prevent excessive myocardial O_2 consumption in the elderly. Intravenous thyroxine (300 to 400 µg) is used in the rare instances of myxedema coma. Its metabolic effects are sufficiently rapid to be more effective than oral thyroxine, and it avoids the marked direct cardiac stimulatory effects of I.V. liothyronine sodium (Cytomel).

The antiarrhythmic drug amiodarone can alter thyroid function by inhibiting the peripheral conversion of T_4 to T_3 and because of its high iodine content, can result in inhibition of thyroid organification. Thus, depending on the state of iodine intake, it can produce either hypothyroidism or hyperthyroidism. These effects can persist for months because of the prolonged half-life of amiodarone.

Other endocrinopathies that affect the heart will be mentioned only briefly. Acromegaly and Cushing's disease are conditions associated with hypersecretion of hormones from the pituitary gland. Increase in growth hormone can produce acromegaly with increased bone growth and enlargement of the viscera, including the heart. Many such patients also have hypertension, coronary disease, and diabetes.[32] Even without these associated conditions, a primary cardiomyopathy may be seen with acromegaly. Echocardiography may reveal concentric hypertrophy.[33]

Cushing's syndrome is associated with cortisol excess. Clinically such patients have a paper-thin, easily ecchymotic skin, moon facies, abdominal striae, truncal obesity, and osteoporosis. Hypertenson, cardiomegaly, and failure can occur.

Parathyroid disorders do not directly affect the heart. The hypercalcemia of hyperparathyroidism can produce hypertension and arrhythmias. The ECG can show a very short Q-T inverval. The hypocalcemia of hypoparathyroidism can aggravate the heart failure due to associated cardiac problems. The Q-T interval is prolonged with hypocalcemia at the expense of the ST segment, not due to widening of the T wave as noted with hypokalemia.

The pancreas can be related to heart disease because of diabetes mellitus. Such diabetic patients have premature coronary disease and also may develop a cardiomyopathic picture with cardiomegaly and failure, yet the epicardial arteries (depicted on coronary arteriography) are normal, and there is intramural small-arteriole changes.[34]

Primary hyperaldosteronism and pheochromocytoma have been discussed in Chapter 5.

OBESITY AND THE HEART

Obesity is an independent predictor of cardiovascular disease, especially in women.[35] Risk factors as hypertension, abnormal lipids, and diabetes are more frequent in the obese and may be worsened by obesity. Blood pressure positively correlates with the degree of overweight. Cardiac output, preload and afterload, and total peripheral resistance are increased in the obese hypertensive, and they develop dilatation and hypertrophy of the left ventricle.[36] In the normotensive obese, cardiac output, left and right end-diastolic pressures, and pulmonary artery and pulmonary artery wedge pressures are high and peripheral vascular resistance may be reduced. Blood volume is increased. Left ventricular function is impaired and a cardiomyopathy develops.

Alexander[37,38] describes a syndrome of chronic circulatory dysfunction in obese patients, leading to heart failure. Such patients have a history of obesity (twice the predicted ideal weight) for 10 years or longer. Progressive dyspnea, orthopnea, and somnolence are present. Eventually findings of heart failure are detected. In this group of patients, these findings occur because of chronic volume overload superimposed on the decreased diastolic ventricular compliance caused by left ventricular hypertrophy (diastolic dysfunction). Blood volume and cardiac output are increased in other obese patients. Pulmonary and systemic vascular congestion develop as a consequence of the chronic volume overload. Myocardial hypertrophy is inadequate and ventricular wall stress is increased and left ventricular systolic dysfunction is superimposed in this group. In a few patients with marked obesity, hypoventilation, hypoxemia, and respiratory acidosis can develop (Pickwickian syndrome, described in Chapter 9). Echocardiography can demonstrate left ventricular dysfunction. Weight reduction should be encouraged, but often is difficult for such patients. Weight reduction improves cardiac function and reduces risk factors. MacMahon[39] showed a reduction of 20% in left ventricular wall mass by echocardiography after weight reduction. Weight loss should be gradual for cardiac arrhythmias or sudden death can occur. Torsade de pointes has been reported in patients on a collagen-based liquid protein diet. Wiring of the jaw, gastric balloon, and stapling operations may be considered in the morbidly obese if results are not significant with a supervised low-calorie diet adequately supplemented with other nutrients.

TUMORS OF THE HEART

Tumors of the heart may be primary or metastatic or encroach on the heart from the surrounding tissues. Metastatic tumors are more common than primary. Primary tumors, such as myxomas, fibromas, lipomas, angiomas, mesothelioma of the AV node, teratomas, and rhabdomyomas, are benign; sarcomas and mesotheliomas are malignant. The metastatic tumors originate from leukemia, Hodgkin's disease, reticulum cell sarcoma, bronchogenic carcinoma, carcinoma of the breast, and many other causes. Melanomas metastasize to the heart in more than 50% of the cases. The cardiac findings of tumors depend on whether the pericardium, myocardium, or endocardium is invaded. Sudden cardiac tamponade can occur.

Myxoma is the commonest[40] primary tumor and can develop in either atrium. Left atrial myxoma is usually most common and is misdiagnosed as mitral valve disease or as bacterial endocarditis.

Tumor emboli can occur, at times as the presenting findings, and diagnosis is made from the material extracted by embolectomy. Fever, anemia, clubbing of the fingers, sudden hemiparesis or a cold extremity, Raynaud's phenomenon, elevated sedimentation rate, and hyperglobulinemia may be present. Varying apical systolic or diastolic murmurs and syncope, especially with changes in body position, are important clues. A third heart sound ("tumor plop") may be mistaken for an opening snap. Atrial fibrillation is rather rare with atrial myxoma. Echocardiography may detect the tumor (Fig 14–2). Two-dimensional echocardiography has demonstrated such tumors and their motion very clearly (Fig 14–3). In fact, this procedure is so diagnostic in some

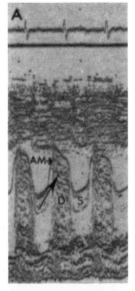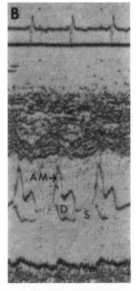

Fig 14–2. Echocardiogram in left atrial myxoma. **A,** preoperative. Multiple echoes (*arrow*) during diastole (D) behind anterior mitral valve leaflet (AM) due to the myxoma. **B,** postoperative. Note clearing of echoes during diastole following removal of the atrial myxoma.

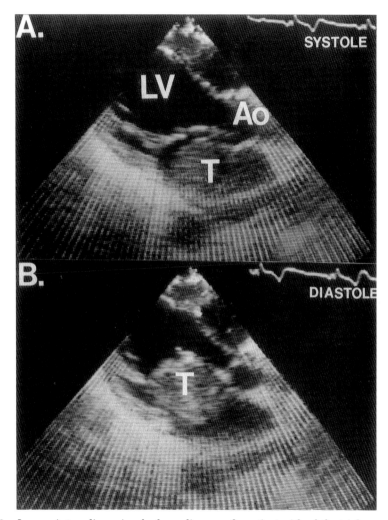

Fig 14-3. Long-axis two-dimensional echocardiogram of a patient with a left atrial myxoma. The tumor (T) can be seen in the left atrium during systole (A) and in the left ventricle during diastole (B). LV = left ventricle; Ao = aorta; T = tumor. (Courtesy of Dr. L. Earl Watts.)

cases that operation can be recommended without invasive procedures. These tumors can also be detected by radionuclide studies, computed tomography (CT), or magnetic resonance imaging (MRI). Diagnosis is confirmed, if necessary, by cineangiocardiography, which reveals the filling defect in the left atrium. Surgical excision should be performed, using cardiopulmonary bypass (Fig 14-4).

Right atrial myxoma should be suspected if there are chronic heart failure, syncopal attacks, prominent A venous waves, and variable tricuspid murmurs. Emboli can occur to the lungs. The diagnosis is made by echocardiography and angiocardiography, and surgery should be performed.

Myxomas were multiple in 5% of patients reported by McAllister.[40] The majority are attached to the atrial septum, have a short, broad-based attachment, and are pedunculated, gelatinous, soft, and polypoid (see Fig 14-4). Myxomas may be familial and transmitted as autosomal dominant.

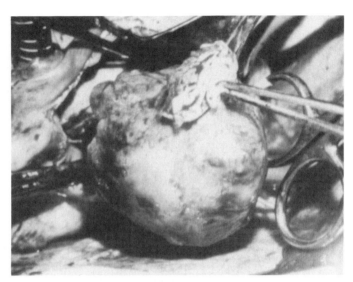

Fig 14–4.   Left atrial myxoma (same case as in Fig 14–2) shown just as it was surgically removed from the left atrium. Note its pedicle, which is held by forceps.

The carcinoid syndrome is associated with carcinoid tumors (most often of the ileum and appendix) which have metastasized to the liver. Serotonin, kinins, and other substances secreted by the tumor which have not been inactivated by the liver have been implicated in the pathogenesis of the cardiac lesions. These substances are inactivated by the lungs; therefore, left-sided cardiac involvement is rare, unless there is a right-to-left shunt or, rarely, if the tumor arises in the bronchus. This syndrome is characterized by episodic or permanent violaceous flushing of the skin (affecting the face, neck, and upper chest), bronchospasm with wheezing, diarrhea, and right-sided fibrotic endocardial lesions. Pulmonic stenosis, tricuspid stenosis or insufficiency, and right-sided heart failure are the most important cardiac changes. Cardiac failure can occur without the valvular lesions. The diagnosis of this syndrome depends on the clinical picture and markedly elevated urinary levels of 5-hydroxyindoleacetic acid (5-HIAA). Echocardiography may show right atrial and ventricular enlargement and thickening of the tricuspid and pulmonic valves. Chemotherapy may aid some with marked liver metastases, or large hepatic metastatic lesions can be removed. Removal of extraportal tumors may be helpful and α-adrenergic blockers and serotonin antagonists may block some of the clinical symptoms. Valve replacement may become necessary.

TRAUMA AND THE HEART

Trauma to the heart may be due to penetrating or nonpenetrating wounds of the chest. Penetrating wounds may produce hemorrhagic pericarditis with cardiac tamponade, pneumopericardium, myocardial contusion, and damage to coronary vessels, the septum, or the valves. Large contusions may lead to true or false ventricular aneurysms. Penetrating injuries are often due to bullet or knife wounds. The clinical picture may be that of pericardial effusion, congestive heart failure, arrhythmias, valvular defects, arteriovenous fistulas, or intracardiac shunts. At times, none of these features are present and there are only ECG changes such as bundle branch block, T wave inversion or even those of an infarction that suggest cardiac damage. Nonpenetrating wounds can produce very similar changes, except rarely, when fistulas or shunts are seen. For medicolegal purposes, frequent ECGs should be taken, because these may be the only clues to trauma of the myocardium. Echocardiography has been helpful in detecting hemopericardium, valvular damage, and a true or false aneurysm. Immediate surgery is indicated for hemopericardium to confirm the diagnosis and to repair the myocardial laceration. Patients with murmurs, valvular defects, or shunts should have heart catheterization studies prior to surgical consideration. Late sequelae may be a ventricular aneurysm, constrictive pericarditis, or the pericardiotomy syndrome. False ventricular aneurysms can rupture, but this rarely occurs in the true types. Ventricular aneurysms can produce heart failure, arrhythmias, and mural thrombosis with embolism, and in view of these complications, should be resected. Constrictive pericarditis and the pericardiotomy syndrome have been discussed in Chapter 13.

ATHLETE'S HEART

High levels of exercise produce physiologic adaptations in the cardiovascular system that can simulate organic heart disease.[41] This does not represent heart disease as was once thought, but does represent an appropriate physiologic adaptation to exercise. Such patients have resting sinus bradycardia and cardiac enlargement (increase in cardiac mass). Right and left ventricular hypertrophy may be present in the electrocardiogram. In addition, sinus bradycardia, junctional rhythm, idioventricular rhythm, first degree AV block, occasionally periods of Wenckebach second degree AV block, and repolarization changes may be noted. Echocardiography demonstrates wall thickness and increase in chamber size. Sudden death is rare in athletes. In those over age 30, it is often related to coronary artery disease.

REFERENCES

1. Mulholland H.C., Boyle McC.: The effect of posture on the cardiac output during the last six weeks of pregnancy. *Am. Heart J.* 76:291, 1968.
2. Metcalfe J., Ueland K.: Maternal cardiovascular adjustment to pregnancy. *Prog. Cardiovasc. Dis.* 16:363, 1974.
3. Hytten F.E., Robertson E.G.: Maternal water metabolism in pregnancy. *Proc. R. Soc. Med.* 64:1072, 1971.
4. Rogers M.C., Willerson J.T., Goldblatt A., et al.: Serum digoxin concentrations in the human fetus, neonate and infant. *N. Engl. J. Med.* 287:1010, 1972.
5. Leman R.B., Assey M.E.: Heart disease and pregnancy. *South. Med. J.* 74:944, 1981.
6. Mendelson C.L.: *Cardiac Disease in Pregnancy.* Philadelphia, F.A. Davis Co., 1960.
7. Etheridge M.J.: Heart disease and pregnancy. *Med. J. Aust.* 2:1172, 1968.
8. Adams J.Q.: Management of pregnant cardiac patients. *Clin. Obstet. Gynecol.* 11:910, 1968.
9. Szekely P., Smith L.: *Heart Disease and Pregnancy.* Edinburgh, Churchill-Livingstone, Inc., 1974.
10. Gladstone G.R., Hordof A., Gersony W.M.: Propranolol administration during pregnancy: Effects on the fetus. *J. Pediatr.* 86:962, 1975.
11. Cottrill C.M., McAlister R.G., Gettes L., et al.: Propranolol therapy during pregnancy, labor, and delivery: Incidence of transplacental drug transfer and impaired neonatal drug disposition. *J. Pediatr.* 91:812, 1977.
12. Hill L.M., Malkasian G.D., Jr.: The use of quinidine sulfate throughout pregnancy. *Obstet. Gynecol.* 54:366, 1979.
13. Pettifor J.M., Benson R.: Congenital malformations associated with the administration of oral anticoagulants during pregnancy. *J. Pediatr.* 86:459, 1975.

14. Harrison E.C., Roschke J., Ferenczi G., et al.: Managing pregnant patients with a heart valve prosthesis. *Contemp. Obstet. Gynecol.* 11:82, 1978.
15. Shub C.: Pregnancy in patients with valvular prostheses—Management. *Learning Center Highlights* 3:16, 1987.
16. Schaefer G., Ardite L.I., Soloman H.A., et al.: Congenital heart disease and pregnancy. *Clin. Obstet. Gynecol.* 11:1148, 1968.
17. Ueland K.: Cardiovascular disease complicating pregnancy. *Clin. Obstet. Gynecol.* 21:429, 1978.
18. Goodwin J.F.: Pregnancy and coarctation of the aorta. *Clin. Obstet. Gynecol.* 4:645, 1961.
19. Deal B.S., Wooley C.F.: Coarctation of the aorta and pregnancy. *Ann. Intern. Med.* 78:706, 1973.
20. Chesley L.C.: *Hypertensive Disorders in Pregnancy.* New York, Appleton-Century Crofts, 1978.
21. Brinkman C.R., Woods J.R.: Effects of cardiovascular drugs during pregnancy. *Cardiovasc. Med.* November 1976.
22. Rubin P.C.: Beta-blockers in pregnancy. *N. Engl. J. Med.* 305:1323, 1981.
23. Mann J.I., Vessey M.P., Thorogood M., et al.: Myocardial infarction in young women with special reference to oral contraceptive practice. *Br. Med. J.* 1:241, 1975.
24. Data on file at Pfizer Laboratories, New York, N.Y.
25. DeSilva R.A., Grayboys T.B., Podrid P.J., et al.: Cardioversion and defibrillation. *Am. Heart J.* 100:881, 1980.
25a. McAnulty J.H., Morton M.J., Ueland K.: The heart and pregnancy. *Curr. Probl. Cardiol.* 13:595, 1988.
26. Sandler G., Wilson G.M.: The nature and prognosis of heart disease in thyrotoxicosis. *Quart. J. Med.* 28:347, 1959.
27. Cavallo A., Joseph C.J., Casta A.: Cardiac complications in juvenile hyperthyroidism. *AJDC* 138:479, 1984.
28. Buccino R.A., Spann J.F., Jr., Pool P.E., et al.: Influence of thyroid state on the intrinsic contractile properties and energy stores of the myocardium. *J. Clin. Invest.* 46:1169, 1967.
29. Wildenthal K: Studies of isolated fetal mouse hearts in organ culture. Evidence for a direct effect of triiodothyronine in enhancing cardiac responsiveness to norepinephrine. *J. Clin. Invest.* 51:2702, 1972.
30. Refetoff S.: Thyroid hormones transport, in Degrott L., Cahill G., Martini L., et al. (eds.): *Endocrinology.* New York, Grune & Stratton, 1979 p. 351.
31. Vanhaelst L., Neve P., Chailly P., et al.: Coronary disease in hypothyroidism. *Lancet* 2:800, 1967.
32. McGuffin W.L., Sherman B.M., Roth J., et al.: Acromegaly and cardiovascular disorders: A prospective study. *Ann. Intern. Med.* 81:11, 1974.
33. Smallridge R.C., Rajfer S., Davis J., et al.: Acromegaly and the heart: An echocardiographic study. *Am. J. Med.* 66:22, 1979.
34. Hamby R.I., Zoneraich S., Sherman L.: Diabetic cardiomyopathy. *JAMA* 229:1749, 1974.
35. Hubert H.B., Feinleib M., McNamara P.M., et al.: Obesity as an independent risk factor for cardiovascular disease: A 26-year follow-up of participants in the Framingham heart study. *Circulation* 67:968, 1983.
36. Bray G.A.: Obesity and the heart. *Mod. Conc. Cardiovasc. Dis.* 56:67, 1987.
37. Alexander J.K.: Obesity and the heart. *Curr. Probl. Cardiol.* 5:6, 1980.
38. Alexander J.K.: The cardiomyopathy of obesity. *Prog. Cardiovasc. Dis.* 27:325, 1985.
39. MacMahon S.W., Wilcken D.E.L., Macdonald G.J.: The effect of weight reduction on left ventricular mass: A randomized controlled trial in young, overweight hypertensive patients. *N. Engl. J. Med.* 314:334, 1986.
40. McAllister H.A.: Primary tumors and cysts of the heart and pericardium. *Curr. Probl. Cardiol.* 4:8, 1979.
41. Park R.C., Crawford M.H.: Heart of the athlete. *Curr. Probl. Cardiol.* 10:1, 1985.

Chapter 15

ARRHYTHMIAS

Before considering the various arrhythmias, it is best to review some facts pertaining to their genesis and also the mechanisms of action of the commonly used antiarrhythmic drugs. Pacemaker cells are present in the sinus node, specialized atrial fibers, distal portion of the AV node, bundle of His, bundle branches, and Purkinje fibers. Normal atrial and ventricular cells do not have pacemaker cells. The pacemaker cells have the ability to initiate self-excitation (automaticity) and do not require external stimuli. The action potential curve of a pacemaker cell, as shown in Figure 15–1, can be recorded with a microelectrode. The inside of the cell is negative to the extracellular fluid, and this resting transmembrane voltage in the Purkinje fiber is about −90mV. On excitation, this negative potential rapidly changes to a positive value (phase 0). Rapid depolarization (phase 0) is the main determinant of conduction velocity or membrane responsiveness and depends on the movement of positively charged sodium ions across the cell membrane and the magnitude of the transmembrane potential immediately before excitation. The greater the magnitude, the steeper is the slope of phase 0. As the inward sodium current subsides there is a period of initial rapid depolarization (phase 1) when negatively charged chloride ions enter the cell, followed immediately by a period of slow or plateau repolarization (phase 2), during which there is an influx of positive calcium and sodium ions. During rapid repolarization (phase 3), there is an increase in membrane permeability to potassium with an efflux of potassium. The effective refractory period extends to phase 3 at about −55 mV, when the cell begins to regain its ability to respond. After full repolarization, there is no steady state as seen in the action potential curve of myocardial cells, but a slow spontaneous diastolic depolarization (phase 4) develops. When phase 4 reaches the threshold potential (TP), the cell is re-excited (automaticity). Thus the shape of the cardiac action potential determines several properties, namely conductivity, refractoriness, and automaticity, which are related to the development of arrhythmias. Arrhythmias can occur as a result of an abnormality of conduction velocity, a refractory period, impulse formation (automaticity), or a combination of these or other less known mechanisms (Table 15–1). Re-entry accounts for the majority of tachyarrhythmias. For re-entry to occur, there must be two conducting pathways which are connected proximally and distally. One pathway must have a longer refractory period and the other a shorter refractory period and slower conduction. Re-entry can produce arrhythmias in the normal or abnormal heart.[1] This can occur at several locations in the heart, such as the SA node (PABs, re-entrant

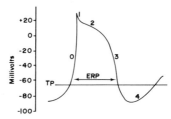

Fig 15–1. Diagrammatic representation of action potential curve from a Purkinje fiber with the various phases (0 to 4). TP = threshold potential; ERP = effective refractory period. (Modified after Hoffman B.F., Singer D.H.: Effects of digitalis on electrical activity of cardiac fibers. *Prog. Cardiovasc. Dis.* 7:226, 1964. By permission of the author and publisher.)

tachycardia), the atria (PABs, atrial flutter or fibrillation), the AV node (re-entrant tachycardia) and the ventricles (PVBs or ventricular tachycardia). Re-entry is the mechanism for supraventricular arrhythmias due to the Wolff-Parkinson-White (WPW) syndrome involving the normal conducting pathway and the accessory pathway. The tachyarrhythmias due to re-entry often require an initiating beat. Another mechanism of arrhythmia formation is abnormality of impulse formation as alteration of normal automaticity or abnormal enhanced automaticity[2,3] (phase 4). This can produce atrial tachycardia with or without AV block, accelerated junctional, accelerated ventricular rhythm, or parasystole. The sinus node is usually the controlling automatic pacemaker. Its activity is enhanced by sympathetic discharge and suppressed by vagal discharge. If the sinus node is suppressed physiologically or due to pathologic states, latent pacemakers take over the automatic function at the junctional tissue. Subsidiary pacemakers may accelerate because of an abnormal state or drugs and take over as the automatic pacemaker. Another mechanism for abnormal impulse formation is the recently discovered triggered activity.[4] Triggered activity does not arise spontaneously. It requires a preceding stimulus that causes early or late after-depolarizations, which cross the threshold and produce arrhythmia. Some arrhythmias may have several mechanisms.

Re-entry and automaticity can produce arrhythmias because of autonomic neurohumoral mediators and a variety of conditions such as ischemia, hypoxia, electrolyte disorders, drugs, and so on. Triggered activity produces arrhythmias when repolarization is delayed, and early after depolarizations (during phase 3 of the action potential curve) occur secondary to hypokalemia or a class

Table 15–1. Mechanisms of Arrhythmias

1. Disorders of impulse formation
   A. Abnormal enhanced automaticity
   B. Triggered activity
      a. Early after-depolarizations
      b. Delayed after-depolarizations
2. Disorders of impulse conduction
   A. Re-entry
   B. Conduction delay and block
3. Combinations of above

1A drug such as quinidine. This could be the explanation for polymorphic ventricular tachycardia (torsades) that can occur when the Q-T interval is prolonged. Delayed after depolarizations occur early in phase 4 and can be caused by increased intracellular calcium, digitalis toxicity, and increased catecholamine stimulation. They may produce premature ectopy or sustained tachyarrhythmias.

Re-entrant arrhythmias can often be abolished by increasing or decreasing conduction velocity (phase 0) and prolonging or shortening the effective refractory period (includes phases 0, 1, and 2) relative to the total action potential duration. Automatic arrhythmias can be abolished by decreasing the slope of diastolic depolarization (phase 4), raising the level (less negative) of the threshold potential, or decreasing the level (more negative) of the resting potential. Early after-depolarization arrhythmias can be treated by correcting the prolonged Q-T interval and delayed after-depolarization arrhythmias respond to verapamil.

ANTIARRHYTHMIC DRUGS

The classification of antiarrhythmic drugs[5] is still controversial, but for clinical purposes they can be classified as shown in Table 15-2. All of the drugs to a certain degree decrease the slope of phase 4 (decreased automaticity) and thus can suppress the automatic arrhythmias. Inhibition of sympathetic excitation can also suppress automatic arrhythmias. Re-entry arrhythmias can be suppressed by depression of the fast response (inward sodium depolarization current), prolongation of the action potential duration, and inhibition of the slow response (inward calcium depolarization current). The different classes of drugs have several of these actions. The dominant action of each class is as follows: class 1 drugs depress the fast inward sodium current; class 2 drugs reduce the sympathetic excitation to the heart; class 3 drugs prolong the action potential duration; and class 4 drugs block the slow calcium channel response. Class 1A drugs moderately depress phase 0 (slow conduction velocity) and lengthen the action potential duration which prolongs repolarization and increases refractoriness. This action can prolong the QRS and Q-T intervals. Class 1B drugs mildly depress phase 0 and shorten the action potential duration and repolarization. Therefore, they cause no QRS or Q-T interval changes. Class 1C drugs markedly depress phase 0 and affect the action potential duration and repolarization very little. They prolong the P-R and QRS intervals. The Q-T interval will be affected because of QRS prolongation and not a repolarization effect. Class 2 drugs are β-adrenergic receptor blockers; they slow conduction and refractoriness in the AV node, prolong the P-R interval, and do not change the Q-T interval. Class 3 drugs prolong the action potential duration, increase refractoriness, and thus prolong the Q-T interval. Class 4 drugs prolong AV conduction and refractoriness and so prolong the P-R interval.

Pharmacodynamic and Pharmacokinetic Effects of Antiarrhythmic Drugs

Quinidine has a half-life of 6 to 8 hours, and is usually given orally every 6 hours to achieve a steady state in about 48 hours. It is well absorbed, has its peak level in about 4 hours, and is partially metabolized by the liver; and 20% is excreted unchanged in the urine. It should be given cautiously in the pres-

Table 15–2. Classification of Antiarrhythmic Agents

Class	Agent	I.V. (mg)	Oral (mg)	Dominant Action
1A	Quinidine		200–400 q6h	Inhibition of the fast inward sodium current
	Procainamide (Pronestyl)	Loading 50 mg/min up to 1 g, then 2 to 6 mg/min	250–1000 q4–6h	
	Disopyramide (Norpace)		100–300 q6–8h	
B	Lidocaine (Xylocaine)	Loading 200–300 mg, then 1–4 mg/min		
	Tocainide (Tonocard)		400–600 q8–12h	
	Mexiletine (Mexitil)		150–300 q6–8h	
	Phenytoin (Dilantin)	Loading 100 mg q 5 min up to 500 mg	300–500 q24h	
C	Flecainide (Tambocor)		100–200 q12h	
	Encainide (Enkaid)		25–75 q6–8h	
	Propafenone (Rythmol)		150–300 q8–12h	
II	β-blocker (Propranolol)	.25–.50 mg q 5 min for up to 0.20 mg/kg	10–60 q6h	Inhibition of sympathetic excitation
III	Bretylium (Bretylol)	Loading 5–10 mg/kg over 10–20 min then 1–2 mg/min		
	Amiodarone (Cardarone)		Loading 800–1600 daily × 2 wk. Then 200–600 daily	
	Sotalol		160–320 mg q12h	
IV	Calcium channel blockers			
	Verapamil (Calan, Isoptin)	5–10 mg over 2 min	80–120 q6–8h	Inhibition of the slow inward calcium current

ence of renal or hepatic disease. It is 80 to 90% bound to proteins. Therapeutic levels are usually between 2 and 6 μg/ml. Quinidine can produce a rash, thrombocytopenia, fever, and GI tract symptoms. About 30% of patients have nausea, vomiting, or diarrhea. Excessive doses can produce cinchonism (blurred vision, tinnitus, and GI tract symptoms). Quinidine may directly prolong the AV conduction and His-Purkinje conduction time. However, its anticholinergic effect and reflex sympathetic stimulation effect resulting from alpha-adrenergic blockade that produces peripheral vasodilatation can override its direct effect on AV conduction and result in a shortening of AV conduction time. Widening of the QRS complex can occur, and this should be monitored periodically, especially if bundle-branch block is present before therapy. Quinidine syncope[6] (syncopal attacks occurring with paroxysmal ventricular arrhythmias—usually torsades de pointes) is usually noted when quinidine produces a long Q-T interval. It is not yet clear to what degree of QRS widening or Q-T interval prolongation warrants discontinuing therapy. However, most agree that if the QRS widens by more than 30% or the Q-T interval corrected for rate becomes greater than 0.55 seconds, the plasma level should be checked and the dosage reduced. Quinidine may elevate the serum digoxin level by decreasing its renal and nonrenal clearance and its volume of distribution.

Procainamide (Pronestyl) has a half-life of 3 to 5 hours. It is well absorbed, has a peak level in about 1 hour, and is excreted by the kidneys. N-acetyl procainamide (NAPA) is one of its metabolites produced by acetylation in the liver, and it has an antiarrhythmic effect. Therapeutic levels of procainamide are usually between 3 and 8 μg/ml, but do not take into account the antiarrhythmic effect of NAPA. Procainamide is only 15% protein-bound. It may have to be given orally every 4 hours; however, in some instances, because of the antiarrhythmic effect of NAPA, it can be given every 6 hours. It is important to measure both procainamide and NAPA levels, especially in patients with renal disease. It can also be given I.V. and I.M. A prolonged release form of procainamide is available. A systemic, lupus-like syndrome (fever, arthralgia, pneumonitis, pleuritis, pericarditis, and hepatomegaly, but not brain or kidney changes) can occur in patients who are slow acetylators of the drug. Antinuclear antibodies (ANA) develop in about 60% within 1 year of therapy, and approximately one third of these develop the lupus picture. This syndrome clears when the drug is stopped. Procainamide produces the same ECG changes noted with quinidine.

Disopyramide (Norpace) has a half-life of 6 to 8 hours and is well absorbed when given orally. Its peak level occurs in about 3 hours, and it is excreted by the kidneys. Therapeutic levels are usually between 2 and 5 μg/ml. The incidence of GI side effects is much smaller than with quinidine. Urinary retention and dry mouth can occur because of its anticholinergic effect. Because it is excreted by the kidneys, in the presence of kidney disease it should be given cautiously and in smaller doses. Because of its negative inotropic effect, it should not be given in the presence of heart failure. As yet it has not been shown to increase the serum digoxin level, as can occur with quinidine. It can produce the same ECG effects noted with quinidine.

A recent study[7] concluded that class 1A drugs (quinidine, procainamide, disopyramide) associated ventricular fibrillation is an early event (median of 3 days) and that left ventricular dysfunction and concomitant therapy with digitalis and diuretic agents may predispose patients to this complication. No evidence of a relation between drug-induced prolongation of the Q-T and the occurrence of drug-associated ventricular fibrillation without torsades was found. In addition, there may be an increased risk of its recurrence with subsequent trials of these antiarrhythmic drugs.

The distributional half-life of lidocaine (Xylocaine) I.V. is 8 minutes, and that of the elimination phase is 108 minutes. Accordingly, the result may be a significant fall in blood level between the peak serum level from the initial bolus (rapid distribution) and the subsequent steady state from the constant infusion, which may take up to 5 to 7 hours. Thus, a significant interval can occur during which plasma levels are inadequate. This cannot be corrected by increasing the concentration or the rate of the constant infusion, but can be overcome by giving a loading dose in divided amounts or as an infusion over a 20-minute period along with the constant infusion.[8] Lidocaine is metabolized by the liver and should be given in lower amounts in the presence of shock or heart failure. Therapeutic plasma levels range from 2 to 5 µg/ml. Overdosage can produce CNS symptoms such as confusion, paresthesias, drowsiness, and even convulsions. It usually does not produce ECG changes. However, if there is impaired conduction of the sinus or AV node, it can precipitate sinus arrest or heart block. Myocardial function can be mildly depressed, depending on the degree of cardiac disease.

Tocainide (Tonocord)[9] has electrophysiologic properties similar to Lidocaine. It is rapidly absorbed orally and has a peak level in 2 hours and has an elimination half-life of almost 12 hours. About 40% is excreted unchanged in the urine. It is used primarily for ventricular arrhythmia with significant reduction in 40 to 60% of patients. Therapeutic plasma levels are 4 to 10 µg/ml. If a patient with ventricular arrhythmia responds to Lidocaine, there is a 50% chance of a good response to Tocainide. The most common side effects are gastrointestinal (nausea, anorexia) and neurologic (tremors, dizziness), which occur in about 30 to 40% of patients. Blood dyscrasia, pulmonary fibrosis and lupus syndrome have also been reported.

Mexiletine (Mexitil)[9] is structurally similar to Lidocaine and Tocainide and is used primarily for ventricular arrhythmia. It is effective in 40 to 60% of patients. It reaches its peak concentration in about 2 to 4 hours with an elimination half-life of about 10 hours. Therapeutic levels range from 0.5 to 2 µg/ml. It is metabolized in the liver. Its side effects are similar to those of Tocainide. Upper gastrointestinal symptoms, dizziness, tremor, and incoordination can occur. Rarely blood dyscrasias can develop. No significant change in P-R, QRS, or Q-T intervals are noted.

Diphenylhydantoin (Dilantin) has a half-life of almost 24 hours. Therapeutic plasma levels are between 10 to 20 µg/ml. Overdosage can produce CNS symptoms, skin rashes, megaloblastic anemia, and a pseudolymphoma picture. It is rarely used alone and currently is used primarily for digitalis-induced toxic arrhythmias.

Flecainide (Tambocor)[10] is well absorbed and reaches a peak plasma concentration in 3 to 4 hours. Its elimination half-life is about 14 to 20 hours with 85% being excreted in the urine. Therapeutic plasma levels range from 0.2 to 1 µg/ml. The drug suppresses ventricular arrhythmias in about 70 to 90% of patients. Side effects include central nervous system disturbances (dizziness, blurred vision, headaches) and nausea. In about 7% of patients, it can cause new arrhythmias or worsen the existing ones. The incidence of this pro-arrhythmic effect is highest in patients who have sustained ventricular tachycardia. In addition, it has a negative inotropic effect that can worsen congestive heart failure. Because it markedly depresses phase 0 (conduction velocity), in almost all cases it will widen the QRS complex even at therapeutic levels. It also prolongs the P-R interval. The Q-T interval will be affected because of QRS prolongation and not a repolarization effect.

Encainide (Enkaid)[11] is similar electrophysiologically to flecainide. Active metabolites contribute to its antiarrhythmic effect. Metabolites 0-desmethyl encainide (ODE) and 3-methyl 0-desmethyl (MODE) contribute to the antiarrhythmic effect of the parent drug Encainide. The variable response of encainide during long-term therapy is probably due to the varying concentrations of the active metabolites. Encainide therapy produces a widening of the QRS complex and P-R interval prolongation. After oral administration, the peak plasma level occurs in about 1.5 hours. Effective serum concentration is 0.5 to 1 μg/ml. Encainide is metabolized in the liver and its elimination half-life ranges from 30 minutes to 4 hours. The half-life of ODE and MODE metabolites is much longer. Encainide suppresses ventricular ectopics in 70 to 90% of patients. It does not have a negative inotropic action. The most serious side effect is worsening or new sustained ventricular tachycardia. Other side effects are blurred vision, dizziness, tremors, and nausea.

Pro-arrhythmia occurs more often in patients treated with flecainide or encainide when they are treated for sustained ventricular tachycardia, especially if they prolong the QRS greater than 50%, the dosages are high, and there is severe ventricular dysfunction. Both drugs are contraindicated if the patient has a pre-existing second or third degree AV block or right bundle-branch block associated with a left hemiblock, unless a pacemaker is present to sustain cardiac rhythm if complete heart block occurs.

Propafenone (Rythmol)[12] is not yet available. In addition to depressing the rate of rise of phase 0, it exhibits a weak β-adrenergic and calcium channel blocking action. It is metabolized in the liver. Peak plasma levels occur in almost 2 hours, and it has a half-life of about 2.5 hours. Therapeutic plasma concentrations range from 0.2 to 3 μg/ml. It is useful for ventricular and supraventricular arrhythmia. Gastrointestinal and CNS symptoms are the most common extracardiac side effects. Propafenone may worsen AV block and it has a negative inotropic effect.

Propranolol (Inderal) is most often used when it is desirable to use a β-blocker as an antiarrhythmic agent. Propranolol has an antiarrhythmic effect because of its β-adrenergic blockade action. In high concentrations, it can have a quinidine-like effect (depression of maximum rate of depolarization). However, this latter effect is considered to play an insignificant part clinically. It does decrease the slope of phase 4 depolarization, but has little effect on the action potential duration. It increases the effective refractory period of the AV node. The half-life of propranolol is about 3 to 6 hours and peak levels occur in about 2 to 4 hours after oral administration. It is over 90% protein-bound. It is metabolized by the liver, and the first-pass effect is so great that bioavailability is low and increasing dosage may be necessary to get an effective amount in the systemic circulation.[13] Therapeutic plasma levels are between 50 and

100 ng/ml. Side effects include excessive bradycardia, bronchoconstriction, hypoglycemia, worsening of peripheral vascular insufficiency, skin rash, diarrhea, insomnia, and heart failure (in view of its negative inotropic effect). It can produce sinus bradycardia and AV block, but does not widen the QRS complex, and it may shorten the Q-T interval.

Bretylium tosylate (Bretylol), an antiadrenergic agent, lengthens the action potential duration and thus prevents the development of ventricular arrhythmias. Currently it is available only for I.V. and I.M. use. It is excreted by the kidneys, with an elimination half-life of 6 to 10 hours. It can produce postural hypotension, nausea, and vomiting.

Amiodarone (Cordarone),[14] a benzofuran derivative, markedly prolongs the action potential duration and refractoriness but has little effect on conduction. The half-life of the drug is 10 to 45 days and a loading dose becomes effective in 7 to 14 days. It is metabolized in the liver. Therapeutic concentrations range between 0.75 and 3.5 µg/ml. It is effective in both supraventricular and ventricular arrhythmias. It suppresses ventricular arrhythmias in up to 60 to 80% of patients and sustained life-threatening ventricular arrhythmias in 30 to 80%. Long-term therapy has many adverse effects, such as microdeposits in the cornea, liver function abnormalities, neuromuscular disorders, bluish-gray skin discoloration, thyroid abnormalities, gastrointestinal disorders, and pulmonary pneumonitis and fibrosis. Many of these are dose-related. Pulmonary toxicity is one of the most serious complications and may be irreversible. After baseline studies, serial chest x rays and pulmonary function tests should be done during long-term therapy. Torsades de pointes, as associated with a long Q-T interval, following amiodarone has been reported.

Sotalol[15] is a noncardioselective beta-adrenergic blocking drug with class 2 and 3 antiarrhythmic effects but is not yet available. About 75% of the dose is excreted in the urine and the half-life is 14 to 20 hours. It reaches peak plasma levels in 2 to 3 hours. It is effective in most supraventricular and ventricular arrhythmias. Therapeutic plasma concentrations range from 1 to 3 µg/ml. The major side effects are hypotension and prolongation of the Q-T interval that may be associated with torsades. Sotalol and its d-isomer are promising new antiarrhythmic drugs which are not yet available.

Verapamil hydrochloride (Calan, Isoptin) blocks the slow calcium channel response. It has little effect on phase 0, depresses phases 1 and 2, and also depresses phase 4 (especially if it is slow-channel-dependent). It prolongs the effective refractory period and conduction through the AV node and is most effective for re-entrant arrhythmias involving the AV node. It lengthens the P-R interval, but has no effect on the other ECG intervals. At present it is available for I.V. and oral use. It has an elimination half-life of 2 to 5 hours and is about 70% excreted by the kidneys. Peak plasma concentration is reached in 1 to 2 hours and effective plasma concentrations range from 0.10 to 0.15 µg/ml. It has a negative inotropic effect, which is offset to a certain degree by its peripheral vasodilation (reduction in afterload). Preferably it should not be given or should be used cautiously with a β-adrenergic-blocking drug or disopyramide. It can produce hypotension and bradycardia.

Diltiazem has electrophysiologic action similar to verapamil but is used primarily for angina.

Drug efficacy for ventricular arrhythmias vary. Morganroth[16] reported the

Table 15–3.   Drug Efficacy for Ventricular Arrhythmias

Drug Class	Benign and Potentially Lethal—% Responding on Holter Recording	Lethal—% VT Not Initiated
IA	50–70	15–25
IB	40–60	10–20
IC	70–90	20–30
II	50–60	5–10
III	60–80	15–30

VT = ventricular tachycardia
(From Morganroth, J.: Ambulatory Electrocardiographic Monitoring of New Antiarrhythmic Drugs. *Circulation* 73:11–92, 1986.)

percentage of patients responding to therapy (Table 15–3) who had benign PVCs, potential lethal ventricular arrhythmias (nonsustained ventricular tachycardia with left ventricular dysfunction) and lethal ventricular arrhythmias (sustained ventricular tachycardia). Holter monitoring was used to follow the benign and potentially lethal arrhythmias. Response was defined as a greater than 75% reduction of frequency of PVCs. Electrophysiologic testing was done for sustained ventricular tachycardia and is reported in the table as percent, showing lack of initiation of the arrhythmia to stimulation.

It is important to be familiar with certain phenomena for interpretation and understanding arrhythmias. These are listed in Table 15–4. They will be explained and demonstrated and it will be shown how they apply to many arrhythmias as these are discussed.

SUPRAVENTRICULAR ARRHYTHMIAS

Sinus tachycardia is present when the rate is over 100 beats per minute. Sinus bradycardia is considered when the rate is below 60 beats per minute. Sinus arrhythmia is a fluctuation of the rate of the sinus node and can vary with respirations (the rate increases with inspiration and decreases with expiration).

Table 15–4.   Arrhythmia Phenomena

Type I (Wenckebach or Mobitz I), Type II (Mobitz II) AV blocks

Aberration

Exit block

Concealed conduction

AV dissociation

Dual or reciprocating conduction

Supernormality and vulnerability

Fascicular block

Automaticity

Capture beats

Fusion beats

Escape beats

Premature Atrial Beats

These arise in different parts of the atria and produce a P wave different from that which originates in the sinus node. The P wave configuration depends on where the ectopic beat originates in the atria. For instance, if the premature beat originates low in the atria and has to travel upward to stimulate the atria, the P wave of the premature beat will be inverted in leads II, III, and aV$_F$ because it has an axis close to -90 degrees. After stimulating the atria, the ectopic beat stimulates the ventricles by the normal pathway, and the resultant QRS complex resembles that of a normal conducted beat. At times PAB occurs early after a normal conducted beat and is blocked because it finds the ventricle refractory. Therefore it is not followed by a QRS complex, or, if it is conducted, the QRS complex may have an aberrant configuration caused by partial refractoriness of the ventricles. Because PABs interfere with the sinus mechanism, they do not produce compensatory pauses; that is, the interval from the beat preceding the ectopic beat to that following it is usually not equal to two sinus beat intervals. Figure 15–2 depicts a variety of PABs. The patient may not be aware of these premature beats or experiences skipping, palpitations, or a variety of other precordial, neck, or upper epigastric sensations.

Atrial premature beats are usually not treated in the otherwise normal person. Precipitating agents such as tobacco and coffee should be eliminated. In the presence of cardiac disease, these premature beats may be the forerunners of supraventricular tachycardias. Therefore, if they occur frequently in diseased states, they should be treated. The drug of choice is quinidine sulfate, usually in a dosage of 200 to 300 mg every 6 hours. Procainamide and diso-

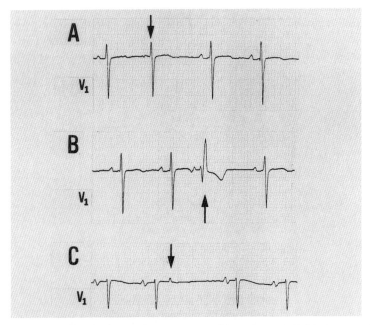

Fig 15–2. Atrial premature beats. A, Premature atrial beat (arrow). B, Premature atrial beat with ventricular aberration (arrow). C, Blocked premature atrial beat (arrow).

pyramide are less effective. If heart failure is present, digitalis should be given.

Supraventricular Tachycardia

Sinus Nodal Re-entrant Tachycardia. This arrhythmia[17] accounts for about 5% of the supraventricular tachycardias. It may be initiated by an atrial premature beat. Because the re-entry is in the SA node, the atria are depolarized in the same direction as during sinus rhythm, and so the P-wave morphology is identical to that of the sinus P-wave. For this reason, it may be difficult to differentiate this from sinus tachycardia. Its abrupt onset and termination are the main determining factors (Fig. 15–3). The rate is usually between 100 and 160 beats per minute. It is most often noted in older patients with heart disease. Atrioventricular block can occur during the tachycardia. Vagal maneuvers can abruptly terminate it, whereas with sinus tachycardia, the rate only slows and then speeds up again when the vagal influence is stopped. Vagal maneuvers, digitalis, verapamil, and propranolol may terminate the tachycardia. These drugs and quinidine may prevent attacks.

Intra-atrial Reentrant Tachycardia. This arrhythmia[17] is rare and is difficult to differentiate from ectopic automatic atrial tachycardia. The re-entry path is in the atria. It is usually more regular than the ectopic type. Vagal maneuvers do not interrupt the tachycardia but produce AV block in both types. Intra-atrial re-entrant tachycardia responds to type 1A drugs.

Atrioventricular Nodal Reentrant Tachycardia. This is the most common of the paroxysmal supraventricular tachycardias and accounts for over 50% of them.[17] The re-entry path is within the AV node. In the past, this was called

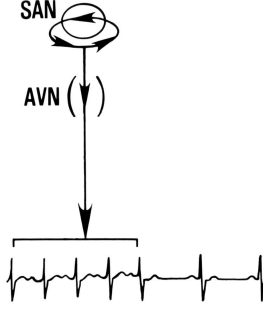

Fig 15–3. Sinus nodal re-entrant tachycardia. The abrupt termination of the tachycardia (arrow) is a factor in differentiating it from sinus tachycardia. SAN = sinoatrial node; AVN = atrioventricular node.

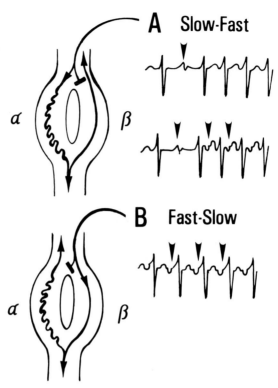

Fig 15–4.   Atrioventricular nodal re-entrant tachycardia. A, Slow–fast type conducts antegrade by way of the α pathway and retrograde by way of the β pathway. Note (arrow) that a premature atrial beat with long P-R interval initiates the tachycardia. The P waves are not visible during the tachycardia. Second tracing shows P waves immediately after the QRS complexes (second and third arrows) during the tachycardia (RP interval < 0.07 seconds). B, Fast–slow type conducts antegrade by way of the β pathway and retrograde by way of the α pathway. Note P waves (arrows) occurring late after the QRS complexes with long RP intervals.

paroxysmal atrial tachycardia before its mechanism was known. The AV node, electrophysiologically, appears to have longitudinal dissociation[18] (Fig. 15–4) and has two pathways. The α pathway conducts slowly and has a short refractory period, and the β pathway conducts fast and has a long refractory period. A sinus beat conducts down both pathways to the ventricles, but a PAB can be blocked in the β pathway (unidirectional block), because of its longer refractory period, and conducts slowly down the α pathway and thus has a long P-R interval. This delay can allow the impulse to conduct not only downward to the ventricles, but also retrograde to the atria if the β pathway has recovered its excitability. If this re-entry continues, a re-entrant supraventricular tachycardia occurs. Often the P waves cannot be seen, for they are buried within the QRS for the atria and ventricles are depolarized simultaneously (Figs. 15–4,A, top ECG strip). In some cases, the retrograde P waves can be seen just after the QRS complex (Fig. 15–4,A, bottom ECG strip). Rarely, the conduction can initially go down the β pathway and retrograde by the α, and the P waves occur late after the QRS (Fig. 15–4,B). It is difficult to differentiate this latter type from the intra-atrial re-entrant or automatic types without electrophysiologic studies.

AV nodal reentrant tachycardia occurs and ends abruptly, and the patient is aware of palpitation. The atrial and ventricular rates are often 140 to 200 beats per minute. The ECG reveals normal-width QRS complexes unless aberration or bundle-branch block is present. Therapy for AV node re-entrant tachycardia can be decided by using drugs that act on the antegrade slow pathway (α) or the retrograde fast pathway (β). Digitalis, verapamil, diltiazem, β-blockers, and amiodarone affect the antegrade pathway, and class 1A drugs and amiodarone affect the retrograde pathway.

If the attacks of re-entrant supraventricular tachycardia are infrequent and short, no therapy is indicated. Prolonged attacks may be terminated by vagal stimulation. Carotid sinus pressure can be tried and, if not effective, a cholinergic drug such as physostigmine (1 ml subcutaneously of a 1:2000 solution) or edrophonium (Tensilon), 5 to 10 mg I.V., can be given. The vagus also may be stimulated by raising the diastolic pressure with a pressor amine such as phenylephrine (1 to 2 mg I.V.). Formerly, such measures were taken and, if regular sinus rhythm was not restarted, digoxin was given I.V. However, it now appears that I.V. verapamil (Calan, Isoptin) is the drug of choice. Five to 10 mg is given over 2 minutes and repeated if necessary in 30 minutes (Fig. 15–5). After the first dose, carotid pressure can be tried again before the second dose. Recently, intravenous flecainide (2 mg/kg over 5 to 10 minutes) was used successfully to terminate AV nodal reentrant tachycardia in 30 of 34

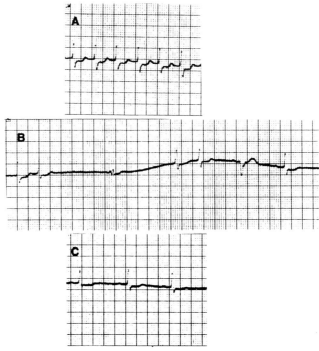

Fig 15–5. A, Paroxysmal supraventricular tachycardia. B, Right carotid pressure was initially unsuccessful, but several minutes after 5 mg of verapamil I.V., light carotid pressure produced ventricular and junctional escape beats and sinus rhythm. C, Sinus rhythm. (From Gazes, P.C.: Atrioventricular nodal reentrant tachycardia, in the Knoll Series of Unusual Arrhythmias. Whippany, N.J., Kroll Pharmaceutical Co., 1982, by permission of the Knoll Pharmaceutical Company.)

patients.[19] However, it has not been approved for this use. Propranolol I.V. (0.1 mg/kg) given at a rate of 1 mg every minute has been used successfully. If heart failure ensues or there is a fall in BP, dc shock may be instituted. If the attacks occur frequently, the patient should be maintained on digitalis. If this is not successful in preventing attacks, quinidine, 300 mg every 6 hours, should be added. Other drugs used prophylactically are verapamil and β-blockers. Class 1C drugs (encainide and flecainide)[20] have been reported effective but have not been approved for use in supraventricular arrhythmias.

    Atrioventricular Re-entrant Tachycardia. This type of AV re-entrant tachycardia is seen in the WPW syndrome with AV bypass tracts which may be manifested or concealed.[21] These are also referred to as reciprocating or circus movement tachycardias and account for 20 to 30% of the supraventricular tachycardias. In at least 90% of patients, conduction is downward through the AV node and returns retrograde through the accessory pathway to the atrium (orthodromic) (Fig. 15–6A). Less than 10% conduct in the reverse (antidromic), and in such cases the QRS complexes manifest the widening seen with the WPW syndrome (Fig. 15–6B). The regular tachycardias usually have a rapid rate of 190 to 250 beats per minute, the P waves are behind the QRS, and the RP interval is greater than 0.07 seconds (Fig. 15–6). A premature beat is usually the initiating mechanism for the development of the arrhythmia. The accessory pathway has a long refractory period and faster conduction as compared to the AV node. Therefore, a critically timed premature beat can block the accessory pathway, conduct down the AV node, and return to the atria by the accessory pathway. Occasionally, block can occur in the right or left

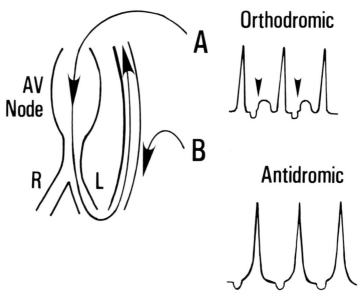

Fig 15–6. Atrioventricular re-entrant tachycardia. A, Conduction antegrade by way of the AV node and retrograde by way of the accessory pathway (orthodromic). Note normal QRS complex's width with P waves (arrows) after the QRS complexes (RP interval > 0.07 seconds). B, Conduction antegrade by way of the accessory pathway and retrograde by way of the AV node (antidromic). Note that QRS complexes have the WPW configuration and P waves are after the QRS (RP interval > 0.07 seconds). AV = atrioventricular.

bundle, and if the block is on the same side as the accessory pathway, the tachycardia is slower than when the block is absent because the impulse takes longer to reach the accessory pathway.

A concealed accessory pathway may be present, allowing retrograde conduction but not antegrade conduction. Therefore, the WPW type of complex is not seen. One should suspect this when the tachycardia has negative P waves 0.07 seconds or greater after the R wave and when the rate is rapid.

This type of circus movement or atrioventricular re-entrant tachycardia responds to vagal maneuvers. Intravenous verapamil by blocking the AV node, or intravenous procainamide by blocking the accessory pathway, can stop the arrhythmia. Recently, intravenous flecainide was reported to be effective, but has not been approved for this use.[19] If these are unsuccessful, then dc shock should be performed. Class 1A drugs and amiodarone can be used for prophylaxis. I would not recommend class 1C drugs at present because they have not been approved for supraventricular arrhythmias.

Automatic or Ectopic Atrial Tachycardia. Ectopic atrial tachycardia is another cause of paroxysmal supraventricular tachycardia.[17] This rhythm is enhanced automaticity or caused by triggered activity but not by re-entry. An atrial focus has spontaneous phase 4 depolarization at a more rapid rate (100 to 200 beats per minute) than the sinus node (Fig. 15–7). The ectopic focus can have a warm-up period, with the rate increasing in the first several beats, and before termination it may slow (Fig. 15–7A).[22] In addition, all of the P waves are the same, whereas in the re-entry type, the initial ectopic P wave differs from the subsequent retrograde P waves. A premature beat may stop the re-entry type, but resets the ectopic atrial tachycardia. Ectopic atrial tachycardia can occur with various degrees of AV block (Fig. 15–7B). In about 50% of cases, it is due to digitalis toxicity, usually with a 2:1 AV block.

Ectopic atrial tachycardia responds best to a class 1A antiarrhythmic agent, such as quinidine, procainamide, or disopyramide, which suppress the rate of phase 4 diastolic depolarization. Encainide and flecainide have also been reported to be effective but have not been approved for this use. Vagal maneuvers or drugs such as digitalis or verapamil may increase the AV block. If it is

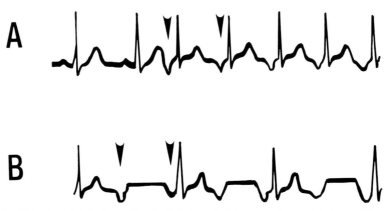

Fig 15–7. Ectopic atrial tachycardia. A, Note inverted P waves (arrows) before QRS complexes. Tachycardia starts slowly and the rate increases. B, Ectopic atrial tachycardia with 2:1 AV block (arrows point to P waves).

due to digitalis, the drug should be stopped and potassium given, especially if there is hypokalemia. Such cases may also respond to the phenytoin and propranolol.

Multifocal atrial tachycardia[17] is of ectopic origin or triggered activity and is most often noted with chronic lung disease. Theophylline may be a precipitating factor. Several atrial foci are present and competing. The P waves are of different morphology (three or more types) and the P-P interval and P-R interval vary (Fig. 15–8). Verapamil is the drug of choice. The response to digitalis is poor. Propranolol can be used to slow the heart rate, but should be used cautiously, for it may aggravate or precipitate bronchospasm. Quinidine may be effective. The underlying lung disease should be treated; clearing hypoxia and stopping or reducing theophylline may resolve the arrhythmia.

Atrial Flutter

Features of atrial flutter indicate that the arrhythmia may be due to a re-entry circuit established in the atrial tissue.[23]

This arrhythmia usually has an atrial rate of 280 to 350 beats per minute (Fig. 15–9A). The gray zone, around 250 atrial beats per minute, may be caused by either atrial ectopic tachycardia or flutter. Usually with atrial flutter there is a 2:1 AV node response producing a ventricular rate half that of the atrial rate. It is usually associated with disease and is rarely seen in a normal person. The atrial waves in flutter usually appear as saw-tooth waves simulating the motion produced by a pebble thrown in water. Carotid sinus pressure decreases AV conduction and brings out the flutter waves, which are commonly inverted in the inferior leads. This is a good diagnostic procedure. The QRS complex is of normal width unless there is aberrant conduction or bundle-branch block. Digitalis is the drug of choice. However, because there is usually only minimal physiologic AV node block due to concealed conduction, high doses of digitalis are necessary. Quinidine should not be used initially because it may enhance AV conduction through its vagolytic effect and its direct slowing effect on the atria and thus increase the ventricular rate. Therefore, before the use of quinidine, digitalis should be given. If regular sinus rhythm is not restored, dc shock can be tried. Because atrial flutter is sensitive to low energies of shock (25 to 50 joules), some consider dc shock the preferable initial mode of therapy, especially if there is associated congestive heart failure, shock, or a 1:1 AV conduction. Rapid atrial pacing has been used with great success, especially in the postoperative cardiac patient in whom temporary atrial pacing wires were inserted and if it is of the slow type I atrial flutter which has an atrial rate of 280 to 320 per minute. Type 2 atrial flutter has an atrial rate above 320 per minute and does not respond often to atrial pacing. Verapamil converts recent onset atrial flutter in about 30% of cases to normal

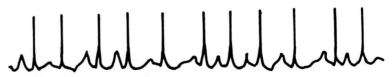

Fig 15–8.   Multifocal atrial tachycardia. Note P waves of different morphology, varying rate, and varying P-R intervals.

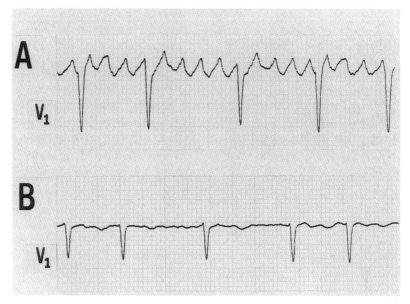

Fig 15–9. Atrial flutter and fibrillation. A, Atrial flutter with primarily a 4:1 AV conduction. Atrial rate is 375 beats per minute. B, Atrial fibrillation. Note irregular ventricular rhythm and absence of P-waves (replaced by atrial fibrillatory waves).

sinus rhythm. Because digitalis or verapamil can shorten the refractory period of the accessory pathway of WPW, these drugs should not be used for atrial flutter in such cases for 1:1 AV conduction can occur.

Quinidine is often used prophylactically to prevent attacks. Verapamil or propranolol may also sometimes be effective.

Atrial Fibrillation

The mechanism of atrial fibrillation has not been definitely proved. However, it appears that it may result from multiple concurrent re-entrant excitation wave fronts.[24]

This arrhythmia produces rapid fibrillatory F waves, often up to a rate of 650 beats per minute, which bombard the AV node with usually less than 200 getting through to stimulate the ventricles (Fig. 15–9B). The QRS complexes are usually normal unless there is aberration or bundle-branch block. Aberrant ventricular conduction can occur and be interpreted as a ventricular arrhythmia. Aberration is usually suggested by the complexes having a right bundle-branch appearance (rsR' in V_1) and the Ashman's phenomenon (after a long cycle, there is a normally conducted complex followed by a short cycle beat which is aberrantly conducted). Runs of aberrant beats may simulate ventricular tachycardia. The F waves may be coarse when atrial fibrillation is due to rheumatic heart disease and thyrotoxicosis, and fine when due to ischemic or hypertensive heart disease.[25] Atrial fibrillation occurs in about 0.4% of the general population. This figure does not include the paroxysmal type. Atrial fibrillation is usually associated with cardiac disease but may occur with no evidence of heart disease, in which case it is classified as lone or idiopathic. Table 15–5 lists some of the causes. It is seen most frequently with coronary

Table 15–5.   Etiology of Atrial Fibrillation

Coronary artery disease
Hypertensive heart disease
Lone atrial fibrillation
Rheumatic heart disease
Cardiomyopathy
Pulmonary emboli
Pericarditis
Thyrotoxicosis
Congenital
Cor pulmonale
Alcohol

artery disease. It can follow an alcoholic binge in healthy individuals (holiday heart). The patient is frequently aware of palpitations. The Framingham study[26] showed that patients with atrial fibrillation, on long-term follow-up, have almost a six times higher incidence of stroke than individuals without atrial fibrillation. It was a significant contribution to stroke at all ages. When it was associated with rheumatic heart disease, there was a 17-fold increase in strokes. In addition, the Framingham study showed that chronic atrial fibrillation shortens life.[27] Another study[28] concluded that lone atrial fibrillation in patients who are under age 60 at diagnosis is associated with a low risk of stroke. It can be stated that up to 30% of individuals with a recurrent or sustained atrial fibrillation will at some time have at least one embolus. Especially prone are those who are going in and out of the arrhythmia.

Digitalis is the drug of choice for this arrhythmia. A recent study[29] reported that digitalis has no effect on the likelihood of reversion to regular sinus rhythm in atrial fibrillation of recent onset. A randomized, open-label, single-blind comparative trial[30] of the ultra short-acting β-blocker, esmolol with verapamil, digoxin, and placebo in the acute treatment of recent onset atrial fibrillation showed that esmolol converted 48%, verapamil 20%, digoxin 15% and placebo 11% to sinus rhythm. Esmolol was given in a loading dose of 10 or 20 mg I.V. bolus and then 2 to 16 mg per minute in increment doses for 10 minutes each. Digoxin was given as a single bolus of 0.5 mg and verapamil was given in 5 or 10 mg I.V. boluses in two titration steps 30 minutes apart. Even though digitalis may not revert the rhythm to normal sinus, it is effective in slowing the ventricular rate and may be of benefit if there is associated heart failure. Because of the considerable physiologic block due to the many impulses that travel into the AV node and decrement producing concealed conduction, it usually does not take as much digitalis to slow the ventricular rate in atrial fibrillation as it does for atrial flutter. Once the rate is slowed and the urgency is over, the underlying condition should be treated. If digitalis alone does not slow the ventricular rate, adding a β-blocker or verapamil is often effective. In some instances, for example with hyperthyroidism, digitalis will not be effective until the associated condition is under control. In addition, a decision has to be made, regardless of the cause, as to whether an attempt to revert the rhythm to regular sinus rhythm should be undertaken. During the past few years, electric cardioversion has practically replaced the use of quinidine for this purpose. Initially, there was much enthusiasm with dc cardioversion, and practically all cases of atrial fibrillation, acute or chronic, were cardioverted. However, regular sinus rhythm was difficult to maintain, and atrial fibrillation recurred in almost 50% of patients within 1 year. At present we reserve dc shock for patients with recent atrial fibrillation (less than 12 months), patients in shock, patients who have sustained an embolism, patients with postoperative mitral valve surgery, and patients with intractable failure in whom restoration of the atrial function increases cardiac output up to about 30%. In addition, dc shock can be used in patients with atrial fibrillation and hyperthyroidism, pericarditis, pulmonary emboli, or any other treatable condition if regular rhythm is not restored after these conditions are controlled (Table 15–6).

However, before considering cardioversion, left atrial size should be measured by echocardiography. Henry et al.[31] have shown that, if the left atrial dimension by echocardiography exceeds 45 mm, cardioversion may be initially successful, but it is unlikely that the regular sinus rhythm can be maintained for at least 6 months. Therefore, we reserve cardioversion for patients with left atrial size of 45 mm or less, consider at least one cardioversion if the left atrial size is between 45 and 50 mm, and do not advise cardioversion if the left atrial size exceeds 50 mm except in a life-threatening situation in which the patient will benefit from immediate restoration of regular sinus rhythm. Patients with a slow ventricular response, in the absence of drug therapy, should not be cardioverted because they may have a sick sinus node or AV node disease. In addition, patients with digitalis toxicity, the elderly, and those who cannot tolerate antiarrhythmic drugs are unfavorable candidates. Idiopathic "lone" atrial fibrillation in the young is a relative contraindication for DC shock because such patients often have sinus node dysfunction. Sinus rhythm occurs only with high energy, complications are high, and sinus rhythm persists only for a short period of time. Likewise, we must be cautious in the elderly because atrial fibrillation may be a manifestation of the tachycardia phase of the bradycardia–tachycardia syndrome and DC shock may produce complete asystole (Table 15-7).

Formerly digoxin was withheld 48 to 72 hours before electrical cardioversion to prevent postcardioversion arrhythmias, but this is not necessary because such arrhythmias do not occur if the serum digoxin level is within therapeutic range and there is no clinical evidence of toxicity.[31a] However, I would reduce the maintenance to half because I usually try quinidine 300 mg every 6 hours before DC shock. With only this program, regular sinus rhythm will be restored in approximately 20% of patients. At the 48-hour period, if atrial fibrillation is still present, dc shock is performed with light anesthesia or diazepam (Valium). An anesthetist should be present, especially if the patient has severe heart dysfunction. Often we have used Valium in increments of 5 mg every 5

Table 15–6. Atrial Fibrillation—Favorable Candidates for DC Shock

1. Less than 12 months' duration
2. Embolic episodes
3. After underlying conditions treated
4. Benefit hemodynamically
5. Normal size atria

Table 15–7. Atrial Fibrillation—Unfavorable Candidates for DC Shock

1. Elderly patients
2. Digitalis toxicity
3. Sinus or AV node disease
4. Large left atrium
5. Antiarrhythmic drugs not tolerated or sinus rhythm not maintained
6. Before surgery
7. Lone atrial fibrillation

minutes until the patient begins to sleep, but still can be aroused. Seldom does one have to use over 30 mg of Valium. The patient may groan with a shock, but later remembers little. The anesthetists often prefer thiopental sodium (Pentothal) or methohexital (Brevital). We usually start with 50 joules of energy shock and increase this with repeated shocks up to 400 joules using anterior-posterior paddles. With restoration of regular sinus rhythm, emboli may occur in up to 2% of cases. Bjerkelund and Orning[32] reported that 2 of 186 patients (1.1%) receiving an anticoagulant and cardioversion had an embolism compared with 11 of 162 patients (6.8%) who were not taking the anticoagulant. Ideally, an oral anticoagulant should be given to all cases. It should be started at least 2 weeks prior to cardioversion and continued for 4 weeks afterward. If this is not feasible in all instances, then individuals in a high risk group (atrial fibrillation of more than 1 week's duration, mitral valve disease, prosthetic mitral valve, prior embolic phenomena, congestive heart failure or cardiomegaly) should be given priority for anticoagulation. The prothrombin time should be maintained at least 1.5 to 2.0 times the normal value. Beside emboli and other major arrhythmias, further complications of dc shock are serum enzyme elevations and ECG changes. However, the MB fraction of creatinine kinase (ck) usually does not rise.[33] The ECG may show ST and T wave abnormalities postcardioversion. Rarely, acute pulmonary edema may occur because the right atrium recovers before the left atrium. The lung fields are flooded because the poorly functioning left atrium cannot receive the increased output from the right side. It may take up to 2 weeks for the left atrium to regain its function because it is most often the atrium that is diseased and associated with the atrial fibrillation. Complications are more frequent with higher energy DC shocks. We usually maintain the patient on 200 to 400 mg of quinidine every 6 hours plus digitalis, or digitalis alone after cardioversion. Disopyramide, procainamide, β-blocker and verapamil have also been used. Class 1C[34] drugs have been reported to be effective for prophylaxis and in intractable problems; amiodarone may be used. However, I would not recommend a class 1C drug because they have not been approved for this use. If normal sinus rhythm is not maintained for more than 6 months, we would not repeat dc shock unless the patient has an urgent need such as intractable heart failure, hypotension, an uncontrolled ventricular rate, or emboli.

If cardioversion is not successful or not attempted, the patient's ventricular rate is controlled with digitalis. In the event that an adequate ventricular rate cannot be achieved, a β-blocker or verapamil can be added. Table 15–8 lists the indications for long-term anticoagulation for patients with chronic atrial fibrillation. As yet there are no good data that aspirin can replace long-term anticoagulation.

Table 15–8.   Long-term Anticoagulation for Chronic Atrial Fibrillation

1. Rheumatic mitral valve disease
2. Coronary artery disease if patient had one embolism
3. Cardiomyopathy
4. Hypertrophic cardiomyopathy
5. Atrial fibrillation with sick sinus syndrome

Endocardial catheter fulguration to ablate the AV node or section of AV node by surgery can be used to control the ventricular rate. These patients require a permanent ventricular pacemaker. Another surgical procedure that is being studied is using an isolated strip of right atrial muscle between the SA and AV node to allow a regular "sino-ventricular rhythm" while the remainder of the atria continues to fibrillate.[24] Table 15–9 summarizes the therapy for atrial fibrillation.

Atrial fibrillation in WPW syndrome usually conducts down the accessory pathway, which does not have decremental conduction properties, and as a result the ventricular rate may be rapid, 250 to 300 beats per minute (Fig. 15–10). Atrioventricular reciprocating tachycardia can degenerate into atrial fibrillation, or atrial fibrillation may occur unrelated to atrioventricular reentry. This can be a serious arrhythmia leading to ventricular fibrillation.[21] Digitalis and verapamil may shorten the refractory period of the accessory pathway and further increase the ventricular rate and may produce ventricular fibrillation. Often such patients require dc shock. If stable, the drug of choice is I.V. procainamide at 50 mg per minute up to 1 g. Intravenous encainide or flecainide have also been reported to be effective but I would not currently recommend these for they have not been approved for this use.[19,20] Class 1A and amiodarone can be given prophylactically. The patients should have electrophysiologic studies, and if the shortest preexcited R-R interval during induced atrial fibrillation is less than 250 msec (but lacks specificity), then surgical division of the accessory pathways should be performed.

AV Junctional Rhythm and Arrhythmias

Pacemaker cells are found in the distal portion of the AV node and its junction with the His bundle and in the His bundle itself. Beats originating in these sites are referred to as AV junctional. If the sinus node is temporarily depressed, a junctional escape beat can occur, or if the depression is prolonged, an AV junctional rhythm can develop usually at a rate of 40 to 60 beats per minute (Fig. 15–11A). The ECG shows normal-width QRS complexes (unless there is bundle-branch block) and inverted P waves preceding or after the QRS complexes. The P waves at times may not be visible if they are embedded in the QRS complexes. When the P waves occur before the QRS complex, the P-R

Table 15–9.   Treatment of Atrial Fibrillation

1. Search for precipitating cause
2. Control ventricular rate: Digitalis, β-Blocker, Verapamil, Diltiazem
3. Cardioversion: Quinidine, electrical cardioversion
4. Anticoagulation prior to cardioversion
5. Prevention: Digoxin, Type 1A, β-blocker, Verapamil, or Amiodarone
6. Surgery

I

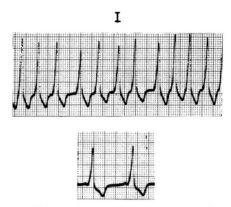

Fig 15–10. *Top tracing,* Wolff-Parkinson-White syndrome and atrial fibrillation simulating ventricular tachycardia. Conduction is by way of the accessory pathway. *Lower tracing,* return to regular sinus rhythm with WPW syndrome. Note short P-R interval and initial slurring of QRS (delta wave).

interval is usually 0.10 seconds or less. The term "wandering pacemaker" has been used, referring to the pacemaker shifting from the SA node to an atrial site or to the AV junctional tissue. The change usually occurs gradually over several beats. Often this occurs in normal persons with increased vagal tone, especially the young and athletes. Persistent AV junctional rhythm can occur with heart disease and usually requires no therapy.

AV junctional premature beats may have similar P wave positions as noted with AV junctional rhythm (Fig. 15–11B). These are treated in the same way as was discussed for PABs.

In addition to AV junctional premature beats, one can have paroxysmal ectopic AV junctional tachycardia with a rate of 140 to 250 beats per minute. This is rather rare in adults and may be associated with AV dissociation. It may be difficult to distinguish this from AV nodal re-entrant tachycardia if the P waves are after the QRS (Fig. 15–11C) or from ectopic atrial tachycardia if the P waves precede the QRS. It may respond to beta blockers or amiodarone or AV node ablation may be necessary if it is incessant.

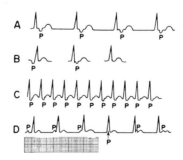

Fig 15–11. AV junctional arrhythmias. **A,** AV junctional rhythm with rate of 55 beats per minute. **B,** three types of AV junctional premature beats. In the third complex the P wave coincides with the QRS complex and is not seen. **C,** paroxysmal AV junctional ectopic tachycardia (190 beats per minute) with P waves after the QRS complexes. **D,** nonparoxysmal AV junctional tachycardia with atrioventricular dissociation. The ventricular rate is 94, and the atrial rate is 83 beats per minute.

Another arrhythmia that can occur in the AV junction is nonparoxysmal AV junctional tachycardia. This is due to enhanced automaticity in the AV junction and has a rate of 70 to 130 beats per minute. The P waves can be positioned as mentioned for AV junctional rhythm or premature beats. This arrhythmia is often associated with AV dissociation where the ventricular rate from the junctional focus is more rapid than the sinus rhythm which activates the atria (Fig. 15–11D). There is retrograde block to the atria, but the sinus node at its slower rate may at times capture the ventricles. Often the P waves can be seen gradually approaching the QRS complex and then following it. At times the atria and ventricles may be firing at the same rate. This is referred to as synchronization or accrochage. Atrial flutter or fibrillation may be present (instead of sinus rhythm controlling the atria) with nonparoxysmal AV junctional tachycardia. Nonparoxysmal AV junctional tachycardia is most often seen with digitalis toxicity, acute inferior infarction, acute carditis, chronic obstructive lung disease, and after open heart surgery. It usually clears and requires no specific therapy. Therapy should be directed at the underlying heart disease or condition.

VENTRICULAR ARRHYTHMIAS

Ventricular arrhythmias can be classified as noted in Table 15–10. This classification is useful for the management of arrhythmias. It is important to recognize that ventricular arrhythmias are frequently detected on routine electrocardiograms or on Holter monitoring in otherwise asymptomatic persons. Table 15–11 shows the percentage of prevalence for such arrhythmias in healthy subjects according to age as compiled from several studies.[35]

Premature Ventricular Beats

These usually appear as bizarre QRS complexes with a compensatory pause (Fig. 15–12,A). At times the PVB may retrograde conduct to the atria and the QRS is followed by inverted P wave. This may be confused with an AV junctional premature beat with aberration and retrograde P wave conduction. The R-P interval may help in the differentiation. The R-P interval with the PVB is usually more than 0.1 of a second, whereas with the junctional premature beat it is equal to or less than this. Premature ventricular beats can be unifocal or multifocal. In addition, the unifocal types can produce responses with differing

Table 15–10. Classification of Ventricular Arrhythmias

1. Benign PVBs

2. Complex PVBs ⟨ without cardiac disease / with cardiac disease ⟨ without ventricular dysfunction / with ventricular dysfunction (potentially lethal)

3. Malignant (lethal)
   a. Sustained ventricular tachyarrhythmia and unsustained with syncope
   b. Torsades de pointes
   c. Ventricular fibrillation

Table 15–11. Prevalence of PVBs in Healthy Subjects

Age	Percentage
20–59	34
15–59	46
55 (Average)	60
>60	69–100
Complex forms	
20–60	<10
60–85	36

QRS configurations (multiformity). Therefore, multiformity of the QRS configuration should not be used synonymously with multifocality. Premature ventricular beats can be found in persons without heart disease, patients with organic heart disease, and patients with diseases other than those of the heart, such as from anoxia, reflexes arising from the GI or genitourinary tract, certain drugs, electrolyte imbalance, and disturbed psychologic states.

Premature ventricular beats that are benign usually are five or less per hour and unifocal on Holter monitoring. Those that have the configuration of left bundle-branch block usually originate from the right ventricle and most often are benign. These are seen in normal persons, according to Rosenbaum,[36] especially if the initial forces are directed anteriorly, producing a slowly inscribed R in the PVB in V_1, and the premature beats in the limb leads have their main forces directed inferiorly producing an axis between +60 and 120 degrees. Rosenbaum believes that these arise from the anterior wall of the right ventricle, and because the initial part of QRS is inscribed slowly, these originate from the myocardium rather than from the Purkinje tissue. He postulated that perhaps stretching of the anterior papillary muscle of the right ventricle during mechanical activity under certain circumstances triggers such benign PVBs.

Complex premature ventricular beats (greater than 10 to 30 per hour) are frequent and include those that occur early on the T-waves (R on T phenomenon), multifocal pairs, and salvos. They may occur in subjects with or without cardiac disease.[37] Those that occur in patients without heart disease may possibly be due to the autonomic nervous system, biochemical abnormalities,

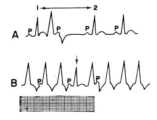

Fig 15–12. PVB and ventricular tachycardia. **A,** PVB with compensatory pause shown between complexes 1 and 2. **B,** ventricular tachycardia. The ventricular rate is 150, and atrial rate is 75 beats per minute. *Arrow* points to capture beat.

or patches of myocarditis. Those that occur with left ventricular dysfunction are potentially lethal.

Many are not aware of benign PVBs, and it may be wiser in some individuals not to direct their attention to the ectopic beats if they have no evidence of heart disease because cardiac neurosis can develop. However, in some cases it may be preferable to mention these beats and explain their insignificance so that the patient will not be alarmed should he become aware of them. Their frequency may be diminished by reduction or elimination of smoking, excessive coffee or tea, alcohol, and certain drugs such as thyroid extract, amphetamine, ephedrine, and analgesics with caffeine. Attention and therapy should be given to symptomatic patients experiencing fear and anxiety who describe palpitations, jumping, skipping, knife-like pain over the precordium, or a sensation of stoppage of the heart. They should avoid stress factors and tensions, and a regulated amount of daily physical exercise should be encouraged. Mild sedation may be beneficial. If all general measures fail, the patient is still emotionally disturbed, and symptoms interfere with the quality of life, an antiarrhythmic drug can be given for a few weeks to allow the patient to regain tranquility. After this, the patient can take one of these for a few days intermittently if the PVBs occur frequently and are bothersome. A class II β-blocker can be given initially. The β-blockers are especially effective if the PVBs increase with higher rates. For many years it was thought that if PVBs were produced by exercise, they were associated with a cardiac abnormality. However, they are frequently found in subjects doing exercise who have no evidence of cardiac disease.[38] Other drugs that can be used are Class 1A or B drugs but never Class III. The class B (tocainide or mexilitine) are preferred to type 1A drugs such as quinidine. The starting doses are those listed in Table 15–2. Often the knowledge that medications are available is reassuring in itself to the patient.

Complex premature ventricular beats in those with no evidence of heart disease are treated if the patient is symptomatic, in the same manner as the benign types. However, if cardiac disease is present, especially if there is left ventricular dysfunction (potentially lethal), antiarrhythmic drugs should be included in the therapy. Reversible factors producing arrhythmias should be removed before drug therapy. One can begin with a class 1A, 1B drug or proceed to a combination of 1A and 1B if necessary.[39,40] Class III drugs should not be given unless all other drugs fail. Often one has to try several drugs before achieving the required response. The usual starting doses are listed in Table 15–2. Plasma concentrations of antiarrhythmic drugs are used to determine compliance, detect drug interactions, assess increasing the dose, and avoid drug reactions. Most guidelines are based on "trough" plasma sampling measured after steady-state equilibrium has been achieved.[40a] Holter monitoring and exercise testing are often used to evaluate drug efficacy and identify potentially serious toxic drug effects. It should be recognized that, even though drug therapy is used, there have been no large control studies demonstrating improved survival.

Ventricular Tachycardia

The mechanism may be automaticity or re-entry. This arrhythmia is present when three or more PVBs occur in succession, usually at a rate of 140 to 250 beats per minute (Figs. 15–12B, 15–13A). It is referred to as sustained if it lasts longer than 30 seconds or requires termination because of hemodynamic instability. The nonsustained types last less than 30 seconds and stop spontaneously. The sustained or nonsustained with hemodynamic instability are referred to as malignant arrhythmias along with torsades de pointes and ventricular fibrillation. These are usually seen in patients with cardiac disease. In the sustained type, in most instances AV dissociation is present; therefore, intermittent cannon A waves in the jugular pulse can be seen when the P waves occur after the QRS complexes. This finding at the bedside may help to distinguish ventricular tachycardia from the supraventricular varieties. The ECG will manifest widened bizarre QRS complexes. In only about 40% of the cases is one certain of the diagnosis because supraventricular tachycardia with aberration or bundle-branch block must be excluded. The diagnosis can be suspected if P waves are seen at a slower rate, independent of the QRS complexes, or if capture beats or fusion beats are present. Capture beats are noted

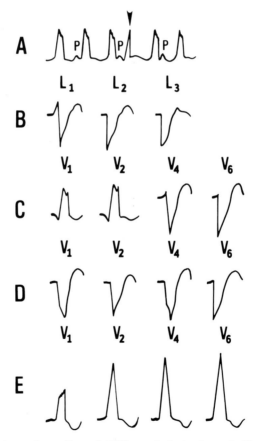

Fig 15–13. Ventricular tachycardia and QRS morphologic clues. A, Ventricular tachycardia. Note widened QRS complexes, capture beat (arrow) with normal contour, and atrioventricular dissociation (independent P waves). B, Marked left axis deviation in frontal plane with widened QRS complexes. C, Biphasic widened QRS complexes with initial small Q waves in V_1 and V_2 and deep S waves in V_4 and V_6. D, Concordant negative widened QRS complexes in V_1 through V_6. E, Concordant positive widened QRS complexes in V_1 through V_6.

when a sinus beat is conducted to the ventricles displaying a normal QRS (Figs. 15–12B, 15–13A), or fusion beats occur when a conducted beat fuses with a ventricular ectopic focus. The configuration of the QRS complexes in the tachycardia may aid in diagnosis (in up to 90% of cases) as described by Wellens.[41,42] A right bundle-branch block configuration of the QRS complexes (best noted in V_1) suggests a supraventricular arrhythmia with aberration. A QRS width of more than 0.14 seconds, QRS in V_1 is monophasic or qR configuration, concordant positive or negative QRS complexes in all precordial leads; a frontal plane axis between -90 and -180 degrees suggests ventricular tachycardia (Fig. 15–13B through E). Also, ventricular tachycardia is suggested if, in the V_6 position, the morphology is rS, QS, or QR. Marriott's coronary care nurses consider ventricular ectopy if in V_1 the left "rabbit ear" is taller than the right when the QRS is bifid.[43] If left bundle-branch morphology is present, ventricular tachycardia can be suspected if the R wave duration in V_1 or V_2 is greater than 30 msec and a notch is present on the downstroke of the S waves in V_1 or V_2, or greater than 70 msec to the S wave nadir in V_1 or V_2, or Q waves in V_6.[42] Before or after the tachycardia, PVBs similar to those in the paroxysm indicate a ventricular origin. Rarely, ventricular tachycardia has retrograde conduction to the atria and the QRS complexes are followed by inverted P waves. This simulates a re-entrant supraventricular tachycardia with aberration of the QRS complexes and P waves after the QRS complexes. At times ventricular tachycardia can be irregular, with grouping of QRS complexes indicating exit blocks, often of the Wenchebach type.

If ventricular tachycardia is sustained and does not cause hemodynamic instability, lidocaine in a bolus of 100 mg I.V. is given and repeated in a few minutes. After this, procainamide, 50 mg/minute I.V., can be given up to 500 mg. If this routine is not successful or if the patient's condition deteriorates, dc shock should be used. If this procedure is not available, then I.V. propranolol (0.5 to 1 mg) or dilantin (100 to 200 mg) can be given. At times a sharp blow to the chest can terminate an attack of ventricular tachycardia. However, this may also precipitate ventricular fibrillation or asystole. Underlying conditions should be treated, such as raising the BP by vasopressors or replacing electrolytes before giving antiarrhythmic drugs. Prevention of recurrences may be difficult. Usually class 1A, 1B, 1CIII, or a combination of class 1A and 1B drugs are tried empirically (see Table 15–2 for dosage). In patients with such malignant arrhythmias, class 1C drugs are not used as the first choice because of the higher incidence of proarrhythmia.[39] The FDA has released a report halting the use of class 1C drugs (encainide and flecainide) in non-life-threatening arrhythmias. The NHLBI Cardiac Arrhythmia Suppression Trial (CAST), a multicenter double-blind, placebo-controlled trial in postmyocardial infarction patients with asymptomatic ventricular arrhythmias reported that encainide and flecainide had a higher rate of total mortality and non-fatal cardiac arrest compared to a matched placebo group. This rate was 40 of 415 patients (9.6%) for encainide and 15 of 416 patients (3.6%) for the matched placebo group. The rate for flecainide was 16 of 315 patients (5.1%) and for its matched placebo group 7 of 309 patients (2.3%). Similar findings were noted for rates of sudden death and nonfatal cardiac arrests and the findings were consistent across a variety of subgroups. Therefore, it is recommended that encainide or flecainide be used only in patients with life-threatening arrhythmias such as sustained ventricular tachycardia. Amiodarone is tried as a last resort (see Table 15–2 for dosage). The patient's condition may dictate which drug should be tried. For example, if heart failure is present, it is best not to use drugs with negative inotropic effects such as disopyramide or flecainide and class 1B drugs are best if the Q-T interval is prolonged. Serum drug blood levels should be followed. Effective therapy may require electrophysiologic studies.[44,45] The percentage of patients in whom complete suppression of inducible ventricular tachycardia or ventricular fibrillation is achieved during electrophysiologic testing with antiarrhythmic drugs, and in whom no spontaneous arrhythmia occurs at 1- to 2-year follow-up ranges between 80 and 95%.[45a]

Intracardiac recording at different sites within the heart and programmed stimulation have offered means of studying ventricular tachycardia and its therapy. Programmed stimulation provides the means of studying conduction and refractoriness. By this method re-entrant circuits can be initiated and terminated. In most instances in patients with recurrent ventricular tachycardia, this arrhythmia can be produced by regular right ventricular pacing and the introduction of properly timed ventricular stimuli. Occasionally, ventricular tachycardia can be induced from only the left ventricle. Effective antiarrhythmic therapy can be determined by giving drugs and noting whether they can prevent induced ventricular tachycardia. Ventricular pacing can also be used to terminate ventricular tachycardia. The site of origin of induced ventricular tachycardia and the activation sequence may be evaluated by endocardial electrode-catheter mapping, by epicardial mapping, or by both.[46,47] Many newer forms of therapy are being investigated for drug-resistant sustained ventricular arrhythmias. They include new antiarrhythmic drugs, antitachycardia surgery, antitachycardia pacing, catheter ablation techniques, and implantable devices for cardioversion and defibrillation. A fully automatic implantable cardioverter-defibrillator (AICD) has improved the prognosis for such patients by preventing recurring cardiac arrest. It was developed by Mirowski in the 1970s, and was first implanted in a human in the 1980s.[48] It has been approved for the following high-risk patients: those who have had a single episode of ventricular fibrillation or hemodynamically unstable ventricular tachycardia without acute myocardial infarction and incomplete protection by antiarrhythmic drugs as determined by arrhythmia inducibility during electrophysiologic testing or stress testing, or on Holter monitoring. Contraindications to its use include limited life expectancy due to noncardiac disease, ingestion of drugs known to influence electrical activity, frequent sustained or nonsustained ventricular tachycardia (device continually discharging) that cannot be suppressed with antiarrhythmic drugs, uncontrolled congestive failure, lack of access to follow-up, and patient anxiety about the device. Studies indicate a 1-year arrhythmic mortality between 27 and 66% for patients with such malignant ventricular arrhythmias that can be reduced by the currently used AICD to 2% or less. Complications can occur early or late with such devices.[49] Early complications are related to implantation and late complications include accelerated battery depletion such as from firing for other arrhythmias (supraventricular that exceed the rate cut off of the pulse generator), and from oversensing P waves, T waves, and myopotentials of various causes.

POLYMORPHIC VENTRICULAR TACHYCARDIA

Torsade de Pointes

This malignant arrhythmia was first described in 1966 and appears to be transitional between conventional ventricular tachycardia and ventricular fibrillation.[50] The ECG shows cycles of alternating electric polarity so that the peaks of the QRS complexes appear to be twisting about the isoelectric lines, and at times there are periods of uniform morphology and polarity (Fig. 15–14). It usually terminates spontaneously, but continues to recur. Most often it occurs in subjects who have severe myocardial disease and a long Q-T interval (over 0.60 seconds).[51] When it is associated with a long Q-T interval, it is referred to as torsade de pointes.[50] Usually drugs for ventricular arrhythmias, such as quinidine, procainamide, or disopyramide, that prolong the Q-T interval can precipitate or aggravate attacks, even though their blood levels are not in the toxic range. Other causes of Q-T interval prolongation, such as electrolyte imbalance (hypokalemia, hypomagnesemia), CNS lesions, congenital Q-T interval syndromes, high-grade AV heart block, psychotropic drugs (phenothiazines, tricyclics), and intrinsic heart disease can produce the arrhythmia.[52] Therapy is directed at removing the predisposing cause if the Q-T interval is prolonged. Isoproterenol (Isuprel) infusion has been used successfully in emergency situations. Overdrive suppression with atrial or ventricular pacing is often used until the predisposing cause of the Q-T interval prolongation can be corrected. Intravenous magnesium sulfate has been effective.[53] A 1 to 2 g bolus is given initially, followed by a continuous infusion of 2 to 7 mg per minute for several hours. If the Q-T interval is normal, magnesium sulfate is ineffective

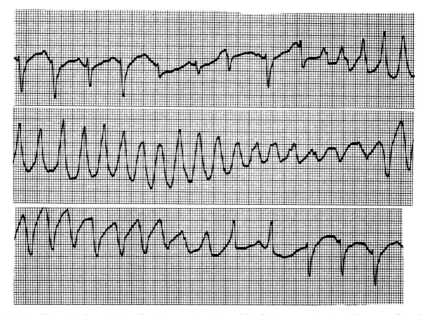

Fig 15–14. Torsade de pointes: Continuous tracing of lead 2 in a patient with severe hypokalemia. In normal conducted beats, the Q-T interval is prolonged. Ventricular ectopic beats occurred, followed by torsade de pointes at end of top strip.

and standard antiarrhythmic therapy should be given. Patients with congenital long Q-T interval syndrome may require left/sided cervicothoracic sympathetic ganglionectomy, which interrupts the stellate ganglion and the first four thoracic ganglia.

OTHER TYPES OF VENTRICULAR TACHYCARDIA

Monomorphic Ventricular Tachycardia

This is a repetitive type of ventricular tachycardia occurring often in the young without evidence of significant heart disease. Abnormal automaticity or triggered activity is thought to be the mechanism. Usually there are three or more premature ventricular complexes with identical configuration that are interrupted by normal sinus beats. This continues in a repetitive fashion and is often incessant. Unless cardiac disease is present, these are treated only if symptomatic.

Bidirectional Ventricular Tachycardia

This is an uncommon tachycardia most often secondary to digitalis toxicity. The QRS complexes have a right bundle-branch block pattern and in the frontal plane the polarity alternates from -60 to -90 degrees to $+120$ to $+130$ degrees. When this is due to digitalis, the drug should be stopped and if lidocaine, potassium, dilantin, or propranolol are not effective, digibind should be tried.

Parasystole

This is an ectopic rhythm (usually ventricular) that is independent of the primary rhythm, protected, and so uninterrupted. The ectopic beats of the parasystolic rhythm have varying coupling intervals with the basic primary rhythm and the interectopic intervals have a common denominator. At times, exit block can occur to produce an irregular rhythm such as Wenchebach exit block. The manifest rate of the parasystolic focus is usually slow (20 to 60 beats per minute), but can be more rapid. The significance of ventricular parasystole has not been determined. One study[54] showed that it seldom leads to sudden death in the late postinfarction period.

Accelerated Idioventricular Rhythm

This has been discussed in Chapter 4, since it occurs in up to 20% of patients with myocardial infarction (especially inferior). This is a slow ventricular ectopic rhythm of 50 to 100 beats per minute, and frequently there are fusion beats with the sinus rhythm in the first few complexes (see Fig. 4–19). Generally this is a benign arrhythmia that has also been noted in children and young adults who apparently have no cardiac disease.[55] Therapy is often not required. If it occurs with ventricular tachycardia or hemodynamic instability is present, it should be treated. Therapy is the same as discussed for ventricular tachycardia. Atropine or atrial pacing have also been effective.

Ventricular Flutter and Fibrillation

Ventricular flutter presents as regular oscillations at a rate usually above 200 and ventricular fibrillation presents as irregular undulations of varying contour and configuration with no discernible QRS, ST, or T waves (Fig. 4–21). These occur in a number of conditions, but primarily with coronary disease. Holter monitoring may show the R on T premature ventricular complexes before the development of ventricular fibrillation. In the presence of coronary disease, it can occur as a primary ventricular fibrillation or secondary to hypotension and heart failure. Patients with an anteroseptal infarction who develop bundle-branch block can later develop ventricular fibrillation. Treatment of ventricular fibrillation will be discussed at the end of this chapter under "Cardiac Arrest."

PRE-EXCITATION SYNDROME (WOLFF-PARKINSON-WHITE)

The true incidence of the Wolff-Parkinson-White (WPW) syndrome is unknown but has been reported to vary from 0.1 to 3 per 1,000 ECGs.[56] In this syndrome, in addition to the AV node, there is an accessory pathway (bundle of Kent) connecting the atria and ventricles, which is the most common cause of pre-excitation (atrio-ventricular connection). When conduction is through the accessory pathway, the ECG will show a short P-R interval (0.1 second or less) and slurring of the initial portion of the QRS complex producing a delta wave with a change in QRS morphology. Activation of the ventricles over two pathways produces a fusion QRS complex whose configuration depends on the contribution of each of the two activation paths. Therefore, the classical QRS complex resembling the Eiffel Tower may not always be present. Traditionally, three types (A, B, and C) are described depending on the direction of the accessory pathway. Types A and B are most common. Type A (left-sided or septal connection) has upright QRS complexes in all the precordial leads and type B (right-sided connection) has a negative QRS complex in V_1 and a positive QRS complex in V_6 (Fig. 15–15). Type C (left lateral wall connection) has a positive QRS complex in V_1 and a negative QRS complex in V_6. A patient can have more than one accessory pathway. The QRS morphology can vary intermittently from that due to normal conduction to that of the various types of

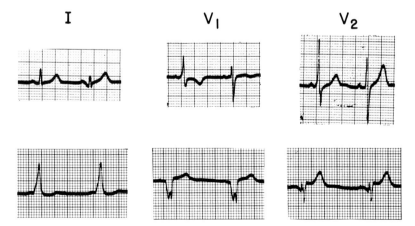

Fig 15–15. Wolff-Parkinson-White (WPW) syndrome. Top tracing shows alternating normal conducted beats with those of the WPW syndrome. The WPW beats are type A. Note short P-R interval and prominent R in V_1 in the WPW beat. Bottom tracing shows WPW syndrome type B. Note absence of R in V_1 and initial Q in V_2, simulating an anteroseptal infarct.

WPW. Type A can be mistaken for right bundle-branch block, a true posterior infarction, or an inferior infarction (see Fig. 3–12); type B for an anteroseptal infarction (Fig. 15–15), inferior infarction, left ventricular hypertrophy, or left bundle-branch block; and type C for right ventricular hypertrophy. In addition, there are often ST-T changes at rest or produced by exercise, giving a false-positive stress test (see Fig. 4–5). The WPW syndrome is often noted in patients without other evidence of heart disease. The incidence of tachyarrhythmia is as yet unknown, but has been reported to vary from 12 to 80%.[56] Earlier in this chapter, tachycardias associated with WPW syndrome were discussed.

The European study group[57] suggested standardizing the nomenclature for the pre-excitation syndrome by using "tract" to describe accessory pathways that insert into specialized conduction tissue and "connection" when pathways end into the myocardium. Other pre-excitation syndromes besides the accessory atrioventricular connection (Kent) are the Lown-Ganong-Levine syndrome (LGL), in which the bypass tract from the atria enters the His bundle (atriofascicular tract), the Mahaim fibers that connect the lower AV node, bundle of His, or upper bundle branches (nodoventricular or fasciculoventricular connections) to the ventricular myocardium and the James fiber that connects the atrium to the AV node (intranodal bypass tract). The LGL syndrome has a short P-R interval (less than 0.12 second) with a normal-width QRS complex. Enhanced AV nodal conduction (EAVN) has been used to describe this short P-R syndrome.[21] An anatomic small AV node or rapid AV node conduction are other mechanisms suggested besides a bypass tract. Various tachyarrhythmias have been noted with this syndrome. It may be difficult to distinguish LGL from a lower atrial or AV junctional rhythm. The latter rhythms usually have inverted P waves in the inferior leads (leads II, III, or aV_F). Mahaim fibers produce a normal P-R interval with a QRS having a delta wave (WPW morphology) or a bundle-branch block pattern depending on the site of insertion. The incidence of arrhythmias in this condition is not known.

REGULAR TACHYCARDIAS

Sinus, SA node re-entrant, ectopic atrial, AV nodal and atrioventricular re-entrant supraventricular tachycardias, atrial flutter, with a 2:1 response, and ventricular tachycardia must be differentiated. Table 15–12 compares the diagnostic features of these regular tachyarrhythmias.

SINUS NODAL DISORDERS

Sinus Tachycardia

Sinus tachycardia is defined as a rate usually from 100 to 180 beats per minute and at times faster during exercise. It can be produced by stresses, diseases, or drugs. Chronic sinus tachycardia without a cause has been noted in patients with a hyperdynamic beta-adrenergic circulatory state.[58] Such patients have cardiac awareness and often systolic hypertension. At times it may be difficult to distinguish sinus tachycardia from a regular supraventricular tachycardia if the P waves are not seen. Vagal maneuvers will slow the rate which gradually returns to its previous rate after the vagal influence is removed. The underlying condition responsible for the sinus tachycardia should be treated. Beta-blockers have been effective in those with the hyperdynamic beta-adrenergic circulatory state.

Sinus Bradycardia

In adults, if the sinus node discharges at a rate of 60 beats per minute or less, this is referred to as sinus bradycardia. It can occur in normal persons and especially in the well-trained athlete. It can occur with excessive vagal stimulation or decrease in sympathetic tone. Frequently during sleep, the normal heart rate may decrease to 30 to 40 beats per minute and sinus pauses can occur of 2 seconds or longer. Sinus bradycardia can be the result of a brain lesion, myxedema, obstructive jaundice, fibrodegenerative changes, myocardial infarction (more often inferior) and drugs (β-blockers, calcium blockers, amiodarone, clonidine and others). It usually is benign and requires no therapy except removing or correcting the underlying condition. In acute instances, atropine is often effective. Electrical pacing may be necessary if the patient is symptomatic with chronic sinus bradycardia and has congestive failure, syncope, or presyncope.

Sinoatrial Pause and Sinoatrial Exit Block

When the SA node fails to discharge, it is referred to as a sinus pause or arrest which differs from SA exit block in that the duration of the pause is variable and is not a multiple of the usual sinus P-P interval (Fig. 15–16A). During SA exit block the impulse forms in the SA node normally, but its conduction to the atria is blocked. Different degrees of SA exit block can occur, such as 2:1 in which every other heartbeat is dropped (type II). This can be mistaken for severe sinus bradycardia (which may be physiologic) unless there are periods when the rate doubles. Sinoatrial exit block also can occur as a Wenckebach block (type I) (Figs. 15–17; 15–19D) and is recognized by the Wenckebach groupings, as will be described later with AV block. The P-R interval remains constant in SA node Wenckebach groupings.

These types of SA node disorders, namely, failure of the sinus node to form impulses or failure of the impulses to reach the atria (exit block), can occur from coronary disease, nonspecific fibrosis, rheumatic fever, and drugs such as digitalis, quinidine, verapamil, diltiazem, and beta-adrenergic-blocking agents. Sinus arrest and SA exit block can occur because of a hypersensitive carotid sinus. Sinus node abnormalities often coexist with abnormalities in the lower conducting system because both are often involved with the same fibrotic or sclerodegenerative process.

Sick Sinus Syndrome (SSS)

This term is used to describe the above disorders of the sinus node with a broad spectrum of clinical symptoms and findings. Such patients may be asymptomatic or have dizziness, light-headedness, syncope, or palpitations. The ECG or Holter monitor may show marked sinus bradycardia, sinus node pauses (arrest) or exit block, AV junctional escape beats or rhythm, and atrial fibrillation or flutter. The "bradycardia-tachycardia" syndrome has been used interchangeably with SSS if there are intermittent periods of bradycardia (SA exit block or pauses, slow AV junctional rhythm, or marked sinus bradycardias) and tachycardia with rapid ventricular rate (atrial fibrillation or flutter

Table 15-12. Differentiation of Regular Tachycardias

	Ventricular Rate per Minute (usual)	Jugular Venous Pulse	Heart Sounds	Carotid Sinus Pressure	ECG Features*	Therapeutic Response
Sinus tachycardia	Below 160	Normal	Normal	Gradual slowing with rapid return	Normal P waves preceding QRS complex or superposition of P and T waves; normal QRS width	Treat underlying condition
Sinus nodal re-entrant tachycardia	100–160	Normal	Normal	Abrupt end of paroxysm or no effect	Same as sinus tachycardia; normal QRS width	Vagal maneuvers, digitalis, verapamil, propranolol
Ectopic atrial tachycardia	100–200	Normal	Normal	May slow ventricular rate due to AV block	All P waves (different from sinus) identical preceding QRS complexes and first few beats progressively increase in rate; premature beat resets ectopic pacemaker; normal width QRS	Class 1A anti-arrhythmia drugs
AV nodal re-entrant supraventricular	140–220 (very regular)	Retrograde P waves produce cannon A waves with each beat	Normal	Abrupt end of paroxysm or no effect	Initial ectopic P wave (PR long) differs from others which are in QRS or retrograde;	Vagal maneuvers, verapamil, diltiazem, digitalis, beta-blocker, dc shock

Table 15–12. *Continued*

	Ventricular Rate per Minute (usual)	Jugular Venous Pulse	Heart Sounds	Carotid Sinus Pressure	ECG Features*	Therapeutic Response
					premature beats stop tachycardia; normal QRS width	
Atrioventricular re-entrant tachycardia (WPW)	190–250	Retrograde P waves produce cannon A waves with each beat	Normal	Abrupt end of paroxysm or no effect	P waves .07 sec or more after the R wave; normal QRS width	Vagal maneuvers, verapamil, procainamide, dc shock
Atrial flutter with 2:1 response	150–180	Rapid A waves more frequent than apical rate	First sound may vary in intensity	Temporary slowing of ventricular rate with jerky return	Usually P waves at rate of 300/min as sawtooth oscillations; normal QRS width	Digitalis, verapamil, dc shock, atrial pacing
Ventricular tachycardia	140–250	Occasional cannon A waves; constant if retrograde atrial activation	Varying intensity of first heart sound and wide splitting of sounds	No effect	Widened QRS complexes with slower independent P waves; ventricular capture or fusion beats; at times retrograde P waves; QRS morphologic clues	Lidocaine procainamide, propranolol, dilantin, dc shock

*It may be difficult to differentiate ventricular tachycardia from the supraventricular types with aberration.

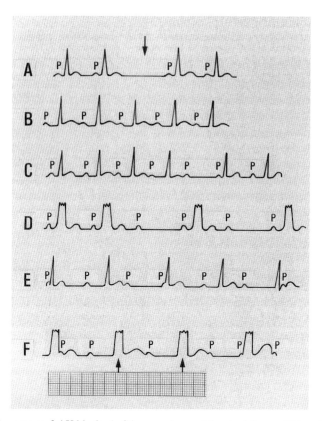

Fig 15–16. SA pause and AV block. A, SA pause (arrow) due to failure of SA node to discharge. B, First-degree AV block; P-R interval prolonged to 0.3 sec. C, Second-degree AV block of the Wenckebach type (Mobitz type 1). Note progressive lengthening of the P-R interval until a sinus beat is not conducted. Then sequence restarts. D, Second-degree AV block (Mobitz type II). Note that the P-R interval remains constant in the beats before nonconducted sinus beats and the QRS complexes are widened. E, Third-degree AV block. Note normal width QRS complexes indicating block is high in AV junction. Ventricular rate is 50, and atrial rate is 72 beats per minute. F, Third-degree AV block with widened QRS complexes indicating that block is in the right and left bundles (trifascicular block). Ventricular rate is 43, and atrial rate is 86 beats per minute.

or both). However, the "bradytachy" syndrome is one of the common manifestations of the SSS and should not be considered as a separate entity. Patients with the bradycardia-tachycardia component are more prone to cerebral emboli.[59] The SSS may also be suspected if there is a 3-second or greater pause with carotid sinus pressure, after cardioversion for a tachyarrhythmia the sinus rhythm is unstable, or the patient has chronic atrial flutter or fibrillation with a slow ventricular response (not due to drugs). In fact, some consider that lone atrial fibrillation is caused by a sick sinus node.

The diagnosis is clear if the patient has any of the above ECG findings on routine tracings or ambulatory Holter monitoring. However, the sinus node may have intermittent dysfunction which may become manifest with provocative tests. After 1 to 2 mg of atropine I.V., if the rate fails to increase beyond 90 beats per minute, or after atrial pacing (90 beats/minute and increasing by 10 beats every 2 to 4 minutes up to 150/minute) the sinus node recovery time

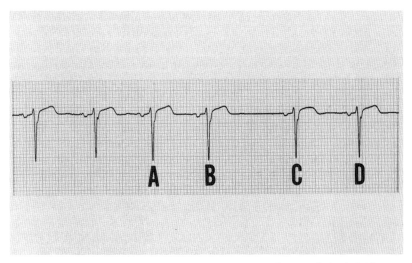

Fig 15-17. Sinoatrial Wenckebach (Type 1) exit block. Note the Wenckebach QRS grouping; the QRS complexes approach each other and BC is less than twice the preceding R-R interval AB and interval AB is less than the R-R interval CD. The P-R interval is constant as would occur with SA node Wenckebach exit block.

(SNRT) is prolonged, SSS should be considered.[60] However, the SNRT may be normal in the presence of SSS. Corrected sinus node recovery time (CSRT) is the difference between the postpacing pause and the resting sinus P-P cycle.[61] This corrected method is used to reduce the variability of the recovery time due to the intrinsic heart rate. Normal maximum CSRT is 525 msec or less. Electrode catheters passed into the right atrium via the right femoral vein are used for this study. The SA conduction time (SACT) is measured by atrial extrastimulus techniques,[62] but is a less sensitive test of sinus node dysfunction. During spontaneous sinus rhythm, single premature atrial stimuli are introduced by stimulating electrodes late in diastole after each sixth to eighth beat. The following intervals are measured: spontaneous cycle length immediately preceding the stimulated atrial complex (A_1A_1); coupling interval of stimulated atrial beat to preceding beat (A_1A_2); the interval from the stimulated atrial beat to the next conducted beat or the post extrasystolic pause (A_2A_3).[62] The SACT is calculated by the following equation: SACT $= (A_2A_3 - A_1A_1)/2$. The maximum normal reported for the CSRT is 120 to 150 msec. However, the SACT, as was the case for the CSRT, may be normal in the presence of the SSS. The sensitivity of the CSRT in patients with symptomatic sinus node disease is about 45%, for the SACT about 51%, and when combined about 68%. The specificity of the procedures when combined is about 88%.[45] The predictive value is low. Therefore, indications for these tests are infrequent and the potential candidate is a patient with unexplained symptoms and a high probability of sinus node disease. They should be used only as supporting evidence in the clinical decision.

Before considering management of the SSS, drugs that may have precipitated or aggravated this syndrome should be stopped. These include β-adrenergic blockers and others. Once this has been clarified, a pacemaker should be inserted if the patient is symptomatic or if he is asymptomatic with bradytachyarrhythmias present because the drugs used to treat the tachyarrhythmia may aggravate the brady component. After implantation of a permanent pacemaker, the atrial tachyarrhythmias can be controlled with drugs such as digitalis, quinidine, disopyramide, procainamide, verapamil, diltiazem, or β-adrenergic blocking agents.

Sinus bradycardia, as has been mentioned, is common in many healthy subjects, especially athletes, and is secondary to drugs such as digitalis and β-adrenergic blockers. In addition, one study[63] showed that patients with sleep-induced obstructive apnea may have marked sinus bradycardia (less than 30 beats/minute), periods of sinus pauses up to 6.3 seconds, and other arrhythmias. These arrhythmias were considered to be caused by increased parasympathetic tone produced by hypoxia and hypercarbia, especially because they cleared with atropine or tracheostomy.[63] Such causes of bradyarrhythmias in normal subjects should be excluded before labeling subjects as having the SSS.

Atrioventricular Heart Block

For many years this was considered primarily to be due to coronary artery disease. However, studies indicate that nonspecific fibrosis is a common cause. The fibrosis may be around the conducting system (Lev's disease) or sclerodegenerative changes in the conducting system (Lenegre's disease).[64] Sarcoidosis should be considered a cause in patients under 40 years of age. The AV block may be congenital or associated with rheumatic heart disease or rheumatoid arthritis. First-degree and second-degree (type 1) AV block are often noted in atheletes.

Atrioventricular block can indicate a conduction defect in the AV node, bundle of His, or bundle branches. The block is often characterized as first-, second-, or third-degree AV block. If the P-R interval is longer than 0.2 second, first-degree AV block is present (Fig 15–16B). In the past, in such situations we considered the block to be in the AV node. However, since the advent of His bundle studies, we now know that this delay could be in the AV node, bundle of His, or any of the bundle branches.

Second-degree AV block is present when one or more sinus beats is not conducted to the ventricles. The P-R interval may gradually increase with each beat until a QRS is nonconducted, and then the P-R interval returns to normal and the sequence again is repeated. This sequence is referred to as the typical Wenckebach phenomenon or Mobitz type I block (Fig 15–16C). If the P-R remains constant and there are one or more nonconducted QRS complexes, this is referred to as Mobitz type II block (Fig 15–16D) which is usually associated with bundle-branch block. In the typical Wenckebach structure, the QRS complexes approach each other as the P-R interval lengthens until a sinus beat is not conducted. The interval with the nonconducted QRS complex is less than twice the preceding R-R interval. In addition, this latter interval is less than the R-R interval after the nonconducted QRS complex (Figs 15–16C and 15–18). If only two beats are conducted before the nonconducted QRS, a 3:2 block (three atrial and two ventricular complexes) is produced. This gives a Wenckebach grouping of QRS complexes in pairs followed by a pause (Fig 15–19A). This is referred to as a pseudobigeminy. Knowing these groupings, one can suspect Wenckebach block even if the P waves are not visible, such as

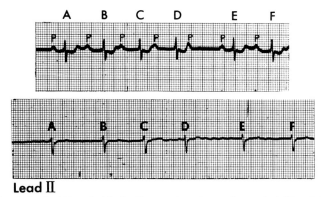

Lead II

Fig 15–18. Wenckebach AV node block. *Top tracing* shows the typical Wenckebach structure. The QRS complexes approach each other as the P-R interval lengthens until a sinus beat is not conducted. The interval with the nonconducted QRS complex DE is less than twice the preceding R-R interval CD. In addition, interval CD is less than the R-R interval EF after the nonconducted QRS complex. *Lower tracing* shows atrial fibrillation with AV dissociation and nonparoxysmal junctional tachycardia with a Wenckebach exit block below the junctional focus. Even though P waves are not seen the grouping of the QRS complexes indicates a Wenckebach AV block. (QRS complexes approach each other; DE is less than 2 CD and EF is greater than CD.)

with atrial fibrillation with AV dissociation and nonparoxysmal junctional tachycardia. Below the junctional focus there is a Wenckebach exit block that produces the QRS groupings (see Figs 15–18 and 15–19C). These groupings apply only to the typical Wenckebach structure and not to the atypical varieties. At times with a Wenckebach there may be a 2:1 response with the P–R interval constant in the conducted beats which have a normal QRS width. This is not a Mobitz II type block where the QRS usually shows a bundle branch block. Frequent recordings in such cases also show the more typical Wenckebach groupings.

Third-degree AV block can occur in the AV node, bundle of His, or as blocks in the bundle branches (trifascicular block). When the block is high in the AV junction, the QRS complexes are normal width and the rate will usually range between 40 and 55 beats per minute (Fig. 15–16E). When bilateral bundle-branch block occurs (trifascicular block), producing AV block, the QRS complexes are widened and the ventricular rate is usually below 45 (Fig 15–16F). This type of block may be preceded by isolated right or left bundle-branch block and at times as alternating right and left bundle-branch blocks. Rosenbaum and associates[64] described conduction impairment in the three main branches (right bundle-branch and two divisions of the left). The right bundle and the left anterior superior branch of the left bundle are long, thin, and vulnerable, whereas the posterior inferior branch of the left bundle is short, thick, and less vulnerable. In addition, the right bundle and the anterior division of the left are nourished only by the perforating branches of the anterior descending artery, whereas the posterior division gets a blood supply from the anterior descending and posterior descending coronary arteries. Bilateral bundle-branch block with resulting AV block may be impending if right bundle-branch block occurs with left axis of about −45 degrees or more to the left or right axis of about +120 degrees or more to the right, especially if such axes occur intermittently in the same patient. The left axis indicates block of the

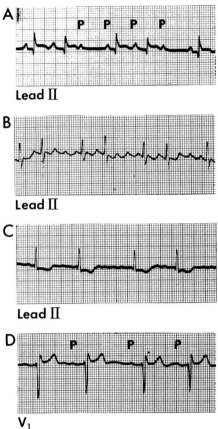

Fig 15–19. SA and AV node Wenckebach with 3:2 block. These are characterized by the QRS complexes occuring in pairs followed by a pause. **A,** sinus rhythm with 3:2 AV node Wenckebach block (three atrial and two ventricular complexes). **B,** atrial flutter with 3:2 AV node Wenckebach block. **C,** atrial fibrillation with AV dissociation and nonparoxysmal junctional tachycardia with a 3:2 Wenckebach exit block below the junctional focus. **D,** sinus rhythm was 3:2 SA node Wenckebach block.

left anterior superior branch of the left bundle (left anterior hemiblock; Fig. 15–20), and right axis indicates block of the left posterior inferior branch of the left bundle (left posterior hemiblock, Fig. 15–21).

Indications for Permanent Pacemakers

Morgagni (1761), Adams (1827), and Stokes (1846) described patients with abnormally slow pulses who had periodic fainting spells without warning. Hubbard[65] suggested the term "Adams-Stokes disease." Opinions vary concerning the exact definition of Adams-Stokes disease and of Adams-Stokes syndrome. While the terms are commonly used synonymously, Zoll et al.[66] and others have said that Adams-Stokes disease implies association of attacks with complete AV block, whether constant or intermittent. Adams-Stokes syndrome refers to attacks associated with cardiac arrhythmia, whether or not AV block is present.

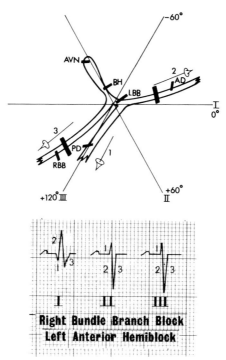

Fig 15–20. Right bundle-branch block with left anterior hemiblock. Vectors 1, 2, and 3 show the path of the impulse and derivation of leads I, II, and III. AVN = atrioventricular node; BH = bundle of His; LBB = left bundle branch; AD = anterior division of left bundle; RBB = right bundle branch; PD = posterior division of left bundle. *Heavy wide lines* show areas of blocks in the bundles. (Modified after Gazes P.C.: Adams-Stokes syndrome: Indications for permanent pacemaker. *Postgrad. Med.* 50:199, 1971.)

Dizziness is a common complaint. One study[67] showed that disorders of the vestibular system accounted for the dizziness in 38% of all patients who had this complaint. Among the vestibular disorders, benign positional vertigo was the most common cause of dizziness. Cardiovascular disorders accounted for dizziness in only 4%. In addition to dizziness, light-headedness and syncope are common symptoms, particularly in older people. Formerly these patients were casually examined and dismissed or were considered to have a neurologic lesion rather than a cardiac one, since isolated ECGs often showed a regular sinus rhythm. Since the advent of continuous ECG monitoring, many cardiac arrhythmias (namely, heart block) have been discovered to account for some of these symptoms. Whereas several years ago these patients were admitted to the neurologic service, today they are often referred to the cardiology service.

The history as given by the patient or someone who has witnessed the attack is helpful in making a diagnosis. An Adams-Stokes attack is initiated by acute cerebral ischemia due to a sudden change in cardiac rhythm. The symptoms produced by this cerebral ischemia may be dizziness, faintness, syncope, or unconsciousness, depending on the period of asystole, which is usually longer than 5 to 10 seconds. There may be momentary giddiness with a sudden pallor of the face or partial loss of consciousness. The loss of consciousness may be

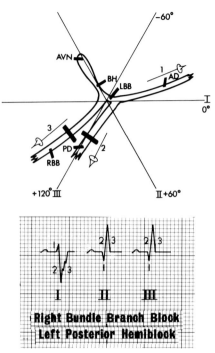

Fig 15–21. Right bundle-branch block with left posterior hemiblock. Vectors 1, 2, and 3 show the path of the impulse and derivation of leads I, II, and III. Abbreviations: Same as for Figure 15–20. (Modified after Gazes P.C.: Adams-Stokes syndrome: Indications for permanent pacemakers. *Postgrad. Med.* 50:199, 1971.)

complete, with or without convulsions and urinary and fecal incontinence. Breathing may be labored. Neurologic findings are usually absent, but may occur as focal phenomena in prolonged attacks. Differentiation from a primary neurologic seizure disorder may be difficult. However, the patient's mental state is usually clear immediately after an Adams-Stokes seizure, unless the attack is prolonged.

Because Adams-Stokes attacks are the main indication for use of a permanent cardiac pacemaker, careful examination of the routine or monitored tracings for ECG changes is necessary. Holter monitoring (magnetic tape recording of the ECG for 24 hours) allows the patient to assume his normal activities. In some cases electrophysiologic studies may be helpful in evaluating patients for pacemaker therapy, if routine ECG tracings or Holter monitoring show no significant findings. His-bundle electrograms (Fig 15–22) can be recorded by right heart catheterization using a tripolar catheter positioned fluoroscopically across the tricuspid valve. Depending on the purpose of the study, more than three catheter electrodes may be necessary. As mentioned previously, sinus node recovery time (SNRT) and sinus node conduction time (SACT) can be measured following atrial pacing and premature atrial stimulations for evaluating SA node function. The AV node and distal conduction system function can also be evaluated. Measurement of the AV nodal conduction time (A-H interval) and His-Purkinje conduction time (H-V interval) can be obtained and, if normal, can be repeated after atrial pacing to demonstrate latent

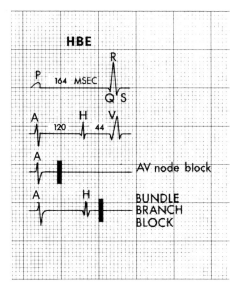

Fig 15–22. His bundle electrogram. Top complex is surface ECG. Below is a corresponding normal His bundle recording. AH interval represents AV nodal conduction and the H-V interval His-Purkinje conduction. Prolongation of the A-H interval would indicate first-degree AV node block and of the H-V interval, delay in a bundle branch. The third recording shows a high-grade AV node block, since the A wave is not followed by a conducted H potential. The bottom recording shows bilateral bundle branch block since the H potential is not followed by a conducted QRS complex. HBE = His bundle electrogram; A = atrial electrogram; H = His bundle electrogram; V = ventricular electrogram. *Heavy lines* show areas of block.

conduction disease. The A-H interval normally ranges from 60 to 130 msec and the H-V interval from 35 to 55 msec. However, such sophisticated studies may not be available and clues must be sought only in the routine or monitored ECG. AV block and SA block are considered diagnostic features in patients with typical Adams-Stokes attacks. However, these may be transient, and frequently a regular sinus rhythm is constantly noted. This necessitates a search for other ECG clues. The following changes may suggest that the dizziness or syncope is cardiac in origin provided noncardiac causes are excluded.

1. AV block of first, second, or third degree can be considered a strong indicator that the attacks are of cardiac origin. This is especially true for the higher-grade blocks (see Fig. 15–16). As mentioned previously, in the presence of atrial arrhythmias the grouping of the QRS complexes can indicate a Wenckebach block (see Figs. 15–18 and 15–19).
2. Bilateral bundle-branch block recently has been implicated as a frequent cause of AV block. Bilateral bundle-branch block with resulting AV block may be impending if right bundle-branch block occurs with left axis (about −45 degrees) or right axis (about +120 degrees), especially if such axes occur intermittently in the same patient. These have been described earlier (see Figs. 15–20 and 15–21).
3. Right bundle-branch block with a normal axis or left bundle-branch block may be a diagnostic finding if associated with some degree of AV block. However, in the presence of a regular sinus rhythm with no AV block or abnormal axis, it is a clue that the attacks may be cardiac in origin. Even

if AV block is present, the routine ECG cannot differentiate the location of this block, since the P-R interval represents conduction time of the cardiac impulse as it traverses from the SA node through the atria, the AV node, and the bundle of His to the bundle branches until the onset of the initial septal depolarization. Therefore a long P-R interval with left bundle-branch block could represent a conduction delay anywhere from the SA node to the right bundle. His bundle electrograms may aid in localizing the block. Figure 15–23 depicts the surface ECG with left bundle-branch block and first-degree AV block. This surface tracing does not localize the AV block. The His bundle electrogram shows that the H-V interval is prolonged, suggesting delayed conduction in the right bundle branch. The A-H interval would be prolonged if the conduction delay were in the AV node. Without His bundle studies, statistically one can predict that the long P-R interval in the presence of left bundle-branch block is due to delay in the right bundle rather than in the AV node.

4. Left axis (about −45 degrees) or right axis (about +120 degrees) as an isolated finding is a weak clue which may be more important if the axes alternate in the same patient on the same or different occasions.

5. Sinoatrial exit block, severe sinus bradycardia, or sinus pause (arrest) indicates the cardiac origin of the attacks (see Fig 15–16A). In some cases

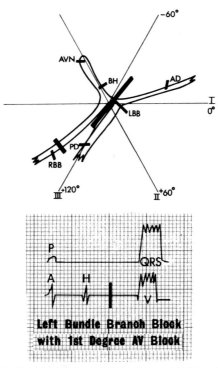

Fig 15–23. Left bundle-branch block with first-degree AV block. The surface ECG (*top tracing*) shows first-degree AV block but does not localize the block. The His bundle electrogram (*lower tracing*) shows that the first-degree AV block is due to delay distal to the His bundle in the right bundle, since the H-V interval is prolonged. Abbreviations: Same as in Figures 15–20 and 15–22. (Modified after Gazes P.C.: Adams-Stokes syndrome: Indications for permanent pacemakers. *Postgrad. Med.* 50:199, 1971.)

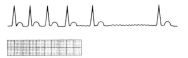

Fig 15–24. Atrial fibrillation with rapid ventricular rate and sudden ventricular standstill followed by a junctional (nodal) escape beat (tachybrady component of sick sinus node syndrome).

these may be associated with periods of rapid atrial arrhythmias. There may be periods of rapid atrial tachycardia and flutter or fibrillation followed by periods of severe sinus bradycardia, sinus pauses, or junctional (nodal) bradycardia. These are referred to as the "tachy-brady" component of a sick sinus node syndrome (Fig 15–24). Treatment in such cases is difficult; cardioaccelerator drugs such as atropine or isoproterenol (Isuprel) given for the "brady" periods may precipitate tachycardia, while antiarrhythmic drugs such as digitalis, quinidine, and propranolol given for the "tachy" periods can accentuate the bradyarrhythmias and produce syncope. The combination of a pacemaker to prevent bradyarrhythmias and antiarrhythmic drugs to control the tachyarrhythmias is often considered the best approach to this problem.

6. Drug-resistant ventricular and supraventricular tachyarrhythmias in the absence of AV block have been noted.

7. Hypersensitive carotid sinus reflex can produce dizziness and syncope, as demonstrated by light carotid sinus pressure. In some cases the sensitive structure may be the heart rather than the carotid sinus. Syncopal attacks due to carotid sinus hypersensitivity are best treated with a DDD or rate-responsive VVI pacemaker.

8. A normal ECG is unusual in patients with Adams-Stokes attacks. However, this can occur and make the decision difficult regarding insertion of a pacemaker. In such cases every effort should be made to monitor an attack. I have followed such cases for several months before documenting an arrhythmia or some other ECG clue (Fig. 15–25). Electrophysiologic studies may be of aid.

SUMMARY OF INDICATIONS FOR PACEMAKERS

Patients with dizziness or syncope or both who have ECG evidence (persistent or intermittent) of bradyarrhythmias, namely, Mobitz type II or third-degree AV block or a sick sinus node, should have a permanent pacemaker. Recordings during syncope in patients with third-degree AV block show ventricular asystole or ventricular tachycardia or ventricular fibrillation. Other ECG features mentioned above, namely, chronic bifascicular block (right bundle-branch block with left anterior hemiblock or left posterior hemiblock and left bundle-branch block) that may be noted in patients with dizziness or syncope are not specific indicators that the attacks are cardiac in origin, unless they are associated with bradyarrhythmias. Much controversy exists as to the

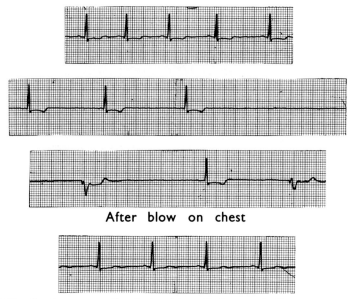

After blow on chest

Fig 15–25. Continuous recording during Adams-Stokes attack. *Top tracing* reveals normal sinus rhythm. *Second tracing* shows slow junctional rhythm and cardiac standstill. After blow on the chest, ventricular and junctional escape beats appeared, followed by regular sinus rhythm (*fourth tracing*). This patient had many Adams-Stokes attacks. Before the recording of this attack, tracings were normal.

frequency with which patients with such chronic bifascicular blocks develop complete heart block, syncope, or both, and sudden death. Some prefer (especially if the symptoms are equivocal) that His bundle studies be performed and a pacemaker implanted only if the H-V interval is prolonged.[68] One study showed that patients with chronic bifascicular block with a prolonged H-V interval have a greater incidence and severity of organic heart disease and higher total and sudden death mortalities, but the incidence of spontaneous trifascicular block is small.[69] Another study concluded that a markedly prolonged H-Q interval ($\geq$100 msec) may detect spontaneous AV block, but prophylactic pacing is of no value to relieve symptoms or prolong life.[70] These authors and others[71,72] recommend permanent pacing only in patients with chronic bifascicular block and documented symptomatic bradyarrhythmia. However, if other causes for dizziness and syncope have been thoroughly excluded and patients have recurrent attacks (especially those with hazardous jobs), we recommend permanent pacing in symptomatic patients with chronic bifascicular block, especially if the H-V interval is prolonged, even though bradyarrhythmia cannot be documented. Even more controversial is what to do with the asymptomatic patient with chronic bifascicular block and a markedly prolonged H-V interval. However, if such patients have spontaneous second- or third-degree infra-His block, even though they are asymptomatic, pacemaker insertion may be advisable. We consider the use of permanent pacemakers for the following patients, even when they are not having presyncope or syncope:

1. Patients who have heart block with heart failure, angina, cerebral insuf-

ficiency, renal insufficiency, widened QRS complexes, a ventricular rate below 40 beats per minute, or an R-R interval of 3 seconds or more. After insertion of the pacemaker, patients with heart block and failure can be digitalized. Elderly patients often become confused or have renal changes with heart block; these conditions as well as angina can improve with the use of a pacemaker.

2. Patients with right bundle-branch block and left anterior or posterior hemiblock and periods of second-degree (Type II) or higher grades of AV block or an H-V interval greater than 90 msec with or without pacing or procainamide.

3. Patients with right bundle-branch block and left anterior or posterior hemiblock with frequent ventricular arrhythmias requiring antiarrhythmic drugs.

4. Patients with drug-refractory tachyarrhythmias may benefit from antitachycardia pacing.

5. Patients with tachy-bradyarrhythmias associated with SSS that cannot be controlled by drugs.

In summary, permanent pacing is indicated in patients with symptomatic proven bradycardia, regardless of its type, if it is not associated with an acute transient event, such as acute myocardial infarction, or a drug, or an electrolyte imbalance. The most common causes are the SSS (with maximum R-R interval of 3 or more seconds or a minimum heart rate below 40 beats per minute) with or without tachycardia and bradycardia, and high-grade atrioventricular block. In asymptomatic patients with persistent bradycardia, the decision is more difficult. Generally, if there is a persistent bradycardia with a maximum R-R interval of more than 3 seconds or with a minimum heart rate of 40 beats per minute, Mobitz type II second-degree AV block, or marked infranodal conduction disturbance with the H-V interval >90 msec or this degree of prolongation by pacing or procainamide, a permanent pacemaker is indicated. Adherence to these criteria[73,74] will reduce the number of unnecessary implants.

TYPES AND MODES OF PACING

Pacing has become so complex that many are specializing in this area. However, the practicing physician should have some knowledge about the indications and types of pacemakers. The type of pacemaker used depends on the type of symptomatic bradyarrhythmia and the expected hemodynamic response that should be achieved. Inappropriate pacemaker selection can produce problems such as the pacemaker syndrome.

Lithium-powered pacemakers have become popular during the past few years because this power source increases the pacemaker lifespan up to 5 to 10 years. Nuclear-powered pacemakers (with plutonium-238 as the energy source), which were introduced because of their longevity, have been made unnecessary by the lithium type. Programmable pacemakers have been developed in an attempt to achieve the ideal pulse generator. Programmable pacemakers allow changes in pacing rate, energy output (voltage, current pulse width), refractory period, hysteresis, and sensing function noninvasively after implantation of the pacemaker.[75] Some pacemakers have telemetry that at

any time can give a readout of these parameters. Negative hysteresis is
present in some pacemakers when the escape interval is longer following a
sensed QRS than the automatic set pacing interval. Positive hysteresis has an
escape interval following a sensed beat that is shorter than the escape interval
following the paced beat. All pacemakers have a pulse generator (power
source) and electrodes to transmit the paced impulse to the endocardium or
myocardium. The pacemaker impulse can be delivered by the electrode catheter passed intravenously into the heart or by the use of epicardial leads. The
transvenous route is predominantly used today, and the epicardial method is
used only when the leads cannot be placed properly intravenously. Single- and
dual-chamber pacemakers are now available with different modes of pacing.
Pulse generators are now categorized according to their mode and site of function and these pacing modalities are given an identification code as follows:[76]
the chamber-paced (V for ventricle, A for atrium, and D for both); the chamber-
sensed (V for ventricle, A for atrium, D for both, and O for not applicable); and
the mode of response (I for inhibited, T for triggered, D for both, and O for not
applicable; Fig. 15–26). These three-position pacemaker codes are most often
used, but two others have been added to include special programmable functions and anti-tachycardia features. Physiologic cardiac pacing allows improved cardiac hemodynamics (properly timed atrial contractions increase cardiac output and reduce filling pressure), control of some ectopic or re-entrant
arrhythmias, and physiologic rate control (when atrial synchronous pacing is
used). Some of the various modes of pacing are as follows: atrial pacing and
sensing, inhibited mode (AAI); ventricular pacing and sensing, inhibited mode
(VVI); atrial and ventricular pacing and ventricular sensing, inhibited mode
(DVI); atrial pacing and sensing, triggered mode (AAT); ventricular pacing
and sensing, triggered mode (VVT); ventricular pacing and atrial sensing,
triggered mode (VAT); atrial pacing, no sensing (AOO); ventricular pacing, no
sensing (VOO); and atrioventricular pacing, no sensing (DOO). The latter
three are now obsolete. Some of these features can be combined to give complex

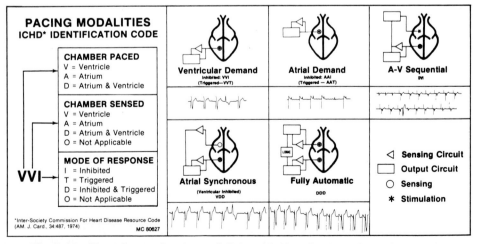

Fig 15–26.   Most often used pacing modalities with identification codes and representative ECG
findings. (Courtesy of Medtronic, Inc., Minneapolis, Minn.)

pacing modalities as VAT and VVI combined to give VDD; and AAI, VDD and DVI combined to give a universal modality DDD which can sense both chambers and can be atrial triggered or ventricular inhibited. During abnormal sinus node function with normal AV conduction, the DDD functions as an atrial demand pacemaker (AAI); during impaired AV conduction and normal sinus node function as an atrial synchronous pacemaker (VDD); and during impaired AV conduction and abnormal sinus node function as an AV sequential pacemaker (DVI). In the inhibited types, the chamber's activity is sensed, and if not detected, the pulse generator sends out a stimulus after a certain preset, fixed interval. In the triggered types the stimulus is sent out synchronously with the natural activity of the chamber and the stimulus artifact is seen on the ECG in the early refractory periods of the QRS complex or P wave. The atrial modes are important for improving or maintaining cardiac hemodynamics by properly timed atrial transport; therefore, such types should not be used in the presence of chronic atrial fibrillation or flutter. The only pacemaker available with rate-adaptivity is the VVI type.[77] The rate varies with body activity or motion. Beside physical activity, rate adaptivity is being studied with other body requirements such as respiratory rate and changes in minute ventilation, venous O_2 saturation, venous pH, central venous temperature and other parameters. The VVI rate-adaptive type can be used in the atria as an AAI rate-adaptive type. A dual-chamber pacemaker (DDD) rate-adaptive type is now undergoing investigation in several institutions, including ours. The algorithm (Fig. 15–27) shows indications for the three most common type pacemakers.[78] The symptomatic patient with sinus node disease and normal AV conduction should have an AAI pacemaker. The AV conduction is considered adequate if atrial pacing produces AV node Wenckebach at a rate greater than 130 beats per minute. A rate-responsive VVI pacemaker could be used in the atria if the sinus rate does not appropriately increase with exercise to at least 75% of the maximum heart rate (chronotropic incompetence). A DDD pacemaker should be used if there is an associated abnormal AV conduction and a chronotropically competent SA node or a rate-responsive one when it becomes available in the future, if the SA node is chronotropically incompetent. The patient with variable or complete heart block and sinus rhythm should receive a DDD pacemaker or a VVI type. A rate-responsive type is best for the chronotropically incompetent patient. If a DDD pacemaker is producing reciprocal tachycardia that cannot be reprogrammed so that this

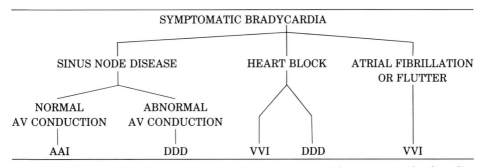

Fig 15–27. Algorithm for pacemaker selection for patients with symptomatic bradycardia.

will not occur, it should be programmed to the DVI mode. The patient with bradyarrhythmia and chronic atrial fibrillation or flutter should receive a standard VVI pacemaker. However, if the patient does not have an appropriate increase in rate with exercise, a rate-adaptive VVI should be used. Figure 15–28 depicts a patient with a DDD pacemaker that has been programmed to show the various pacing modes.

At times, noninvasive electric pacing can be used when temporary cardiac stimulation is indicated.[79] The Zoll noninvasive temporary pacemaker consists of a demand pulse generator, a two-trace nonfade ECG monitor scope, and a strip chart recorder. Two pacing electrodes are placed on the back and precordium. It is used for pacing in conscious or unconscious patients for up to 2 hours as an alternative to endocardial stimulation. It usually is used for resuscitation from standstill or bradycardia of any cause, as a standby when standstill or bradycardia might be expected, or for suppression of tachycardia. It can produce some discomfort or unavoidable skeletal muscle contraction.

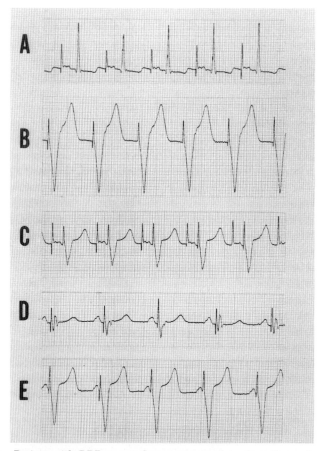

Fig 15–28. Patient with DDD pacemaker programmed to show the various pacing modes. A, Atrial demand pacing (AAI). B, Ventricular demand pacing (VVI). C, A-V sequential pacing (DVI). D, Atrial-synchronous pacing (VDD) with A-V interval of 120 msec with ventricular fusion beats. E, VDD pacing with A-V interval of 80 msec eliminates the fusion beats.

PACEMAKER MALFUNCTION

Sophisticated pacemakers require follow-up for detection of malfunction and reprogramming when necessary to meet patients' physiologic needs. Many institutions have a surveillance clinic or office follow-up with scheduled visits after implantation. The frequency of pacemaker surveillance is now dictated in most institutions by the medical reimbursement schedule.[79a] During the visit, an ECG is taken for determination of capturing and sensoring and, with appropriate equipment, pacemaker parameters are measured and recorded and reprogramming is done if necessary. In addition to the office or clinic visits, in-between telephone monitoring of the patient's electrocardiogram, pacing rate, and duration of stimulus can be done. The ECG is most useful for detecting malfunction as inadequate sensing, capture, changes in heart rate, and changes in QRS configuration or axes of the paced beats (suggesting electrode displacement). It also confirms the mode of pacing. If the patient's intrinsic rhythm inhibits the pacemaker, a magnet over the pacemaker will convert the unit to an asynchronous operation so that capture can be detected. Carotid massage may reduce the intrinsic rate and allow pacing to take over. X rays of the chest may detect lead position, fractures, or disconnection. The pacemaker programmer can evaluate many functions such as pacing rate, refractory period, stimulus strength, amplifier sensitivity, and pacing modes. Systems can also provide telemetry for evaluating the lead systems or recording programmed settings for comparison with expected performance. Malfunction can be due to failure to capture, sensing, oversensing, change in rate, or changes due to infections or external sources (Fig. 15–29). Failure to capture occurs if the system fails to deliver a stimulus, as occurs with a broken lead wire, inappropriate programming of strength of pacemaker stimulus, or if the stimulus is delivered during the refractory period of the myocardium. Failure to

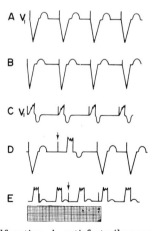

Fig 15–29. Pacemaker malfunction. **A,** satisfactorily paced rhythm with QRS complexes in V₁ having a left bundle-branch block appearance, indicating pacing is from right ventricle. **B,** decrease in amplitude of impulse spike due to decrease in pacer output. **C,** paced rhythm; however, QRS configuration in V₁ has changed to that of right bundle-branch block indicating catheter has changed pacing sites. The catheter may have perforated the septum or right ventricle and paced the left ventricle, or the catheter is in the coronary sinus. **D,** normal sensing, but intermittent failure to capture (*arrow*). **E,** failure to sense QRS complexes.

sense can occur and is often caused by lead displacement, although there are many other causes. Oversensing can occur, for example sensing of the T wave or electromagnetic signals from radio, television transmitters, or other electrical sources. Weapon detection devices and microwave ovens are no longer a problem with the newer pacemakers. Electrocautery or defibrillation paddles near the pulse generator may produce damage to the system. Incorrect pacing modes may produce pacemaker-mediated tachyarrhythmias or the pacemaker syndrome.[80] Patients with the pacemaker syndrome complain of weakness, lightheadedness, dizziness, dyspnea, chest discomfort, or palpitations. The symptoms occur with the onset of ventricular (VVI) pacing. The blood pressure can drop, cannon "A" waves in the neck are noted, and pulmonary congestion and regurgitant murmurs can occur. Restoration of atrioventricular synchrony with a dual-chamber (DDD) pacer usually eliminates the syndrome. One must be familiar with the types of pacing modes and the programmed parameters to properly interpret the ECG recordings. Some pacemakers have hysteresis with the escape interval of the first pacemaker stimulus (interval between last normal beat and first paced beat) exceeding the set pacing interval and allowing the patient a longer interval for normally conducted beats. A pacemaker may have a committed mode (DVI device) with a pacemaker committed to deliver a ventricular stimulus after stimulating the atrium regardless of spontaneous ventricular activity.

Patients with pacemakers should resume all their activities, and their limitations depend on the underlying cardiac problem. It is important that the patient tell the physician about his activities and hobbies so that placement of the pulse generator will not interfere with these.

ECG CLUES FOR DETECTION OF COMPLEX ARRHYTHMIAS

Many complex arrhythmias have been clarified recently by electrophysiologic studies. However, these are often unavailable, or because of the emergency state, one cannot wait for them to be performed. Therefore, clinical judgment and the ECG findings must be relied on heavily. Fortunately, many of the arrhythmias can be identified in the ECG if one will memorize a few patterns and groupings of the complexes. Some of these are as follows:

1. Ventricular ectopic beats may be confused with those of supraventricular origin with aberration. If there is a long pause, a normal conducted beat, and then the ectopic beat, a supraventricular beat with aberration should be suspected (Fig. 15–30A). In addition, if this beat has a right bundle-branch configuration (rSR'), aberration should be suspected because ventricular ectopy usually has a monophasic R or a qR. A ventricular ectopic beat can conduct retrograde and activate the atria. This beat can be confused with a junctional premature beat with aberration and retrograde conduction to the atria. The latter is probably present if the R-P interval is 0.1 second or less.

2. In the presence of a regular tachycardia with widened QRS complexes, a sudden normal conducted beat (capture beat; see Fig. 15–30B) or one that does not resemble those of the tachycardia (fusion beat) suggests that the tachycardia is ventricular in origin rather than supraventricular with aberration or bundle-branch block.

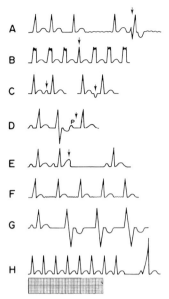

Fig 15–30. Complex arrhythmias. **A,** atrial fibrillation. *Arrow* points to aberrant conducted beat which resembles right bundle-branch block, and follows a short cycle preceded by a long cycle. **B,** ventricular tachycardia. *Arrow* points to capture beat which confirms the tachycardia is of ventricular rather than supraventricular origin with bundle-branch block. **C,** sandwiched P waves between two QRS complexes. Upright P waves indicate atrioventricular dissociation with ventricular capture. Inverted P waves indicate junctional rhythm with retrograde conduction to atria and progressive increase in R-P interval until ventricles can respond to antegrade conduction (reciprocal beat). **D,** long P-R interval after interpolated ventricular extrasystole because of retrograde conduction into the AV node, blocking antegrade sinus conduction (concealed conduction). **E,** blocked PAB. Note that the second QRS complex has a higher T wave (*arrow*) than the preceding beat, indicating a hidden P wave. **F,** atrial fibrillation and regular ventricular response (100 beats per minute) indicating AV dissociation with nonparoxysmal junctional tachycardia. **G,** accelerated idioventricular rhythm (75 beats per minute) after first normal conducted beat. **H,** supraventricular tachycardia (normal conduction) with sudden return to regular sinus rhythm and the WPW syndrome.

3. At times a P wave may be sandwiched between two QRS complexes with no P wave preceding the first QRS complex. If this P wave is upright, one should consider junctional rhythm or nonparoxysmal AV junctional tachycardia with AV dissociation with a capture beat (Fig. 15–30C). If the P wave is inverted, junctional rhythm with retrograde conduction is present (Fig. 15–30C). In this latter situation, the R-P interval may progressively lengthen to a point when the ventricle has recovered from its previous stimulation and can respond to antegrade conduction (reciprocal beat). This sequence is often referred to as a retrograde Wenckebach block.

4. Sudden prolongation of the P-R interval in an occasional beat with prompt return to normal in the other normal sinus beats suggests concealed conduction. A PVB may retrograde conduct into the AV node and delay the next normal conducted beat so that the P-R interval is prolonged. This is most often seen with interpolated ventricular extrasystoles, which occur between two normal conducted beats where the basic rate has not changed (Fig. 15–30D). In addition, occasional P-R interval pro-

longation can indicate concealed conduction due to a His bundle premature (junctional) beat with antegrade and retrograde block so that it is not seen in the surface ECG. However, this blocked beat will cause sudden P-R interval prolongation by producing a delay in antegrade conduction of the next normal sinus beat. In fact, because of this, high-grade blocks can occur and are referred to as pseudo-AV blocks.[81] This should be particularly suspected if an occasional conducted junctional beat is noted.

5. Usually, if two QRS complexes are similar in configuration, the repolarization T waves also should be alike. If this is not the case, a P wave is probably hidden in the T wave as seen with a blocked PAB (Fig. 15–30E). This can be mistaken for a sinus pause.
6. The typical Wenckebach groupings have been previously discussed (see Figs. 15–16C, 15–18, 15–19). Those of the SA node can be mistaken for sinus arrhythmia, and those of the AV node with atrial fibrillation or flutter may be mistaken as the expected AV response.
7. Sudden, regular ventricular rhythm in the presence of atrial fibrillation should suggest third-degree AV block if the rate is below 50 beats per minute, or AV dissociation with nonparoxysmal AV junctional tachycardia if the rate is between 70 and 130 beats per minute (FIg. 15–30F).
8. A sudden burst of slow, widened QRS complexes (60 to 100 beats per minute) is not slow ventricular tachycardia (Figs. 15–30G, 4–17), is usually benign, and is referred to as accelerated idioventricular rhythm. It often appears with an inferior infarction and may even occur in normal persons.
9. Individuals with tachyarrhythmias may have the WPW syndrome (Fig. 15–30H). In fact, some of these patients cannot conduct antegrade via the accessory pathway and so do not show the WPW morphology at any time. Yet such patients can develop reentrant tachycardia because the bypass pathway can conduct retrograde. Such cases are said to have a concealed WPW syndrome[82] that can be detected only by electrophysiologic studies. Arrhythmias can occur in some persons who have only short P-R intervals (Lown-Ganong-Levine syndrome).

SUDDEN CARDIAC DEATH

Sudden cardiac death has become an important subject because many persons are being resuscitated today and preventive measures are being established. It is frequently due to coronary artery disease, and, unfortunately, may be its first manifestation.[83] Sudden cardiac death is usually defined as death within 1 hour of collapse. About 25% of these cases have had no known prior cardiac disease.[84] In addition, sudden death has been noted in congenital abnormalities, obstructive and nonobstructive cardiomyopathies, mitral valve prolapse, and other valvular disease, and rarely in the apparently normal heart. Any type of coronary event such as angina, myocardial infarction, or arrhythmia without chest pain can produce sudden death. It has also been related to hereditary, prolonged Q-T interval syndromes, such as the Romano-Ward syndrome[85,86] (no associated deafness) and the Jervell and Lange-Nielsen syndrome[87] (associated deafness). Rarely, sudden death can occur with the Wolff-Parkinson-White (WPW) syndrome. Conduction down the accessory pathway can be rapid with atrial fibrillation, and this alone or with digitalis (which shortens refractory period of accessory pathway, further increasing ventricular response) can lead to ventricular fibrillation. Maron et al.[88] have reported that hypertrophic cardiomyopathy is a frequent cause of sudden death in the athlete. The most likely precipitating mechanism is an arrhythmia, namely ventricular tachycardia and fibrillation.[89] Supraventricular arrhythmias may also be a factor because such patients lose the atrial contribution to diastolic filling. Sudden death is more common in aortic stenosis than in other types of valvular disease. It is rare in mitral valve prolapse. Swartz et al.[90] reported 8 instances of sudden death in 589 patients with mitral valve prolapse and associated arrhythmias. Factors that favor the occurrence of sudden death in mitral valve prolapse are female gender, unexplained syncope or presyncope, long Q-T interval, or nonspecific ST-T changes, murmur of mitral insufficiency, malignant ventricular arrhythmias at rest or with exercise, and a family history of sudden death. Sudden death has also been reported in individuals in whom no evidence of cardiac disease was ever noted, and even autopsy studies could not disclose a cause.

How do we identify patients at high risk for sudden death? This is an important question, and equally important is how sudden death can be prevented. Clinical profiles for many conditions, as mentioned for mitral valve prolapse, are surfacing. Patients with coronary artery disease should have any associated major tachyarrhythmias or bradyarrhythmias treated. In has been shown that patients with ventricular arrhythmias occurring during the first few days of an acute myocardial infarction have a better prognosis than if the arrhythmia occurred late postinfarction.[91] It also has been shown that individuals not known to have coronary artery disease who developed cardiac arrest due to ventricular fibrillation and were resuscitated have a mortality of up to 30% during the first year, yet patients resuscitated after ventricular fibrillation developed in acute myocardial infarction have only a 2% mortality for the first year.[92] Coronary arteriography in such patients without known prior disease often shows triple-vessel disease, and such patients have a better prognosis with bypass surgery. Holter monitoring, radionuclide function studies, and a limited stress test (in uncomplicated cases) postinfarction are being used to detect the high-risk patient. It has been shown that the prognosis is worse if patients have complex arrhythmias, left ventricular dysfunction, or a positive stress test.[93,94] Programmed ventricular extrastimulation in the right ventricular apex has resulted in reproducible initiation of ventricular tachycardia.[95] Such techniques have been used to evaluate antiarrhythmic therapy and in certain instances to localize the arrhythmia for a surgical approach.[96] However, much conflicting data exists as to the significance of inducible sustained ventricular tachycardia or ventricular fibrillation as a marker.[97] Studies by Ruberman et al.[98] and Schulze et al.[93] demonstrated that the risk of dying is greater if complex PVBs and reduced ventricular function are present. However, the PVBs alone have an independent contribution. Bigger et al.[99] performed 24-hour Holter recordings before hospital discharge in 430 patients who survived an acute myocardial infarction. Fifty patients (11.6%) had ventricular tachycardia (3 or more consecutive ventricular complexes). This tachycardia group had a 38% 1-year mortality compared with 11.6% in the group without tachycardia. The same investigators[100] analyzed 24 hours of ECG recordings on 500 patients shortly before hospital discharge after sustaining an acute myocardial infarction and related their findings to the 1-year mortality. The overall 1-year mortality was 14%; patients with PVBs greater than 10 per hour had a mortality of 25%; patients with pairs or ventricular tachycardia had a mortality of 25%. Multiform or R on T premature beats did not have a significant increased rate. Many use the classification of Lown et al.[101] (Table 15–13); increasing grades have increasing risks of sudden death. This classification originated from monitoring patients with acute myocardial infarction.

Signal-averaged ECG can identify late potentials which are low-level electrical signals detected on the body surface that occur after the normal QRS and represent delayed conduction in damaged or diseased myocardium.[102] These late potentials can be the harbinger of serious ventricular arrhythmias because they represent delayed conduction, which sets up re-entry. Late potentials cannot be seen on a normal ECG and are recorded from the body surface using high resolution electrocardiography. This technique combines low noise amplification, high gain, and signal averaging to reduce background noise. Fast-Fourier transform analysis is applied to the signal-averaged ECG to enhance the identification and quantification of the late potentials. Signal-averaging ECG is being used to identify late potentials and quantitate these as markers for risk of ventricular tachycardia and fibrillation especially in postinfarction patients, in those with syncope of unknown origin, in asymptomatic complex ectopy, and in those with nonsustained ventricular tachycardia.[103] It is also being investigated as a method to screen patients for invasive electrophysiologic studies and to identify cardiac transplant rejection.[104,105]

In summary, there are many studies of the hypothesis that ventricular arrhythmias represent an independent predictor of sudden cardiac death. However, none have shown that these increase the risk of sudden death in subjects without heart disease. In patients with coronary disease, it has been shown that left ventricular dysfunction and complex ventricular arrhythmias are independent predictors of both total mortality and sudden cardiac death. However, this does not indicate that there is a cause and effect relationship with

Table 15–13. Classification of Premature Ventricular Contractions (PVCs)*

Grade	PVC Occurrence
O	None
Simple	
1A	<1/min
	<30/hr
1B	>1/min
	<30/hr
2	>30/hr
3	Multiform
4A	Couplets
Complex	
4B	≥3 in a row
5	R on T phenomenon

*From Lown B., Graboys T. B.: Sudden death: An ancient problem newly perceived. *Cardiovasc. Med.* 2:219, 1977. (Used by permission.)

the ventricular arrhythmias and sudden cardiac death. A survey by Surawicz[35] suggests that in patients with well-preserved ventricular function, therapy is not likely to reduce the incidence of sudden death. The incidence and complexity of ventricular arrhythmias increases with the severity of heart disease and myocardial dysfunction and with these the incidence of sudden death. Although these are treated as of this date, antiarrhythmic therapy has made no impact on the incidence of sudden death. The NHLBI is currently conducting a large multicenter trial in an attempt to answer the question as to whether antiarrhythmic therapy can alter the incidence of sudden death in the postinfarction patients[106] (see page 427 for preliminary results of cast study).

Some cases of long Q-T interval syndrome and malignant ventricular arrhythmias have responded to unilateral cervicothoracic sympathetic ganglionectomy.[107] Patients with the WPW syndrome and arrhythmias who do not respond to medical treatment should have mapping and surgical resection of the pathway. If there are major arrhythmias or a family history of sudden death in patients with hypertrophic cardiomyopathy (HCM), the patients should be given propranolol, even though there is no evidence that propranolol prevents sudden death. Future studies with calcium blockers such as verapamil may show effective preventive action. Digitalis, nitrates, diuretics, and strenuous exercise should be avoided in such cases of HCM, for they can produce sudden death. The patients with aortic valve stenosis who are prone to sudden death are those who have left ventricular hypertrophy and a high systolic gradient across the valve. These patients should have valve replacement.

In all types of conditions, sympathetic neural factors and psychologic stress may be important in sudden death.

MANAGEMENT OF CARDIAC ARREST

Cardiopulmonary resuscitation (CPR) is the basic life support for cardiac arrest. Kouwenhoven et al.[108] in 1960 demonstrated the effectiveness of closed-chest cardiac massage. Before this, external ac cardiac defibrillation was reported by Zoll and associates,[109] and later Lowen et al.[110] showed that dc defibrillation was the preferred mode. Every physician should be well trained in CPR. Other medical and paramedical personnel are also being trained, accounting for the many successful cases resuscitated. The first step in training paramedical personnel is the recognition of cardiac arrest, which is characterized by a loss of carotid pulses, heart sounds, respirations, and the development of unconsciousness. Cardiopulmonary resuscitation can be performed by either one person or a team. Usually a team approach is preplanned in the hospital setting or in such emergency units as the mobile coronary care or emergency medical care units. It is also important to know that certain types of patients, such as those with terminal disease (e.g., cancer), are not candidates for CPR. The ABCs of therapy are: A, open airway; B, begin breathing; and C, restore circulation. These patients should be placed in the supine position, and the head is tilted back by placing one hand on the forehead and the other behind the neck. This lifts the tongue away from the back of the throat. Any foreign bodies or dentures should be removed, and one should listen for breathing with the ear over the victim's mouth while observing the chest. If breathing does not start after these maneuvers, one should begin ventilation by mouth-to-mouth, mouth-to-nose, and bag-and-mask (if available). The mouth-to-mouth procedure is the most common nonhospital method. With the head tilted backward, the nostrils are pinched closed with the hand, and the resuscitator, after a full inspiration, places his mouth tightly over that of the victim and exhales into it. After inflation, the resuscitator removes his mouth to allow for exhalation. The ventilator pause should be 1.5 seconds to allow adequate ventilation. Cardiac massage should be started with ventilation. The resuscitator places the heel of one hand over the lower third of the sternum. The other hand is placed on the top and the sternum is depressed 3 to 5 cm. The elbows should be stiff and the arms straight and compression should be vertical, not bouncing. The rate of compressions should be 80 to 100 per minute. If only one rescuer is present, each series of 15 cardiac compressions should be followed by two lung inflations. If there are two rescuers, one lung inflation should follow each series of 5 cardiac compressions without any interruptions. Periodically, rescuers should check for return of pulse and spontaneous breathing. They should know a local emergency system telephone number.

Until recently, it was thought that external cardiac massage produced ventricular compression between the sternum and spine and thus propelled blood forward through the systemic circulation. However, studies[111,112] have shown that vascular pressures and flow recorded during chest compression depend on the generated intrathoracic pressure (thoracic pump) rather than on ventricular compression. Selective flow to the brachiocephalic vascular bed occurs because of the arteriovenous gradient produced by closure of the venous valves at the thoracic inlet. This arteriovenous gradient is augmented during chest compression with sustained lung inflation. The left heart acts as a conduit during CPR and not as a pump.

Complications such as rib and sternum fracture, laceration of lung or liver, pulmonary or cerebral fat emboli, cardiac tamponade, hemothorax, and pneumothorax have been reported. It is important that basic life support be started immediately, for any delay may result in failure of resuscitation, or resuscitation can be established but the patient can be left with brain damage.

Once CPR is started and is effective, advanced life support should follow. Advanced life support includes optimizing ventilation, starting an I.V. line, cardiac defibrillation, monitoring rhythm and BP, administering drugs to stabilize these, and postresuscitation care. Naturally, the setting in which the cardiac arrest occurs often determines the initial therapy. For example, in the coronary care unit, often dc shock is the first procedure for ventricular fibrillation, even before basic life support. Many mobile units (including helicopters) are now equipped for advanced life support and have well-trained paramedical personnel who are allowed to perform many of the procedures. Often the ECG is transmitted by telemetry to the base hospital. Such mobile units should have the I.V. drugs and solutions that are usually available in the coronary care units; a battery-operated oscilloscope for monitoring, a battery-operated ECG recorder; a dc defibrillator; and oxygen supply with Ambu bags, endotracheal tubes, and suction apparatus. Some units, especially the helicopter types, have external noninvasive temporary pacemakers. If one witnesses the event, an immediate sharp thumb on the chest can be given before starting CPR. Direct-current shock is given if ventricular fibrillation is present. Blind defibrillation can be performed if there is delay in obtaining a satisfactory

ECG recording. The electrode paddles should be coated with electrode gel or saline solution, and firm contact should be made between the skin and paddles. The paddles can be placed diagonally across the anterior chest (usually one electrode at the second right intercostal space next to the sternum and the other at the fifth intercostal space at the mid-axillary line) or in the AP position, with the flat posterior paddle positioned at the angle of the left scapula. Studies have shown that lower-energy shocks such as 200 joules are as effective as high-energy shocks and are safer. In addition, because transthoracic impedance declines with repeated shocks, greater current flows result from the second shock. In addition to defibrillation, the sequence for the treatment of ventricular fibrillation recommended by the 1985 National Conference on Cardiopulmonary Resuscitation (CPR) and Emergency Cardiac Care (ECC) is presented in Figure 15–31.[113] It should be noted that treatment with sodium bicarbonate is no longer recommended except for selected patients because CO_2 and lactate accumulate in the venous system, and bicarbonate, by generating CO_2, can worsen the venous respiratory acidemia. Thus, cardiac and CNS function may deteriorate. Therefore, arterial blood gases may not reflect the true state of acid-base abnormalities in the tissues. Epinephrine is the pressor agent of choice in cardiac arrest. Its alpha effect produces peripheral vasoconstriction and raises the aortic diastolic pressure. If there is a delay in starting an intravenous line, epinephrine can be given by the endotracheal tube. Lidocaine and atropine can also be given by this route. Recent studies[114] have shown no difference in outcome when bretylium and lidocaine were compared.

Recently a study[115] was reported of the use by firefighters of an automatic external defibrillator which is a relatively simple device that requires only a modest amount of training to use. Firefighters were instructed to use the device until paramedics arrived and continued care with standard defibrillator-monitors, tracheal intubation, and medications as needed. Of 276 patients who were initially treated with the automatic defibrillator, 30% survived to hospital discharge; and of 228 patients in whom it was not used and who were given only basic cardiopulmonary resuscitation but awaited defibrillation after arrival of the paramedic team, only 19% survived.

Patients with severe sinus bradycardia with hypotension, second- or third-degree AV block with slow ventricular rates, hypotension, or Stokes-Adams attacks should be given atropine I.V. or have a pacemaker inserted. Ventricular asystole noted in some patients with cardiac arrest is often associated with pump failure. Atrial activity may or may not be present. At times it may actually be fine ventricular fibrillation, and when there is doubt, dc shock should be used. After a sharp blow to the chest, if the heartbeat is not restored, CPR should be started. The algorithm of Figure 15–32 can be used as a guide for the management of asystolic arrest as recommended by the National Conference on CPR and ECC.[113] Calcium chloride is no longer recommended; in fact at high levels it can be detrimental. However, there may be subsets where it is of value. Urban et al.[116] obtained blood ionized and total calcium levels in patients with out-of-hospital cardiac arrest and compared these with levels of in-hospital arrest when the levels were obtained in 3 minutes of cardiac arrest. Severe ionized hypocalcemia (total serum calcium was normal) was noted in the out-of-hospital group, and the conclusion was that hypocalcemia appears to

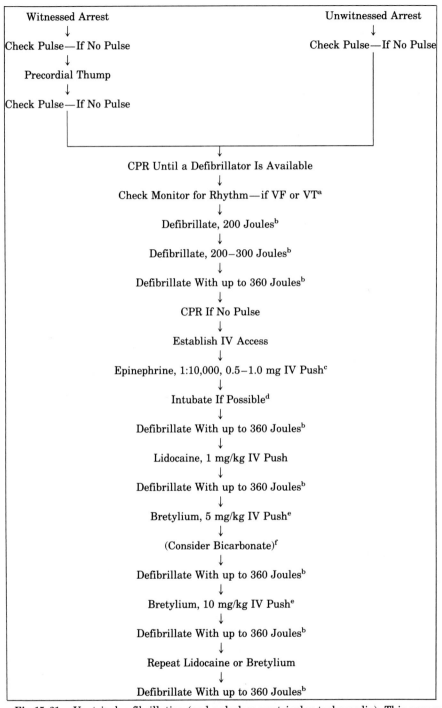

Fig 15–31. Ventricular fibrillation (and pulseless ventricular tachycardia). This sequence was developed to assist in teaching how to treat a broad range of patients with ventricular fibrillation (VF) or pulseless ventricular tachycardia (VT). Some patients may require care not specified herein. This algorithm should not be construed as prohibiting such flexibility. Flow of algorithm presumes that VF is continuing. CPR indicates cardiopulmonary resuscitation.

[a]Pulseless VT should be treated identically to VF. (*Legend continues on facing page.*)

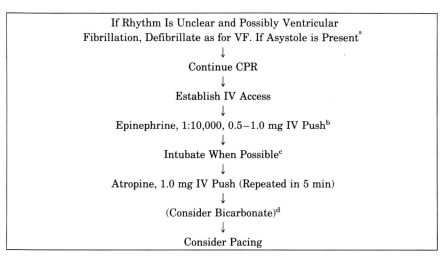

If Rhythm Is Unclear and Possibly Ventricular
Fibrillation, Defibrillate as for VF. If Asystole is Present[a]
↓
Continue CPR
↓
Establish IV Access
↓
Epinephrine, 1:10,000, 0.5–1.0 mg IV Push[b]
↓
Intubate When Possible[c]
↓
Atropine, 1.0 mg IV Push (Repeated in 5 min)
↓
(Consider Bicarbonate)[d]
↓
Consider Pacing

Fig 15–32. Asystole (cardiac standstill). This sequence was developed to assist in teaching how to treat a broad range of patients with asystole. Some patients may require care not specified herein. This algorithm should not be construed to prohibit such flexibility. Flow of algorithm presumes asystole is continuing. VF indicates ventricular fibrillation; IV, intravenous.

[a]Asystole should be confirmed in two leads.

[b]Epinephrine should be repeated every 5 minutes.

[c]Intubation is preferable; if it can be accomplished simultaneously with other techniques, the earlier the better. However, cardiopulmonary resuscitation (CPR) and use of epinephrine are more important initially if patient can be ventilated without intubation. (Endotracheal epinephrine may be used.)

[d]Value of sodium bicarbonate is questionable during cardiac arrest, and it is not recommended for the routine cardiac arrest sequence. Consideration of its use in a dose of 1 mEq/kg is appropriate at this point. Half of original dose may be repeated every 10 minutes if it is used. (From Standards and Guidelines for Cardiopulmonary Resuscitation (CPR) and Emergency Cardiac Care (ECC). *JAMA* 255:2905, 1986. Copyright 1986, American Medical Association.)

be time-dependent and further work is needed to determine whether patients benefit from calcium administration.

Electromechanical dissociation is present when there is evidence of electrical activity on the ECG, but there is failure of effective myocardial contraction. In such instances, the measures shown in the algorithm of Figure 15–33 should be done.[113]

Cardiopulmonary resuscitation should be terminated if appropriate cardiac

Fig. 15–31 continued   [b]Check pulse and rhythm after each shock. If VF recurs after transiently converting (rather than persists without ever converting), use whatever energy level has previously been successful for defibrillation.

[c]Epinephrine should be repeated every 5 minutes.

[d]Intubation is preferable. If it can be accomplished simultaneously with other techniques, the earlier the better. However, defibrillation and epinephrine are more important initially if the patient can be ventilated without intubation.

[e]Some may prefer repeated doses of lidocaine, which may be given in 0.5-mg/kg boluses every 8 minutes to a total dose of 3 mg/kg.

[f]Value of sodium bicarbonate is questionable during cardiac arrest, and it is not recommended for routine cardiac arrest sequence. Consideration of its use in a dose of 1 mEq/kg is appropriate at this point. Half of original dose may be repeated every ten minutes if it is used. (From Standards and Guidelines for Cardiopulmonary Resuscitation (CPR) and Emergency Cardiac Care (ECC). *JAMA* 255:2905, 1986. Copyright 1986, American Medical Association.)

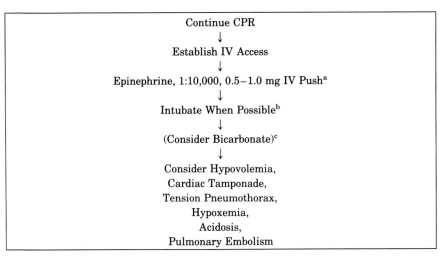

Fig 15–33. Electromechanical dissociation. This sequence was developed to assist in teaching how to treat a broad range of patients with electromechanical dissociation. Some patients may require care not specified herein. This algorithm should not be construed to prohibit such flexibility. Flow of algorithm presumes that electromechanical dissociation is continuing. CPR indicates cardiopulmonary resuscitation; IV, intravenous.

[a]Epinephrine should be repeated every 5 minutes.

[b]Intubation is preferable. If it can be accomplished simultaneously with other techniques, the earlier the better. However, epinephrine is more important initially if the patient can be ventilated without intubation.

[c]Value of sodium bicarbonate is questionable during cardiac arrest, and it is not recommended for routine cardiac arrest sequence. Consideration of its use in a dose of 1 mEq/kg is appropriate at this point. Half of original dose may be repeated every 10 minutes if it is used. (From Standards and Guidelines for Cardiopulmonary Resuscitation (CPR) and Emergency Cardiac Care (ECC). *JAMA* 255:2905, 1986. Copyright 1986, American Medical Association.)

rhythm and adequate pump performance cannot be restored or if there is evidence of severe irreversible cerebral damage. If the patient is successfully resuscitated, postresuscitation care should be instituted. It is important to assess the diagnosis and any factors that may have precipitated the cardiac arrest. Johnson et al.[117] reviewed 552 patients in whom CPR was attempted. They found the cause to be coronary artery disease in 239, respiratory failure in 55, pulmonary embolism in 18, Adams-Stokes syndrome in 11, cardiomyopathy in 7, reaction to angiography in 6, and uremia in 32 patients. The remaining patients had a variety of causes. If the patient is having chest pain, morphine should be given and the usual management of acute myocardial infarction begun in a coronary care unit. If pulmonary insufficiency is present, ventilation should be adequate, and blood gases should be monitored. Any postresuscitation arrhythmias should be treated appropriately. Electrophysiologic testing may be required to assess proper therapy if the arrest was due to ventricular tachycardia or fibrillation. The patient's neurologic status should be carefully observed and, if cerebral edema is suspected, a steroid should be given. Studies[118] have shown that approximately 30% of patients who undergo CPR are discharged from the hospital. The management of patients who survive cardiac arrest involves establishing a diagnosis and designed long-term management.[119]

Cardiac arrest can be prevented in certain instances when there is complete airway obstruction and the victim is conscious or unconscious. The conscious patient may be sitting or standing. If the patient cannot speak, the rescuer should deliver four sharp, rapid, forceful blows between the shoulder blades while supporting the victim's chest with the other hand. As a single method, this is not as effective as the Heimlich maneuver, which should be performed if the patient does not respond. The rescuer should stand behind him wrapping his arms around the patient's waist. One fist should be grasped by the other hand and the thumb side of the fist placed in the midline between the waist and rib cage of the victim. The fist is pressed into the victim's abdomen with quick inward and upward thrusts. In certain cases, it is best to give four chest thrusts with the thumb side of the fist on the breastbone. If the patient is unconscious and unresponsiveness is established, the head should be tilted with one hand on the forehead, the neck lifted with the other, and ventilation attempted. If the airway remains obstructed, the head should be repositioned and another attempt at ventilation made. If there are no results, the victim should be rolled toward the rescuer and four forceful, rapid blows delivered to the back between the shoulder blades. Next, four quick upward abdominal thrusts (heel of one hand above the navel and below the xiphoid and the second hand directly on top of the first) can be tried with the rescuer's knees positioned close to the patient's hips. The finger should be used to check for foreign bodies with the patient's head turned to the side. Ventilation should be attempted again. These procedures should be repeated as is necessary.

OFFICE EMERGENCIES

Most patients in emergency today do not go to the physician's office, and many who do reach the office do not require immediate therapy. However, there are still some conditions in which immediate therapy may be life-saving or may prevent later complications. The following is a list of such emergencies, with the drugs that should be available and the initial procedures that should be done before transferring the patient to the hospital.

1. Acute myocardial infarction. Demerol, 50 to 100 mg or morphine sulfate, 4 to 10 mg I.M. or I.V. for pain. Oxygen. Thrombolytic therapy started if patient meets criteria and there are no contraindications.
2. Atrial fibrillation. Digoxin, 0.5 mg I.V. if the ventricular rate is rapid and severe heart failure or hypotension is present.
3. Ventricular tachycardia. Lidocaine, 100 mg bolus I.V. If unstable, dc shock if defibrillator is available.
4. Cardiac arrest. Elevate legs. Give sharp blow to the chest. Mouth-to-airway ventilation or Ambu bag. External cardiac massage. Blind dc shock if defibrillator is available. If an ECG recording is available and ventricular fibrillation is noted, dc shock is used; if ventricular asystole is noted, give 5 ml of 1:10,000 solution of adrenalin.
5. Heart block with Adams-Stokes attacks. Isuprel, 0.02 mg, and atropine, 0.6 mg, I.V.
6. Acute pulmonary edema. Oxygen, sublingual nitroglycerin, and morphine, 2 to 5 mg I.V.

If an ECG machine is not available and the patient with a provisional diagnosis of acute myocardial infarction has a tachyarrhythmia (rate over 120 beats per minute) or an irregular rhythm over 55 beats per minute, give 100 mg bolus of lidocaine IV or 400 mg I.M.[120] On the other hand, if a bradyarrhythmia (rate below 55 beats per minute) is present and the patient is symptomatic, give 0.6 mg atropine I.V. Physicians who are seeing many office emergencies and performing exercise stress tests should have a dc defibrillator available.

Success in the treatment of cardiac emergencies depends on trained individuals being promptly available and ready with necessary equipment and drugs prepared in advance.

One should become familiar with the report of the 1985 National Conference on Cardiopulmonary Resuscitation (CPR) and Emergency Cardiac Care (ECC), which represents an update of the standards and guidelines that were published in 1974 and updated once since, in 1980. Deviation from the standards and guidelines may occur if a trained physician in CPR and ECC feels that it is in the patient's best interests.[113]

REFERENCES

1. Wit A.L., Rosen M.R.: Cellular electrophysiology of cardiac arrhythmias. Part II. Arrhythmias caused by abnormal impulse conduction. *Mod. Concepts Cardiovasc. Dis.* 50:7, 1981.
2. Wit A.L., Rosen M.R.: Cellular electrophysiology of cardiac arrhythmias: Part I. Arrhythmias caused by abnormal impulse generation. *Mod. Concepts Cardiovasc. Dis.* 50:1, 1981.
3. Vassale M.: Automaticity and automatic rhythms. *Am. J. Cardiol.* 28:245, 1971.
4. Cranefield P.F.: *The Conduction of the Cardiac Impulse.* Mount Kisco, New York, Futura Publishing Co., 1975.
5. Vaughn Williams E.M.: A classification of antiarrhythmic actions reassessed after a decade of new drugs. *J. Clin. Pharmacol.* 24:129, 1984.
6. Selzer A., Wray H.W.: Quinidine syncope. *Circulation* 30:17, 1964.
7. Minardo J.D., Heger J.J., Miles W.M., et al. Clinical characteristics of patients with ventricular fibrillation during antiarrhythmic drug therapy. *N. Engl. J. Med.* 319:257, 1988.
8. Woosley R.L.: Lidocaine Therapy: Application of clinical pharmacokinetic principles. *Cardiac Impulse* 8(2):1, 1987.
9. Woosley R.L., Funck-Bretano C.: Overview of the clinical pharmacology of antiarrhythmic drugs. *Am. J. Cardiol.* 61:61A, 1988.
10. Roden D.M., Woosley R.L.: Flecainide. *N. Engl. J. Med.* 315:36, 1986.
11. Woosley R.L., Wood A.J.J., Roden D.M.: Encainide. *N. Engl. J. Med.* 318:1107, 1988.
12. Antman E.M., Friedman P.L.: Propafenone hydrochloride: A unique new antiarrhythmic. *Primary Cardiology* 14:24, 1988.
13. Conolly M.E., Kesting F., Dollery C.T.: The clinical pharmacology of beta-adrenoreceptor-blocking drugs. *Prog. Cardiovasc. Dis.* 19:203, 1976.
14. Mason J.W.: Amiodarone. *N. Engl. J. Med.* 316:455, 1987.
15. Anderson J.L., Askins J.C., Gilbert E.M., et al.: Multicenter trial of sotalol for suppression of frequent complex ventricular arrhythmias: A double-blind randomized placebo-controlled evaluation of two doses. *J. Am. Coll. Cardiol.* 8:752, 1986.
16. Morganroth J.: Ambulatory electrocardiographic monitoring in the evaluation of new antiarrhythmic drugs. *Circulation* 73:II−92, 1986.
17. Manolis A.S., Estes N.A.M.: Supraventricular tachycardia. *Arch. Intern. Med.* 147:1706, 1987.
18. Peters R.W., Scheinman M.M.: Emergency treatment of supraventricular tachycardia. *Med. Clin. North Am.* 63:73, 1979.
19. Hellestrand K.J.: Intravenous flecainide acetate for supraventricular tachycardias. *Am. J. Cardiol.* 62:16D, 1988.
20. Pool P.E.: Treatment of supraventricular arrhythmias with encainide. *Am. J. Cardiol.* 58:55C, 1986.
21. Prystowsky E.N.: Diagnosis and management of the preexcitation syndromes. *Curr. Probl. Cardiol.* 13:231, 1988.
22. Goldreyer B.N., Gallagher J.J., Damato A.N.: The elctrophysiologic demonstration of atrial ectopic tachycardia in man. *Am. Heart J.* 85:205, 1973.
23. Han J.: The concepts of reentrant activity responsible for ectopic rhythms. *Am. J. Cardiol.* 28:253, 1971.

24. Olshansky B., Waldo A.L.: Atrial fibrillation: Update on mechanism, diagnosis, and management. *Mod. Concepts Cardiovasc. Dis.* 56:23, 1987.
25. Culler M.R., Boone J.A., Gazes P.C.: Fibrillatory wave size as a clue to etiological diagnosis. *Am. Heart J.* 66:435, 1963.
26. Wolf P.A., Abbott R.D., Kannel W.B.: Atrial fibrillation: A major contributor to stroke in the elderly. *Arch. Intern. Med.* 147:1561, 1987.
27. Kannel W.B., Abbott R.D., Savage D.D., et al.: Epidemiologic features of chronic atrial fibrillation. *N. Engl. J. Med.* 306:1018, 1982.
28. Kopecky S.L., Gersh B.J., Phil C.B.D., et al.: The natural history of lone atrial fibrillation. A population-based study over three decades. *N. Engl. J. Med.* 317:669, 1987.
29. Falk R.H., Knowlton A.A., Bernard S.A., et al.: Digoxin for converting recent-onset atrial fibrillation to sinus rhythm. *Ann. Intern. Med.* 106:503, 1987.
30. Platia E.V., Waclawski S.H., Pluth T.A., et al.: Management of acute-onset atrial fibrillation/flutter: Esmolol vs. verapamil vs. digoxin vs. placebo. *Circulation* 76 (Suppl. II):4, 1987.
31. Henry W.L., Morganroth J., Pearlman A.S., et al.: Relation between echocardiographically determined left atrial size and atrial fibrillation. *Circulation* 53:273, 1976.
31a. Mann DL, Maisel AS, Atwood JE, et al.: Absence of cardioversion-induced ventricular arrhythmias in patients with therapeutic dogixin levels. *J.A.C.C.* 5:882, 1985.
32. Bjerkelund C.J., Orning O.M.: The efficacy of anticoagulant therapy in preventing embolism related to D.C. electrical conversion of atrial fibrillation. *Am. J. Cardiol.* 23:208, 1969.
33. Reiffel J.A., Gambino S.R., McCarthy D.M., et al.: Direct current cardioversion: Effect on creatine kinase, lactic dehydrogenase and myocardial isoenzymes. *JAMA* 239:122, 1978.
34. Chouty F., Coumel P.: Oral flecainide for prophylaxis of paroxysmal atrial fibrillation. *Am. J. Cardiol.* 62:35D, 1988.
35. Surawicz B.: Prognosis of ventricular arrhythmias in relation to sudden cardiac death: Therapeutic implications. *J. Am. Coll. Cardiol.* 10:435, 1987.
36. Rosenbaum M.B.: Classification of ventricular extrasystoles according to form. *J. Electrocardiol.* 2:289, 1969.
37. Kennedy H.L., Whitlock J.A., Sprague M.K., et al.: Long-term follow-up of asymptomatic healthy subjects with frequent and complex ventricular ectopy. *N. Engl. J. Med.* 312:193, 1985.
38. Ekblom B., Hartley L.H., Day W.C.: Occurrence and reproducibility of exercise-induced ventricular ectopy in normal subject. *Am. J. Cardiol.* 43:35, 1979.
39. Morganroth J.: Choosing drugs for ventricular arrhythmia. *Cardiol.* May, 1988, pg 86.
40. Duff H.J., Roden D., Primm R.K., et al.: Mexiletine in the treatment of resistant ventricular arrhythmias: Enhancement of efficacy and reduction of dose-related side effects by combination with quinidine. *Circulaton* 67:1124, 1983.
40a. Woosley R.L.: Role of plasma concentration monitoring in the evaluation of response to antiarrhythmic drugs. *Am. J. Cardiol.* 62:9H, 1988.
41. Wellens H.J.J., Bar F.W.H.M., Lie K.I.: The value of the electrocardiogram in the differential diagnosis of a tachycardia with a widened QRS complex. *Am. J. Med.* 64:27, 1978.
42. Wellens H.J.J., Brugada P.: The approach to the patient with ventricular tachycardia. *Cardiac Impulse* 9:1, 1988.
43. Gozensky C., Thorne, D.: Rabbit ears: An aid in distinguishing ventricular ectopy from aberration. *Heart Lung* 3:634, 1974.
44. Rahimtoola S.H., Zipes D.P., Akhtar M., et al.: Consensus statement of the conference on the state of the art of electrophysiologic testing in the diagnosis and treatment of patients with cardiac arrhythmias. Part I. *Mod. Concepts Cardiovasc. Dis.* 56:55, 1987.
45. Rahimtoola S.H., Zipes D.P., Akhtar M., et al.: Consensus statement of the conference on the state of the art of electrophysiologic testing in the diagnosis and treatment of patients with cardiac arrhythmias. Part II. *Mod. Concepts Cardiovasc. Dis.* 56:61, 1987.
45a. Kuchar D.L., Garan H., Ruskin J.N.: Electrophysiologic evaluation of antiarrhythmic therapy for ventricular tachyarrhythmias. *Am. J. Cardiol.* 62:39H, 1988.
46. Kastor J.A., Horowitz L.N., Harken A.H., et al.: Clinical electrophysiology of ventricular tachycardia. *N. Engl. J. Med.* 304:1004, 1981.
47. Horowitz L.N., Harken A.H., Kastor J.A., et al.: Ventricular resection guided by epicardial and endocardial mapping for treatment of recurrent ventricular tachycardia. *N. Engl. J. Med.* 302:598, 1980.
48. Mirowski, M.: The automatic implantable cardioverter-defibrillator: An overview. *J. Am. Coll. Cardiol.* 6:461, 1985.
49. Borbola J., Denes P., Ezri M.D., et al.: The automatic implantable cardiometer-defibrillator: Clinical complications, and follow-up in 25 patients. *Arch. Intern. Med.* 148:70, 1988.
50. Dessertenne F.: La tachycardia ventriculaire à deux foyers opposés variables. *Arch. Mal. Coeur.* 59:263, 1966.

466   *Arrhythmias*

51. Keren A., Tzivoni D., Gavish D.: Etiology, warning signs and therapy of torsade de pointes. *Circulation* 64:1167, 1981.
52. Gallagher J.J.: "Les torsades de pointes": An unusual ventricular arrhythmia. *Ann. Intern. Med.* 93:578, 1980.
53. Tzivoni D., Keren A., Cohen A.M., et al.: Magnesium therapy for torsades de pointes. *Am. J. Cardiol.* 53:528, 1984.
54. Kotler M.N., Tabatnick B., Mower M.M., et al.: Prognostic significance of ventricular ectopic beats with respect to sudden death in late postinfarction period. *Circulation* 47:595, 1973.
55. Gaum W.E., Biancaniello T., Kaplan S.: Accelerated ventricular rhythm in childhood. *Am. J. Cardiol.* 43:162, 1979.
56. Wellens H.J.J., Brugada P., Penn O.C.: The management of preexcitation syndromes. *JAMA* 257:2325, 1987.
57. Anderson R.H., Becker A.E., Brechenmacher C., et al.: Ventricular preexcitation: A proposed nomenclature for its substrate. *Eur. J. Cardiol.* 3:27, 1975.
58. Frolich E.D., Tarazi, R.C., Dustan H.P.: Hyperdynamic β-adrenergic circulatory state. *Arch. Intern. Med.* 123:1, 1969.
59. Rubenstein J.J., Schulman C.L., Yurchak P.M., et al.: Clinical spectrum of the sick sinus syndrome. *Circulation* 46:5, 1972.
60. Chung E.K.: Sick sinus node syndrome: Current views. *Mod. Concepts Cardiovasc. Dis.* 49:67, 1980.
61. Narula O.S., Samet P., Javier R.P.: Significance of the sinus node recovery time. *Circulation* 45:140, 1972.
62. Breithardt G., Seipel L., Loogen F.: Sinus node recovery time and calculated sinoatrial conduction time in normal subjects and patients with sinus node dysfunction. *Circulation* 56:43, 1977.
63. Tilkian A.G., Guilleminault C., Schroeder J.S., et al.: Sleep-induced apnea syndrome. *Am. J. Med.* 63:348, 1977.
64. Rosenbaum M.B.: The hemiblocks: Diagnostic criteria and clinical significance. *Mod. Concepts Cardiovasc. Dis.* 39:141, 1970.
65. Johansson B.W.: Adams-Stokes syndrome: A review and follow-up study of forty-two cases. *Am. J. Cardiol.* 8:76, 1961.
66. Zoll P.M., Linenthol A.J., Normal L.R., et al.: External electric stimulation of the heart in cardiac arrest: Stokes-Adams disease, reflex vagal standstill, drug-induced standstill, and unexpected circulatory arrest. *Arch. Intern. Med.* 96:639, 1955.
67. Drachman D.A., Hart C.W.: An approach to the dizzy patient. *Neurology* 22:323, 1972.
68. Scheinman M., Weiss A., Kundel F.: His bundle recordings in patients with bundle branch block and neurologic symptoms. *Circulation* 48:322, 1973.
69. Dhingra R.C., Palileo E., Strasberg B., et al.: Significance of the HV interval in 517 patients with chronic bifascicular block. *Circulation* 64:1265, 1981.
70. Scheinman M.M., Peters R.W., Morady F., et al.: Electrophysiologic studies in patients with bundle branch block. *PACE* 6:1157, 1983.
71. McAnulty H.H., Rahimtoola S.H., Murphy E.S., et al.: A prospective study of sudden death in "high-risk" bundle-branch block. *N. Engl. J. Med.* 299:209, 1978.
72. McAnulty J.H., Rahimtoola S.H., Murphy E., et al.: Natural history of "high-risk" bundle-branch block. Final report of a prospective study. *N. Engl. J. Med.* 307:137, 1982.
73. Greenspan A.M., Kay H.R., Berger B.C., et al.: Incidence of unwarranted implantation of permanent cardiac pacemakers in a large medical population. *N. Engl. J. Med.* 318:158, 1988.
74. Frye R.L., Collins J.J., DeSanctis R.W., et al.: Guidelines for permanent cardiac pacemaker implantation, May 1984: A report of the joint American College of Cardiology/American Heart Association Task Force in assessment of cardiovascular procedures (subcommittee on pacemaker implantation). *J. Am. Coll. Cardiol.* 4:434, 1984.
75. Vera Z., Klein R.C., Mason D.T.: Recent advantages in programmable pacemakers, consideration of advantages, longevity and future expectations. *Am. J. Med.* 66:473, 1979.
76. Parsonnet V., Furman S., Smyth N.P.D.: Implantable cardiac pacemakers: Status report and resource guideline. *Am. J. Cardiol.* 34:487, 1974.
77. Benditt D.G., Mianulli M., Fetter J., et al.: Single-chamber cardiac pacing with activity-initiated chronotropic response: Evaluation by cardiopulmonary exercise testing. *Circulation* 75:184, 1987.
78. Rediker D.E., Harthorne J.W.: Symptomatic bradycardia: How to select the appropriate pacemaker. *Cardiac Impulse* 8:1, 1987.
79. Zoll P.M., Zoll R.H., Falk, R.H., et al.: External noninvasive temporary cardiac pacing: Clinical trials. *Circulation* 71:937, 1985.
79a. Vallario L.E., Leman R.B., Gillette P.C., et al.: Pacemaker follow-up and adequacy of Medicare guidelines. *Am. Heart J.* 116:11, 1988.
80. Ausubel K., Furman S.: The pacemaker syndrome. *Ann. Intern. Med.* 103:420, 1985.

81. Rosen K.M., Rahimtoola S.H., Gunnar R.M.: Pseudo A-V block secondary to premature nonpropagated His bundle depolarizations: Documented by His bundle electrocardiography. *Circulation* 42:367, 1970.
82. Neuss H., Schlepper M., Thormann J.: Analysis of re-entry mechanism in three patients with concealed Wolff-Parkinson-White syndrome. *Circulation* 51:75, 1975.
83. Kannel W.B., Doyle J.T., McNamara P.M., et al.: Precursors of sudden coronary death: Factors related to incidence of sudden death. *Circulation* 51:608, 1975.
84. Lown B.: Sudden cardiac death: The major challenge confronting contemporary cardiology. *Am. J. Cardiol.* 43:313, 1979.
85. Romano C., Gemme G., Pongiglione R.: Aritmie cardiache rare dell'eta pediatrica. *Clin. Pediat.* 45:656, 1963.
86. Ward O.C.: A new familial cardiac syndrome in children. *J. Irish Med. Assoc.* 54:103, 1964.
87. Jervell A., Lange-Nielsen F.: Congenital deaf mutism, functional heart disease with prolongation of Q-T interval and sudden death. *Am. Heart J.* 54:59, 1957.
88. Maron B.J., Roberts W.C., McAllister H.A., et al.: Sudden death in young athletes. *Circulation* 62:218, 1980.
89. Nicod P., Polikar R., Peterson K.L.: Hypertrophic cardiomyopathy and sudden death. *N. Engl. J. Med.* 318:1255, 1988.
90. Swartz M.H., Teichholz L.E., Donoso E.: Mitral valve prolapse: A review of associated arrhythmias. *Am. J. Med.* 62:377, 1977.
91. Moss A.J., Decamilla J.J., Davis H.P., et al.: Clinical significance of ventricular ectopic beats in the early post-hospital phase of myocardial infarction. *Am. J. Cardiol.* 39:635, 1977.
92. Cobb L.A., Baum R.S., Alvarez H. III, et al.: Resuscitation from out-of-the hospital ventricular fibrillation: 4 years follow up. *Circulation* 51 and 52: (Suppl. 3):223, 1975.
93. Schulze R., Strauss H., Pitt B.: Sudden death in the year following myocardial infarction. *Am. J. Med.* 62:192, 1977.
94. Theroux P., Waters D.D., Halphen C., et al.: Prognostic value of exercise testing soon after myocardial infarction. *N. Engl. J. Med.* 301:341, 1979.
95. Ruskin J.N., DiMarco J.P., Garan H.: Repetitive response to single ventricular extra stimuli in patients with serious ventricular arrhythmias: Incidence and clinical significance. *Circulation* 63:767, 1981.
96. Horowitz L.N., Josephson M.E., Farshidi A., et al.: Recurrent sustained ventricular tachycardia: 3. Role of the electrophysiologic study in selection of arrhythmic regimens. *Circulation* 58:986, 1978.
97. Josephson M.E.: Treatment of ventricular arrhythmias after myocardial infarction. Current Views. *Circulation,* July 1986–June 1988, pg. 162.
98. Ruberman W., Weinblatt E., Goldberg J.D., et al.: Ventricular premature beats and mortality after myocardial infarction. *N. Engl. J. Med.* 297:750, 1977.
99. Bigger J.T., Jr., Weld F.M., Rolnitzky L.M.: Prevalence, characteristics and significance of ventricular tachycardia (three or more complexes) detected with ambulatory electrocardiographic recording in the late hospital phase of acute myocardial infarction. *Am. J. Cardiol.* 48:815, 1981.
100. Bigger J.T., Jr., Weld F.M., Rolnitzky L.M.: Which ventricular arrhythmias should be treated in the post hospital phase of myocardial infarction: Abstracted, No. 1176, *Circulation* 64 (Part 2):IV–307, 1981.
101. Lown B., Graboys T.B.: Sudden death: An ancient problem newly perceived. *Cardiovasc. Med.* 2:219, 1977.
102. Berbari E.J., et al.: Recording from the body surface of arrhythmogenic ventricular activity during the S-T segment. *Am. J. Cardiol.* 41:697, 1978.
103. Kuchar D.L., et al.: Signal-averaged electrocardiograms for evaluation of recurrent syncope. *Am. J. Cardiol.* 58:949, 1986.
104. Nalos P.C., et al.: The signal-averaged electrocardiogram as a screening test for inducibility of sustained ventricular tachycardia high risk patients: A prospective study. *J. Am. Coll. Cardiol.* 9:539, 1987.
105. Haberl R., et al.: Frequency analysis of the surface electrocardiogram for recognition of acute rejection after orthotopic cardiac transplantation in man. *Circulation* 76:101, 1987.
106. Caps Investigators: The cardiac arrhythmia pilot study. *Am. J. Cardiol.* 57:91, 1986.
107. Moss A., McDonald J.: Unilateral cervicothoracic sympathetic ganglionectomy for the treatment of the long Q-T interval syndrome. *N. Engl. J. Med.* 285:903, 1971.
108. Kouwenhoven W.B., Jude J.R., Knickerbocker G.G.: Closed-chest cardiac massage. *JAMA* 173:94, 1960.
109. Zoll P.M., Paul M.H., Linenthal A.J., et al.: The effects of external electric currents on the heart. *Circulation* 14:745, 1956.
110. Lown B., Neuman J., Amarasingham R., et al.: Comparison of alternating current with direct current electroshock across the closed chest. *Am. J. Cardiol* 10:223, 1962.

111. Ewy G.A.: Current status of cardiopulmonary resuscitation. *Mod. Concepts Cardiovasc. Dis.* 53:43, 1984.
112. Weisfeldt M.L., Halperin H.R.: Cardiopulmonary resuscitation: Beyond cardiac massage. *Circulation* July 1986–June 1988, pg 231–236.
113. Standards and guidelines for cardiopulmonary resuscitation (CPR) and emergency cardiac care (ECC). *JAMA* 255:2905, 1986.
114. Haynes R.E., Copass M.K., Chinn T.L., et al.: Randomized comparison of bretylium and lidocaine in resuscitation of patients from out-of-hospital ventricular fibrillation. *Circulation* (Part 2) 58:II–177, 1987.
115. Weaver W.D., Hill D., Fahrenbruch C.E., Copass M.K., et al.: Use of the automatic defibrillator in the management of out-of-hospital cardiac arrest. *N. Engl. J. Med.* 319:661, 1988.
116. Urban P., Scheidegger D, Buchmann B, et al.: Cardiac arrest and blood ionized calcium levels. *Ann. Intern. Med.* 109:110, 1988.
117. Johnson A.L., Transer P.H., Ulan R.A., et al.: Results of cardiac resuscitation in 552 patients. *Am. J. Cardiol.* 20:831, 1967.
118. Cobb L.A., Hallstrom A.P.: Community-based cardiopulmonary resuscitation: What have we learned? *Ann. NY Acad. Sci.* 182:330, 1982.
119. Myerburg R.J., Kessler K.M.: Management of patients who survive cardiac arrest. *Mod. Concepts Cardiovasc. Dis.* 55:61, 1986.
120. Koster R.W., Dunning A.J.: Intramuscular lidocaine for prevention of lethal arrhythmias in the prehospitalization phase of acute myocardial infarction. *N. Engl. J. Med.* 313:1105, 1985.

Chapter 16

CARDIAC FAILURE IN ADULTS

Heart failure is not a diagnosis, and its cause should be carefully sought. The symptoms and findings of congestive heart failure usually develop because of decreased myocardial contractility with systolic dysfunction. As a result, the cardiac output, regardless of its level, is inadequate to maintain blood flow to body organs and tissues. In addition the atrial pressures are increased. The cardiac output is most often depressed with common forms of heart failure, but it can be elevated in conditions such as hyperthyroidism, anemia, and others (high-output failure). The decreased cardiac output causes a decrease in renal blood flow and release of renin, which interacts with angiotensinogen to liberate angiotensin I, which in turn interacts with angiotensin-converting enzyme to yield angiotensin II, which is a potent pressor substance that increases peripheral vascular resistance and also acts on the adrenal cortex, stimulating the release of aldosterone, which effects an increase in salt and water retention, with increase in blood volume, venous hypertension, and edema. The increased venous pressure can produce transudation of fluid from the capillaries and decreased effective blood volume and increased aldosterone secretion. It also can cause liver congestion with impaired breakdown of aldosterone. In addition, the decreased glomerular filtration associated with the inadequate cardiac output results in increased sodium reabsorption, further contributing to the edema. Various neurohumoral mechanisms are also activated that result in inappropriate vasoconstriction and further depression of cardiac function and include, as mentioned above, the sympathetic nervous system with release of norepinephrine, stimulation of the renin-angiotension-aldosterone system, sodium retention resulting from multiple mechanisms, including vasopressin activity, and enhanced smooth muscle tone in the vascular tree secondary to calcium. Heart failure can occur with no abnormality of myocardial function when the normal heart is exposed to a load that exceeds its capacity or when ventricular filling is impaired. In addition, there are conditions that have congestive state findings (abnormal salt and water retention), but the cardiac function is normal.

Cardiac functional abnormalities can be classified on a pathophysiologic basis as follows:

1. Primary disturbances of ventricular contractility, as occurs in ischemic heart disease and cardiomyopathies.
2. Pressure or volume overloading of the ventricles, as occurs in valvular disease and congenital heart disease. Pressure load can be produced on the left ventricle by aortic stenosis or systemic hypertension and on the

right ventricle by pulmonary stenosis, pulmonary hypertension, left ventricular failure, or chronic lung disease. Volume load on the left ventricle is caused by valvular lesions, such as aortic or mitral insufficiency, and by congenital heart defects, such as patent ductus arteriosus and ventricular septal defect. Volume load on the right ventricle can be caused by an atrial septal defect. Increase in cardiac output can produce a volume load on the entire heart, as in anemia, thyrotoxicosis, beriberi, and arteriovenous fistula.

3. Restriction of diastolic filling of the heart, as occurs in pericardial disease, hypertrophic cardiomyopathy, with certain types of myocardial changes, and mitral stenosis. Some patients in this category may have symptoms and signs of congestive heart failure, but their hearts appear small on x ray (mitral stenosis, pericardial constriction, or an acute process). Usually patients with congestive heart failure have cardiomegaly. Impaired systolic function (jugular venous distention, cardiomegaly, rales, S_3 gallop, edema) is most often emphasized in heart failure. However, heart failure can also occur from incomplete myocardial relaxation and therefore impaired filling—abnormal diastolic function. Most patients who have systolic dysfunction probably have some element of diastolic dysfunction. Conditions that produce hypertrophy and fibrosis can cause impairment in diastolic function. Patients with heart failure and a normal ejection fraction often have primarily left ventricular diastolic dysfunction (with or without intermittent systolic dysfunction), and often the failure is due to ischemic heart disease or hypertension.[1] At the bedside, clinical distinction between heart failure associated mainly with systolic versus diastolic dysfunction may not always be possible. Patients with diastolic dysfunction often have normal systolic function as measured by parameters like the ejection fraction. The treatment of heart failure caused by diastolic dysfunction at present is not clear. However, it should be stressed that the usual standard therapy for systolic dysfunction may be harmful for diastolic dysfunction.

When these functional cardiac abnormalities occur, compensatory mechanisms which can support the resting cardiac output are called into play, such as an increased adrenergic activity, overactivity of the renin-angiotensin axis, ventricular dilatation (Frank-Starling principle), and ventricular hypertrophy. Two of the earliest of these mechanisms are increased adrenergic, arginine vasopressin, and renin-angiotensin activity, manifested by an increase in heart rate and systemic vascular resistance. These neural and humoral vasoconstrictors limit blood flow to the skin, kidneys, splanchnic vessels, and nonexercising muscle. Systemic arterial blood pressure is maintained so that the heart and brain can maintain normal perfusion.[1a] While the increase in heart rate may normalize the resting cardiac output, even in the face of a reduced stroke volume, the afterload added to the left ventricle by peripheral vasoconstriction may eventually worsen cardiac function.

The Frank-Starling principle (Fig 16–1) explains how the failing heart attempts to maintain its resting pump requirements through ventricular dilatation. By increasing the end-diastolic fiber length, the stroke volume in the subsequent systole is enhanced. This is the most important of the compensatory mechanisms. It was first demonstrated on frog myocardium by Frank[2] in

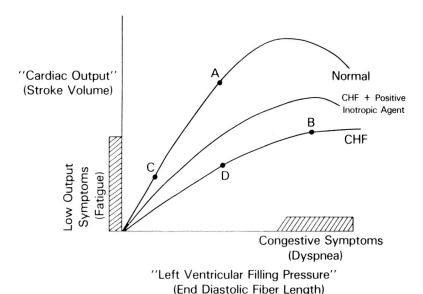

Fig 16–1. Ventricular function curves showing normal and abnormal Frank-Starling relationships. CHF = Congestive heart failure. (Modified by Gazes P.C., Assey M.E., from Mason D.T.: Regulation of cardiac performance in clinical heart disease: Interactions between contractile state, mechanical abnormalities, and ventricular compensatory mechanisms. *Am. J. Cardiol.* 32:437–448, 1972. Used by permission.)

1895 and described by Starling[3] 20 years later in the following way: "The energy of contraction, however measured, is a function of the length of the muscle fiber." Braunwald and associates[4] have shown the applicability of this principle to the human heart.

As Figure 16–1 demonstrates, a ventricular function curve can be constructed by plotting stroke volume, or any systolic parameter of ventricular function, over a range of filling pressures, whether measured as the pulmonary capillary wedge pressure, left ventricular end-diastolic pressure, or direct angiographic left ventricular end-diastolic volume.[5] The patient with congestive heart failure due to an intrinsic disturbance of ventricular contractility has a lower stroke volume for any given filling pressure when compared with the normal, resulting in a flat ventricular function curve (downward and rightward shift). Point B is located on the flattest portion of the depressed ventricular function curve, creating a situation in which resting cardiac output is maintained only at the expense of congestive symptoms. The left ventricular filling pressure is usually above 18 mm Hg. Although point C is on the normal ventricular function curve, it represents low-output symptoms (such as fatigue) due to an inadequate filling pressure, as occurs with hypovolemic shock or diuretic misuse. This situation should in no way be misconstrued as heart failure, since contractility is normal. When a more optimal Frank-Starling relationship is restored with volume expansion, stroke volume normalizes and symptoms disappear. Point D represents low-output symptoms resulting from depressed contractility as well as a relatively low filling pressure. In this situation, unlike point C, volume expansion "unmasked" the congestive state.

There is a limit to this compensatory mechanism. If cardiac fibers are stretched beyond a certain length, interactions between the actin and myosin myofilaments are compromised, thereby decreasing cardiac performance. This is demonstrated by the descending limb of the normal ventricular function curve in Figure 16–1. Controversy exists as to whether or not there actually is a descending limb of the Frank-Starling curve in man. An alternative explanation is that, as the preload limit is reached (that is, the peak sarcomere stretch), any additional volume only increases wall tension (afterload), thereby decreasing stroke volume.

Another compensatory mechanism is ventricular hypertrophy, commonly seen in chronic pressure and volume overload states. According to the law of La Place, myocardial thickening tends to limit the stress which the heart must generate to empty itself. Hypertrophy may be concentric or eccentric, depending on the type of stimulus. When the stimulus to hypertrophy is a pressure overload, such as hypertension or aortic stenosis, there is an increased peak systolic tension that results in sarcomere replication in parallel, manifested as wall thickening at the expense of chamber size (concentric hypertrophy). Volume overload as from aortic regurgitation results in an increased end-diastolic diameter and increased diastolic tension that stimulates sarcomere replication in series, resulting in chamber enlargement as well as wall thickening (eccentric hypertrophy). Both types of hypertrophy result in the failing heart using less oxygen with each contraction as it meets the metabolic needs of the body, and both types are particularly important in chronic cardiac decompensation.[6] Gaasch[7] emphasized the importance of "appropriate" hypertrophy in chronic aortic insufficiency and congestive cardiomyopathy. Field et al.[8] showed that the degree of hypertrophy is an indicator of survival in patients with congestive cardiomyopathy, independent of the left ventricular ejection fraction. Although from a mechanical standpoint appropriate cardiac hypertrophy appears to be beneficial, many investigators have proposed that in cardiac hypertrophy are laid the seeds of cardiac failure. Before any reduction in left ventricular contractility, the hypertensive heart exposed to a chronic pressure overload may demonstrate depletion of myosin adenosine triphosphatase (ATPase) activity. Because this enzyme system is important in supplying energy not only for contraction, but for cardiac relaxation, abnormalities of left ventricular diastolic function are not infrequently observed. Newman and Webb have demonstrated an inadequate response of contractility to positive inotropic agents early in the course of ventricular hypertrophy.[9] Finally, there may be an inadequate increase in coronary blood flow under stress in certain types of left ventricular pressure overload states, such as aortic stenosis.[10]

The heart, when it fails, does not directly cause symptoms, but it does produce abnormal physical findings. As the heart's compensatory mechanisms (mentioned previously) become inadequate (overshoot and become deleterious), even though they may maintain the resting cardiac output, eventually symptoms occur from the secondarily altered organs; namely, the lungs, liver, and kidneys. Recent work suggests that central hemodynamic abnormalities (elevated left atrial pressure and reduced cardiac output) are not the sole determinants of symptoms.[11] Other factors that can contribute to the genesis of symptoms are impaired vasodilation and altered metabolism in skeletal muscle, circulating metabolites, and pulmonary ventilation-perfusion mismatch with consequent increased physiologic dead space. Careful examination of the heart, arteries, and veins is extremely important, not only for diagnosis, but also for finding abnormalities of myocardial dysfunction before congestive phenomena develop in other organs. Evidence of myocardial dysfunction may be cardiomegaly, S_3 or S_4 gallops, pulses alternans, abnormal neck vein distention, x-ray evidence of interstitial edema, or ECG evidence of left or right ventricular hypertrophy.

SYMPTOMS

Symptoms are often described as those due to left-sided or right-sided heart failure. Even though there are many factors against such a division, and symptoms of both types overlap, the classification is helpful.

Left-Sided Heart Failure

The symptoms of failure of the left side of the heart can be overt or occult. Fatigability, exertional dyspnea, paroxysmal nocturnal dyspnea, orthopnea, cough, insomnia, hemoptysis, and restlessness are among the common complaints. Each symptom must be carefully reviewed with the patient to appreciate its true significance. Most patients will answer "yes" when asked about shortness of breath. Often this complaint is not dyspnea but inability to get enough air and is characterized by slow, deep, sighing respiration. In fact, these patients will demonstrate this type of breathing as they give their history and state, "See, I have it now." Cardiac dyspnea is usually characterized by rapid, shallow respiration.

Paroxysmal nocturnal dyspnea occurs after the patient has been asleep for a few hours and suddenly awakens with dyspnea. Many precipitating factors have been considered in its production, such as the reabsorption of dependent edema that has developed during the day and elevation of thoracic blood volume and diaphragm on recumbency. The left ventricle will not tolerate this increased volume. In addition, nocturnal depression of the respiratory center and reduced adrenergic drive to the left ventricle are factors. Orthopnea refers to the type of dyspnea which occurs when the patient is recumbent, and as a result the patient uses two or more pillows to prop himself up to avoid dyspnea.

Cough may be an early finding of left-sided heart failure. It often occurs nocturnally and is dry and nonproductive. The fact that the cough clears when the patient sits up or stands may aid in differentiating it from the cough of lung disease. This is not an absolute indicator of cardiac origin, since patients with chronic obstructive lung disease may be awakened at night coughing because of bronchial secretions accumulating while they are recumbent. However, this cough is usually productive.

Insomnia associated with heart failure often is due to Cheyne-Stokes respiration (characterized by rapid deep breathing and periods of apnea). The patient is restless during the hyperpneic phase. This symptom is most common in the elderly, especially when they have been sedated. It is probably due to decreased blood flow to the respiratory center.

Nocturnal angina may be a manifestation of heart failure, occurring either with paroxysmal nocturnal dyspnea or as the only symptom. It often responds to treatment for heart failure.

Acute pulmonary edema (acute cardiac decompensation) can develop suddenly, with extreme dyspnea and frothy, blood-tinged sputum. It most often follows myocardial infarction or a hypertensive crisis. Hemoptysis and dyspnea can be due to pulmonary emboli, which often occur in patients with heart failure.

Right-Sided Heart Failure

Symptoms of failure of the right side of the heart occur relatively late. The patient complains of pitting edema of the ankles, unexplained weight gain, upper abdominal pain due to liver congestion, nocturia, excessive sweating (increased adrenergic activity of failure), extreme weakness, anorexia and nausea (edema of bowel), and abdominal distention.

Water retention is noted early because of weight gain or nocturia rather than because of pitting edema. The latter becomes obvious only after retention of at least 10 lb fluid. In early heart failure, the kidneys retain fluid because of the inadequate cardiac output during daytime activities. At night, the cardiac output improves with rest, and diuresis occurs (nocturia).

The fatigue of heart failure can be due to insomnia, nocturia, dyspnea, cough, low cardiac output, or the catabolic effect of chronic failure.

PHYSICAL FINDINGS

The physical findings of cardiac failure can be separated into the cardiovascular findings and the secondary congestive phenomena.

Cardiovascular Findings

Myocardial dysfunction in heart failure may be subtle and often occurs before secondary congestive phenomena are noted in the lungs, liver, kidneys, or tissues. Cardiomegaly is usually a prerequisite for heart failure with systolic dysfunction; however, the heart can be of normal size in acute myocardial infarction, cor pulmonale, mitral stenosis, constrictive pericarditis, acute renal failure, and acute infection or damage of the valves or myocardium.

X ray is commonly used as a reliable method of detecting cardiomegaly, but at times clinical findings may be superior, especially in detecting concentric hypertrophy, which may not be evident on x ray. Left ventricular dilatation usually produces a diffuse visible apical impulse. The apical impulse of predominant hypertrophy may be difficult to see but can be detected by palpation. The lift of left ventricular hypertrophy is usually slow and sustained throughout systole. It is due to a resistant load, such as that which results from aortic stenosis or systemic hypertension. A diffuse, active apical lift is usually produced by a volume load that causes more dilatation than hypertrophy. Such lifts are seen with aortic or mitral insufficiency. A sustained right ventricular lift is often due to a resistant load, as is seen in pulmonary stenosis; a vigorous, brisk lift can be produced by a volume load, as is seen in atrial septal defect.

A ventricular (S_3) or an atrial (S_4) gallop may be the first sign of myocardial dysfunction. An atrial gallop has assumed importance, since physiologic studies have shown that in the absence of a long P-R interval it indicates impaired ventricular filling due to an elevated end-diastolic pressure or to reduced ventricular distensibility (compliance). There are varying opinions as to how frequently it occurs in the absence of any other signs or symptoms of cardiac disease. S_4 gallops are frequent in the elderly[12] and are not in themselves a priori evidence of heart failure. Although an S_3 gallop is strong evidence of congestive heart failure in patients older than 25 years, it may be a normal finding in younger people, and it may have a different significance in patients with left ventricular volume overloads and increased transmitral flow (as in mitral or aortic insufficiency). Gallops originating in the left ventricle are heard best during expiration, whereas those originating in the right ventricle are most distinct during inspiration, unless the ventricle is so badly diseased that it cannot generate enough cardiac output.

In heart failure the heart rate is usually rapid, especially when an S_3 gallop is present. Left ventricular dysfunction also can produce paradoxical splitting of the second sound with expiration. It may be difficult to distinguish between an S_3 gallop, an S_4 gallop, and a splitting of the heart sounds. However, the important point is to recognize that an extra sound is present and, particularly, that it was not present previously. Functional mitral or tricuspid insufficiency murmurs may appear with cardiac failure. The peripheral pulse is often overlooked but may be an important clue to the presence of left ventricular failure. In addition to a rapid rate and decreased amplitude, pulsus alternans (a beat-to-beat variation in systolic BP) may be observed. This often can be noted following PVBs. The mechanism of pulsus alternans is poorly understood, even though it was initially described by Traube[13] over a century ago. Cohn et al.[14] have suggested that the cause is multifactorial, reflecting alterations in ventricular end-diastolic volume (Starling mechanism) as well as alterations in ventricular contractility without changes in volume. On occasion, pulsus alternans can be seen in normal subjects during or just after termination of a tachyarrhythmia.

The extremities can be cold and at times there can be cyanosis of the digits because of the increased adrenergic activity, which is a compensatory mechanism to support the blood pressure.

The neck veins should be examined with the patient in a position 45 degree from horizontal. In early cardiac failure, the pulsations of the deep internal jugular vein rise above the clavicles when sustained pressure is applied over the liver or abdomen (positive hepatojugular reflux). Later, these pulsations will be visible without compression. As the congestion increases, the pulsations ascend and may reach the earlobes. The pulsations become less visible when the veins are tensely distended from the high venous pressure of congestive heart failure or pericardial constriction. Eventually, the external jugular veins become visible.

Obstruction of the superior vena cava or the innominate veins may produce unilateral or bilateral venous distention without pulsations. Unilateral left venous distention can occur when an atherosclerotic aorta compresses the innominate vein against the sternum. As the physician's acumen in clinical evaluation of neck veins has improved, the need for venous pressure determinations has decreased.

Congestive Phenomena

Congestive phenomena cause heart failure symptoms and produce findings that can be detected by examination. Bilaterally moist basilar rales are usually present in pulmonary congestion secondary to increased pulmonary venous pressure but may be absent in interstitial edema in which fluid has not

extravasated into the alveoli. In chronically ill patients with low colloid oncotic pressures, rales can develop at lower than expected pulmonary capillary
wedge pressures. It should be recognized that rales are not specific for heart
failure and also can be due to a variety of bronchorespiratory diseases. Too
often the emphasis is on rales; yet these are the least reliable signs of heart
failure. Rales can be predominantly on one side of the chest (usually the right)
but rarely occur unilaterally. In differentiating pulmonary causes from cardiac
rales, the chest x ray (in the upright position) is useful because, by the time
rales due to left heart failure are present, other signs of pulmonary venous
congestion, such as cephalization of flow, will be seen. As further pulmonary
congestion develops, interstitial pulmonary edema with wheezing may be
noted. Wheezing is most often associated with bronchitis, but can be caused by
the bronchial edema of heart failure.

Paroxysmal nocturnal dyspnea may occur for months before being brought
to the physician's attention, because if the patient is not seen during an attack,
the lungs later may clear, eliminating the evidence.

Pulmonary edema produces extensive rales, coughing, wheezing and frothy,
blood-tinged sputum. Gas exchange may become impaired, leading to hypoxemia and cyanosis, and hypotension can occur.

Pleural effusion (hydrothorax) may be bilateral or unilateral but usually
occurs in the right pleural cavity. This proclivity toward the right side has
never been satisfactorily explained, but may be due to the additional drainage
of the azygos vein, a large right pleural space or the preference of most heart
patients for sleeping on the right side. The sleeping preference is probably due
to increased awareness of the heartbeat when lying on the left side and to the
possibility of left lateral decubitus dyspnea. The mechanism for this type of
dyspnea (trepopnea) is not clearly understood but may be due to the lower
cardiac output and poor coronary perfusion that result from the heart shift in
accommodating a recumbent left-sided position.

Pleural effusion is usually associated with right-sided heart failure but may
be present with left-sided heart failure, as the pleural venous drainage is into
both the pulmonary and systemic veins. The visceral pleura empties into the
pulmonary veins and the parietal pleura, into the systemic veins. The fluid is
nonhemorrhagic unless associated with or due to pulmonary infarctions.

Hepatomegaly occurs when the central venous pressure (CVP) increases.
The liver is not considered enlarged unless the distance between its dull upper
edge and palpable lower edge is more than 11 cm. When the diaphragm is low,
the liver may have descended into the right pelvis and yet be of normal size.
Upper right quadrant tenderness may be overlooked as hepatitis or cholecys-
titis rather than rapid distention of the liver from heart failure. In chronic
congestion with fibrotic changes, the liver is usually nontender. Hepatomegaly
may also be caused by many noncardiac disorders. Splenomegaly can occur in
heart failure, especially in cases associated with secondary tricuspid insufficiency.

Subcutaneous edema does not occur until at least 10 lb of fluid has accumulated, usually in dependent areas such as the feet and ankles and then generalized throughout the body (anasarca). The left lower extremity frequently
shows edema first because the common iliac artery partially compresses the
left common iliac vein, increasing the venous pressure in the left leg. Bedrid-

den patients will accumulate edema fluid initially in the presacral area. Ascites (effusion of fluid into the abdominal cavity) disproportionate to other findings may occur with tricuspid disease or constrictive pericarditis and is related to portal venous engorgement. Because edema occurs late in heart failure and has many noncardiac causes, it is not a reliable sign.

Peripheral edema is most unusual in heart failure unless cardiomegaly, neck vein distention, and hepatomegaly are present. However, chronic left-heart failure with decreased cardiac output, can manifest edema; yet the systemic venous pressure may be normal or mildly elevated. Peripheral edema is more common in obesity; venous stasis, varicosities, and other venous disease; menopause; and psychogenic or cyclic, hepatic, and renal disease. Often patients are digitalized and given diuretics when the cause of the edema is noncardiac. Even normal persons can lose up to 3 lb in weight when given a diuretic. Before excluding heart failure as a cause, particularly when the physician who made the initial examination was uncertain, I prefer to forego administering drugs and to observe the patient for a few weeks.

X-RAY EXAMINATION AND OTHER TESTS

Left ventricular failure and mitral stenosis can produce elevated pulmonary venous pressure and passive congestion of the lungs. Interstitial edema may not be heard but may be seen on the x ray as haziness in the lung fields extending to the periphery. As the pulmonary venous pressure rises, the central pulmonary arteries and the superior pulmonary veins become dilated. To avoid false suggestions of pulmonary venous hypertension, the film should be taken in the upright position. The arteries and veins in the lower lobe constrict, giving the engorged superior veins an antler-like appearance. The superior vena cava and azygos vein may become prominent. The hilar markings often are hazy, and congestion of the pulmonary lymphatics with thickened interlobar septa due to interstitial edema produces B lines of Kerley when the pulmonary capillary pressure exceeds 20 to 25 mm Hg. Pleural effusions due to extravascular transudate may simulate tumors in the interlobar spaces that clear with therapy (phantom tumors). The hilar areas can be markedly congested (intra-alveolar edema) in cases of acute pulmonary edema (pulmonary capillary pressure is usually over 25 mm Hg), producing a butterfly-like, cloudy, or "bat wing" appearance.

The results of pulmonary function studies may be altered, showing depressed ventilatory function, specifically in determinations of total and timed vital capacity and maximum breathing capacity (maximum volume ventilation).

Hepatic congestion can alter the results of liver function tests. Serum bilirubin seldom goes above 2 mg/100 ml. However, it may be much higher with acute hepatic venous congestion or necrosis. Serum transaminase is frequently elevated. Reports[15] have described marked elevation of serum enzymes in occasional patients with heart failure, leading to an initial diagnosis of viral hepatitis. Autopsy examination or liver biopsy in such patients has shown centrizonal necrosis. Serum albumin levels are ordinarily normal, but occasional patients with severe chronic congestion of the intestine may have hypoalbuminemia caused by protein-losing enteropathy and impaired albumin synthesis associated with chronic cardiac cirrhosis.

Congestive changes may develop in the kidney and are manifested by elevated BUN and specific gravity and by albuminuria.

The ECG does not aid in detecting heart failure but can aid in the diagnosis of its cause.

M-mode, two-dimensional echocardiography, and Doppler have provided the physician with a noninvasive means of establishing the pathophysiologic basis and etiology of congestive heart failure in some patients. Based on the clinical picture and echocardiographic findings, the physician has a more sound basis for appropriate and specific medical or surgical interventions.

Radionuclide studies (^{99m}Tc pyp imaging and thallium scintigraphy) have become important in providing clues as to the presence and etiology of cardiac failure. Gated radionuclide angiocardiography is able to provide information on ejection fraction and wall motion, and in addition to its diagnostic value is useful in the longitudinal follow-up of patients with heart failure and in the assessment of medical and surgical interventions.

Central venous pressure is commonly normal when there is left heart failure. The Swan-Ganz catheter can give a pulmonary capillary wedge pressure which is helpful in evaluating left ventricular failure.

DIASTOLIC DYSFUNCTION

Patients with heart failure and a normal ejection fraction often have primarily left ventricular diastolic dysfunction. In the past, disease states such as hypertrophic cardiomyopathy and restrictive cardiomyopathy were considered in this category. However, diastolic dysfunction may occur with common conditions such as hypertension or ischemic heart disease with a normal ejection fraction. Clinical examination may not differentiate those patients with congestive heart failure with classic systolic dysfunction from those with primarily diastolic dysfunction. The assessment of diastolic function is usually divided into three components: chamber stiffness, ventricular relaxation and myocardial stiffness. Investigators do not agree on the optimal variables of diastolic functional indexes and on load dependence on these indexes. Invasive methods of measuring diastolic function have limitations and are not practical for clinical use. Noninvasive assessment of diastolic function has been done by the use of Doppler echocardiography and radionuclide angiography. Doppler echocardiography depicts left ventricular inflow velocities which with diastolic dysfunction show a reduced initial diastolic filling (E point) and an increased filling velocity secondary to atrial contraction (A point). However, the E/A ratio reduction can be influenced by many factors such as age, preload, afterload, heart rate and left ventricular and atrial compliance. Therefore, the precise role of these noninvasive methods remains to be determined.

DIAGNOSTIC PROBLEMS

Congestive heart failure is frequently confused with primary pulmonary disease, and often both exist in the same patient.

Left ventricular failure must be differentiated from bronchitis, which is often associated with chronic obstructive emphysema. Bronchitis is usually characterized by many years of coughing, wheezing, and dyspnea. Paroxysmal nocturnal dyspnea or orthopnea with little wheezing favors left-sided heart failure. During an attack of dyspnea, a cardiac patient can be relieved by sitting up, but this may not be true of the patient with lung disease. Palpable apical impulse, gallops, or pulsus alternans favors heart failure. When in doubt, it is best to administer aminophylline and oxygen (beneficial in both heart failure and pulmonary disease) rather than morphine (helpful in acute heart failure) or epinephrine (helpful in bronchial asthma).

Right-sided heart failure also is often misdiagnosed. The lower edge of the liver may be palpable in the right pelvis because of flattening of the diaphragm rather than because of congestion, and the peripheral edema may be gravitational due to venous stasis associated with the patient's inactivity or other noncardiac causes.

A history, physical examination, and chest x ray are usually adequate, without recourse to highly technical studies, in detecting heart failure.

TREATMENT OF HEART FAILURE

Patients with heart failure should be hospitalized to permit thorough diagnostic studies (to determine its cause and the contribution of diastolic dysfunction) and a therapy regimen guided by frequent observation and to ensure several days of proper emotional and physical rest. Bed rest is important, but when prolonged, it predisposes to thromboembolism. After hospital discharge, the patient should resume, insofar as possible, preillness activities, particularly work. Activities producing symptoms should be restricted, and emotional problems should be openly discussed.

Therapy for heart failure is directed at reducing the workload of the heart and manipulating the various factors that control cardiac performance, namely, heart rate, contractility, and wall tension (including preload and afterload). The treatment of heart failure can be outlined as shown in Table 16–1.

Attempts should be made to normalize cardiac rhythm and heart rate. From the point of view of cardiac performance, a patient is much better off in sinus rhythm than in atrial fibrillation. Many early studies using various methods to measure cardiac output showed an average increase of up to 40% in forward cardiac ouput when patients were converted from atrial fibrillation to normal sinus rhythm. Quinidine was the method of cardioversion used in these patients, and the studies were criticized because of poor technique and the possibility that the increase in cardiac output was in part due to the vasodilator effect of quinidine. Morris et al.[16] studied 12 patients who were converted from atrial fibrillation to normal sinus rhythm by electric cardioversion. In 7 of the

---

TABLE 16–1. Outline of Treatment of Heart Failure

1. Identify causes and contribution of diastolic dysfunction
2. Reduce the work load of the heart (reduce activity, weight loss, control hypertension and other contributing factors)
3. Sodium restriction
4. Digitalis and other inotropic agents
5. Diuretics
6. Water restriction (if hyponatremia is present)
7. Vasodilator therapy

11 patients studied at rest, cardiac output increased 0.6 L/min or more, with an average increase in cardiac output of 34%. Furthermore, 5 patients were studied at exercise, in which case sinus rhythm resulted in an average increase of 17% in the cardiac output.

A more recent study of the atrial contribution to cardiac output[17] showed a 25% increase in cardiac output with atrial pacing compared with ventricular pacing, which has no coordinated atrial contribution. However, the investigators showed an inverse relationship between ventricular filling pressure and atrial contribution to cardiac output, as well as an attenuated effect of atrial contractility in patients with poor left ventricular function who were on the flat portion of the ventricular function curve. These findings do not argue against the value of coordinated atrial contraction, but do underscore the greater importance of the Frank-Starling relationship, and wall tension in general, in determining the cardiac ouput of the failing heart.

Uncontrolled tachycardia not only increases myocardial oxygen consumption, but also limits diastolic filling time, thereby preventing the heart from fully utilizing its Frank-Starling relationship. Heart rates above 120 beats per minute are usually not well tolerated in the older age group, although this may be associated with an increase in the cardiac output of younger patients and in those with more normally compliant ventricles.

Patients with bradyarrhythmias may present with congestive heart failure and require a pacemaker for any of several reasons. Atrial pacing and AV sequential pacing should be considered in these patients who might benefit from preserving the atrial contribution to cardiac output. If atrial pacing is used in patients with underlying conduction disease, electrophysiologic studies should be performed to evaluate junctional and infra-His conduction.

Contractility, independent of loading, is an important intrinsic mechanism for determining stroke volume and cardiac output.

Preload refers to the left ventricular fiber length at the end of diastole, and in essence is the venous return. As mentioned, the Frank-Starling mechanism shows that as the left ventricular fiber length increases, the subsequent stroke volume will be greater, up to a point. Clinically, it is difficult to measure left ventricular fiber length, so we rely on measurements of left ventricular end-diastolic pressure or pulmonary capillary wedge pressure, which have a relationship to the left ventricular end-diastolic fiber length as determined by the compliance of the ventricle. As pulmonary artery pressure monitoring became popular, several different groups of investigators found that in patients with abnormally compliant ventricles, a pulmonary capillary wedge pressure of 18 mm Hg was needed to maximize the Frank-Starling compensatory mechanism. Increasing preload above this point causes an increase in myocardial oxygen consumption without any improvement in cardiac systolic performance. Furthermore, because of low colloid oncotic pressures of various causes, not all patients are able to maximize their left ventricular filling by increasing the pulmonary capillary wedge pressure to 18 mm Hg. Patients with a decreased total serum protein value, such as those with chronic liver disease or nephrotic syndrome, have lower colloid oncotic pressures and in some cases cannot tolerate even "normal" pulmonary capillary wedge pressures without developing pulmonary vascular congestion. Patients with adult respiratory distress syndrome and those with leaky pulmonary capillaries are also unable to tolerate otherwise normal pulmonary capillary wedge pressure (in an attempt to maximize the Frank-Starling compensatory mechanism) without developing pulmonary interstitial and alveolar edema.

Afterload refers to the tension that has to be generated in the wall of the left ventricle to open the aortic valve and discharge a certain stroke volume into the systemic circulation. Although LaPlace's law shows that afterload is proportional to the systemic arterial pressure and ventricular radius, it is determined not only by the peripheral vascular resistance, but also the aortic impedance and, in the face of congestive heart failure, the incompletely understood factor of reflected waves (reflectance).

Contractility, independent of loading, is an important intrinsic mechanism for determining stroke volume and cardiac output. This determinant of cardiac function is difficult to define and measure. It refers to the force of cardiac contraction, or the speed at which tension is generated during ventricular systole. Given a constant preload and afterload, any increase in the contractility results in a higher stroke volume and cardiac output. Changes in ventricular preload result in metabolic changes within the cardiac fibers that directly affect contractility. Additionally, mechanical stretch on cardiac fibers may cause a reduction in intracellular potassium and an increase in calcium concentrations. The transmembrane flux of calcium is intimately related to contractility by its ability to stimulate or inhibit intracellular enzyme systems.

DIGITALIS THERAPY

Digitalis has been used for over 200 years and is still a valuable agent in the treatment of heart failure. Some[18] have considered that digitalis has no value in patients who are in cardiac failure and in sinus rhythm. A long-term study by Arnold et al.[19] has shown that digitalis improves left ventricular function in heart failure. Patients were studied (hemodynamically and by radioangiographic methods) during long-term digoxin therapy, after withdrawal of the drug, and 6 hours after readministration. Upon withdrawal of digoxin, left ventricular function deteriorated, and acute readministration restored the hemodynamic values to those observed during long-term digoxin therapy. The improvement was also observed during exercise. Another study[20] suggests that long-term digoxin therapy is clinically beneficial in patients with heart failure unaccompanied by atrial fibrillation whose failure persists despite diuretic treatment and who have a third heart sound. The results of such studies should be evaluated in the light of the patient population selected (especially regarding the degree and type of ventricular dysfunction), which probably accounts for the variable results. At present, it is agreed that patients with systolic dysfunction (dilated failing heart often with an S_3 gallop) improved with digitalis, but those with elevated filling pressures caused by reduced ventricular compliance (diastolic dysfunction) and normal systolic function do not improve unless there is an associated supraventricular tachyarrhythmia.

Action

Although many details of its action are not completely established, digitalis appears to increase myocardial contractility at the cellular level by binding to and inhibiting Na, K-ATPase. This increases intracellular sodium concentration, which in turn increases intracellular calcium by the sodium-calcium exchange mechanism. Thus, more free ionized calcium is available for the contractile process.[21] This finding and a study of electrophysiologic effects have confirmed three major clinical cardiac actions produced by digitalis: increased contractility, AV node block, and sensitization of the vagus nerve.

Digitalis is one of the most important of a group of drugs that increase myocardial contractility. It is used in all types of heart disease in which heart failure is present, such as that due to ischemia, valvular disease, hypertension, congenital defects, cardiomyopathies, or cor pulmonale. The increase in contractility also has been demonstrated in the nonfailing heart, even though in such cases the cardiac output may be unchanged or even decreased due to adjustments of the peripheral circulation. The increased contractility will increase myocardial oxygen consumption; however, in the failing heart the reduction of the ventricular radius will reduce the wall tension and counterbalance this deleterious effect.

Digitalis may act on the AV node directly or indirectly through the vagus nerve, decreasing conduction and prolonging the refractory period of the node. Vagal stimulation produces the initial effects, and the direct effects become prominent at full digitalization. These effects prolong the P-R interval and may even block conduction of impulses, thus reducing the ventricular rate as with atrial fibrillation or flutter. Also, the vagal effect of digitalis on the SA node may produce bradycardia and the effect on the atrium (shortening of the refractory period) may produce rapid atrial arrhythmia or increase the rate of a pre-existing arrhythmia. These autonomic nervous system effects of digitalis have been confirmed by the fact that they are not noted in the denervated transplanted heart.[22]

Although cardioactive glycosides are numerous and diverse, they have a basically similar pattern of action. No difference has been found in their toxic-therapeutic ratios, but individual differences do exist in their speed and persistence of action, stability, absorption rates, and absolute doses. Thus, familiarity with the details of at least one preparation, rather than a general knowledge of several, is important. Digoxin (Lanoxin), an intermediate-acting agent, is the most widely used of these preparations. Digoxin solution in capsules (Lanoxicaps) has been demonstrated to be 90 to 100% absorbed from the gastrointestinal tract and is associated with reduced variability in steady-state serum concentrations between patients and within individual patients. However, physicians also should become acquainted with digitoxin and digitalis leaf, because they are still prescribed occasionally. Digitoxin is well absorbed and is not affected by renal function as is digoxin. It is a long-acting drug with a half-life of 6 days compared with only 1.6 days for digoxin.

Determining Optimal Dose

The trial-and-error method of digitalization (loading dose) has been used for many years. Pharmacokinetic data (namely, from Jelliffe et al.[23,24]) and methods for measuring cardiac glycoside blood levels have given a more specific method of prescribing digitalis with less possibility of toxicity. Older recommendations for dosage were entirely too high. This in part was explainable by unreliable bioavailabilities of various digitalis preparations.[25] Digitalis bioavailability is today much more uniform. In addition, we now know that the effect of digitalis is linear and that the degree of increase in myocardial contractility is dose-dependent. Consequently, lower dosages can be used in patients with mild congestive failure or those at high risk of toxicity. An "all or none" approach or "usual digitalizing dose" should be avoided. For rapid oral digitalization, Ogilvie and Ruedy[26] suggest 0.0075 mg (7.5 μg) of digoxin per lb of lean body weight, given usually in three divided doses at 6-hour intervals. Larger doses may be necessary for supraventricular arrhythmias to achieve the proper chronotropic effects. It is important to use lean body weight in the calculation of dosage rather than total body weight. It has been shown that digoxin levels and pharmacokinetics are essentially the same before and after loss of large amounts of adipose tissue by obese persons.[27] Rapid digitalization should be avoided if previous digitalis status is unknown.

Many prefer slow oral digitalization in the nonurgent cases by giving only a maintenance dose daily and not beginning with a loading dose. This method takes approximately 5 to 7 days for digitalization. This is based on the fact that a steady state for any drug will be reached after a period four times longer than the serum half-life, if no loading dose is given and a constant elimination is assumed. The calculated maintenance dose depends on renal function, especially since at least 80% of the most commonly used preparation, digoxin, is excreted by the kidney. Kidney function can be assessed more accurately by the creatinine clearance than by the serum creatinine or urea nitrogen. Often in the elderly the blood urea nitrogen (BUN and creatinine are normal, yet the creatinine clearance is significantly reduced. However, it is not always practical to perform creatinine clearances, and we must rely on stable values of BUN or creatinine. Table 16–2 gives the daily maintenance dose as percent of loading dose depending on stable values of BUN as suggested by Ogilvie and Ruedy's[26] modification of pharmacokinetic data from Jelliffe et al. For example, a person with a lean body weight of 150 lb would receive an approximate loading dose of 1.125 mg (0.0075 mg × 150) and a maintenance dose of 0.37 mg (33.3% off 1.125 mg) if the BUN is less than 20 mg/100 ml. Usually the average-sized person with good renal function can take a maintenance dose of approximately 0.25 mg digoxin daily. Since accurate creatinine clearances are not often immediately available, Smith, using figures from the Jelliffe study groups, suggests the use of a stable serum creatinine to determine daily loss by the expression shown in the following page.

Table 16–2. Daily Maintenance Dose of Digoxin as % of Loading Dose When the BUN is Stable*

BUN, mg/100 ml	Daily Maintenance Dose as % of Loading Dose
<20	33.3
30	30.0
40	27.0
50	24.0
60	21.0
70	18.0
>80	15.0

*Source: Ogilvie R.I., Ruedy J.: An educational program in digitalis therapy. JAMA 222:50, 1972.

$$\% \text{ daily loss (men)} = 11.6 + \frac{20}{\text{creatinine}}$$

and

$$\% \text{ daily loss (women)} = 12.6 + \frac{16}{\text{creatinine}}.$$

This value for daily percent loss multiplied by the loading dose gives an approximation of the daily maintenance dose.

Table 16–3 gives the approximate average dosage of digitalis used for therapeutic inotropic effect. Table 16–4 gives a comparison of digoxin and digitoxin.

To change from digitoxin to digoxin, one should stop the longer-acting agent and start digoxin 3 days later without a loading dose to avoid glycoside toxicity. This recommendation is based on the work of Bigger and Strauss,[28] who showed that a maximum cumulative effect occurs between the fourth and seventh day if digoxin is started at the same time that digitoxin is discontinued.

Because studies have shown no differences in serum levels of digitoxin in normal volunteers compared with patients with abnormal renal function,[29] digitoxin might appear to be the glycoside of choice in renal failure. However, we favor digoxin, even in this setting, for several reasons. First, the kinetics of digoxin in renal failure have been well worked out and the use of digoxin nomograms[30] or frequent checks of the serum creatinine level allow for rational drug use in this setting. Second, a certain amount of digitoxin (12-hydroxydigoxin) is normally converted to digoxin, and in the setting of renal failure, the degree of conversion is enhanced. Thus, when digitoxin is used, an unknown amount of digoxin is similarly added to the patient. Third, digitoxin is highly protein-bound, and in patients with renal failure, particularly those with the nephrotic syndrome, serum protein levels are quite variable. Finally, if toxicity does occur, digitoxin is more of a problem because of its extended half-life.

Heart rate cannot be used in gauging digitalis dosage unless atrial fibrillation is present. When sinus rhythm is present, the response is judged by relief from the usual signs and symptoms, such as dyspnea, orthopnea, rales, hepatomegaly, and peripheral edema. The end point of adequate digitalis dosage is difficult to recognize when the signs of heart failure are mild or subtle. Furthermore, many drugs, such as diuretics, add to the confusion. When sinus rhythm is present, the physician should never instruct the nurse to continue digitalis therapy until the heart rate is below 65 beats per minute as was

Table 16–3. Average Doses of Commonly Used Digitalis Agents

Drug	Onset of Action (Oral)	Peak Effect (Oral)	Loading Dose		Daily Maintenance Dose (Oral)
			Oral	IV or IM	
Digoxin	1–2 hr	1½–5 hr	0.75–1.5 mg	0.75–1.0 mg	0.125–0.5 mg
Digitoxin	2–4 hr	8–12 hr	0.7–1.4 mg	1 mg	0.1–0.15 mg
Digitalis leaf	2–6 hr	8–24 hr	0.8–1.2 g	—	0.1 g

Table 16–4. Comparison of Digoxin and Digitoxin

	Digoxin	Digitoxin
GI absorption	80%	90%–100%
Onset of action (IV)	15–30 min	25–120 min
Peak effect (IV)	1½–5 hr	4–12 hr
Half-life of elimination	36 hr	4–6 days
Protein-binding	25%–30%	85%–95%
Fat-binding	Poor	High
Renal metabolism	+ + + +	+
Hepatic metabolism	+	+ + + +

advised many years ago. The heart rate may decrease if the increased sympathetic tone of congestive failure is reduced with improvement in compensation.

After administration of the average loading dose, additional digitalis may be necessary. Conversely, if toxic signs appear, digitalis may have to be withheld for a few days. It is not wise to increase the dosage of the drug until toxicity occurs to establish an end point.

When atrial fibrillation is present, the apex rate can be used as a dosage guide. In such cases, AV node blocking, as well as increased contractility, is important and may require more than the usual amount of digitalis that is required for patients with a regular sinus rhythm and congestive failure. A reduction in apical rate to about 70 beats per minute is usually desirable; however, when the atrial fibrillation is associated with infections or thyrotoxicosis, a satisfactory rate is about 100 to 110 beats per minute. Larger doses are usually required in atrial flutter to block the AV node, since concealed conduction, due to many impulses being stored in the AV node, does not occur to the degree that it occurs in atrial fibrillation. Digitalis may convert supraventricular tachyarrhythmias to normal sinus rhythm in the course of digitalization.

The fallacy that the ECG can be used as a guide to an optimal dose should be corrected. At therapeutic levels of digitalis, some (but not all) patients have S-T segment depression or T wave inversion or both, which does not correlate with the loading dose, toxic effects, or need for digitalis. Clinical acumen is the best guide to judging clinical response.

After an optimal or a loading dose has been achieved, a daily maintenance dose should be initiated to replace daily losses and in many cases should be continued indefinitely and adjustment made based on frequent observation of the patient. In some patients, especially the elderly on digitalis chronically, the drug could be withdrawn without ill effects.

Precautions

Certain cases of heart failure require extra precaution in administering digitalis. Some examples follow and are listed in Table 16–5.

In severe heart disease the therapeutic-toxic ratio is narrow and toxicity often occurs. Sometimes, ascertaining the presence of toxicity or the need for additional digitalis may be difficult. Unless the situation is urgent, it is best to withhold the digitalis and to allow time to resolve the problem. I do not advise

Table 16–5.   Conditions Prone to Digitalis Toxicity*

1. Severe heart disease
2. Elderly patients
3. Thyroid disease
4. SA and AV block
5. Mitral stenosis
6. Acute myocardial infarction
7. High-output failure
8. Hypoxic states
9. IHSS and WPW syndromes
10. Electrolyte disturbances
11. Renal insufficiency
12. Multiple drug therapy

*IHSS = idiopathic hypertrophic subaortic stenosis; WPW = Wolff-Parkinson-White syndrome.

giving small increments of acetylstrophanthidine I.V. or using dc shock to determine the need for digitalis, even though some physicians have used these methods successfully.

Elderly patients tolerate digitalis poorly and often have excess vagal effects, with marked sinus bradycardia or sinus pauses, or both, before an optimal dose is reached. They also have decreased skeletal muscle mass and may have impaired renal function (decrease in creatinine clearance), even when creatinine and BUN levels are normal, which will decrease the urinary excretion of digoxin.[31]

Patients with hypothyroidism have an increased sensitivity to digitalis. Morrow et al.[32] showed that the increase in contractile force of the right ventricular myocardium following the administration of ouabain was significantly greater in dogs that were made hypothyroid compared with euthyroid and hyperthyroid dogs. Patients with hyperthyroidism have a lower steady state level of digoxin than those who have hypothyroidism or are euthyroid. Some investigators found a close correlation between serum levels and an enhanced glomerular filtration rate and a shorter half-life,[33] but an increased volume of distribution in hyperthyroid states was suggested in other studies.[34] Today there is no longer any need to administer excessive doses of digitalis to control the rapid ventricular response to atrial fibrillation seen in thyrotoxicosis, since β-blocking agents are available.

A study[35] has demonstrated that digitalis can be safely used in patients with sinus node dysfunction. In fact, some patients demonstrate improved sinus node function following the addition of digitalis. However, other studies[36] have shown that digitalis is not well tolerated even at low dosage. We are cautious with these patients, who are usually elderly and consequently are at higher risk of digitalis toxicity, even independent of their diseased conduction system. Ambulatory Holter monitoring after starting digitalis would appear prudent in patients manifesting clinical or electrophysiological evidence of sinus node dysfunction. The patient with first-degree AV block and heart failure can be given digitalis if the P-R interval is not excessively prolonged (that is, if it is less than 0.28 second). However, if the block increases or the patient has second-degree or third-degree AV block, a pacemaker may be necessary before digitalization can be safely employed.

Mitral stenosis with normal sinus rhythm usually does not improve with digitalis therapy unless right ventricular failure is present; in fact, some physicians consider digitalis beneficial in these cases only when atrial fibrillation is present.

Some investigators feel that the use of digitalis in the setting of an acute myocardial infarction is contraindicated, because the drug's positive inotropic effect will increase myocardial oxygen consumption and thereby extend the infarction. Varonkov et al.[37] found that digitalis (acetylstrophanthidine) I.V. increased CPK levels when given to patients within 15 hours after the onset of symptoms. However, none of the patients in this study was in clinical heart failure, and the extension of the infarction, if this is what the elevated CPK levels represented, may have been due to the direct peripheral vasoconstrictor effect of the intravenous digitalis preparations.[38] Other investigators have shown favorable hemodynamic responses to digitalis when used in the setting of an acute myocardial infarction. Lesch[39] feels that after the initial 24 hours, digitalis can be used as with any other situation, because the infarct is probably complete and the digitalis may be helpful in the subacute phase. I feel that digitalis is indicated if clinical heart failure, as evidenced by an S_3 gallop, pulmonary rales or pulmonary congestion by x ray (Killip class 2), and cardiomegaly are present, in which case the reduction in left ventricular wall tension and heart rate overrides the increase in myocardial oxygen consumption resulting from enhanced contractility. Digitalis is not recommended for mild or moderate congestive heart failure, which can be managed with diuretics and careful use of vasodilators. Morrison and co-workers[40] have shown that digitalis increases the ejection fraction in patients with acute myocardial infarction with moderate to severe heart failure (Killip class 2), and this was accomplished without evidence of a decrease in myocardial perfusion or an increase in infarct size. Because such patients are more sensitive, the loading dose should be reduced to one half to three fourths of the usual. Intravenous digitalis should be given slowly because it can increase peripheral vascular resistance before its inotropic effect and so impair left ventricular function and decrease cardiac output.[41] However, systemic vascular resistance is already high as a result of the congestive heart failure so that the peripheral vasoconstrictor effect of digitalis could be blunted. In patients with cardiogenic shock, in whom up to 40% of the myocardium is usually infarcted, I avoid using digitalis. In this case, the therapeutic/toxic ratio is low, and more reliable and more easily controllable agents such as dopamine and dobutamine are available should a positive inotropic agent be required.

Atrial fibrillation with a rapid ventricular response is an indication for digitalization even in the presence of an acute infarction. Digitalis is always administered slowly, and a reduced loading dose is given. If this reduced dose is inadequate in controlling the ventricular response, we favor propranolol, verapamil, or dc shock.

High-output failure associated with anemia, thyrotoxicosis, cor pulmonale, and other conditions often presents with a rapid heart rate. A tendency to increase digitalis in an attempt to slow the heart rate often results in toxicity. Arterial hypoxemia, particularly when acute, increases the sensitivity to digitalis, perhaps due to an increase in circulating catecholamines. Chronic obstructive pulmonary disease, particularly when complicated by acute respiratory decompensation, often presents with the arrhythmia of multifocal atrial tachycardia, which, although superficially resembling atrial fibrillation, is particularly resistant to digitalis therapy and carries a high risk of digitalis toxicity. Wang et al.[42] observed this arrhythmia in 41 seriously ill patients, with 88% suffering from acute respiratory distress. Digitalis was ineffective in controlling the rapid ventricular response, but propranolol was helpful in all cases where it was used. Verapamil, because it does not produce bronchoconstriction, is a better choice for controlling the ventricular response.

Hypertrophic subaortic stenosis, Wolff-Parkinson-White (WPW) syndrome, and constrictive pericarditis are relative contraindications to the use of digitalis. The inotropic effect of digitalis may increase the muscular subvalvular obstruction in idiopathic hypertrophic subaortic stenosis (IHSS) and worsen the heart failure. In patients in whom this disorder is complicated by supraventricular arrhythmias, digitalis may have a role, since slowing the ventricular rate is crucial to allow time for adequate ventricular filling. However, propranolol and verapamil would appear to be superior agents. In addition to slowing the ventricular rate by increasing AV block, the negative inotropic effect of these drugs reduces the dynamic left ventricular outflow tract obstruction.

In the presence of WPW syndrome, atrial fibrillation may develop with conduction down the accessory pathway at fast rates. Digitalis is dangerous in this situation because it can shorten the refractory period of the accessory pathway, thereby speeding the ventricular rate and possibly inducing ventricular fibrillation. Sellers et al.[43] have suggested that patients with WPW syndrome and atrial fibrillation in whom the shortest R-R interval is less than 300 msec cannot be safely treated with digitalis, since a high percentage will have conduction rapidly down the accessory pathway resulting in ventricular fibrillation. In patients with atrial fibrillation and the WPW syndrome, dc shock is indicated for hemodynamic instability, i.v. procainamide for less urgent situations, and quinidine, procainamide, or amiodarone for long-term management.

Constrictive pericarditis does not usually improve with digitalis unless the myocardium is also involved in the disease process.

Acute hypokalemia may result in increased digitalis sensitivity[44] and less so with chronic hypokalemia.[45] This enhanced digitalis sensitivity may be due to an increased rate of uptake and associated increase in the inhibition of the Na, K ATPase.[46] Metabolic and respiratory acidosis can produce hyperkalemia. Hyperkalemia, by blocking receptor sites otherwise available to digitalis, may diminish the inotropic effect of the glycoside, and as a result high doses may be given. When the acidosis clears with treatment, then the masked digitalis effect can appear, producing toxicity.

Other electrolyte disturbances may occur in patients with heart failure, particularly those receiving diuretics. Hypomagnesemia may be associated with an increased sensitivity to digitalis and may occur with diuretic use and following myocardial infarctions. In a study by Beller et al.,[47] hypomagnesemia was present in 21% of patients thought to have digitalis toxicity on the basis of serial ECGs. Hypermagnesemia was also more frequent in patients with digitalis toxicity compared with those who were not, but this appeared to be related to abnormal renal function. Thus, hospitalized patients with congestive heart failure being treated with powerful diuretics may develop digitalis toxicity secondary to hypomagnesemia, but magnesium replacement must be done judiciously in patients with abnormal renal function.

Hypercalcemia may increase the risk of digitalis intoxication, although Nola et al.[48] found this to be true only at high serum calcium levels (greater than 15 mEq/L). Calcium can enhance the vasoconstrictor effect of digitalis thus increasing systemic vascular resistance. Furthermore, since the combination of calcium and digitalis may precipitate ventricular arrhythmias, one must be careful in administering calcium salts to patients during a cardiac arrest if they are on maintenance digitalis.

The maintenance dose of digoxin must be decreased in patients with renal failure. Less well appreciated is the fact that the loading dose of digoxin should also be decreased in this setting. This is because azotemia reduces the volume of distribution of the drug,[49] possibly due to a reduced affinity of the cell membrane receptor for digoxin, and such patients have less muscle mass because of their illness.

Premature beats are often present with heart failure and may clear or decrease with digitalis therapy. Treatment must be given cautiously, however, because the premature ventricular or atrial beats may increase before an optimal dose is reached. In fact, these premature beats may lead to runs of ventricular tachycardia or atrial arrhythmias. When this occurs, antiarrhythmia drugs may be needed with the digitalis.

Certain drugs increase the sensitivity or resistance to digitalis. Often such drugs have to be discontinued to achieve proper response to digitalis. (Later in this chapter these drugs will be discussed further.)

DIGITALIS TOXICITY

The incidence of digitalis toxicity is 15 to 20% in hospitalized patients and is increasing daily with wider use of the drug, especially in the elderly. Preventing toxicity is difficult in patients with advanced heart disease and in those with severe renal impairment. The highly potent crystalline glycosides are easily overused because they do not readily produce the warnings signs of anorexia, nausea, and vomiting. These symptoms (probably of CNS origin) also are often masked by the use of tranquilizers with antiemetic effects. Other extracardiac symptoms of toxicity may be fatigue, dizziness, facial pain, headache, visual (such as objects appear yellow), or even psychoses. These are rather uncommon. Rarely, bilateral or unilateral gynecomastia or mesenteric venous occlusion with hemorrhagic necrosis of the bowel can occur.[50]

As previously mentioned, toxicity is precipitated by many factors, especially hypokalemia, decreased kidney function, and certain drugs. It is important to remember that intracellular potassium can be low in spite of a normal serum level. Myocardial hypokalemia sometimes may be detected by ECG findings rather than by the serum potassium level.

When it is uncertain whether a patient has received digitalis, small doses should be administered cautiously. Determining whether arrhythmias are due to toxicity or to the underlying heart disease also is difficult in some cases.

The most important toxic effects of digitalis are the arrhythmias, which are best detected by electrocardiography. Unfortunately, these usually precede the extracardiac findings. However, the arrhythmias may be suspected clinically when the rhythm becomes irregular, slow, or very rapid. Toxic arrhythmias may be those of tachyarrhythmia, acceleration of lower pacemakers, or AV block. Among the toxic arrhythmias are PVBs, ventricular bigeminy, multifocal PVBs, ventricular tachycardia, bidirectional tachycardia, AV heart block, SA block or sinus pauses with or without escape rhythms, atrial tachycardia with block, and nonparoxysmal junctional (nodal) tachycardia with AV dissociation.

Premature ventricular beats are often present with heart failure and may clear with digitalis. In fact, digitalis has been successfully used in the treatment of ventricular ectopy even without clinical evidence of congestive heart failure.[51] This may be due to the enhancement of vagal tone seen with digitalis. However, any arrhythmia developing while the patient is receiving digitalis should be considered a potentially digitalis toxic arrhythmia until proved otherwise.

Premature ventricular beats may occur as unifocal type (often as bigeminy), multifocal, or ventricular tachycardia. Rarely, bidirectional tachycardia develops. The bidirectional tachycardia may be ventricular or junctional in origin, and has been shown to be due either to different ventricular foci or, as in the case of supraventricular origin, alternating bundle-branch blocks or hemiblock. Acceleration of the junctional pacemaker can produce nonparoxysmal junctional tachycardia with AV dissociation with, at times, capture beats. This arrhythmia is not third-degree AV block, since the ventricular rate is usually 70 to 130 per minute and the atrial rate is slower.

The classic supraventricular arrhythmia described with digitalis toxicity has been atrial tachycardia with 2:1 AV block. However, in at least 50% of cases, this arrhythmia is not due to digitalis but is associated with the inherent heart disease. In the study of Beller et al.[52] that utilized serum digoxin and digitoxin levels in the diagnosis of digitalis toxicity, only 2 of 55 definitely digitalis-toxic arrhythmias were paroxysmal atrial tachycardia with AV block. Ventricular bigeminy or trigeminy, junctional escape rhythm, and nonparoxysmal junctional tachycardia composed two thirds of the toxic arrhythmias.

At times atrial fibrillation can be due to digitalis toxicity; however, we are reluctant to diagnose this arrhythmia as secondary to digitalis toxicity unless there is a slow ventricular response (less than 50 beats per minute) as well as PVBs. Any patient in atrial fibrillation who is being given digitalis should be observed for the development of nonparoxysmal junctional tachycardia with AV dissociation. The heart rate in these patients will be regular at 70 and 130 beats per minute and consequently this is sometimes misinterpreted as a conversion to normal sinus rhythm. If a regular rhythm develops in a patient with atrial fibrillation on digitalis, an ECG should be recorded to document the underlying arrhythmia. While nonparoxysmal junctional tachycardia with AV dissociation strongly suggests digitalis toxicity in those patients taking the drug, it is also seen following cardiopulmonary bypass, as a complication of inferior myocardial infarction, and occasionally in normal children. It should also be appreciated that digitalis in the presence of atrial fibrillation can produce AV dissociation and nonparoxysmal junctional tachycardia with a

Wenckebach exit block below the junctional focus. In view of this, all patients with atrial fibrillation receiving digitalis should be observed carefully to be certain that the QRS complexes do not show Wenckebach groupings (see Figs 15–18 and 15–19C).

Any degree of AV node block can occur with digitalis. Usually, if third-degree AV block occurs, an idiojunctional rhythm will be present with an adequate ventricular rate.

A clinically important concept that has evolved from studies[53] of the electrophysiology of digitalis and digitalis intoxication is that of oscillating after-potentials (also called delayed after-depolarizations). These transient oscillations in membrane potential may be induced by digitalis and can, under appropriate situations, attain threshold and initiate spontaneous action potentials.[54] The clinical corollary is the repetitive ventricular response, in which the induction of a single premature ventricular beat in the digitalized heart may result in ventricular tachycardia.[55] The calcium antagonist verapamil decreases the magnitude of the oscillating action potential and thus appears to be a promising agent in such digitalis-induced arrhythmias.

Therapy of Digitalis Toxicity

The precise role of the serum digitalis level in the diagnosis of digitalis toxicity is unclear.[56] While some investigators have found it helpful in recognizing what we now know to be a common clinical problem, other work disputes this claim. Certainly the therapeutic effect of digitalis is somewhat related to the serum digitalis level. However, because we do not know the amount of binding to cell membrane ATPase or to the plasma protein in any given patient, these levels are only helpful in the broad sense. Radiotracer studies have shown that the usual myocardial to serum level ratio is 40:1 at a steady state concentration of the drug.[57] When one considers this, as well as the fact that the drug levels are measured in extremely small quantities (ng/ml), it is no wonder that the validity of this laboratory test varies significantly. There is overlap in serum digitalis concentrations between toxic and nontoxic values. Generally, a level of 0.5 to 1.5 ng/ml is therapeutic, and above 2.5 ng/ml is toxic. However, in the range of 1.5 to 2.5 ng/ml, the patient may be in either the therapeutic or toxic range. In addition, for tachyarrhythmias such as atrial fibrillation, one may have to give doses that produce a higher level than 3 ng/ml to slow the ventricular response.[58]

The use of serum digitalis levels appears indicated when there is the suspicion of drug intoxication and in assessing the status of digitalization, as long as one realizes the pitfalls of measurement and interpretation, such as the timing of drug levels and the marked variation in patient sensitivity to the drug. For digoxin, it takes 6 hours for a steady state (between the serum and myocardial tissue) to be reached after an oral dose, and 2 hours after an I.V. dose. Serum digoxin levels drawn prior to this will reflect high, nonsteady-state levels that do not correlate with electrophysiologic or clinical toxicity.[59]

When digitalis toxicity occurs, the drug must be withheld rather than given in reduced dosage. This is the only treatment required in most cases, such as first-degree AV block, occasional PVBs, sinus bradycardia, nausea, vomiting, or sudden loss of appetite. Conditions such as hypoxia that decrease digitalis tolerance should be corrected.

Potassium salts can suppress the arrhythmias, especially when hypokalemia is present. Potassium chloride can be given initially by slow I.V. infusion, 40 to 80 mEq in 250 ml glucose in water under constant ECG monitoring, and then given orally, 20 mEq three times daily. A large intake of carbohydrates may cause an intracellular shift of potassium with a decrease of serum potassium and worsen the digitalis toxicity or precipitate it. Although the antiarrhythmic effect of potassium is mainly extracellular and dextrose may increase the potassium intracellularly, use of saline often is unwise. Potassium should not be used in AV block of second degree or higher because it can further depress the AV nodal and junctional tissue; however, atrial tachycardia with 2:1 AV block is an exception. Also, potassium should be used cautiously in cases of associated renal disease.

Of the many drugs that have been used for non-AV block types of digitalis arrhythmias (tachyarrhythmias), diphenylhydantoin (Dilantin) and β-adrenergic blocking agents such as propranolol (Inderal) and lidocaine are the most promising. Diphenylhydantoin may be given initially in a dose of 100 to 200 mg IV and then 100 mg orally four times daily. Because studies indicate that diphenylhydantoin facilitates AV conduction, it may be used in the presence of first-degree AV block for tachyarrhythmias induced by digitalis, but it is not recommended if AV block of second degree or higher is present. Lidocaine should be used for ventricular ectopy, especially for ventricular tachycardia or prevention of recurrent ventricular fibrillation. Propranolol may be given initially in a dose of 1 to 2 mg slowly I.V. and then 10 mg or more orally four times daily. It should be used cautiously, because it may produce depression of conduction or contractility. Procainamide (Pronestyl) is not used as often today for digitalis toxicity.

Cardioversion is used only when other measures fail, because it can induce more serious arrhythmias in the presence of digitalis toxicity. Complete heart block due to digitalis does not require treatment unless the patient is symptomatic and has a heart rate of less than 40 beats per minute, or the QRS complex is widened, and then a temporary transvenous pacer should be inserted. Fortunately, in most cases the block is high in the AV node and the ventricular rate is adequate with a normal QRS width. Thus, these patients seldom have Adams-Stokes attacks, which commonly occur in complete AV block from other causes. Atropine may be beneficial if the vagal contribution to the block is significant.

Until recently, there have been only a few isolated cases of reversal of advanced digoxin intoxication with digoxin specific antibodies.[60] At present, many patients with life-threatening digitalis intoxication have received Digibind, a digoxin immune fab (ovine).[61] Patients treated with this digoxin-specific antibody are those judged highly unlikely to respond to usual measures for massive intoxication. Therapeutic response has been rapid, usually within 30 minutes with complete response in 3 to 4 hours. The average dosage is about 520 mg, with a range from 4 to 1600 mg.[62] The drug is administered I.V. over a 15- to 30-minute period. The dosage is calculated to be equimolar to the amount of digoxin in the patient's body. Total digoxin load is estimated from the medical history or from determination of serum digoxin level. Potency tests of Digibind show that each 40 mg vial is capable of neutralizing approximately 0.6 mg of digoxin. Thus, one method to calculate the dose would be to divide the total body load of digoxin by 0.6 mg to determine the number of vials necessary for the patient. There have been no unexpected side effects. Potassium concentrations usually fall after administration of the antibody fragments, indicating reversal of digitalis-induced inactivation of the Na^+ K^+ pump.

Hemodialysis is not useful for digoxin overdose, for it does not remove substantial amounts of digoxin because of high tissue- and protein-binding. Charcoal hemoperfusion coupled with hemodialysis, in a recent case report, showed no significant effect on digoxin elimination,[63] even though other limited studies suggested that it might be of value.

A few patients cannot tolerate any amount of digitalis. Because small amounts of the drug often cause nausea in the elderly, other means of controlling the heart failure may be required. Several other inotropic agents are being studied for use in heart failure.

DIURETICS

When restricted activity, digitalis, and low salt intake can control heart failure, diuretics should be withheld. These should be added to the regimen, however, if heart failure persists or if a more palatable, less rigid salt-restricted diet will improve the patient's morale. I usually advise patients to avoid excessively salty food and to use only enough salt in cooking to make food palatable. This alone may reduce the sodium to near 2 g per day. Salt substitutes can be used, but some patients complain that these agents have a brassy taste.

Although in most cases of congestive heart failure there is no intrinsic renal abnormality, sodium and water retention plays a prominent role in the production of signs and symptoms of congestive heart failure. The reduction in left ventricular stroke volume occurring with congestive heart failure ("forward failure") activates certain hemodynamic, hormonal, and neural compensatory mechanisms that result in salt and water retention by the kidneys. Although the exact stimuli that activate these compensatory mechanisms are poorly understood, it seems likely that a decrease in the effective arterial plasma volume plays a significant role.[64–66] The sympathetic nervous system[67] and renin-angiotensin-aldosterone system[68,69] are activated in an attempt to maintain arterial blood pressure and blood flow to vital organs, namely, the brain and heart. The decrease in renal blood flow resulting from the overall reduction in cardiac output, as well as shunting of flow to the vital organs, initially causes postglomerular arteriolar vasoconstriction. The glomerular filtration rate is thereby maintained or only slightly decreased, but at the expense of a decreased blood pressure and increased colloid oncotic pressure in the peritubular capillaries. The resulting increase in filtration fraction (that is, the ratio of glomerular filtration rate to renal blood flow) is an important factor in promoting sodium reabsorption. Intrarenal blood flow is redistributed, with the juxtamedullary nephrons receiving an increased share of the renal blood flow. This redistribution also results in enhanced reabsorption of sodium and water, because these nephrons have large glomeruli and a relatively higher filtration rate.

More important in sodium and water retention is tubular reabsorption, which is markedly increased in congestive heart failure, even in mild cases in which the glomerular filtration rate is unchanged. Some 60 to 70% of the filtered load of sodium is reabsorbed in the proximal convoluted tubule (the result of active transport), 20% in the ascending limb of Henle's loop (result of active chloride transport), and the remainder in the distal convoluted tubule and collecting duct (partially under the control of aldosterone). Because the bulk of this tubular reabsorption is proximal, hormonal factors (aldosterone, antidiuretic hormone) are not considered to play an important role in sodium and water reabsorption.

Hyperaldosteronism has been demonstrated in congestive heart failure states.[70] This results from the enhanced activity of the renin-angiotensin system as well as from a decreased hepatic metabolism. The latter is particularly prominent in the presence of right-sided congestive heart failure. Enhanced renin activity further contributes to the pathophysiologic abnormality by increasing the level of circulating angiotensin I, which is converted to the powerful vasoconstrictor angiotensin II (increases afterload). Angiotensin II is a known stimulus for the antidiuretic hormone arginine vasopressin, which is increased in congestive heart failure. However, its increase is less than that of the norepinephrine and plasma renin activity. This may contribute to the decrease in secretion of a water load, but its exact degree of involvement in edema formation is unclear. Atrial natriuretic peptide (ANP) is increased in patients with heart failure (partly regulated by right and left atrial pressures).[71] This may be an appropriate physiologic response to produce natriuresis and reduce preload and afterload in the presence of myocardial dysfunction. However, its action may be overridden by the more powerful effect of the sympathetic and renin-angiotensin system in heart failure.

The diuretics act at various sites to interrupt or retard the enhanced sodium and water reabsorption, thereby directly reducing the edematous state. Indirectly, they reduce ventricular preload and, by decreasing left ventricular volume, diminish left ventricular afterload. The resulting improvement in ventricular function serves to further reduce or eliminate the sodium and water overload.

A convenient way to classify the diuretics is by their site of action at the renal tube (Fig 16–2). Many types of diuretics are available: mercurials, carbonic anhydrase inhibitors, thiazides and related drugs, so-called loop diuretics, and the potassium-sparing diuretics. Mercurial diuretics, which require parenteral administration, are now seldom used. These drugs prevent absorption of sodium, chloride, and water chiefly in the ascending limb of Henle's loop and partly in the proximal tubule. Hypochloremic alkalosis is a common side effect of the mercurials; therefore, the regimen for reestablishing diuresis often includes intermittent administration of ammonium chloride or a carbonic anhydrase inhibitor such as acetazolamide (Diamox). Since the mercurials have been replaced by oral diuretics, these are now used primarily when a patient is refractory to other forms of therapy because of excess body water (dilutional hyponatremia). The water diuresis that may be produced by mercurial diuretics may be beneficial.

The carbonic anhydrase inhibitor acetazolamide (Diamox) acts predominantly on the proximal tubule, where carbonic anhydrase is found along the brush border of the tubules, but it also has some effect at distal sites (see Fig 16–2). Since carbonic anhydrase catalyzes the hydration of CO_2 and H_2O with

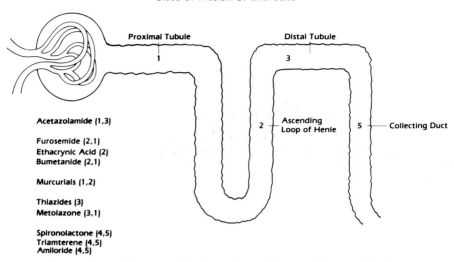

Fig 16–2. Commonly used diuretics. Numbers indicate the sites of action of the diuretics in the tubules. (From Gazes P.C., Assey M.E.: The management of congestive heart failure. *Curr. Probl. Cardiol.* 4:1, 1984).

a resultant increase in hydrogen ions, inhibiting the enzyme decreases sodium reabsorption in exchange for hydrogen ions, and this results in a sodium bicarbonate diuresis. The action of Diamox is self-limited, and tolerance to the drug develops in a few days. As bicarbonate is excreted chloride tends to be retained, and attendant volume depletion leads to the development of hyperchloremic acidosis. In the presence of liver abnormalities, Diamox can cause drowsiness or mental confusion. Its duration of action is about 6 to 8 hours. Therefore, it should be given in divided doses three times per day. It is most valuable when used in conjunction with the more potent loop diuretics.

The major site of action of the thiazide diuretics and related preparations is at the early distal tubule, where they probably have a direct effect on active sodium and the accompanying passive chloride transport, as well as impairing urinary dilution (Fig 16–2). The action of most of these persists from 6 to 12 hours and thus can be given in divided doses twice per day. Some, such as chlorthalidone (Hygroton), may be effective for 18 to 48 hours. It is pharmacologically similar to the thiazides, although it is chemically unrelated. These agents, by blocking the reabsorption of sodium, present it distally where it may be exchanged for potassium, and hypokalemia can develop (Fig 16–3). Other side effects include skin rash, hyperuricemia, hyperglycemia, vasculitis, blood dyscrasias, lipid abnormalities (increased total cholesterol, low-density lipoproteins, and triglycerides), and occasionally hypercalcemia. The hypercalcemia is minor, but can be deleterious in patients with pre-existing hypercalcemia such as in hyperparathyroidism. In susceptible individuals the hyperuricemia may precipitate gout. These diuretics also can produce hemolysis in patients with glucose-6-phosphate dehydrogenase (G-6-PD) deficiency and neonatal jaundice (if thiazides are used during pregnancy).[72] The thiazides are relatively ineffective in patients with impaired kidney function (GFR less than 30 ml/min).

HYPOKALEMIA

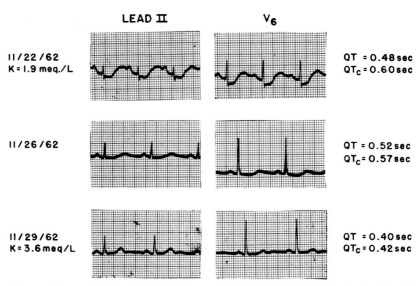

Fig 16–3. A 65-year-old woman with severe weakness due to hypokalemia. She had been on chlorothiazide for 2 months. *Top tracing* reveals characteristic ECG changes of hypokalemia (ST-T changes and prolonged Q-T interval). Serum potassium of 1.9 mEq/L. *Bottom strip* shows ECG and serum potassium returning toward normal after potassium replacement. QT_c, Q-T interval corrected for rate.

Metolazone (Zaroxolyn, Diulo) is a sulfonamide, like the thiazides, which acts primarily to inhibit sodium reabsorption on the early distal tubule and possibly at the proximal tubule as well. At maximum therapeutic dosage, its diuretic potency approximates that of the thiazides. However, it can produce diuresis in the presence of poor renal function (unlike the thiazides), and, in addition, is able to produce a marked diuresis when given with furosemide. Metolazone's action can persist for 24 hours and it is usually given in a dosage of 5 to 10 mg daily. Because of the drug's potent diuretic effect when used concomitantly with furosemide, this regimen should be initiated in the hospital, where intravascular volume and electrolyte balance can be closely monitored.

The "loop" diuretics, ethacrynic acid (Edecrin), furosemide (Lasix), and bumetanide (Bumex), are potent, and diuresis may be massive. Both drugs act on the thick ascending limb of the loop of Henle to prevent reabsorption of sodium and chloride, and both dilution and concentration of the urine are impaired (see Fig 16–2). In addition, furosemide has a slight carbonic anhydrase inhibitor effect on the proximal tubule and bumetanide induces mild phosphaturia, which indicates an additional action at the proximal tubule. The loop diuretics appear to retain their efficacy in patients with impaired renal function. When either of these two drugs is given orally, action begins within 30 minutes and continues for 6 to 8 hours. They are usually given as one early morning dose or twice per day. With I.V. administration, action begins in a few minutes and is maximal in 1 hour. When furosemide is used in congestive heart failure following an acute myocardial infarction, clinical and hemodynamic improvement precedes the diuretic effect of the drug.[73] This is due to its venodilating effect, which is manifested as a reduction in pulmonary capillary wedge pressure. The actual clearing of the excess lung water may take several hours and may be related to the degree of reduction in wedge pressure or perhaps the amount of pre-existing left ventricular dysfunction. These can precipitate hyponatremia, hypokalemia, hypochloremic alkalosis, hyperglycemia, and hyperuricemia. "Rebound" sodium retention may occur. Acute hearing loss, vertigo, and tinnitus can occur with ethacrynic acid or furosemide in large doses, usually over 200 mg, especially in patients with renal disease and azotemia. On occasion, interstitial nephritis and serious hypovolemia may develop.

The potassium-sparing diuretics such as spironolactone (Aldactone), triamterene (Dyrenium), and amiloride (Midamor) act at the distal sodium-hydrogen-potassium exchange sites in the late distal tubule and collecting duct (see Fig 16–2). Spironolactone inhibits the action of aldosterone on the distal renal tubule and thereby increases excretion of sodium and decreases potassium and hydrogen ion secretion. Triamterene and amiloride do not require the presence of aldosterone to produce the same effect. It takes 2 to 3 days before spironolactone has its maximal action, 12 to 16 hours for triamterene, and 6 to 10 hours for amiloride. The delay in spironolactone effect results from the aldosterone already present and active at the receptor site when the drug is started. These drugs are often administered with diuretics that promote potassium loss, such as the thiazides or "loop" diuretics. In this setting they have their greatest usefulness. In thiazide-fast states, renewed diuresis may be produced by addition of these agents. Secondary hyperaldosteronism is often mild to moderate in cardiac failure, and spironolactone may not be effective; therefore triamterene or amiloride should be used. Because of their potassium-retaining effect, they should be used with caution in the presence of renal diseases and excessive intake of foods or salt substitutes with large amounts of potassium because hyperkalemia can be produced. In addition, they should not be prescribed with potassium supplements. Triamterene and amiloride exert an effect even in the absence of aldosterone and thus are more prone to produce hyperkalemia. Spironolactone, a steroid, can produce gynecomastia and occasionally nausea and vomiting. Patients who develop gynecomastia have been wrongly diagnosed as having angina because of the soreness and fullness in the chest. Triamterene and amiloride do not produce this side effect. Potassium-sparing diuretics can cause skin rash.

Table 16–6 lists the usual daily dosage of the various diuretics. These are often given in divided amounts. Diuretics may be required intermittently or daily. One should avoid daily use when intermittent use is adequate to avoid refractoriness and electrolyte depletion. The dosage schedule is determined by the patient's daily weight, clinical symptoms, and physical findings. Because of the different sites of action and effects of various diuretics (see Fig 16–2), combined use of complementary agents often may be necessary to achieve maximal efficacy. Thiazides, ethacrynic acid, furosemide, and acetazolamide are less effective after a few days; intermittent use or periodic withholding for a day or two allows for recovery of action. However, spironolactone is effective only when used continuously. By correcting hypochloremia, acetazolamide and ammonium chloride can restore the effectiveness of the other diuretics.

Hypokalemia can be prevented by using diuretics intermittently, observing

Table 16–6. Daily Dosage of Commonly Used Diuretics

Diuretic	Dose (mg)
Acetazolamide (Diamox)	750
Furosemide (Lasix)	40–160
Ethacrynic acid (Edecrin)	50–150
Bumetanide (Bumex)	0.5–10
Hydrochlorothiazide (Hydrodiuril, Esidrix, Oretic)	25–100
Chlorthalidone (Hygroton)	25–100
Metolazone (Diulo, Zaroxolyn)	2.5–10
Spironolactone (Aldactone)	75–100
Triamterene (Dyrenium)	50–200
Amiloride (Midamor)	5–10

symptoms, electrolyte values and diet and by giving potassium supplements if necessary. However, potassium supplements should be given continuously (if at all) when the patient is receiving a potassium-sparing drug or has underlying renal disease. In such situations, hyperkalemia can occur, which is a more serious threat to the cardiac patient than hypokalemia. Many food items have potassium and are listed in Table 16–7. Supplements of 40 to 60 mEq/day can be achieved by eating some of these foods. However, dietary potassium alone is not effective if hypochloremia and hypokalemia are present. In such situations, potassium drug supplementation should be given. If the patient has a low serum potassium or has evidence of hypokalemic changes in the ECG, potassium drug supplement may be given (Fig 16–3). Kassirer et al.[74] have shown that diuretic-induced hypochloremia and attendant metabolic alkalosis are often present with or without hypokalemia; therefore, in addition to potassium it is necessary to replace chloride ions. Potassium can best be given in the form of chloride (20 mEq of potassium two or three times daily). Enteric-coated potassium chloride tablets have been associated with small-bowel ulcerations and should be avoided. At times, hypokalemia may be prevented when a potent diuretic is being given by adding a potassium-sparing diuretic

Table 16–7. Potassium Dietary Supplements

Quantity	K Content (mEq)
Orange juice, 8 oz.	12.7
Tomato juice, 8 oz	14.0
Prune juice, 8 oz	14.4
Banana, 1 medium	16.1
Cauliflower, 10 oz	12.8
Figs, 7 small dried	20.0
Peaches, 4 oz dried	28.2
Wheat germ, 4 oz	18.9
Meat, chicken, fish, 4 oz	8.2
Skimmed milk, 8 oz	8.0

rather than giving a potassium supplement. Angiotensin-converting enzyme (ACE) inhibitors retain potassium. Potassium-sparing diuretics and potassium supplementation should be discontinued in patients receiving ACE inhibitors. In addition to hypokalemia, hypomagnesemia may occur when high doses of potent diuretics are given. It is wise to check serum potassium and magnesium levels frequently in patients taking diuretics, especially the elderly.

Drug interactions are frequently encountered with diuretic use. For example, thiazide diuretics increase the reabsorption of lithium given for manic-depressive psychosis and may precipitate confusion and toxic psychosis. Indomethacin, probably due to its inhibition of prostaglandin synthesis, may antagonize the effects of furosemide.[75] Furosemide may increase the risk of nephrotoxicity due to cephalothin when the two drugs are taken together. Salicylates (as little as 10 gr/day) can markedly reduce the natriuresis produced by spironolactone. The simultaneous use of furosemide and salicylates may lead to unusually high salicylate levels, producing toxicity.

VASODILATOR THERAPY

The treatment of congestive cardiac failure has been dramatically improved by the introduction of short- and long-term vasodilation therapy. This has given us a new approach to patients with heart failure, especially those refractory to conventional treatment. In fact, some physicians prefer vasodilator therapy as an initial treatment for heart failure in view of the frequent toxicity involved with the use of digitalis and diuretics.

In 1956 Burch[76] administered hexamethonium to patients in congestive heart failure for the purpose of increasing venous capacitance and thereby decreasing pulmonary congestion. At the same time Johnson et al.[77] used nitroglycerin to relieve dyspnea in patients with congestive heart failure secondary to left ventricular failure. Despite these early studies, and the widely accepted fact that systemic and venous resistance were increased in heart failure, it took many years for vasodilator therapy in normotensive heart failure to be clinically accepted. Mason[78] attributes this therapeutic lag to the preoccupation of traditional cardiology with contractility and preload as the major determinants of cardiac function. Patients with normal contractility operate on a point on the Frank-Starling curve that is preload-dependent, and in which case systemic vascular resistance (afterload) offers little, if any, inhibition to cardiac performance. However, the patient with myocardial dysfunction operates on the flat portion of the ventricular function curve and cardiac emptying (stroke volume, cardiac output, ejection fraction) becomes impedance-dependent (afterload). This "afterload mismatch" results from the activation of multiple neurohumoral factors which cause systemic and venous resistance to increase, resulting in abnormal cardiac hemodynamics, manifested as low output and congestive symptoms.

The arterial blood pressure is the product of the cardiac output and systemic vascular resistance. The cardiac output is determined by the stroke volume and heart rate. Left ventricular stroke volume is in turn determined by preload, contractility, and afterload. The patient with a reduced stroke volume due to an abnormality of cardiac contractility must adjust for the resultant drop in stroke volume and arterial blood pressure. Vasoconstrictor mechanisms are activated which increase heart rate and systemic vascular resistance, thereby maintaining arterial blood pressure and perfusion of the vital organs. Unfortunately, however, this same vasoconstriction increases left ventricular afterload, which further depresses the already abnormal cardiac performance. The increased activity of the sympathetic nerve system resulting in venous and systemic vasoconstriction is inappropriate in this setting. Arterial vasoconstriction reflexly decreases stroke volume by adding afterload to the already compromised ventricle, and (inappropriate) venoconstriction only worsens the already present pulmonary and systemic congestion. Because the ventricle is operating on a flat portion of the Frank-Starling curve, cardiac stimulation does not result in an increase in contractility. Finally, renal vasoconstriction results in further limitations of urine output and more circulatory congestion.

For whatever reason, in congestive heart failure various neurohumoral mechanisms are activated that result in inappropriate vasoconstriction and further depression of cardiac function. These neurohumoral mechanisms include, as mentioned above, the sympathetic nervous system with release of norepinephrine, stimulation of the renin-angiotensin-aldosterone system, sodium retention resulting from multiple mechanisms, including vasopressin activity, and enhanced smooth muscle tone in the vascular tree secondary to calcium. Vasodilator therapy and selection of the appropriate vasodilator are aimed at blocking or attenuating the vasoconstrictive effect of whatever neurohumoral mechanism is inappropriately activated in a given patient with heart failure. The sympathetic nervous system overactivity can be opposed by the administration of α-blocking drugs such as prazosin. Angiotensin-converting enzyme (ACE) inhibitors as captopril, enalapril, and lisinopril antagonize the renin-angiotensin-aldosterone system at the level of enzymatic conversion of angiotensin I to angiotensin II. This system can also be antagonized by drugs that reduce renin and by specific diuretics, such as spironolactone. The enhanced vascular tone secondary to calcium can be blocked by administration of systemically active calcium channel-blocking agents. In addition to these examples, vasodilation can result from drugs that directly relax smooth muscle tone in the walls of the inappropriately constricted venous and arterial beds, such as nitrates and hydralazine.

Table 16–8 lists the various vasodilators used for the treatment of heart failure. It is convenient to classify these agents on the basis of their principal site of action: preload reducing agents (venous-capacitance vasodilators), afterload reducing agents (arterial-resistance vasodilators), and combinations of preload and afterload reducing agents. Table 16–9 represents another type of classification, in which the vasodilator is classified according to its mechanism rather than site of action.

Nitrates are primarily venodilators that reduce preload and thereby aid in the alleviation of symptoms of pulmonary congestion and dyspnea. Since they reduce left ventricular volume, afterload is also reduced (according to LaPlace's law), and they also have a mild effect on reducing systemic vascular resistance.

The short-acting nitrate, sublingual nitroglycerin, directly relaxes smooth muscle of the systemic venous system. This results in pooling of blood in the capacitance vessels, decreasing preload, and reducing left ventricular size. The clinical corollary of these hemodynamic effects is a reduction in pulmonary

Table 16–8. Classification of Vasodilators According to Site of Action

Venous (capacitance) vasodilators
  Nitroglycerin (I.V., sublingual, transdermal)
  Isosorbide dinitrate (oral)

Arterial (resistance) vasodilators
  Hydralazine
  Minoxidil
  Phentolamine
  Nifedipine
  Diazoxide

Mixed (capacitance and resistance) vasodilators
  Sodium nitropursside
  Captopril, enalapril, lisinopril
  Prazosin
  Trimazosin

congestion (dyspnea) and, since left ventricular volume is decreased, myocardial oxygen consumption decreases and angina may be alleviated in patients with coronary artery disease. An increase in coronary blood flow, secondary to enhanced collateral flow or direct dilatation of ischemic coronary arteries, is another effect of nitroglycerin, making this drug a valuable agent for patients with ischemic heart disease and congestive failure. Unfortunately, the hemodynamic effects of sublingual nitroglycerin are short-lived, lasting less than 30 minutes.

The long-acting nitrates, such as isosorbide dinitrate, are available both sublingually and orally. Many studies have shown that the long-acting nitrates are effective in reducing left ventricular filling pressure, thereby improving symptoms of pulmonary congestion and alleviating angina. These favorable hemodynamic effects are seen for 5 to 6 hours following 20 to 40 mg of oral isosorbide dinitrate, and for up to 2 hours following 5 to 10 mg if given sublingually. Isosorbide dinitrate and related compounds are also available as

Table 16–9. Classification of Vasodilators According to Mechanism of Action

Direct vasodilators
  Nitroglycerin
  Isosorbide dinitrate
  Sodium nitroprusside
  Minoxidil
  Diazoxide

Sympathetic nervous system blockade
  Prazosin
  Trimazosin
  Phentolamine

Angiotensin-converting enzyme (ACE) inhibitors
  Captopril
  Enalapril
  Lisinopril

Calcium channel blockade
  Nifedipine

time-release capsules that may show an effect up to 8 to 12 hours.[79] These long-acting agents may be less reliable than the sublingual or cutaneous compounds, but have the advantage of better patient acceptability and drug compliance. Cutaneous forms of nitroglycerin have become popular. Nitrol ointment (2% strength) is applied at about 1 in. every 8 hours initially, but this can be increased in strength according to the patient's need and tolerance. Several transdermal methods (tranderm-nitro, nitro-dur, and nitro-disc) have made the delivery of nitroglycerin easier and much less messy by using a patch resembling an adhesive bandage. As yet, the exact dose of these transdermal patches for congestive heart failure is not known. However, it appears that relatively high doses as 60 mg/24 hr may be necessary to achieve good results.[80] A major problem with all sustained action nitrates is the development of tolerance. The mechanism of nitrate tolerance is not clear. Continued nitrate administration may produce a deficiency of reduced sulfhydryl groups and decreased production of nitrosothiols and cyclic GMP.[81] It is best to have the patient off these for several hours (nitrate-free period) per day, i.e., take off the nitro patch at night or omit the oral dose of isosorbide dinitrate at night to allow for recovery from tolerance. The nitrate can also produce headache and postural hypotension. Despite these concerns, the Veterans Administration Cooperative Heart Failure Trial randomly assigned 642 patients with chronic congestive failure with impaired cardiac function and reduced exercise tolerance to placebo, prazosin, or the combination of hydralazine and isosorbide dinitrate.[82] They showed that isosorbide dinitrate and hydralazine, when added to the therapeutic regimen of digoxin and diuretics in patients with chronic congestive heart failure, can prolong life and have a favorable effect on left ventricular function. In this study, this combination reduced mortality at the end of 2 years by 34% and at 3 years by 23% as compared with placebo, whereas prazosin was not different from placebo. However, a later preliminary report revealed that exercise tolerance improved very little with hydralazine and nitrates.[82a]

Because the nitrates have such a limited effect on systemic vascular resistance, they are not generally effective in increasing cardiac output and alleviating low-output symptoms. After diuretics and nitrates have been used to return the patient to his most optimal position on the Frank-Starling curve, hydralazine (afterload reducing agent) can be added to lower systemic vascular resistance and thereby increase cardiac output.[83] One should start with a 25 to 50-mg dose every 6 to 8 hours, but this can be advanced as needed. It is interesting that even at high doses, such as 400 mg per day, hydralazine does not usually cause orthostatic hypotension or reflex tachycardia. This is probably because the decrease in systemic vascular resistance improves left ventricular stroke volume sufficiently to maintain or increase the arterial pressure, thereby removing the stimulus for reflex tachycardia. Furthermore, enhanced adrenergic activity secondary to long-standing heart failure may also blunt the expected reflex tachycardia when vasodilators are used. One report suggests that the response to oral hydralazine is similar to that seen with acute I.V. studies, and that these favorable hemodynamic responses are sustained.[84] However, Packer et al.[85] have shown that drug-specific tolerance may account for the lack of clinical improvement in some patients who receive long-term hydralazine for severe heart failure. Yet, other oral vasodilators were still effective when this occurred. High doses of hydralazine can produce a lupus-like syndrome.

Minoxidil is similar to hydralazine in its ability to dilate the systemic vascular tree, thereby reducing impedance to left ventricular emptying and improving low output symptoms. Franciosa and Cohn[86] have demonstrated the favorable hemodynamic and clinical effects of Minoxidil in patients with severe congestive heart failure. However, this drug is associated with certain side effects, including hirsutism and sodium retention, which may limit its widespread usefulness.

Phentolamine, prazosin, and nitroprusside have a balanced effect on the arterial and venous beds (preload and afterload reducing agents). Clinical improvement results from this balanced action as manifested by alleviation of symptoms of pulmonary congestion as well as enhanced cardiac output (less fatigue). Phentolamine was initially used in 1971 by Majid et al.[87] and was actually the first pharmacologic agent used specifically for impedance reduction in normotensive patients with heart failure. It is an α-adrenergic blocking agent, and clinical experiences with these drugs have mainly been with I.V. administration.

Prazosin was initially classified as a direct-acting vasodilator, but is now known to exert its effect as a result of α-adrenergic blockade. The cardiovascular effects of oral prazosin are virtually identical to those of nitroprusside, suggesting it as the drug of choice for ambulatory use when IV nitroprusside is discontinued.[88] It has a theoretical advantage over other α-adrenergic blockers due to its selectivity for postsynaptic α_1-adrenergic receptors. It has been suggested that the failure of prazosin to block the presynaptic α_2-adrenergic receptor accounts for the relative lack of tachycardia when hypotension is produced. Although its similarity to nitroprusside and its long action (6 hours) make prazosin an attractive agent for ambulatory use, several reports indicate limitations to its effectiveness. One such study indicated that while prazosin increased cardiac output and stroke volume significantly during exercise, these changes were not present at rest.[89] More important, different investigators have reported the development of clinical tolerance (improperly termed tachyphylaxis) to the effects of prazosin resulting in attenuation of its favorable initial response.[90,91] Some feel that the favorable response can be restored with further diuretic administration or omitting it for 1 to 2 weeks. Avan and Mason[92] consider the attenuation of prazosin that occurs in about one third of patients to be of two types. Early subacute attenuation can occur temporarily which they relate to the interaction of the α_1- (blocked by prazosin) and α_2-receptors. With continuous therapy this attenuation is lost. The second type of attenuation, they state, occurs months later and is the result of body salt and water retention that often is noted with all types of vasodilators. They stimulate the renin-angiotensin system and may activate the sympathetic nervous system. This can be abated by captopril or by elevating the diuretic dosage and particularly by the use of spironolactone, thus correcting the secondary hyperaldosteronism due to the increased activity of the renin-angiotensin system, which often accompanies chronic vasodilator therapy in congestive heart failure. Prazosin can produce sudden unexpected hypotension, and has even been reported to cause syncope as a result of interaction with nitroglycerin.[93] I generally administer the first dose (1 mg) at bedtime to minimize this risk.

This first-dose phenomenon has actually been reported only in hypertensive patients and has not been a problem in patients treated with prazosin for congestive heart failure in my experience. The usual maintenance dosage is 2 to 6 mg every 8 hours.

Nitroprusside[94] was used initially for normotensive heart failure in 1972. Since then, it has undergone extensive investigation and continues to be valuable for the treatment of acute heart failure and for acute exacerbations of chronic heart failure. Like phentolamine and prazosin, its hemodynamic effects alleviate symptoms of pulmonary congestion as well as low output. I feel that therapy should be instituted only in an intensive care setting, usually with pulmonary artery and systemic pressure monitoring. I generally start at a low dosage, such as 0.25 μg/kg/min to avoid undesirable excessive falls in BP which could compromise coronary and cerebral perfusion. The left ventricular filling pressure should be lowered to the lowest pressure at which cardiac output is maintained at a normal level. Patients given nitroprusside for longer than 48 hours should have monitoring of serum thiocyanate levels to avoid thiocyanate toxicity, which is a definite threat, particularly if renal function is impaired. Cyanide toxicity is less of a threat because of the rapid conversion of cyanide to thiocyanate in the liver. However, in patients with significant liver disease, as may occur secondary to tricuspid insufficiency, cyanide poisoning could occur. The toxic manifestations range from muscular weakness to nausea, epigastric discomfort, hypothyroidism, convulsions, psychosis, and cyanosis secondary to methemoglobinemia.[95] Should thiocyanate toxicity develop, hemodialysis may be lifesaving, since the thiocyanate ion is readily removed through this process. Other research has shown that infusions of sodium nitrate, thiosulfate, or hydroxocobalamin are helpful and are indicated when stopping the nitroprusside infusion alone is inadequate.[94] A recent report described significant hemodynamic deterioration as a rebound phenomenon after abrupt withdrawal of nitroprusside.[96] This appears to be due to the unopposed activation of reflex vasoconstrictive forces. Therefore, nitroprusside should be tapered when the drug has been used for several hours or at high doses.

It is an oversimplification to describe the compensatory mechanism of enhanced adrenergic tone in congestive heart failure as simply "increased sympathetic tone." As pointed out by Zellis et al.,[97] this sympathetic tone can be primarily neuronally mediated (nerve terminals releasing norepinephrine), hormonally mediated (direct effect of norepinephrine or angiotensin), or enhanced sensitivity of the vasculature to sympathetic tone and circulating hormones. Different types of heart failure tend to utilize these mechanisms to varying degrees. Many of these mechanisms can be treated to reduce peripheral vascular resistance besides smooth muscle dilatation as produced by hydralazine. Angiotensin-converting enzyme (ACE) inhibitors have provided a new approach to treating heart failure. Diuretics and arteriolar vasodilators activate the renin-angiotensin-aldosterone system and thus they may increase the need for ACE inhibitors.

Teprotide (IV) and captopril (orally) inhibit angiotensin-converting enzyme, thereby reducing the elevated systemic vascular resistance present in heart failure. Curtiss et al.[98] used teprotide in 15 patients with severe chronic left ventricular failure and noted a reduction in ventricular filling pressures and an increase in cardiac output, with the most favorable hemodynamic responses noted in patients with the highest peripheral renin activity. This study demonstrated not only the benefit of blocking of angiotensin II for the treatment of congestive heart failure, but also indicates the important role of hemodynamic typing prior to the selection of a vasodilator in the treatment of congestive heart failure. Other investigators[99] studying teprotide found that, although total vascular resistance decreased and cardiac function improved due to the reduction in afterload, the responses were independent of the level of plasma renin activity suggesting that the mechanism of hemodynamic improvement was incompletely understood. More recently, Levine et al.[100] studied resting hemodynamic and neurohumoral measurements (including catecholamine and renin activity levels) in patients with chronic congestive heart failure. Although plasma norepinephrine and plasma renin activity levels were significantly higher than normal, the degree of hemodynamic abnormality did not correlate with plasma renin activity. These findings are consistent with the multiple and complex neurohumoral responses noted in patients with congestive heart failure of various degree and chronicity.

The oral inhibitor of angiotensin-converting enzyme captopril has also been shown to reduce ventricular filling pressures and systemic vascular resistance and so alleviate pulmonary congestion and increase cardiac output. Plasma renin activity has been demonstrated to increase, while plasma norepinephrine and aldosterone levels decrease.[101] Davis et al.[102] have used captopril over a long term in a limited number of patients and demonstrated maintenance of clinical improvement on long-term treatment. In this study, plasma renin activity levels did not correlate with the effect of captopril, suggesting that multiple compensatory mechanisms were involved. Although hypotension was described in the patients treated with captopril during the acute phase, no untoward effects were noted with chronic therapy.

Captopril may be one of the most effective vasodilators for the treatment of advanced congestive heart failure (when the renin-angiotensin-aldosterone system may be active) because it blocks the formation of angiotensin II (thus reducing afterload) and it also inhibits the adrenal release of aldosterone and so inhibits sodium retention that sometimes accompanies the effect of other vasodilator agents. Indirectly, it down-regulates the sympathetic nervous system and stimulates the production of vasodilating prostaglandins. In addition, it produces venodilation (thus reducing preload). The mechanism of its venodilator action is not clear, but it may be due to the fact that it prevents deactivation of bradykinin, which is a potent vasodilator of the venous and arteriolar beds. Packer et al.[103] compared the hemodynamic responses of captopril and nitroprusside, and it appeared that captopril produced less of an effect on reducing venous capacitance, but a greater effect than nitroprusside in reducing left ventricular filling (which indicates an effect on compliance). Furthermore, this study of 15 patients demonstrated the intrinsic negative chronotropic effect of the drug (decreased heart rate) and the ability of captopril to reduce left ventricular compliance. Captopril also may improve renal perfusion, increase the GFR, and reduce prerenal azotemia, which often occurs with heart failure and the use of diuretics. However, it is important to observe for hypotension, which can produce renal dysfunction. Side effects such as proteinuria, loss of taste, hyperkalemia, skin rash, and neutropenia are rare and reversible. However, captopril should be used with caution in patients with impaired renal function or serious autoimmune disease (particularly SLE). The starting dosage is usually 6.5 to 25 mg three times per day.

Enalapril (Vasotec) and lisinopril (Prinivil, Zestril) are also now available.[104] These agents require longer to reach a peak effect. Captopril begins to act in 30 minutes and has a peak effect between 60 and 90 minutes and persists for 6 to 8 hours. Enalapril is a pro-drug ACE inhibitor, in that it is hydrolyzed in the liver to the active form, enalaprilat. It has a slower onset and longer duration of action (12 to 24 hours) than captopril. The dosage ranges between 2.5 to 20 mg b.i.d. Lisinopril also requires longer to peak because of slower absorption. It can be given once daily (usual dosage 2.5 to 20 mg). ACE inhibitors with a prolonged action are more likely to produce renal or cerebral insufficiency in patients with severe chronic heart failure by producing prolonged hypotension.[105] This occurs more in patients with low blood pressure, diabetes, or large diuretic dosages. All ACE inhibitors can be given safely if one observes for hypotension and rising renal function abnormalities and adjusts dosage accordingly.[106] Many studies have documented the acute and long-term hemodynamic improvement, increase in exercise capacity, and alleviation of symptoms in patients with severe heart failure (refractory to diuretics and digitalis). In addition, they have shown benefit in mild to moderate heart failure. A multi-center, double-blind, placebo-controlled study compared the effects of captopril treatment with those of digoxin treatment during maintenance diuretic therapy in patients with mild to moderate heart failure.[107] The captopril group showed improvement in exercise tolerance and the digoxin group in ejection fractions. The number of premature beats decreased 45% in the captopril group and increased 4% in the digoxin group in patients with more than 10 ventricular premature beats per hour. The study concluded that a diuretic alone should not be the treatment of choice for a patient with mild to moderate heart failure and that captopril is an alternative to digoxin therapy. The consensus trial study randomly assigned 253 patients in a double-blind study to receive either placebo or enalapril (2.5 to 40 mg per day) in patients with severe congestive heart failure (NYHA class IV).[108] Conventional treatment for heart failure including the use of other vasodilators was continued in both groups. At the end of 6 months, the crude mortality was 26% in the enalapril group and 44% in the placebo group (a reduction of 40%). Mortality at 1 year was reduced by 31% and by the end of the study up to 20 months, there was a reduction of 27%. The beneficial effect on mortality was due to a reduction in death from the progression of heart failure and not in incidence of sudden cardiac death. A second Veterans Administration trial will compare the effect of enalapril versus hydralazine plus isosorbide dinitrate on the prognosis in congestive heart failure. The Studies of Left Ventricular Dysfunction (SOLVD) trial sponsored by the National Institutes of Health is randomizing a symptomatic congestive heart failure group to an ACE inhibitor or placebo to determine survival in a broader population. In addition, another part of this study includes asymptomatic patients with left ventricular ejection fractions <35% who are randomized to determine if ACE inhibitors prevent progression to more severe chronic congestive heart failure and prolong life. In summary, the evidence indicates that vasodilator therapy not only improves symptoms and cardiac function in patients with heart failure, but also may prolong life.

Calcium antagonists, such as verapamil, nifedipine, diltiazem, and the prostaglandins, are being investigated as vasodilator agents for use in congestive heart failure. Calcium channel blocking agents by inhibiting excitation-contraction in vascular smooth muscle are potent coronary and peripheral artery dilators. The net hemodynamic effect of these agents results from a complex interplay of direct and reflex effects. Nifedipine increases myocardial oxygen supply by coronary vasodilatation and decreases myocardial oxygen demand by decreasing afterload. Cardiac output increases, but there is a variable effect on left ventricular filling pressure, which may increase and cause clinical worsening. Verapamil and diltiazem exert somewhat similar effects (but less so than nifedipine) and also aid in supraventricular arrhythmias.

Calcium channel-blocking agents should be used with caution in patients with abnormal left ventricular systolic function. When the ejection fraction is moderately or severely reduced, verapamil should be avoided, because of this drug's particularly potent in situ negative inotropic effect. Even in normal or mildly compromised ventricles, verapamil should be given carefully or withheld if β-blocker drugs are used. In patients with moderate or severely compromised ventricular function, diltiazem or nifedipine would be drugs of choice, but both must be used with caution. Diltiazem has little effect on the systemic vascular tree, and although it is not a potent vasodilator, it may be used safely in patients with congestive heart failure because of its relatively mild negative inotropic effect. In patients with severely compromised ventricles (ejection fraction less than 25%) we recommend consideration of hemodynamic monitoring (Swan-Ganz catheter) before institution of calcium channel blockers in these patients.

OLD AND NEW POSITIVE INOTROPIC AGENTS

Dopamine (Intropin), dobutamine (Dobutrex), and isoproterenol (Isuprel) are intravenous positive inotropic agents. Oral positive inotropic agents include digitalis preparations (already discussed), amrinone and milrinone (still investigational), sympathomimetic drugs (such as ephedrine), and other drugs (such as terbutaline) not generally thought of as cardiotonic agents.

Dopamine has been the I.V. positive inotropic agent of choice for several years, particularly when the systolic blood pressure is borderline or reduced. Its efficacy in patients with chronic refractory congestive heart failure is well established.[109] At low doses (2 to 5 μg/kg/min), dopaminergic receptors are stimulated resulting in renal and mesenteric vasodilatation. This can result in diuresis even before a positive inotropic effect is demonstrated. The efficacy of diuretics can be enhanced through the concommitant use of dopamine. At high doses, >20 μg/kg/min, dopamine's α-adrenergic actions predominate, in which case BP is maintained at the expense of increased cardiac afterload (vasoconstrictor effect). Activation of the α-receptors in the venous bed causes venoconstriction, with a resulting increase in pulmonary pressures and left ventricular filling pressures. Volume expansion, under the guide of pulmonary artery pressure monitoring, should be done before the institution of dopamine, so that the drug's maximum inotropic effect can be realized at the lowest possible dose, thereby minimizing α stimulation and reducing adverse effects. In addition to the elevation of ventricular filling pressures, significant adverse effects of dopamine are ventricular arrhythmias secondary to direct cardiac stimulation. Rarely, nausea and vomiting limit its usefulness.

Dobutamine is a synthetic derivative of isoproterenol with strong β_1-receptor activity and a minor degree of β_2- and α-receptor stimulation.[110] Unlike with dopamine, this α effect is not clinically important. It directly enhances myocardial contractility, but, importantly, has less of a tendency to induce tachycardia than its parent drug, isoproterenol. Its effect is very similar to that of combined dopamine and nitroprusside; it is often used in cardiogenic shock as a substitute for this combination when the α stimulation of dopamine should be avoided.[111] Francis et al.[112] compared dopamine and dobutamine in acute low-output cardiac failure. Nine patients with acute circulatory collapse were studied, 5 of whom had cardiogenic shock. Although both drugs improved the cardiac index, dopamine produced a greater increase in mean arterial pressure; but left ventricular filling pressure also increased with dopamine, while tending to decrease with dobutamine. Systemic vascular resistance decreased with dobutamine and was unchanged with dopamine. Although stroke work index improved to the same extent with both agents, this occurred with dopamine at a higher filling pressure. Tolerance to dobutamine may occur during continuous, long-term infusion.[113]

Isoproterenol is a pure β-agonist which produces an increase in cardiac output through its positive inotropic as well as peripheral vasodilatory effects. Unfortunately, its marked increased chronotropic and arrhythmogenic effects limit its usefulness particularly in patients with coronary artery disease. I use isoproterenol only when low cardiac output states are complicated by bradyarrhythmias or high-degree AV block, and even then only until temporary cardiac pacing can be achieved. Isoproterenol may be the vasopressor of choice in patients with hypotension or acute right-sided heart failure secondary to pulmonary embolism, since the drug possesses direct pulmonary and bronchial vasodilatory properties.

Amrinone is a bipyridine derivative that has been shown to exert a strong positive inotropic effect in both experimental animals[114] and man. No toxicity was observed when the drug was administered to 8 patients with congestive heart failure already receiving full doses of digitalis.[115] In this study, cardiac index and peak rate of late ventricular pressure rise increased, while ventricular filling pressures decreased and heart rate remained unchanged. Systemic vascular resistance is also reduced. Another study[116] showed that amrinone improved the function of the failing heart at rest and during exercise in patients with chronic heart failure refractory to digitalis, diuretics, and vasodilators. The mechanism of action is due to its inhibition of myocardial and vascular phosphodiesterase. The level of cyclic AMP increases in the myocardium and promotes increased calcium influx and increased contractility. Apparently it does not act through inhibition of the sodium potassium ATPase pump. Sustained beneficial effects on cardiac and renal function have been reported in patients with refractory heart failure given oral doses of 300 to 900 mg per day. However, long-term therapy has been complicated by the occurrence of thrombocytopenia. This appears to be dose-related. Low doses give a positive inotropic effect but have less direct arterial vasodilatory effect. One study[117] showed a beneficial effect of low doses with a hydralazine-amrinone combination without producing thrombocytopenia.

Amrinone has been approved for intravenous use in patients with refractory congestive heart failure. The recommended intravenous dose is 0.5 to 1.5 mg/ kg as I.V. bolus and continuous injection at a rate up to 10 μg/kg/min. It may be used concomitantly with digoxin, diuretics, and vasodilators. It has not been approved for oral use. Baim and colleagues[118] reported the results of using milrinone, a derivative of amrinone, in patients with severe congestive heart failure. Intravenous milrinone resulted in significant decreases in filling pressures and systemic vascular resistance, while cardiac index increased. The positive inotropic effect of the compound was demonstrated by the increase in the peak positive first derivative of left ventricular pressure with a simultaneous decrease in heart rate. Nineteen of 20 patients who received oral milrinone for up to 11 months showed sustained improvement in symptoms of heart failure, and in 10 patients radionuclide ventriculography showed increases in left ventricular ejection fraction. In a subsequent report, they followed 100 patients on oral milrinone for severe congestive heart failure for over 2½ years.[119] Despite hemodynamic and clinical improvements, there was no evidence of improvement in the high baseline mortality of this disorder. Unlike amrinone, the drug did not cause fever or thrombocytopenia. One study randomly assigned 230 patients in sinus rhythm with moderately severe heart failure to treatment with digoxin, milrinone, both, or placebo.[119a] Milrinone increased exercise tolerance and reduced the frequency of worsened heart failure, but it, alone or in combination with digoxin, offered no advantage over digoxin alone. In fact it may aggravate ventricular arrhythmias. At present, studies do not show that milrinone changes the long-term prognosis of patients with severe heart failure, even though they have had a beneficial symptomatic response. It is still under active investigation.

Terbutaline, thought to be predominantly a selective β_2-agonist, has been demonstrated to have a positive inotropic effect when studied by radionuclear angiography in patients with chronic obstructive pulmonary disease and coronary artery disease.[120] The significance of this and similar studies with drugs previously thought to exert little or no significant cardiac effects remains to be determined. However, the clinician must be aware of these potential drug effects and interactions if he is to use cardiac medications rationally in the patient with congestive heart failure. This is particularly true in the subset of congestive heart failure patients with ischemic heart disease in whom the added positive inotropic effect may increase myocardial oxygen demand to the point of inducing angina.

ARRHYTHMIAS IN CONGESTIVE HEART FAILURE

Although survival can be related to the extent of cardiac dysfunction, many patients with congestive heart failure die suddenly. Holter monitoring has revealed a high prevalence of simple and complex arrhythmias. There are many factors predisposing to arrhythmias, such as increased catecholamine and electrolyte abnormalities. Treatment with ACE inhibitors reduces the frequency of ventricular arrhythmias, but as yet it is not known if this will have a favorable impact on mortality or sudden death.[121] The high incidence of sudden death in patients with congestive heart failure suggests that antiarrhythmic agents may be of benefit, but controlled studies are lacking. Dargie et al.[122] in an uncontrolled study showed that amiodarone improved survival.

SUMMARY OF TREATMENT OF CHRONIC HEART FAILURE DUE PRIMARILY TO SYSTOLIC DYSFUNCTION

Although preliminary studies[107] are encouraging for the use of vasodilators as initial therapy in mild to moderate congestive heart failure, I still prefer to use standard therapy (restricted activity, digitalis, and diuretics) in most cases until further data become available. Naturally, if the patient is not responding adequately, vasodilators should be added. ACE inhibitors are an acceptable alternative to digoxin, especially when the latter is not well tolerated. ACE inhibitors may limit potassium loss and in combination with a diuretic may be effective as initial therapy. A diuretic may be the first-line drug if edema is the major factor. Therefore, at present, any of the three drug classes (diuretics, vasodilators, or inotropic agents) can be considered as first-line therapy depending on other factors. For severe heart failure, vasodilators should be used initially with standard therapy. Diuretics should be used properly to avoid electrolyte problems. It is best to start with furosemide administered intermittently and then daily with spironolactone if evidence of congestive heart failure continues. In some instances, triamterene or amiloride may be more effective than spironolactone. Since diuretics act at different sites, they can complement each other. A potent and effective combination is furosemide with metolazone, which requires very close follow-up for electrolyte imbalances. In the event of hypochloremia, acetazolamide given intermittently may restore diuresis, provided that kidney function is good. In some instances, patients have required 160 mg or more of furosemide each day, 50 to 100 mg spironolactone twice per day, metolazone 2.5 to 10 mg daily, and 250 mg of acetazolamide three times per day for 3 days of each week. At times, a slow I.V. infusion of 250 to 500 mg of theophylline ethylenediamide (aminophylline) given 1 hour after a diuretic will potentiate diuresis by increasing the GFR and, by its positive inotropic effect, the cardiac output. Vasodilators have altered the frequent need for such maximum use of diuretics with their potential for toxicity. As mentioned previously, studies have shown that ACE inhibitors prolong life and improve symptoms and a combination of hydralazine and isosorbide dinitrate improve survival but produce little benefit in exercise tolerance.[82,82a] ACE inhibitors also have fewer side effects. Therefore, at present, I prefer ACE inhibitors and use hydralazine and nitrate in combination as an alternatie approach in those who do not respond well or do not tolerate ACE inhibitors because of side effects (namely hypotension).

At times, in severe heart failure, amrinone or dobutamine I.V. for 48 to 72 hours may be useful in the treatment of patients refractory to combination therapy of digitalis, diuretics, and vasodilators. These are especially helpful if there is an acute factor that aggravated the chronic congestive failure and can be reversed. On rare occasions, peritoneal or hemodialysis may be used to remove excessive water and sodium. Such procedures may help restore cardiac decompensation and allow the usual forms of therapy to regain their response.

Several major trials are now in progress in patients with congestive heart failure which may answer more clearly the following important questions: What is the preferable initial therapy? When should vasodilators be used? Which is the preferable vasodilator? Is survival improved with vasodilators in a broader population as compared with earlier trials? Which of the newer vasodilators and inotropic agents are promising? Do antiarrhythmic drugs prevent sudden death in patients with chronic congestive heart failure?

TREATMENT OF HEART FAILURE DUE PRIMARILY TO DIASTOLIC DYSFUNCTION

At present there is no effective treatment for heart failure in all conditions with diastolic dysfunction. Constrictive pericarditis and mitral stenosis can be improved dramatically with surgery. Some patients with hypertrophic cardio-myopathy may benefit from calcium blockers. Hypertensive hypertrophy with impaired ventricular filling can be controlled by the use of antihypertensive agents such as ACE inhibitors, antiadrenergic drugs, or calcium blockers. It is important to realize that the standard therapy for heart failure due to systolic dysfunction such as digitalis, diuretics and vasodilators may be harmful to some patients with diastolic dysfunction and lead to low output or hypotension. However, diuretics and vasodilators may be beneficial in some situations such as hypertensive hypertrophy with diastolic dysfunction, normal ejection fraction, and acute pulmonary edema.

ACUTE PULMONARY EDEMA

Acute pulmonary edema is a dramatic event that may be the initial manifestation of cardiac disease in a patient or may occur in a known cardiac. The usual cause is disease of the left side of the heart, such as aortic stenosis or insufficiency, hypertension, coronary artery disease, mitral valve disease, tachyarrhythmias, or fluid overload of the circulation, but there are many rarer causes. Pulmonary edema is a true, urgent medical emergency and requires initiating therapy immediately.

The patient has labored breathing and is frightened. Pink, frothy sputum may be produced, and wet rales are present. Because of orthopnea, patients prefer to sit or stand. It is best for the legs to be dependent, thus providing internal venesection; of course, a patient in shock should be recumbent.

At times it may be difficult clinically to differentiate acute pulmonary edema from severe asthmatic bronchitis. Measurements of pulmonary capillary wedge pressure by means of a Swan-Ganz catheter usually reveal a pressure exceeding 25 mm Hg in acute pulmonary edema.

Therapy is aimed at reducing left ventricular end-diastolic pressure by increasing myocardial contractility (allowing the heart to produce an increased stroke volume at a lower filling pressure), reducing directly the preload (ventricular filling pressure), and reducing the afterload (peripheral vascular resistance).

Morphine is a most valuable drug for acute pulmonary edema. Three to 5 mg can be given initially by slow I.V. injection and repeated if necessary in 15 minutes. In mild cases 8 to 10 mg can be given subcutaneously. By slowing the respiratory rate and thereby reducing the work on the ventilatory muscles, morphine allows better oxygen exchange. It allays anxiety. It also produces internal venesection by causing venous pooling in the extremities. It reduces preload and afterload by decreasing the central sympathetic outflow which produces venous and arteriolar constriction. The drug should not be used, however, in patients with severe chronic lung disease.

Oxygen by mask or nasal catheter is beneficial. If arterial oxygen tensions cannot be maintained at 60 mm Hg, or progressive hypercapnia occurs, mechanical ventilation may be necessary.

Furosemide has been shown in congestive heart failure following acute myocardial infarction to produce clinical and hemodynamic improvement prior to its diuretic effect. This is due to its venodilatory effect, which is manifested as a reduction in pulmonary capillary wedge pressure.[73] It does very little to elevate cardiac output. It appears to be most helpful for pulmonary edema that occurs during chronic congestive heart failure. The usual dosage is 20 to 80 mg I.V.

Digitalis given I.V. may be useful depending on the etiology of the pulmonary edema. It is especially beneficial for slowing the ventricular rate in patients with atrial fibrillation secondary to mitral stenosis where the short diastolic filling period has increased the left atrial pressure. In other conditions, one must be cautious if the patient has a regular sinus rhythm and has been receiving long-term digitalis therapy. If the patient has not been taking digitalis and has a regular sinus rhythm and has systolic left ventricular dysfunction, digitalis may be beneficial.

Vasodilators reduce pulmonary and systemic vascular pressure and have become important agents in pulmonary edema. They reduce preload and afterload and so reduce pulmonary congestion and increase the cardiac output. Sodium nitroprusside reduces both preload and afterload and can be started intravenously at 20 μg/min and increased accordingly. Arterial pressure should be monitored to avoid hypotension. Nitrates are also useful, since they reduce preload by inducing venodilation. Vasodilators are best for acute pulmonary edema secondary to systemic hypertension.

Theophylline, 5 mg/kg, can be given by I.V. infusion over a 10-minute period followed by a constant infusion of 0.5 mg/kg/hr. Blood levels should be performed to avoid side effects (optimal blood levels range from 10 to 20 mg/liter). It increases myocardial contractility and decreases preload. It is most effective when severe bronchospasm is present. Caution is necessary, since too-rapid administration can cause arrhythmias and vascular collapse.

If the aforementioned measures are not effective in relieving pulmonary edema, attempts should be made to decrease the preload by using tourniquets or venesection. The tourniquets should be applied to three extremities at a pressure that does not impair blood flow and should be moved to a different extremity, in rotation, every 15 minutes. When the pulmonary edema has cleared, the tourniquets should be removed slowly, one at a time; rapid release of all three at the same time may cause recurrence of edema. Tourniquets should not be used when shock is present. Venesection of about 500 ml of blood (rarely necessary) may be beneficial, particularly in patients who are hypertensive or have chronic heart failure with increased blood volume.

In the presence of pulmonary edema, arrhythmias should be treated actively and cardioversion used if necessary. Other precipitating factors, such as myocardial ischemia or infarction, fluid overload, infections, pulmonary emboli, severe hypertension, or severe anemia, should be identified and treated.

Figure 16–4 shows the chest x rays, before and after therapy, of a 36-year-old man with coronary artery disease and acute pulmonary edema.

REFRACTORY HEART FAILURE

If the patient continues in heart failure after receiving every known form of therapy, the problem should be re-evaluated. Often, reviewing the problem

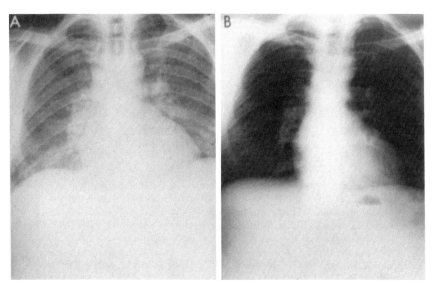

Fig 16–4. 36-year-old man with coronary artery disease and acute pulmonary edema. **A,** x ray during acute pulmonary edema. **B,** x ray after therapy shows clearing of the pulmonary congestion.

unveils overlooked clues. Too often, because of multiple past admissions with many records, we accept past findings. The diagnosis should be firmly established; the dyspnea may be due to underlying lung disease, the edema to venous stasis or renal or hepatic disease. M mode and two-dimensional echocardiography have proved extremely helpful in identifying surgically correctable cardiac lesions such as valvular disease, intracardiac shunts, and left ventricular aneurysms. Radionuclide studies, such as the multigated nuclear angiogram, are also helpful in distinguishing lesions such as left ventricular aneurysm from congestive cardiomyopathy, particularly in patients with technically suboptimal echocardiographic studies. Many studies have confirmed an excellent correlation between this type of cardiac imaging and cineangiography. Precipitating and contributing factors should be sought. Thyrotoxicosis in the elderly may be silent (apathetic hyperthyroidism), except for atrial fibrillation and cardiac decompensation. T_3 thyrotoxicosis may not be detected on routine thyroid function studies and should be ruled out by measuring T_3 by radioimmunoassay technique. Anemia may be a cause of high-output failure, or contribute to coronary insufficiency particularly in elderly patients with coronary atherosclerosis. Rheumatic myocarditis may be the cause of cardiac decompensation in patients with rheumatic heart disease, rather than the more commonly suspected valvular cause. Other types of myocarditis, such as infectious or toxic (alcoholic), can precipitate congestive heart failure. Because most alcoholics deny or seriously underestimate the volume of alcohol intake, family members must be questioned to establish the most accurate history. Recurrent pulmonary emboli may result in pulmonary hypertension with subsequent right heart failure and eventually biventricular failure. This should be suspected in patients with a risk factor profile consistent with deep vein thrombosis, including the otherwise healthy woman taking oral contraceptives as a form of birth control. Although aortic valve endocarditis is usually a fulminant condition presenting with left ventricular failure, mitral valve endocarditis may be much more subtle in its presentation and should not be discounted. During a 3-year period at our institution, only 14% of patients with mitral valve endocarditis presented primarily because of congestive heart failure. The vast majority had constitutional symptoms of fatigue, weight loss, and anemia, despite echocardiographic evaluation revealing prominent left ventricular volume overloading, and occasionally even flail leaflets secondary to destruction produced by the infection. Endocarditis involving the right-sided cardiac valve, particularly the tricuspid valve, is most often secondary to intravenous drug abuse. Although many patients have a chief complaint of fever and other constitutional symptoms, congestive heart failure (particularly right-sided heart failure) may be the most prominent complaint.

Silent coronary artery disease, such as in the diabetic patient unable to experience angina, may precipitate acute congestive heart failure or result in a deterioration in a previously compensated patient. It is not unusual for even nondiabetic patients, however, to have an acute myocardial infarction and pulmonary edema with no complaint of chest pain. In this case, the dyspnea is so much more prominent than the chest pain that the patient does not admit to chest pain that would otherwise indicate the etiology of the cardiac decompensation.

Systemic infections increase the work of the heart, and pulmonary infections add an extra burden by producing arterial hypoxemia. Digitalis toxicity, particularly when complicated by bradyarrhythmias, may be a cause of refractory heart failure. Tachyarrhythmias (such as atrial fibrillation with a rapid ventricular response) or bradyarrhythmias can precipitate or aggravate cardiac decompensation.

Refractory heart failure in renal disease is multifactorial, resulting from anemia, volume overload, electrolyte imbalance, and digitalis intoxication.

Excessive salt intake and dietary indiscretion, generally leading to obesity, is a frequent cause of refractory heart failure. Overactivity may be a problem, particularly in patients in whom denial of heart disease is prominent.

Poorly controlled hypertension increases the work of the heart by increasing left ventricular afterload. Excessive restriction of sodium and diuresis can produce an electrolyte imbalance such as hypokalemia, hypochloremia, or hyponatremia.

In this era of polypharmacy, drug interactions and the use of drugs with negative inotropic effects are not uncommon causes of refractory heart failure (Table 16–10). Prominent among these are propranolol and other β-blockers, which can exacerbate heart failure due to their negative inotropic effect. However, a report showed that propranolol might be safer to use than originally thought.[123] When it was given to 24 patients with severe myocardial dysfunction secondary to congestive cardiomyopathy, myocardial function improved in all treated patients except one, and the survival in 1 year (83%) was twice that of the control group (46%). Obviously one must individualize treatment, but even with propranolol's negative inotropic effect, patients with resting tachycardia may realize an improvement in ventricular function due to a reduction in myocardial oxygen consumption when the heart rate slows. Whether or not β-blocking agents with intrinsic sympathomimetic activity (pindolol) enhance the safety of β-blocker therapy in patients with cardiac failure remains to be

Table 16–10. Drug Interactions With Digitalis

Increase Sensitivity to Digitalis	Increase Resistance to Digitalis
Glucagon	Neomycin
Glucose	Cholestyramine (Cuemid, Questran)
β-blockers	Kaopectate
Reserpine	Aluminum and magnesium
Succinylcholine (Anectine)	hydroxides (Maalox)
Sympathomimetics	Barbiturates*
Calcium	Diphenylhydantoin* (Dilantin)
Corticosteroids	Phenylbutazone* (Butazolidin)
Diuretics	Vasodilators
Antithyroid drugs	
Quinidine	
Spironolactone	
Antibiotics	

*Inhibit effect of digitoxin.

convincingly demonstrated. Similarly, verapamil has been studied in 20 patients without congestive heart failure.[124] Despite concern about the drug's negative myocardial inotropic effect, ejection fraction (measured by contrast radiography) and cardiac output increased, probably due to the drug's reduction in systemic vascular resistance. Disopyramide's and flecainide's negative inotropic effect may aggravate or precipitate heart failure.

Drug interactions are important in terms of increasing or decreasing the sensitivity to digitalis. Certain drugs, such as glucagon, glucose, β-blockers, reserpine, anectine, calcium, corticosteroids, diuretics, antithyroid drugs, sympathomimetics, spironolactone,[125] and quinidine will increase the sensitivity to digitalis.

The interaction of quinidine and digoxin is a fairly recent discovery that is extremely important in view of the frequent co-usage of these two medications. It is well accepted now that the addition of quinidine increases the serum digoxin level and may precipitate toxicity, even while digoxin dosage is maintained at a stable level. Leahy et al.[126] reported this interaction in approximately one third of the patients taking both drugs. It is possible that quinidine displaces digoxin selectively from extracardiac binding sites, producing an increased serum digoxin concentration that will then exert a cardiac effect. Other studies[127] suggest that this is not the case, and show that this effect may be due to quinidine decreasing renal glycoside clearance. Whatever the mechanism, one should expect a doubling of the serum digoxin level within 48 hours after the addition of quinidine. Anticipating this, it may be best to decrease the maintenance dose of digoxin the day after quinidine is started. Some data suggest that digoxin levels may increase in patients taking verapamil or nifedipine. This has not been noted in patients taking disopyramide or procainamide.

Certain drugs decrease the effect of digitalis. Cholestyramine, Kaopectate, and Maalox may prevent the absorption of digitalis. Brown et al.[128] suggest that the decreased digoxin bioavailability seen with hypocholesterolemic agents is related to the dosage as well as the time of drug administration. Patients should not take digoxin within 8 hours of taking these agents. The decreased blood levels seen when digoxin is used with antacids and Kaopectate is not entirely explained by a change in gut transit time or by absorption of these medications.[129] Patients with peptic ulcer disease may therefore have lower digoxin levels with intensive antacid regimens. Furthermore, if gastric outlet obstruction develops, acid hydrolysis of digoxin could further decrease absorption. Interestingly, though, in patients who have undergone Billroth I or Billroth II operations[130] in which much of their intestinal mucosa has been resected, digoxin levels are not decreased. Marcus et al.[131] have shown that the half-life of digoxin is essentially unchanged even after removal of the majority of the small bowel, indicating that the enterohepatic recirculation is not important in digoxin elimination. Acute vasodilator therapy can increase renal clearance of digoxin in patients with congestive heart failure and thus alter the maintenance dosage required for optimal therapy.[132] Barbiturates, phenytoin, and phenylbutazone may in some patients diminish serum digitoxin concentrations through the induction of hepatic microenzymes. Normally, about 8% of digitoxin is converted to digoxin, and with activation of the P-450 microenzymes by these drugs, the digoxin level may actually increase as a result of enhanced digitoxin metabolism. When considering digitalis toxicity in patients taking these drugs and also taking digitoxin, both digoxin and digitoxin levels should be checked.

Changes in the enteric flora (1 in 10 patients) may markedly alter the state of digitalization.[133] In some persons, digoxin is inactivated by gastrointestinal bacteria. The administration of antibiotics in such patients may result in higher serum levels and possible toxicity.

CARDIAC TRANSPLANTATION

Cardiac transplantation should be considered a viable alternative for the patient with congestive heart failure refractory to all conventional therapy and without lesions amenable to more traditional cardiac surgery. Although several institutions now provide the opportunity for cardiac transplantation, in the United States, the pioneering team at Stanford University has the greatest experience.[134] As of June 1987, 448 patients at Stanford had undergone cardiac transplantation. The majority of these patients had coronary artery disease as an underlying etiology for their intractable heart failure, with a large minority having idiopathic cardiomyopathy. This profile may vary among institutions. Survival rates have improved dramatically in patients undergoing transplantation in the last 5 years. In 1987, the 1-year survival rate was 80 to 90%. The 5-year survival rate is now up to 75%. These survival figures are comparable to those for renal transplantations with non-immunologically matched donor and recipient. In addition to the improved technical skills, the use of endomyocardial biopsies to correlate histologic and clinical evidence of rejection, and to guide drug therapy of organ rejection, as well as the use of the immunosuppressive agent cyclosporine have contributed to the improved survival statistics. Basic immunotherapy includes the use of cyclosporine, azothioprine, prednisone, and antithymocyte globulin. Not all patients are candidates for cardiac transplantation. Patients over 57 years of age (with exceptions), those with systemic illnesses that would otherwise limit life expectancy, insulin-requiring diabetics with significant secondary complications, and patients with excessively elevated pulmonary vascular resistance (greater than 640 dyne/sec/cm^{-5}) particularly if unresponsive to vasodilating agents such as nitroprusside, those with mental illness, and those with unresolved pulmonary infarctions are not considered acceptable candidates for cardiac transplantation.[135]

Accelerated coronary atherosclerosis (incidence near 30% at 2 to 3 years) can occur in the transplanted heart, and may be caused by rejection-induced injury to the intima of the coronary arteries. Hypercholesterolemia is a major risk factor and should be aggressively treated.[135,136]

The ability to transplant heart and lungs simultaneously makes transplantation of the heart applicable to patients with severe pulmonary hypertension due to fixed pulmonary vascular resistance (as is the case with primary pulmonary hypertension or Eisenmenger's syndrome). At this time, the number of cases so treated does not allow a fair assessment of the long-term efficacy of this technique.

CIRCULATORY SUPPORT WITH MECHANICAL DEVICES

Intra-aortic balloon counterpulsation and temporary left ventricular assist devices are used for patients in whom there is a possibility of recovering some left ventricular function so that these devices can be removed.

In late 1982, clinicians and researchers at the University of Utah Medical Center implanted a totally artificial heart in a patient who was moribund with no hope for survival. The patient, Dr. Barney Clark, had been preselected on the basis of his end-stage cardiac disease, his age (which disqualified him from consideration of transplantation), and his overall candidacy (including mental status) to become the world's first recipient of a totally artificial heart. The device, implanted by Dr. William DeVries, was the Jarvik-7 and was able to maintain Dr. Clark's life, with one structural problem requiring replacement of a cardiac valve, for 112 days. Since then, several other patients have had total artificial hearts, with survival from 1 month to over 2 years.[137] Serious problems are hemorrhage from anticoagulation and thrombosis of the prosthesis. Many scientific, socioeconomic, and philosophic questions remain unanswered concerning the applicability to the general population of the artificial heart. At present, it is used primarily as a temporary bridge to cardiac transplantation.

The reader is referred to a recent detailed review of the management of congestive heart failure that has been published by Gazes and Assay.[138]

REFERENCES

1. Kessler K.M.: Heart failure with normal systolic function. Update of prevalence, differential diagnosis, prognosis, and therapy. *Arch. Intern. Med.* 148:2109, 1988.
1a. Zelis R., Sinoway L.I., Musch T.I., et al.: Regional blood flow in congestive heart failure: Concept of compensatory mechanisms with short and long time constants. *Am. J. Cardiol.* 62:2E, 1988.
2. Frank O.: Zur Dynamik des Hermuskels. *Z. Biol.* 32:370, 1895.
3. Starling E.H.: *The Linacre Lecture on the Law of the Heart.* London, Longmans, Green & Co., 1915.
4. Braunwald E., Ross J., Sonnenblick E.H.: *Mechanism of Contraction of the Normal and Failing Heart.* Boston, Little, Brown & Co., 1968, p. 77.

5. Mason D.T.: Regulation of cardiac performance in clinical heart disease: Interactions between contractile state, mechanical abnormalities and ventricular compensatory mechanisms. *Am. J. Cardiol.* 32:437, 1972.
6. Ross J., McCollough W.: Nature of enhanced performance of the dilated left ventricle in the dog during chronic volume overloading. *Circ. Res.* 30:549, 1972.
7. Gaasch W.H.: Left ventricular radius to wall thickness ratio. *Am. J. Cardiol.* 43:1189, 1979.
8. Field B.J., Baxley W.A., Russell R.O., et al.: Left ventricular function in cardiomyopathy with depressed ejection fraction. *Circulation* 47:1022, 1973.
9. Newman W.H., Webb J.G.: Adaptation of left ventricle to chronic pressure overload: Response to inotropic drugs. *Am. J. Physiol.* 234:4134, 1980.
10. Marcus M.L., Doty D.B., Hirotza L.F., et al.: Decreased coronary reserve: A mechanism for angina pectoris in patients with aortic stenosis and normal coronary arteries. *N. Engl. J. Med.* 307:1362, 1982.
11. Poole-Wilson P.A., Buller N.P.: Causes of symptoms in chronic congestive heart failure and implications for treatment. *Am. J. Cardiol.* 62:31A, 1988.
12. Spodick D.H., Quarry-Pigott V.M.: Fourth heart sound as a normal finding in older persons. *N. Engl. J. Med.* 288:140, 1973.
13. Traube L.: Ein Fall von Pulsus bigeminus nebst Bemerkungen über die Lebershwellungen bei Klappenfehlern und über acute Leberatrophie. *Ber. Klin. Wochenschr.* 9:185, 1872.
14. Cohn K.E., Sandler H., Hancock E.W.: Mechanisms of pulsus alternans. *Circulation* 36:372, 1967.
15. Cohen J.A., Kaplan M.N.: Left-sided heart failure presenting as hepatitis. *Gastroenterology* 74:583, 1978.
16. Morris J.J., Entman M., North W.C., et al.: The changes in cardiac output with reversion of atrial fibrillation to sinus rhythm. *Circulation* 31:670, 1965.
17. Greenberg B., Chatterjee K., Parmley W.W., et al.: The influence of left ventricular filling pressure on atrial contribution to cardiac output. *Am. Heart J.* 98:742, 1979.
18. Selzer A.: Digitalis in cardiac failure. *Arch. Intern. Med.* 141:18, 1981.
19. Arnold S.B., et al.: Long-term digitalis therapy improves left ventricular function in heart failure. *N. Engl. J. Med.* 303:1443, 1980.
20. Lee D.C., Johnson R.A., Bingham J.B., et al.: Heart failure in outpatients: A randomized trial of digoxin versus placebo. *N. Engl. J. Med.* 306:699, 1982.
21. Smith T.W.: Digitalis. Mechanisms of action and clinical use. *N. Engl. J. Med.* 318:358, 1988.
22. Goodman D.J., Rossen R.M., Cannom D.S., et al.: Effect of digoxin on atrioventricular conduction. Studies in patients with and without cardiac autonomic innervation. *Circulation* 51:251, 1975.
23. Jelliffe R.W.: An improved method of digoxin therapy. *Ann. Intern. Med.* 69:703, 1968.
24. Jellifffe R.W., et al.: An improved method of digitoxin therapy. *Ann. Intern. Med.* 72:453, 1970.
25. Lindenbaum J., Mallow M.H., Blackstone M.O. et al.: Variation in biological availability of digoxin from four preparations. *N. Engl. J. Med.* 285:1344, 1971.
26. Ogilvie R.I., Ruedy, J.: An educational program in digitalis therapy. *JAMA* 222:50, 1972.
27. Ewy G.A., Grover B.M., Ball M.F., et al.: Digoxin metabolism in obesity. *Circulation* 44:810, 1971.
28. Bigger J.T., Strauss H.C.: Digitalis toxicity: Drug interactions promoting toxicity and the management of toxicity. *Sem. Drug Treat.* 2:147, 1972.
29. Rasmussen K., Jewell J., Storstein L., et al.: Digitoxin kinetics in patients with impaired renal function. *Clin. Pharmacol. Ther.* 13:6, 1972.
30. Jellife R.W., Brooker G.: A nomogram for digoxin therapy. *Am. J. Med.* 57:63, 1974.
31. Ewy G.A., Kapadia G.G., Yao L., et al.: Digoxin metabolism in the elderly. *Circulation* 39:449, 1969.
32. Morrow D.H., Gaffney T.E., Braunwald E.: Studies on digitalis: VII. Influence of hyper- and hypothyroidism on the myocardial response to Ouabain. *J. Pharmacol. Exp. Ther.* 140:324, 1963.
33. Croxson M.S., Ibbertson H.K.: Serum digoxin in patients with thyroid disease. *Br. Med. J.* 3:566, 1975.
34. Lawrence J.R., Sumner D.J., Kalk W.J., et al.: Digoxin kinetics in patients with thyroid dysfunction. *Clin. Pharmacol. Ther.* 22:7, 1977.
35. Reiffel J.A., Bigger J.T., Cramer M.: Effects of digoxin on sinus node function before and after vagal blockade in patients with sinus node dysfunction. *Am. J. Cardiol.* 43:983, 1979.
36. Margolis J.R., Strauss H.C., Miller H.C., et al.: Digitalis and the sick sinus syndrome—clinical and electrophysiological documentation of a severe toxic effect on sinus node function. *Circulation* 52:162, 1975.
37. Varonkov Y., Shell W.E., Smirnov V.: Augmentation of serum CPK activity by digitalis in patients with acute myocardial infarction. *Circulation* 55:719, 1977.

38. Balcon R., Hoy J., Sowton E.: Hemodynamic effects of rapid digitalization following acute myocardial infarction. *Br. Heart J.* 30:373, 1968.
39. Lesch M.: Inotropic agents and infarct size: Theoretical and practical considerations. *Am. J. Cardiol.* 37:508, 1976.
40. Morrison J., et al.: Digitalis and myocardial infarction in man. *Circulation* 62:8, 1980.
41. Lipp G., et al.: Hemodynamic response to acute intravenous digoxin in patients with recent myocardial infarction and coronary insufficiency with and without heart failure. *Chest* 63:862, 1973.
42. Wang K., Goldfarb B.L., Gobel F.L., et al.: Multifocal atrial tachycardia: A clinical analysis of 41 cases. *Arch. Intern. Med.* 137:161, 1977.
43. Sellers T.D., Bashore T.M., Gallagher J.J.: Digitalis in the preexcitation syndrome: Analysis during atrial fibrillation. *Circulation* 56:260, 1977.
44. Lown B., Weller J.M., Wyatt N., et al.: Effects of alterations of body potassium on digitalis toxicity (abstr.). *J. Clin. Invest.* 31:648, 1952.
45. Kleiger R.E., Seta K., Vitale J.J., et al.: Effects of chronic depletion of potassium and magnesium upon the actions of acetylstrophanthidin on the heart. *Am. J. Cardiol.* 17:520, 1966.
46. Hall R.J., Gelbart A., Silverman M., et al.: Studies on digitalis induced arrhythmias in glucose and insulin induced hypokalemia. *J. Pharmacol. Exp. Ther.* 201:709, 1977.
47. Beller G.A., Hood W.A., Smith T.S., et al.: Correlation of serum magnesium levels and cardiac digitalis intoxication. *Am. J. Cardiol.* 33:225, 1974.
48. Nola G.T., Pope S., Harrison D.C.: Assessment of the synergystic relationship between serum calcium and digitalis. *Am. Heart J.* 79:499, 1972.
49. Aronson J.K., Graham-Smith D.G.: Altered distribution of digoxin in renal failure: A cause of digoxin toxicity? *Br. J. Clin. Pharmacol.* 3:1045, 1976.
50. Gazes P.C., et al.: Acute hemorrhage and necrosis of the intestines associated with digitalization. *Circulation* 23:358, 1961.
51. Lown B., Grayboys T.B.: Management of patients with malignant ventricular arrhythmias. *N. Engl. J. Med.* 296:301, 1977.
52. Beller G.A., Smith T.W., Abelmann W.H., et al.: Digitalis intoxication—a prospective clinical study with serum level correlations. *N. Engl. J. Med.* 284:989, 1971.
53. Rosen M.R., Wit A.L., Hoffman B.F.: Electrophysiology and pharmacology of cardiac arrhythmias: IV. Cardiac antiarrhythmic and toxic effects of digitalis. *Am. Heart J.* 89:391, 1975.
54. Ferrier G.R., Saunders J.H., Mendez C.: A cellular mechanism for the generation of ventricular arrhythmias by acetylstrophanthidin. *Circ. Res.* 32:600, 1973.
55. Lown B.: Electrical stimulation to estimate the degree of digitalization. *Am. J. Cardiol.* 22:251, 1968.
56. Doherty J.E.: How and when to use the digitalis serum levels. *JAMA* 239:2594, 1978.
57. Doherty J.E., Perkins W.H., Flanigan W.J.: The distribution and concentration of tritiated digoxin in human tissues. *Ann. Intern. Med.* 66:116, 1967.
58. Goldman S., Probst P., Selzer A., et al.: Inefficiency of "therapeutic" serum levels of digoxin in controlling the ventricular rate in atrial fibrillation. *Am. J. Cardiol.* 35:651, 1975.
59. Walsh F.M., Sode J.: Significance of non-steady state serum digoxin concentrations. *Am. J. Clin. Pathol.* 63:446, 1975.
60. Smith T.W., Haber E., Yeatman L., et al.: Reversal of digoxin intoxication with Fab fragments of digoxin specific antibodies. *N. Engl. J. Med.* 294:797, 1976.
61. Smith T.W., Butler V.P., Jr., Haber E., et al.: Treatment of life threatening digitalis intoxication with digoxin-specific fab fragments: Experience in 26 cases. *N. Engl. J. Med.* 307:1357, 1982.
62. Wenger T.L., Butler V.P., Jr., Haber E., et al.: Treatment of 63 severely digitalis-toxic patients with digoxin-specific antibody fragments. *J. Am. Coll. Cardiol.* 5:118A, 1985.
63. Warren S.E., Fannenstill D.O.: Digoxin overdosage: Limitation of hemoperfusion-hemodialysis treatment. *JAMA* 242:2100, 1979.
64. Cannon P.J.: The kidney in heart failure. *N. Engl. J. Med.* 296:26, 1977.
65. Del Greco F.: The kidney in congestive heart failure. *Mod. Concepts Cardiovasc. Dis.* 44:47, 1975.
66. Goldberg M.: The kidney in heart failure, in Fishman A. (ed.): *Heart Failure.* Washington, Hemisphere Press, 1978, p. 261.
67. Kramer R.S., Mason D.T., Braunwald E.: Augmented sympathetic neurotransmitter activity in the peripheral vascular bed of patients with congestive heart failure and cardiac norepinephrine depletion. *Circulation* 38:629, 1968.
68. Watkins L., Burton J.A., Haber E., et al.: The renin-angiotensin-aldosterone system in congestive heart failure in conscious dogs. *J. Clin. Invest.* 57:1606, 1976.
69. Laragh J.H., Sealey J.E.: The renin-angiotensin hormonal system and regulation of sodium,

potassium and blood pressure hemostasis, in Renal Physiology. Section 8, *Handbook of Physiology*. Washington, D.C., American Physiological Society, 1976, p. 831.

70. Wolff H.P., Koczorck K.R., Buchborn E., et al.: Endocrine factors. *J. Chronic Dis.* 9:554, 1959.
71. Raine A.E.G., Phil D., Erne P., et al.: Atrial natriuretic peptide and atrial pressure in patients with congestive heart failure. *N. Engl. J. Med.* 315:533, 1986.
72. Hall W.D.: Clinical use of diuretics in congestive heart failure. *Med. Times* 107:24, 1979.
73. Dikshit K., Vyden J.K., Forrester J.S., et al.: Renal and extrarenal hemodynamic effects of furosemide in congestive heart failure after acute myocardial infarction. *N. Engl. J. Med.* 288:1087, 1973.
74. Kassirer J.P., Beckman P.M., Lawrenz D.R., et al.: The critical role of chloride in the correction of hypokalemic alkalosis in man. *Am. J. Med.* 38:172, 1965.
75. Patak R.U., Mookenjee B.K., Bentzel C.T., et al.: Antagonism of the effects of furosemide by indomethacin in normal and hypertensive man. *Prostaglandins* 10:649, 1975.
76. Burch G.E.: Evidence of increased venous tone in chronic congestive heart failure. *Arch. Intern. Med.* 98:750, 1956.
77. Johnson J.B., Gross J.F., Hole E.: Effects of sublingual nitroglycerin on pulmonary artery pressure in patients with failure of the left ventricle. *N. Engl. J. Med.* 257:1114, 1957.
78. Mason D.T.: Symposium on vasodilator and inotropic therapy of heart failure. *Am. J. Med.* 65:101, 1978.
79. Strumza P., Rigaud M., Rachid M., et al.: Prolonged hemodynamic effects (12 hours) of orally administered sustained-release nitroglycerin. *Am. J. Cardiol.* 43:272, 1979.
80. Jordan R.A., Henry A., Wilen M.M., et al.: Transdermal nitroglycerin in heart failure. *Circulation* 70:114, 1984.
81. Ignarro L.J., Lippton H., Edwards J.C., et al.: Mechanism of vascular smooth muscle relaxation of organic nitrates, nitrites, nitroprusside and nitric oxide: Evidence for the involvement of S-nitrosothiols as active intermediates. *J. Pharmacol. Exp. Therap.* 218:739, 1981.
82. Cohn J.N., Archibald D.G., Ziesche S., et al.: Effect of vasodilator therapy on mortality in chronic congestive heart failure. *N. Engl. J. Med.* 314:1547, 1986.
82a. Cohn J.N., et al.: Effects of vasodilator therapy on peak exercise oxygen consumption in heart failure. V-HeFT (abstr). *Circulation* 76:IV–443, 1987.
83. Chatterjee K., Parmley W.W., Massie B., et al.: Oral hydralazine therapy for chronic refractory heart failure. *Circulation* 54:879, 1978.
84. Fitchett D.H., Marin Neto J.A., Oakley C.M., et al.: Hydralazine in the management of left ventricular failure. *Am. J. Cardiol.* 44:303, 1979.
85. Packer M., Meller J., Medina N., et al.: Hemodynamic characterization of tolerance to long-term hydralazine therapy in severe chronic heart failure. *N. Engl. J. Med.* 306:57, 1982.
86. Franciosa J.A., Cohn J.N.: Effects of minoxidil on hemodynamics in patients with congestive heart failure. *Circulation* 63:652, 1981.
87. Majid P.A., Sharmo B., Taylor S.H.: Phentolamine for vasodilator treatment of heart failure. *Lancet* 2:719, 1971.
88. Awan N.A., Miller R.R., Mason D.T.: Comparison of effects of nitroprusside and prazosin on left ventricular function and the peripheral circulation in chronic refractory heart failure. *Circulation* 57:153, 1978.
89. Rubin S.A., Chatterjee K., Gelberg H.J., et al.: Paradox of improved exercise but not resting hemodynamics with short-term prazosin in chronic heart failure. *Am. J. Cardiol.* 43:810, 1979.
90. Packer M., Meller J., Gorlin R., et al.: Hemodynamic and clinical tachyphylaxis to prazosin-mediated afterload reduction in severe chronic congestive heart failure. *Circulation* 59:531, 1979.
91. Arnold S.B., Williams R.L., Ports T.A., et al.: Attenuation of prazosin effect on cardiac output in chronic congestive heart failure. *Ann. Intern. Med.* 91:345, 1979.
92. Avan N.A., Mason D.T.: Oral vasodilator therapy with prazosin in severe congestive heart failure. *Am. Heart J.* 101:695, 1981.
93. Stokes G.S., Gain J.M., Malony J.F., et al.: Long-term use of prazosin in combination or alone for treating hypertension. *Med. J. Aust.* 2(suppl. 1):13, 1977.
94. Cohn J.M., Burke L.: Nitroprusside. *Ann. Intern. Med.* 91:752, 1979.
95. Bower P.J., Peterson J.N.: Methemoglobinemia after sodium nitroprusside therapy. *N. Engl. J. Med.* 293:865, 1976.
96. Packer M., Meller J., Medina N., et al.: Rebound hemodynamic events after the abrupt withdrawal of nitroprusside in patients with severe congestive heart failure. *N. Engl. J. Med.* 301:1193, 1979.
97. Zellis R., Flaim S.F., Moscowitz R.M., et al.: How much can we expect from vasodilator therapy in congestive heart failure? (editorial). *Am. J. Cardiol.* 59:1092, 1979.
98. Curtiss C., Cohn J.N., Vrobel J., et al.: Role of the renin-angiotensin system in the systemic vasculature of chronic congestive heart failure. *Circulation* 58:763, 1978.

99. Gavras H., Faxon D.P., Berkohen J., et al.: Angiotensin-converting enzyme inhibition in patients with congestive heart failure. *Circulation* 58:770, 1978.
100. Levine T.B., Francis G.S., Goldsmith S.R., et al.: Activity of the sympathetic nervous system and renin-angiotensin system assessed by plasma hormone levels and their relation to hemodynamic abnormalities in congestive heart failure. *Am. J. Cardiol.* 49:1659, 1982.
101. Turini G.A., Gribic M., Brunner H.R., et al.: Improvement of chronic congestive heart failure by oral captopril. *Lancet* 1:1213, 1979.
102. Davis R., Ribner H.S., Keung E., et al.: Treatment of chronic congestive heart failure with captopril, an oral inhibitor of angiotensin-converting enzyme. *N. Engl. J. Med.* 301:117, 1979.
103. Packer M., Meller J., Medina N., et al.: Differences in the responses to captopril and nitroprusside in severe heart failure indicate that captopril has actions independent of its vasodilator effects. *Am. J. Cardiol.* 49:988, 1982.
104. Massie B.M.: Ace inhibitors and other vasodilators for CHF. *Cardio.* (Clinical Overview):117, 1988.
105. Packer M., Lee W.H., Yushak M., et al.: Comparison of captopril and enalapril in patients with severe chronic heart failure. *N. Engl. J. Med.* 315:847, 1986.
106. Uretsky B.F., Shaver J.A., Liang C., et al.: Modulation of hemodynamic effects with a converting enzyme inhibitor: Acute hemodynamic dose-response relationship of a new angiotensin converting enzyme inhibitor, lisinopril, with observations on long-term clinical, functional, and biochemical responses. *Am. Heart J.* 116:480, 1988.
107. The Captopril-Digoxin Multicenter Research Group: Comparative effects of therapy with captopril and digoxin in patients with mild to moderate heart failure. *JAMA* 259:539, 1988.
108. The Consensus Trial Study Group: Effects of enalapril on mortality in severe congestive heart failure. Results of the cooperative north Scandinavian enalapril survival study (consensus). *N. Engl. J. Med.* 316:1429, 1987.
109. Goldberg L.I.: Dopamine—clinical uses of an endogenous catecholamine. *N. Engl. J. Med.* 291:707, 1974.
110. Sonnenblick E., Frishman W.H., Le-Jemetel T.H.: Dobutamine: A new synthetic cardioactive sympathomimetic amine. *N. Engl. J. Med.* 300:17, 1979.
111. Loeb H., Bredakis J., Gunnar R.M.: Superiority of dobutamine over dopamine for augmentation of cardiac output in patients with chronic low output failure. *Circulation* 55:375, 1977.
112. Francis G., Sharma B., Hodges M.: Comparison of dobutamine to dopamine in acute low output cardiac failure (abstr.). *Circulation* 59-60(suppl. 2):183, 1979.
113. Unverferth D.V., Blanford M., Leier C.V.: Tolerance to dobutamine (abstr.). *Circulation* 59-60(suppl. 2):199, 1979.
114. Alouisi A.A., Farah A.E., Lesher G.Y., et al.: Cardiotonic activity of amrinone (WIN 40680): 5-amino-3,4'bipyridin-6(IH)-one. *Fed. Proc.* 37:914, 1978.
115. Benotti J.R., Grossman W., Braunwald E.: Hemodynamic assessment of amrinone–a new inotropic agent. *N. Engl. J. Med.* 299:1373, 1978.
116. Weber K.T., Andrews V., Janicki J.J., et al.: Amrinone and exercise performance in patients with chronic heart failure. *Am. J. Cardiol.* 48:164, 1981.
117. Siegel L.A., et al.: Beneficial effects of amrinone-hydralazine combination on resting hemodynamics and exercise capacity in patients with severe congestive heart failure. *Circulation* 63:838, 1981.
118. Baim D.S., McDowell A.V., Cherniles J., et al.: Evaluation of a new bipyridine inotropic agent—milrinone—in patients with severe congestive heart failure. *N. Engl. J. Med.* 309:748, 1983.
119. Baim D.S., Colucci W.S., Monrad E.S., et al.: Survival of patients with severe congestive heart failure treated with oral milrinone. *J. Am. Coll. Cardiol.* 7:661, 1986.
119a. DiBianco R., Shabetai R., Kostuk W., et al.: A comparison of oral milrinone, digoxin, and their combination in the treatment of patients with chronic heart failure. *New Engl. J. Med.* 320:677, 1989.
120. Slutsky R., Gerber K., Hooper W., et al.: The effect of subcutaneous terbutaline on the left ventricle, evidence for an inotropic effect (abstr.). *Circulation* 50-60(suppl. 2):182, 1979.
121. Cleland J.G., Dargie H.J.: Arrhythmias, catecholamines and electrolytes. *Am. J. Cardiol.* 62:55A, 1988.
122. Dargie H.J., Cleland J.G., Leckie B.J., et al.: Relation of arrhythmias and electrolyte abnormalities to survival in patients with severe chronic heart failure. *Circulation* 75:IV—98, 1987.
123. Swedberg K., Hjalmarson A., Waagstein F., et al.: Prolongation of survival in congestive cardiomyopathy by beta-receptor blockade. *Lancet* 1:1374, 1979.
124. Ferling J., Easthope J.L., Aranow W.S.: Effects of verapamil on myocardial performance in coronary disease. *Circulation* 59:313, 1979.
125. Waldroff S., Anderson J.D., Heeboll-Nielson N., et al.: Spironolactone-induced changes in digoxin kinetics. *Clin. Pharmacol. Ther.* 2:162, 1978.

126. Leahy E.B., Reiffel J.A., Drusin R.E., et al.: Interaction between quinidine and digoxin. *JAMA* 240:533, 1978.
127. Doering W.: Quinidine-digoxin interaction: Pharmacokinetics, underlying mechanism and clinical implication. *N. Engl. J. Med.* 301:400, 1979.
128. Brown D.D., Juhl R.P., Warner S.L.: Decreased bioavailability of digoxin due to hypercholesterolemic interventions. *Circulation* 58:164, 1978.
129. Brown D.D., Juhl R.P.: Decreased bioavailability of digoxin due to antacids and kaolin-pectin. *N. Engl. J. Med.* 295:1034, 1976.
130. Beermann B., Hellström K., Roger A.: The gastrointestinal absorption of digoxin in seven patients with gastric or small intestinal reconstructions. *Acta Med. Scand.* 193:293, 1973.
131. Marcus F.I., Horton H., Jacobs S., et al.: The effects of jejunoileal bypass in patients with morbid obesity on the pharmacokinetics of digoxin in man (abstr.). *Am. J. Cardiol.* 37:154, 1976.
132. Cogan J.J., Humphreys M.H., Carlson C.J., et al.: Acute vasodilator therapy increases renal clearance of digoxin in patients with congestive heart failure. *Circulation* 64:973, 1981.
133. Lindenbaum J., Rund D.G., Butler V.P. Jr.: Inactivation of digoxin by the gut flora: Reversal of antibiotic therapy. *N. Engl. J. Med.* 305:789, 1981.
134. Jamieson S.W., Stinson E.G., Shumway N.E.: Cardiac transplantation in 150 patients at Stanford University. *Br. Med. J.* 1:93, 1979.
135. Copeland J.G.: Cardiac Transplantation. *Curr. Probl. Cardiol.* 13:163, 1988.
136. Nitkin R.S., Hunt S.A., Schroeder J.J.: Accelerated atherosclerosis in cardiac transplant patient. *J. Am. Coll. Cardiol.* 6:243, 1985.
137. Devries W.C., Anderson J.L., Joyce L.D., et al.: Clinical use of the total artificial heart. *N. Engl. J. Med.* 310:273, 1988.
138. Gazes P.C., Assey M.E.: The management of congestive heart failure. *Curr. Probl. Cardiol.* 8:8, 1984.

Chapter 17

NONCARDIAC SURGERY IN CARDIAC PATIENTS

Physicians frequently have to evaluate patients with cardiac disease before they undergo noncardiac surgery because many complications can occur during or after operation. Hunter and associates[1] have reported that 38% of 141 randomly selected surgical patients aged 35 years or older had historic or physical evidence of heart disease, hypertension, or diabetes mellitus in preoperative assessment. Forty-five percent had abnormal preoperative ECGs. Almost 50% of the deaths associated with noncardiac surgery are due to cardiovascular complications. Patients with cardiac disease may have limited ability to respond to the hemodynamic and metabolic stress of surgery and anesthetic agents. Myocardial oxygen demand is increased because of volume loss, the stress of surgery, and the increase of catecholamines secondary to pain. This can cause congestive failure in patients with left ventricular dysfunction and arrhythmias and myocardial ischemia in patients with coronary disease. Consultants should evaluate patients with cardiac disease to estimate the cardiopulmonary reserve before noncardiac surgery because many complications, which can be anticipated, can occur during or after an operation.

PREOPERATIVE EVALUATION

Some factors to be considered before advising noncardiac surgery, especially elective procedures, in cardiac patients are the type and severity of the heart disease, the length and magnitude of the operation, the age of the patient, nutrition, obesity, and the administration of the anesthesia. For example, a herniorrhaphy or transurethral resection is much less of a surgical risk than intrathoracic surgery, gastric resection, cholecystectomy, or other intraperitoneal surgery.[2] Progress in surgery and medicine, particularly in anesthesia, now makes surgery possible in patients who previously would have been considered prohibitive surgical risks.

In addition to the symptoms of heart disease such as chest pain, dyspnea, cough, hemoptysis, palpitations, dizziness, syncope, or edema, the history should include a meticulous review of all drugs the patient is taking. The consultant cardiologist or surgeon often must obtain this information from the attending physician or the pharmacist unless labeled medication bottles are available. An increasing number of drugs have been found to alter the cardiac hemodynamics during and after operation. Furthermore, in congestive heart failure the hepatic congestion can increase and prolong the action of drugs that are detoxified in the liver, such as opiates.

Preoperative Drug Evaluation

Among the drugs that require special attention before surgery are corticosteroids, antihypertensive agents, tranquilizers and antidepressants, hypoglycemic agents, antiplatelet agents and anticoagulants, and specific cardiovascular agents.

Corticosteroids. Adrenal insufficiency may follow withdrawal of corticosteroid therapy due to inhibition of adrenal corticotropin releasing factor and/or adrenal atrophy. Patients who are receiving or have received high doses and long-term corticosteroid therapy any time during the year preceding the operation require the therapy to be supplemented or reinstituted. The oral steroid should be continued to the day before surgery. One hundred milligrams of hydrocortisone can be given I.M. with the preoperative medications. During and after surgery, 100 mg hydrocortisone can be given I.V. and repeated as needed (as much as 500 to 700 mg may have to be given in a few hours).[3] Those who previously had small doses or intermittent therapy should only be observed closely. Some anesthesiologists feel that preparation with steroids is unnecessary at any time, since the associated problems are relatively infrequent, but they do give prompt treatment when hypotension occurs.

Antihypertensive agents. About two million hypertensive patients are anesthetized each year. For many years there were varying opinions as to whether antihypertensive agents should be continued before surgery. However, at present the majority agree that patients with hypertension who are maintained on antihypertensive drugs with good control of their BP have less fluctuation of BP during anesthesia than those who were untreated.[4] In fact, some drugs, such as the β-blockers and clonidine, may cause rebound hypertension or tachyarrhythmia or increase in angina and even myocardial infarction during or after surgery if they are suddenly stopped in patients with coronary artery disease. Propranolol has a half-life of about 6.5 hours, but it is bound tightly to β-adrenergic receptors; therefore, after discontinuing this drug, its negative inotropic effects persist for 12 to 15 hours and negative chronotropic effects up to 36 hours.[5] Supersensitivity to isoproterenol was noted in one study[6] beginning 2 to 6 hours after abrupt drug discontinuation and lasting for 3 to 13 days. In view of these and other studies, we are in agreement with Goldman's[7] recommendations. Propranolol should be maintained up to the morning of surgery, and if the patient is able to resume full-dose oral medications within 12 to 24 hours after surgery, I.V. therapy is not necessary. However, if the patient cannot take oral medications after 24 hours, then 1 to 2 mg of I.V. propranolol should be given every 1 to 6 hours, depending on the patient's response and until the patient can resume full oral dosage. Because intravenous propranolol is more bio-available by avoiding liver extraction, about 1 mg I.V. is roughly equivalent to 20 mg orally. In one study,[8] propranolol was maintained postoperatively by continuous intravenous infusion (3.0 mg/hr) from 1 to 9 days. The propranolol withdrawal syndrome did not occur in any of these patients. Calcium blockers are now used frequently for hypertension and should be continued to time of surgery.

At times, well-controlled hypertensive patients can develop intraoperative or postoperative hypertension. This can be treated with I.V. sodium nitroprusside, and if tachycardia is also present, with 0.25 to 0.5 mg of propranolol I.V. as necessary.

Diuretic agents may deplete body potassium, sodium, chlorides, and total body water and may decrease peripheral vascular resistance. Potassium deficit sensitizes the heart to the toxic effects of digitalis and predisposes to arrhythmias. Body potassium may be depleted in the presence of a normal serum potassium and may be aggravated by I.V. glucose. Metabolic alkalosis predisposes to cardiopulmonary arrest.

Electrolyte disturbances may potentiate the action of muscle relaxants, although this is not a serious threat if ventilation is supported. Hypotension can occur during anesthesia when the blood volume is contracted secondary to hyponatremia. Diuretics also reduce the vascular reactivity to catecholamines and potentiate the hypotensive effect of preganglionic blockage by spinal and epidural anesthesia. The potassium-sparing diuretics (spironolactone, triamterene, amiloride) can produce hyperkalemia and cardiac arrest. Hyperkalemia can also be induced by potassium supplements and angiotensin-converting enzyme inhibitors, especially if renal disease is present.

Before operation, the blood volume should be restored, and any electrolyte imbalance should be corrected.

Antidepressants. Monoamine oxidase inhibitors affect catecholamine uptake and may augment the hypotensive effect of anesthetic agents, surgery, and narcotics and produce ventricular arrhythmias and death.[9] They should be discontinued 10 to 14 days before surgery. Antidepressants such as imipramine (Tofranil), doxepin (Sinequan), amitriptyline (Elavil), fluoxetine (Prozac), maprotiline (Ludiomil), trazodone (Desyrel), and desipramine (Pertofrane) are widely prescribed today. Each of these has a variety of pharmacologic actions such as an anticholinergic effect (produces dryness of the mouth, increase in heart rate), α-adrenoceptor blockade, and quinidine-like effect. These vary in degree for each agent. For example, amitriptyline is most anticholinergic and trazodone the least anticholinergic. High doses can cause cardiovascular abnormalities such as ECG changes, arrhythmias, postural hypotension, and decreased myocardial contractility. Doxepin and fluoxetine may have less cardiotoxicity. One study[10] suggested that in the absence of severe impairment of myocardial performance, depressed patients with preexisting heart disease can be effectively treated with therapeutic doses of imipramine or doxepin without an adverse effect on ventricular rhythm or hemodynamic function. However, ventricular tachyarrhythmias can occur when such drugs are associated with certain anesthetic agents such as halothane and a muscle relaxant such as pancuronium.[11] Preferably such drugs should be discontinued several days before anesthesia is administered.

Hypoglycemic agents. Mildly elevated blood sugar lessens the dangers of hypoglycemia, but ketoacidosis should be avoided. The management of the insulin-dependent diabetic prior to elective surgery depends on his insulin program and the fluid and electrolyte requirements of the surgical procedure. In addition, major surgery can render the patient glucose-intolerant and insulin-resistant.[12] Therefore, many prefer not to use an arbitrary insulin program to control blood glucose during surgery. They suggest that each case should be individualized to maintain plasma glucose in a range between 80 and 120 mg/dl. On the other hand, the following method has been suggested. If the patient is taking a single dose of intermediate-acting insulin (NPH or

Lente), he can usually be maintained on this on the day of surgery, and 5% glucose in water is given in appropriate amounts to replace the carbohydrate in the diet. If the patient is taking more than one daily dose of the intermediate-acting insulin, the preoperative carbohydrate and insulin are divided by four and given every 6 hours as 5% dextrose in water I.V. and regular insulin subcutaneously.[13] Supplemental regular insulin dosage can be given in both methods when necessary, which will vary depending on the duration of the hyperglycemia produced by the stress of the surgery. Oral hypoglycemic agents are discontinued preoperatively, and regular insulin is given depending on blood sugar levels determined at 9 AM and 6 PM. Usually 10 units of regular insulin is given every 8 hours for every 50 mg of elevation of the blood sugar above 150 mg. When the patient can take food orally, the administration of the intermediate-acting insulin or oral hypoglycemic agent can be resumed.

Anticoagulants and anti-platelet drugs. Oral anticoagulants should be omitted before surgery. Some physicians prefer to gradually taper anticoagulants over several days prior to surgery, even though there is no good evidence that rebound hypercoagulability occurs. Oral anticoagulants are no longer used for chronic coronary artery disease; therefore, today this is primarily a problem in patients who have prosthetic valves and are undergoing noncardiac surgery. In one study[14] of 159 patients with prosthetic valves undergoing noncardiac surgical procedures, no thromboembolic complications were noted when the anticoagulant was discontinued an average of 2.9 days (allowing the prothrombin time to return to within 20% of the normal range) preoperatively and restarted 2.7 days postoperatively. Patients with a prior history of emboli and those with valvular prostheses (especially mitral) are at high risk for thromboembolism. Generally, in such patients, warfarin should be discontinued at least 3 days before surgery (prothrombin time should be restored to within 20% of normal), and constant intravenous heparin should be begun (maintaining partial thromboplastin times at about twice control values). The effect of heparin should be reversed immediately before surgery by giving protamine sulfate intravenously. After surgery, when there is no evidence of bleeding, heparin and warfarin should be restarted, and only oral warfarin continued once the prothrombin time is therapeutic.

In emergency operations, the effect of oral anticoagulants can be neutralized with the I.V. administration of vitamin K_1 in initial doses of 10 to 25 mg. If vitamin K_1 is ineffective or insufficient time is available, then fresh blood or plasma should be given. If it is elected to administer oral anticoagulants before, during, or immediately after a dental or surgical procedure, it is recommended that the dosage be adjusted to maintain the prothrombin time at approximately 1½ to 2 times the control level. The operative site should be one that permits effective use of local procedures for hemostasis. If the patient is taking heparin, surgery can be performed several hours after the last dose. Excessive clotting or partial thromboplastin time produced by heparin can be neutralized by slow I.V. administration of 50 to 100 mg of protamine sulfate. The average life span of blood platelets is 9 days. For at least 5 days prior to elective surgery, the patient should avoid taking medications such as aspirin, other nonsteroidal anti-inflammatory agents, or dipyridamole (Persantine) which adversely affect platelet function and may enhance bleeding.

Cardiovascular drugs. Many cardiovascular medications can interact with anesthetics because both groups of agents can alter the peripheral and central sympathetic and parasympathetic tone, depolarize the membranes of the heart, and alter contractility and peripheral vascular resistance directly or indirectly. Digitalis can be continued parenterally during or after surgery. If digitalis toxicity is present, surgery should be postponed, except in emergencies. In patients whose intoxication produces life-threatening arrhythmias which do not respond to usual measures and who require emergency surgery, digoxin-immune fab (Digibind) can be given. Antiarrhythmic drugs should be continued up to the time of surgery. Most supraventricular arrhythmias during or after surgery can be controlled by the use of digitalis, propranolol, verapamil, or a combination of these; ventricular arrhythmias usually can be controlled by a 50 to 100 mg bolus of lidocaine (Xylocaine hydrochloride) followed by an I.V. drip (2 g in 1 L glucose in water) at a rate of 1 ml/min. Ventricular arrhythmias can also be controlled by I.V. propranolol or procainamide if lidocaine is ineffective. In sustained arrhythmias, cardioversion sometimes may be necessary.

Nitrates, β-blockers, calcium blockers, and afterload-reducing agents such as hydralazine, and ACE inhibitors should be continued to the day of surgery.

In addition to the history, a complete physical examination with ECG (at times stress test), chest x ray, urinalysis, and routine blood determinations (CBC, hematocrit, BUN, blood sugar, and electrolytes) is necessary. The results of these procedures may indicate further studies to determine the possible presence of anemia, renal disease, liver disease, or some other abnormality. At times echocardiography, Doppler and nuclear studies may be indicated. In some cases pulmonary function studies and cardiac catheterization may be necessary. After evaluation of the results, recommendations should be made concerning operative survival and the degree of surgical risk. The New York Heart Association's (NYHA) classification "Cardiac Status and Prognosis" is an excellent guide in evaluating the patient's surgical risk. Patients with uncompromised or slightly compromised (classes I and II) cardiac status (arrived at after total assessment of the etiologic, anatomic, and physiologic diagnoses) tolerate surgery well. Those with moderately or severely compromised (classes III and IV) cardiac status are substantial operative risks and may present problems. Goldman et al.[15] have proposed a multifactorial index of cardiac risks in noncardiac surgical procedures. This score system has become popular for assessment of surgical risks. Table 17–1 shows the risk factors and the associated point scores. Based on total points, patients could be separated into four classes of different risks. Class I (0–5 points) and class II (6–12 points) had significantly fewer complications than class III (13–25 points) and class IV (26 points or greater). The authors concluded that only lifesaving procedures be performed on patients in class IV and that patients in class III should have preoperative cardiac consultation. Since 28 of the 53 points are potentially controllable or reversible situations (i.e., a third heart sound, recent myocardial infarction, jugular venous distention, significant aortic stenosis and general medical condition), if possible surgery should be delayed to lower the risks with therapy. In view of the increase in knowledge of cardiac disease and its natural history since the Goldman risk-factor index was devised in 1977, these risk factors should be re-evaluated. For example, Goldman assigned seven points if more than five premature ventricular beats per minute were documented at any time before surgery. One may interpret this as being so even if there is no evidence of cardiac disease. However, note that

Table 17–1. Computation of the Cardiac Risk Index*

Criteria	Points
History	
Age >70 yr	5
MI in previous 6 mo	10
Physical examination	
S_3 gallop or JVD	11
Important valvular aortic stenosis	3
Electrocardiogram	
Rhythm other than sinus or PACs on last preoperative ECG	7
>5 PVCs/min at any time before operation	7
General status	
Po_2 <60 or Pco_2 >50 mm Hg, K <3.0 or Hco_3 <20 mEq/L, BUN >50	
or Cr >3.0 mg/dl, abnormal SGOT, signs of chronic liver disease, or	
patient bedridden from noncardiac causes	3
Operation	
Intraperitoneal, intrathoracic, or aortic operation	3
Emergency operation	4
Total possible	53

*MI = myocardial infarction; JVD = jugular-vein distention; PACs = premature atrial contractions; PVCs = premature ventricular contractions; Po_2 = partial pressure of oxygen; Pco_2 = partial pressure of carbon dioxide; K = potassium; Hco_3 = bicarbonate; BUN = blood urea nitrogen; Cr = creatinine; SGOT = serum glutamic oxalacetic transminase.
From Goldman L., et al.: Multifactorial index of cardiac risk in noncardiac surgical procedures. *N. Engl. J. Med.* 297:845, 1977. Used by permission of author and publisher.

of the 44 patients in that study who had more than 5 PVBs per minute, 43 also had other evidence of serious cardiac disease. This multifactorial index in unselected general surgical patients is a useful way to assess risk, but some subgroups need additional testing such as ECG or radionuclide stress testing or heart catheterization studies for full evaluation of the patient's risk. Detsky et al.[16] devised a modified Goldman approach by using the Bayesian method and developed a normagram.

The American Society of Anesthesiologists uses a classification of physical status which applies not only to patients with heart disease (such as the New York Heart Classification and Goldman's), but also to other types of disease.[17]

The majority of patients should have ECG monitoring, and the poor-risk type may need Swan-Ganz catheter monitoring for pressure measurements in the right atrium, right ventricle, and pulmonary artery, and for measurement of cardiac output. One study[18] recommended such invasive monitoring for preoperative assessment in the elderly (over the age of 65 years) for whom major surgery was planned. They disclosed a high percentage of serious physiologic abnormalities requiring delay or cancellation of surgery in patients who had been cleared for surgery by standard assessment. Elective surgery should be postponed until the patient is stable and does not have problems such as fever, heart failure, electrolytic imbalance, anemia, unstable angina, recent infarction, and other organ system conditions.

The anesthesiologist on the day before surgery should review the patient's record, interview and examine the patient, and explain the anesthetic procedure to the patient. The case should also be discussed with the attending physician. The anesthesiologist should then decide which type of preanesthetic medications and which type of anesthesia should be used. These choices are those of the anesthesiologist; however, the cardiologist or internist as consultants should have some knowledge of the cardiovascular effects of anesthesia.

Preanesthetic medications. Various combinations of preanesthetic medications are prescribed depending on the anesthesiologist's preference. Premedications include sedatives, opiates, tranquilizers, and anticholinergics. Some use diazepam (Valium), or lorazepam (Ativan), plus atropine or scopolamine added to morphine or meperidine hydrochloride (Demerol). Our group prefers to give an I.M. injection of 0.07–0.08 mg/kg of midazolam hydrochloride (Versed) and 0.002 mg/lb of Robinul 1 hour preoperatively.

Meperidine (Demerol) should be used cautiously because its anticholinergic effect may increase the heart rate (for example, increase the ventricular rate in the presence of atrial fibrillation). This is especially true when atropine also has been given. The incidence of sinus arrest or cardiac standstill may be reduced by the administration of atropine sulfate, which blocks the cardiac vagus nerve. The usual dose is 0.6 to 0.8 mg, but it may be necessary to give higher doses, and is repeated every 2 hours, especially during long surgical procedures. Glycopyrrolate (Robinul) has become popular because it is twice as potent as atropine, is longer-acting, and produces less tachycardia. Central stimulation and confusion are lacking because it does not cross the blood-brain barrier. Since the introduction of less irritating inhalation anesthetics, anticholinergics are used primarily for specific indications.

Depending on the cardiac problem, other drugs should be given or be available in the operating room. Nitrol ointment (1 to 2 in.) or a transdermal type is applied on the skin as a prophylactic measure in patients with coronary artery disease, and I.V. nitroglycerin should be available in case it is needed.

Anesthetic agents. More important than the selection of the anesthetic is the manner in which the anesthetic is delivered and the anesthetist's expertise. There is no correlation between the type of anesthetic agent and mortality. Studies have shown that most general anesthetics reduce myocardial contractility, have complex actions on the autonomic nervous system, produce changes in BP, affect the conduction system, and may cause respiratory depression with concurrent hypoxemia, hypercapnia (accumulation of carbon dioxide), and arrhythmias. Such changes can also affect preload and afterload. These responses may be more pronounced in cardiac patients because many cardiovascular drugs also alter the myocardial function and response. However, when used judiciously, they may confer an overall beneficial effect. A specific anesthetic agent may be chosen because of its effects on the autonomic and cardiovascular system depending on the types of cardiac problems and anesthetic requirements. Side effects limit their doses so that they are seldom used alone but are combined with other drugs to achieve satisfactory anesthesia with a lower dose.

Arrhythmias can occur because of the anesthetic agent and surgical manipulations. They occur most often during the period of light anesthesia. Kuner and associates[19] recorded one or more abnormal cardiac rhythms during operation in 95 of 154 consecutive patients (61.7%). The most frequent arrhythmias were wandering pacemaker, AV dissociation, and junctional (nodal) rhythm. The precipitating factors were the type of anesthetic, intubation, hyperventilation, and duration of surgery. An unexpected finding in this study was that the number of arrhythmias in the noncardiac patients was similar to the number in patients with pre-existent heart disease or arrhythmias. However, the arrhythmias may cause more harm in cardiac patients during operation. Cardiac arrhythmias were recorded in 44 of 103 procedures (42.7%) in apparently healthy persons during oral surgery with halothane-nitrous oxide-oxygen anesthesia.[20]

A variety of anesthetic techniques are available, including general inhalation, intravenous, and regional types.

Halothane, enflurane, isoflurane and nitrous oxide are agents in the general inhalation category. All of these exert a direct depressant effect on the myocardial contractility in a dose-dependent fashion. Nitrous oxide decreases cardiac output but because of reflex vasoconstriction does not cause hypotension. Halothane, enflurane, and isoflurane have similar effects on the cardiovascular system. They do not produce sympathetic nervous system stimulation, and cardiovascular depression is noted by a decrease in blood pressure, stroke volume, and cardiac output. These effects are more pronounced if there is significant left ventricular dysfunction, hypovolemia, or concurrent use of vasodilators. Isoflurane produces a greater decrease in systemic vascular resistance and lower blood pressure than halothane or enflurane and has less of a negative inotropic effect. Halothane sensitizes the myocardium to catecholamines and may precipitate arrhythmias, which occurs less often with enflurane or isoflurane.[21] These general anesthetics are rarely used alone, so they may be given at a relatively low dose. Nitrous oxide is most often used in combination with a narcotic or an anesthetic agent such as halothane or enflurane.

Barbiturates such as thiopental (Pentothal) and methohexital (Brevital) are in the intravenous group, along with Ketamine and the narcotics (Fentanyl and Sufenta). Pentothal is most often used to induce anesthesia. It is a mild myocardial depressant, and produces peripheral vasodilation. Compensation may occur by a baroreceptor-mediated sympathetic increase in peripheral vascular resistance. Ketamine is a mild sympathetic stimulating drug which can be used for induction, especially in patients with fixed cardiac output and secondary vasoconstriction, sick sinus syndrome, cardiac tamponade or hypovolemia. However, because it increases myocardial oxygen consumption, it should be given with caution to patients with severe coronary artery disease.

A narcotic-oxygen-relaxant technique is often used in poor-risk patients. Induction is accomplished by sequential input of a narcotic (such as Fentanyl) and controlled ventilation prevents the undesired sequela of narcotic-induced respiratory depression.[22] On a comparable milligram basis, Fentanyl is more potent than morphine and Sufenta is more potent than Fentanyl. Fentanyl can be combined with droperidol, which is a tranquilizer. This combination (Innovar) has a mild cardiodepressant effect.

At times local anesthesia with sedation will be adequate for surgery. However, large doses of lidocaine can produce depression of the myocardium and conduction system and sometimes CNS excitation and convulsions. Often, because of length of surgery and the patient's agitation, it is best that the cardiac patient have general anesthesia.

Caudal, epidural, or low-spinal regional anesthetics (procaine, tetracaine, lidocaine, bipivacaine) may be used for surgery on the lower extremities or pelvic area, especially in patients with coronary artery disease. Sympathetic blockade by these agents can produce hypotension, but this can be treated with vasopressors or intravenous fluids. Brachial plexus blocks or axillary blocks (which are more common) are sometimes used for upper extremity surgery.

Muscle tone can be controlled by use of muscle relaxants to obtain an optimal surgical field. A neuromuscular-blocking agent such as succinylcholine chloride (Anectine), pancuronium (Pavulon), or dimethyl tubocurarine (metocurine) may be given I.V. to provide muscular relaxation. Pancuronium has a vagolytic effect and may increase heart rate and arterial pressure, while dimethyl tubocurarine produces minimal decrease in systemic vascular resistance and increase in cardiac output. Studies have shown that succinylcholine chloride has a digitalis-like effect and can induce arrhythmias, especially when given to a digitalized patient.[23] In one study,[24] arrhythmia occurred in 76% of patients for elective heart surgery who received succinylcholine. In this study, digitalis did not increase the frequency of arrhythmia. Quinidine, procainamide, β-blockers, bretylium, trimethaphan and nitroglycerin may potentiate the action of neuromuscular blocking agents.[25] One of our patients several years ago who was taking digoxin and quinidine had atrial fibrillation and was given thiopental sodium and succinylcholine chloride before cardioversion. Immediately after he had received succinylcholine chloride, ventricular ectopic beats appeared, followed by torsade de pointes (Fig 17–1), which is an unusual ventricular arrhythmia (see Chap. 15). The Q-T interval was prolonged in the normally conducted beats. Quinidine was probably an associated factor, since it prolongs the Q-T interval and may potentiate the action of neuromuscular blocking agents.

With the more recent knowledge of anesthetics and the increasing skills of anesthesiologists, deaths attributable to anesthesia have declined.

PREOPERATIVE MANAGEMENT

Preoperative preparation should include the management of specific types of heart disease, arrhythmias, myocardial dysfunction, and congestive heart failure. An abnormal ECG and the contraindications to elective surgery should be evaluated.

Coronary Atherosclerotic Heart Disease

This condition is the most common type of heart disease and accounts for most of the operative mortality. Knapp et al.[26] evaluated 8984 male surgical patients who were more than 50 years old. Of this group, 8557 had no previous history of coronary artery disease. Postoperative occlusion developed in 59 (0.7%) of these patients, 11 (19%) of whom died. Of the 427 patients with a previous history of coronary artery disease, 26 (6%) had a postoperative occlusion, which was fatal in 15 (58%). When a coronary occlusion had occurred less than 6 months before operation, the incidence of postoperative occlusion was 100%; when it had occurred more than 2 years preoperatively, the postoperative incidence was 12%.

The results of surgery after an acute myocardial infarction depend upon the myocardial reserve and the length of time since the infarction occurred. In a study of 1005 patients with coronary heart disease who were undergoing op-

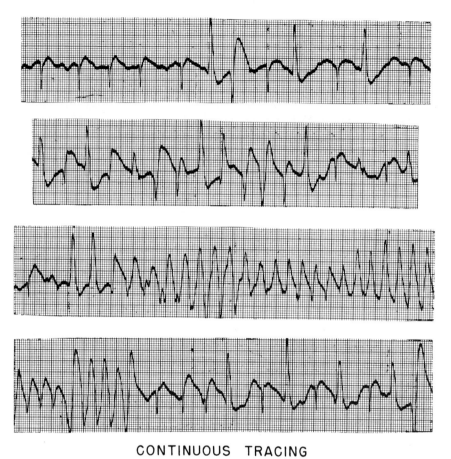

CONTINUOUS TRACING

Fig 17–1.   Continuous tracing of lead II in a patient with atrial fibrillation. Immediately after I.V.
administration of succinylcholine chloride, ventricular ectopic beats occurred, followed by torsade
de pointes. (From Gazes P.C.: Noncardiac surgery in cardiac patients. Part I: Preoperative evaluation. *Postgrad. Med.* 49:170, 1971. Used by permission.)

eration, Arkins et al.[27] reported a mortality of 40% in 27 patients who had had
a coronary occlusion within 3 months preceding operation. However, in a study
of patients who had transurethal prostatectomy within 6 months after infarction, the mortality rate was no greater. In another study reported by Tarhan
et al.[28] patients who were operated on within 3 months of infarction had a 37%
reinfarction rate; within 3 to 6 months, 16%; and after 6 months, remained at
4 to 5%. Fifty-four percent of these patients who had previous myocardial
infarctions died as a result of recurrent myocardial infarction. In this study
operations on the thorax and upper abdomen were followed by three times as
many reinfarctions as operations at other sites. From these studies, it can be
concluded that the shorter the interval between preoperative coronary occlusion and surgery, the greater is the chance that occlusion will recur. Steen et
al.[29] repeated this study at the Mayo Clinic during 1974–1975, using 587
patients who had a prior myocardial infarction and who underwent anesthesia
and surgery. They repeated this study because of improvements in anesthetic
agents and techniques and changes in medical management since the earlier

study. The incidence and severity of reinfarction was statistically unchanged from the earlier period (1967–1968). Thirty-six (6.1%) had a reinfarction, and 25 (69%) died. Those operated on within 3 months of the previous infarction had a 27% reinfarction rate; within 3 to 6 months, 11%; and more than 6 months, 4 to 5%.

In a more recent study,[30] the incidence of reinfarction decreased within the first 3 months postinfarction to 5.7% and between 4 to 6 months to 2.3%. Invasive hemodynamic monitoring and new cardiac drugs probably accounted for this. However, all patients with infarction should not be considered in one group because their prognosis varies according to left ventricular function, arrhythmias, and other factors. Depending on these factors, high-risk and low-risk subgroups can be identified, which will vary the risk of major noncardiac surgery. In general, the standard recommendation is that elective surgery be postponed until at least 6 months following an infarction, unless a life-threatening surgical emergency develops, and then invasive hemodynamic monitoring should be done during surgery. Tachycardia, hypoxemia, hypotension, hemorrhage, and low cardiac output are some of the factors that may precipitate infarction during or after operation. The incidence of myocardial infarction is greater during the third postoperative day.[28] Therefore, the patients should have an increased inspired oxygen tension, and prevention of atelectasis should be aided by coughing and deep-breathing exercises so that the myocardial oxygen is adequate and infarction may be avoided. Patients with a prior history of infarction should be monitored postoperatively in an intensive care area for several days. In addition, complete ECGs should be taken daily for at least 2 to 4 days, and in the event of any hemodynamic instability, serial estimations of serum CK-MB (and radionuclide studies in some cases), since myocardial infarction in the perioperative period often is painless.[28,29]

The risk of surgery in patients with angina pectoris often depends on the frequency of the angina. Patients with chronic stable angina (NYHA Class II) usually tolerate anesthesia and surgery with appropriate monitoring for ischemia. However, it is often best to delineate the coronary anatomy by coronary arteriography, especially before major noncardiac surgical procedures. Patients with unstable angina tolerate surgery poorly and should be considered for myocardial revascularization (bypass surgery or angioplasty) before elective surgery.[31]

Nitrates, β-blockers, and calcium blockers should be continued to the time of surgery. The importance of not abruptly stopping β-blockers has been discussed earlier. Nitroglycerin ointment or patches can be applied before surgery to an area away from the surgical site where it will not be wiped off or removed. Intravenous nitroglycerin should be available in the operating room.

Verapamil should be used cautiously in the presence of left ventricular dysfunction, especially because anesthetic agents also decrease myocardial contractility.

Several studies suggest that coronary bypass grafting can alter the mortality and morbidity of patients having noncardiac surgery. The coronary artery surgery study (CASS) documented the fact that coronary artery bypass grafting in patients with severe coronary artery disease reduced the mortality that can occur during noncardiac surgery.[32]

Hypertensive Cardiovascular Disease

As mentioned previously, controlled hypertension usually does not increase the risk of general anesthesia or major surgery. The antihypertensive agents should be continued up to surgery. Sodium nitroprusside, hydralazine, methyldopa, or trimethaphan given I.V. can control hypertension, if it occurs during or after surgery, until the patient can begin receiving oral medications. Sublingual nifedipine has also been found effective for hypertensive crises.[33] If tachycardia is also present, 0.25 to 0.5 mg or more of propranolol I.V. can be given as necessary. Intraoperative hypotension is more often noted with halothane than during other anesthetic agents in the hypertensive patient.[34]

Valvular Heart Disease

Patients with valvular heart disease whose cardiac status is uncompromised or slightly compromised, NYHA class I or II, usually tolerate surgery as well as noncardiac patients. Those whose cardiac status is moderately or severely compromised, class III or IV, especially those who have critical aortic stenosis or mitral stenosis, often have complications and the worst prognosis. Anesthesia or a sudden decrease in blood volume can precipitate cardiovascular collapse or a lethal ventricular arrhythmia in patients with symptomatic aortic or mitral stenosis.[35] Fluid overload or tachycardia can worsen mitral stenosis. Aortic regurgitation may worsen if the heart rate slows or the peripheral vascular resistance increases. Aortic and mitral regurgitation tolerate vasodilation well (afterload reduction). Patients with significant symptomatic valvular disease should undergo corrective surgery before having elective noncardiac operations. In some cases it may be more feasible to have aortic or mitral balloon valvuloplasty for stenotic lesions. Those with valvular disease (including calcified mitral annulus) or prosthetic valves (very high-risk group for endocarditis) who are undergoing dental or surgical procedures should receive prophylactic antibiotic therapy to prevent bacterial endocarditis[36] (Table 17–2). Those with mid systolic clicks (which indicate mitral prolapse) or ejection sounds (which may indicate aortic or pulmonic valvular stenosis) with or without an associated murmur should also receive prophylaxis. However, some physicians give antibiotic prophylaxis only if these extra sounds are associated with murmurs, possibly ignoring the fact that a murmur may be intermittent. Dental procedures (which are likely to cause gingival bleeding), such as filling, cleaning, root canal work, bridgework, and extraction, can result in bacteremia. This can also ocur with certain procedures in the upper respiratory tract, such as tonsillectomy, bronchoscopy, and any surgical procedure, including biopsy, involving the respiratory mucosa. Bacteremia also can occur in many other procedures, such as surgery or instrumentation of the genitourinary or GI tract, urethral catheterization, cystoscopy, and with obstetric infections. Prophylaxis is also recommended for colonoscopy, esophageal dilatation, and upper GI endoscopy or proctosigmoidoscopy with biopsy. Endocarditis following uncomplicated vaginal delivery is rare, and the necessity for antibiotic prophylaxis has not been established.

The American Heart Association[36] does not recommend prophylaxis for some procedures such as liver biopsy, upper GI endoscopy, barium enema, sigmoidoscopy, or proctoscopy. In addition, uterine dilatation and curettage,

Table 17–2. Prophylaxis Against Bacterial Endocarditis (Adults)

| Procedure | Medications | |
	Before Procedure	After Procedure
Dental and upper respiratory tract	2.0 g penicillin V orally 1 hr before procedure	1.0 g 6 hr after initial dose
	or	
	2 million units of aqueous Penicillin G I.V. or I.M. 30–60 min before procedure	1 million units 6 hr later
	Allergic to Penicillin Erythromycin 1.0 g orally 1 hour before procedure	500 mg 6 hr after initial dose
	Prosthetic Valves and Other Higher Risks Ampicillin 1.0–2.0 g plus gentamicin 1.5 mg/kg I.M. or I.V., both given 30 min before procedure	Penicillin V 1.0 g orally 6 hr later
	Allergic to Penicillin Vancomycin 1 g I.V. over 60 min begun 60 min before procedure	No repeat dose necessary
Gastrointestinal and genitourinary tract surgery and instrumentation	*For Most Patients* Ampicillin 2.0 g I.M., or I.V. plus gentamicin 1.5 mg/kg I.M. or I.V. 30 min before procedure	One follow up dose 8 hr later
	Allergic to Penicillin Vancomycin 1.0 g I.V. given over 60 min plus 1.5 mg/kg gentamicin I.M. or I.V. each 1 hr before procedure	Dose repeated once 8–12 hr later
	For Minor or Repeative Procedures in Low Risk Patients Amoxicillin 3.0 g orally 1 hr before procedure	1.5 g 6 hr after initial dose

Adapted from: Shulman ST et al.: Prevention of Bacterial Endocarditis. American Heart Association Committee Report, *Circulation* 70:1123A, 1984.

insertion of pelvic devices, cesarean section, and therapeutic abortion do not routinely require prophylaxis unless infection is present. However, some physicians recommend prophylaxis in these procedures for patients with prosthetic valves, even though the data do not substantiate this. Prophylaxis is also not recommended for coronary artery bypass surgery.

Rheumatic fever prophylaxis (antistreptococcal) should not be confused with prophylaxis against bacterial endocarditis, which requires extra antibiotic protection.

The majority of patients with prosthetic valves receive long-term anticoagulant therapy to prevent thromboembolism. Management of such patients was previously discussed.

Congenital Heart Disease

Patients who have noncyanotic congenital heart lesions without evidence of heart failure tolerate surgery and have few complications. Cyanotic patients are greater risks, especially in regard to problems of postoperative hemorrhage and vascular thrombosis. Such complications may be reduced in these polycythemic patients if phlebotomy is performed preoperatively to lower the hematocrit to about 55%. Patients with cyanotic heart disease tolerate systemic hypotension poorly. Patients with congential heart disease should receive antibiotic prophylaxis (same schedule as for valvular heart disease) to decrease the risk of bacterial endocarditis. Those with an uncomplicated secundum atrial septal defect repaired with direct sutures without a prosthetic patch and patients who have had ligation and division of a patent ductus arteriosus do not require prophylaxis following a healing period of 6 months after surgery.

Pulmonary Heart Disease

In addition to routine preoperative studies, patients with lung disease should be evaluated by pulmonary function studies and arterial blood gases. Some clinical idea of the patient's pulmonary reserve can be gained by observing the patient walking up several flights of stairs. If he can perform this function without undue dyspnea, surgery is usually well tolerated.

Problems with anesthetics and intraoperative and postoperative complications (hypoxia, hypercarbia, atelectasis, and infections) occur more often in cardiac patients with lung disease. These patients should be prepared preoperatively by using bronchodilators, expectorants, and aerosol with intermittent positive pressure, and by eliminating smoking. Opiates should be avoided, and antibiotics should be used empirically. Alveolar hypoventilation with carbon dioxide retention should be avoided because respiratory acidosis predisposes to arrhythmias, hyperkalemia, myocardial depression, and cardiac arrest. Postoperatively the use of a respirator may be necessary to assist respiration. These patients should have frequent arterial blood gas studies.

Hypertrophic Obstructive Cardiomyopathy (HOCM)

Patients with HOCM should have careful fluid management because hypovolemia may aggravate left ventricular outflow obstruction. β-adrenergic stimulant drugs such as dopamine, isoproterenol, and epinephrine can increase the obstruction. Supraventricular arrhythmias can lead to hemodynamic instability and should promptly be treated. Preoperative insertion of a Swan-Ganz catheter and intra-arterial monitoring are essential for optimal management of such patients.

Preoperative Arrhythmias

Premature atrial or junctional (nodal) beats or rare PVBs do not require therapy. Goldman et al.[15] in their point system for computation of the cardiac risk assigned 7 points if the rhythm was other than sinus or PABs on the last preoperative ECG or if there were more than 5 PVBs per minute documented at any time before operation. It should be noted that of the 44 patients who had a history of more than 5 PVBs per minute, 43 also had other evidence of major cardiac disease. When PVBs occur at more than 5 per minute, multifocal, in runs or pairs, or R-on-T phenomenon, an intravenous drip of 2 to 3 g of lidocaine (Xylocaine) in 1 L of 5% glucose in water, administered at a rate of 1 ml (2 to 3 mg) per minute, is begun preoperatively in patients with cardiac disease (especially those with ischemic heart disease) and continued during the operation. In the person without evidence of cardiac disease, premature ventricular beats are not associated with increased risk and antiarrhythmic therapy is not necessary.[37] Patients with supraventricular tachyarrhythmias should be digitalized and at times cardioverted. Beta-blockers and verapamil have also been used.

Many patients require noncardiac surgery and they have various degrees of sinoatrial pause or block, AV block, or intraventricular conduction abnormalities or combination of these. Insertion of a temporary transvenous pacemaker in such patients prior to surgery has been debated. Most agree that patients with SA pause or block, second- or third-degree AV block or those with a clear history of Stokes-Adams attacks should have a temporary pacer.[38] The need of this in patients with bifascicular block (left bundle-branch or right bundle-branch block with left anterior or posterior fascicular block) has been debated. A study of 30 patients with ECG evidence of bifascicular block indicated that a pacing catheter was not justified in such patients preoperatively.[39] Other studies[15,40,41] came to the same conclusion, and in addition the patients with bifascicular block and prolongation of the P-R interval did not have episodes of complete heart block perioperatively. Most agree now that patients with such asymptomatic bifascicular blocks do not need a prophylactic pacemaker insertion before surgery. However, a noninvasive temporary pacemaker and a pacing catheter should be available in the operating room.

A Swan-Ganz catheter may produce right bundle-branch block, and in a patient who already has left bundle-branch block, this can produce complete heart block.[42] Therefore, in this situation it would be best to use a multipurpose catheter that can be used to measure pressures and cardiac output and has pacing electrodes which allow for atrial, ventricular, or AV sequential pacing.

Congestive Heart Failure

Patients with evidence of systolic dysfunction and congestive heart failure should receive digitalis, diuretics, and vasodilator therapy as indicated. Non-emergency surgical procedures should be delayed until compensation is restored and there is no evidence of side effects from therapy such as electrolyte imbalance or hypovolemia. Digoxin and vasodilators are of no benefit in patients with heart failure caused by diastolic dysfunction. Such patients can respond to judicious use of diuretics, calcium blockers, and β-blockers.

The advisability of routine preoperative digitalization in the absence of signs of overt systolic dysfunction and heart failure or atrial fibrillation or flutter is controversial. Proponents of digitalization base their decision on the facts that most general anesthetics depress myocardial contractility and that oxygen utilization is decreased in patients with enlarged but compensated hearts. Digitalis may prevent the cardiac depressant effects of anesthesia in patients with limited cardiac reserve.[43,44] In addition, digitalization may prevent some arrhythmias, and when those such as atrial fibrillation or flutter (most frequent in the postoperative period) do occur, it provides better control and tolerance.

Guides to optimal digitalization are poor, and postoperative toxicity may be difficult to recognize. In addition, serum potassium levels, metabolic activity, and blood gas measurements may vary perioperatively and alter the digitalis status. Therefore, many physicians prefer not to give prophylactic digitalization. However, I prefer digitalization before major surgery, even when the patient does not show overt evidence of congestive findings, in the following situations:

1. Myocardial systolic dysfunction (moderate or severe cardiomegaly, S_3 gallop, pulsus alternans, abnormal neck vein distention, or interstitial edema by x ray).
2. Paroxysmal attacks of supraventricular tachycardia, most commonly atrial fibrillation or flutter.
3. Prior to thoracotomies (15% postoperative incidence of atrial fibrillation).

Digitalization should be done several days before elective surgery to establish a nontoxic maintenance dose. The proper daily maintenance dose is a percentage of the loading dose, depending on renal function. In the event of emergency surgery, digitalization should be started before the operation and completed afterward.

Abnormal Electrocardiogram

It seems appropriate to take ECGs in all patients 40 years or older and a stress test in those with a history suggestive of ischemic heart disease. A thallium stress may be necessary when the resting ECG is abnormal and at times in females who have chest symptoms. Frequent preoperative tracings, especially in persons over 65 years old, reveal changes even when the patient has no other evidence of heart disease. Nonspecific T waves, bundle-branch blocks, and arrhythmias are the most common findings. Although some of these patients may not require specific therapy, this information, especially the knowledge that the changes did not develop during or after surgery, is important in following the postoperative course. In addition, with control tracings, changes that may appear postoperative are more meaningful. Such changes include P-waves indicating right atrial enlargement may suggest pulmonary emboli, and P-waves indicating left atrial enlargement may indicate left ventricular failure. Mauney et al.[45] reported a prospective study of 365 patients with preoperative electrocardiographic evidence of an old infarction, bundle-branch block, left ventricular hypertrophy or ST-T changes. Thirty patients developed perioperative infarctions with 16 deaths. More recently, Carliner et al.,[46] in a prospective study of 198 patients, found that an abnormal preoperative electrocardiogram (especially ST-T abnormalities and intraventricular conduction delay) was a statistically significant independent predictor of an increased risk of postoperative death or cardiac events.

Contraindications to Elective Surgery

Surgeons and anesthesiologists often ask if the operation has any contraindications. Except for a limited group, most cardiac patients can tolerate operation. Patients with a severely compromised cardiac status (NYHA class IV), regardless of the type of heart disease they may have, should be rejected for surgery except in an emergency. Included in this category are such patients who are unable to carry on any physical activity without cardiac symptoms and who often have symptoms, such as angina and dyspnea, even at rest.

It is important for the physician to decide whether a surgical problem is present or whether the cardiac disorder can explain all the symptoms and findings. For example, an acutely congested liver may simulate an acute abdominal emergency. The life expectancy of the patient should be considered before elective surgery, because performing an operation on the patient who cannot live to enjoy the benefits is foolish.

OPERATIVE PERIOD

During major surgery, patients with heart disease should have continuous ECG monitoring, intra-arterial pressure monitoring, and in addition, in the poor-risk patients, pressures and cardiac output monitoring with a Swan-Ganz catheter. Patients with less severe cardiac disease may need only ECG monitoring, blood pressure measurement by cuff, and application of a chest stethoscope.

Cardiac arrest associated with anesthesia is not common today because anesthesiologists do not allow hypoxia or hypercapnia (carbon dioxide retention) to occur. Cardiac arrest during operation is managed like arrest from other causes (see Chap. 15). A dc defibrillator should be available in the operating room.

In all instances of cardiac arrest, cardiac massage should be performed either externally or internally, and directly if the heart is accessible through the open incision of the left side of the chest or through the diaphragm in an abdominal incision. Adequate oxygenation and elimination of carbon dioxide are necessary for successful resuscitation. Cardiopulmonary resuscitation is discussed in detail in Chapter 15. It should be remembered that epinephrine and lidocaine can be given directly down an endotracheal tube if an I.V. line is not available, rather than lacerating the heart or producing pneumothorax in attempting to give these drugs by intracardiac injection.

When cardiac arrhythmias appear during surgery, the anesthesiologist must determine whether they are produced by the anesthesia, poor oxygenation, carbon dioxide rentention, hypotension, or reflex cardiac stimulation by the surgical maneuvers. If these causes are eliminated and the arrhythmias persist, specific antiarrhythmic therapy should be instituted. Ventricular premature beats or ventricular tachycardia can be controlled with 50 to 100 mg bolus of lidocaine given I.V. and repeated as necessary, with an infusion of 2 g in 1 L of glucose in water continued at 1 ml/minute as maintenance therapy. DC shock may be required for sustained ventricular tachycardia. Digitalis is best for atrial tachyarrhythmias. If the patient has been digitalized preoperatively, small increments may be necessary with continuous monitoring to avoid toxicity. A β-blocker or verapamil may be necessary to further slow the ventricular response in rapid atrial tachyarrhythmias if they do not convert to sinus rhythm. In the presence of heart failure or hypotension, dc cardioversion can prevent further complications.

Sinus bradycardia can be caused by vagal reflexes stimulated by surgery or the anesthetic and can be treated with 0.6 to 1.0 mg of atropine given I.V. A transvenous pacing catheter is inserted for high degrees of heart block. The Zoll noninvasive temporary pacemaker may be used until the transvenous pacer is inserted.

The concurrent replacement of fluid or blood loss is essential during operation, especially in long, difficult operative procedures. Monitoring of central venous pressure (CVP) provides a rough gauge for fluid replacement. Elevation of CVP is usually indicative of right ventricular failure. However, it must be recognized that the CVP may be normal, yet the pulmonary capillary wedge pressure (which reflects left ventricular function) can be elevated. Ideally, the pulmonary artery or the pulmonary capillary wedge pressure also should be monitored. Fluid overload, anesthetic-induced myocardial-depression, myocardial ischemia, and hypertension are some factors that may precipitate pulmonary edema. Pulmonary edema occurs when the hydrostatic pressure in the pulmonary capillaries rises from the normal of 5 to 28 mm Hg or more exceeding the oncotic pressure. It may be treated by elevating the chest, giving I.V. morphine, positive-pressure oxygen, and by giving 20 to 40 mg of furosemide I.V. Preload reducing agents such as nitroglycerin or nitroprusside, which have fewer side effects, may be given as initial therapy. When the patient has not been digitalized, I.V. digitalis should be given, especially if there is an associated atrial tachyarrhythmia. However, digitalis and arterial vasodilators should not be given if there is predominantly diastolic dysfunction.

Many patients today who have permanent pacemakers are undergoing surgery. Inhibition of demand pacemakers by sensing extrinsic electric sources has been recognized for several years. Electrocautery can cause temporary suppression of the unit, in spite of electric shielding of the pacemaker and the introduction of filters. During surgery the electrosurgical tip and the ground plate should be as far away as possible from the pacemaker, and electrosurgery should be limited to intermittent 2- to 3-second periods if any pacemaker suppression is produced.[47] Permanent damage can be caused to the pacemaker if a spark comes into direct contact with it. If necessary by use of the magnet, the pacemaker can be converted to a fixed-rate mode (this can be programmed into the newer pacemakers), which is affected less by the current,[48] yet even this can develop problems. The arterial pulse should be monitored, since electrosurgery interferes with the ECG. Many types of pacemakers are now available, and their response to perioperative interference can be complex.[49]

POSTOPERATIVE MANAGEMENT

After noncardiac surgery, the cardiac patient may have problems of electrolyte disturbances, hypovolemia or hypervolemia, hypotension, oliguria, respiratory depression (hypoxia and hypercarbia), arrhythmias, congestive heart failure, fever, or thrombophlebitis and pulmonary embolism. These complications can be caused by the surgical stress, increase in catecholamines, ACTH, cortisol, antidiuretic hormone, and changes in the acid-base and electrolyte balance, plus other contributing factors.

These complications can be better managed and often prevented by monitoring the BP, pulse and respiratory rates; arterial blood gases; hourly urine output and specific gravity; osmolality of serum and urine; daily weight when feasible; and electrolyte concentrations. Continuous ECG monitoring is advisable when arrhythmias are present, and CVP and pulmonary capillary wedge pressure should be monitored in the presence of hypotension, congestive failure, or other major complications. Patients with coronary disease should have frequent ECGs.

Usually during the first 24 hours postoperatively, or for a longer period after some operations, the patient does not take fluids orally. In addition, fluid is lost by its passage from the blood and extracellular spaces into cells or into inaccessible "third spaces." This fluid must be replaced carefully without producing hypervolemia with congestive heart failure. During the second and third postoperative days, diuresis occurs as fluid is mobilized from the third space. At times during this phase, diuretics may be necessary in the patient with myocardial dysfunction. Initially, glucose can be given, but patients require Ringer's lactate type solutions because they may be glucose-intolerant and insulin-resistant during major surgery. Electrolyte disturbances should be corrected because these disturbances, such as hypokalemia, can produce arrhythmias, especially in digitalized patients. In some major operations (especially abdominal), sudden and unexpected circulatory collapse in the immediate postoperative period may be due to an albumin deficit. In view of the hydration status, the plasma protein levels may be unreliable.

Urinary output should be maintained at 40 ml/hour. A lesser output and electrolyte imbalance often require adjustments in fluid management. However, the stress of surgery, anesthetics, and drugs can reduce renal blood flow and tubular function, and thus it may be misleading just to monitor urine volume for fluid balance. If venous pressure (central) and pulmonary capillary wedge pressure are not being monitored, the neck should be observed at the 45-degree position for abnormal venous distention. In addition, the patient should be observed carefully for signs of left heart failure during fluid administration, since the pulmonary capillary wedge pressure may be elevated to levels near pulmonary edema, yet the CVP may be normal. For this reason, in the patient with left ventricular dysfunction it is best to measure the pulmonary capillary wedge pressure, which reflects left ventricular filling pressure, whereas the CVP reflects filling pressure of the right ventricle. The left ventricular filling pressure differentiates hypotension caused by volume deficit from myocardial failure.

Measuring specific gravity of urine and osmolality of urine and plasma also may be helpful at times in fluid replacement. Osmolality is concerned with the number of particles per unit of solvent, whereas specific gravity reflects particle size. For example, glucose contributes disproportionately more to specific gravity than to osmolality. In the plasma, electrolytes (sodium ions) compose 98% of the osmolality; in urine, electrolytes compose 50% of the osmolality, and the remaining 50% is urea. The measurement of the freezing point depression of a solution is related to its osmotic concentration (osmolality). Based on this principle, the osmolality of a few milliliters of urine or serum can be measured in a few minutes with an osmometer. This measurement estimates the effective number of particles in solution, even though the nature or concentration of the individual substances dissolved in the solution is not known.

Because the osmolality of urine at a given specific gravity varies widely, one must be cautious in predicting urine osmolality on the basis of specific gravity. Specific gravity is not a factor in renal regulation of water and electrolyte balance, which depends on the osmolality of the body fluids. Normal osmolality of plasma ranges from 285 to 290 mOsm, whereas osmolality of urine varies

(250 to 1,200 mOsm in a normal adult) depending on many factors, such as the action of antidiuretic hormone on the distal and collecting ducts of the kidney, ingestion of water, and solute from food degradation. The kidney acts as a selective filter to pass water and hold solute, or vice versa, in controlling the concentration (osmolality) of the blood. The ratio of urine to serum osmolality normally is greater than one.

Electrolyte Disturbances

Electrolyte disturbances can be differentiated by determining serum electrolyte levels and osmolality of serum and urine (Table 17–3). The osmolality of serum and urine is elevated in dehydration and can be corrected by the administration of 5% glucose in water. The glucose is rapidly metabolized, leaving additional pure water. Hypertonic glucose solution should not be used, because water can be drawn from the cells until the glucose is metabolized.

With true sodium depletion (low-salt syndrome), the osmolality of serum and urine is low. Clinically, the salt deficit is usually caused by prolonged vomiting, diarrhea, excessive use of diuretics, gastric suction, or renal failure. This deficit can be corrected by the administration of isotonic saline solution. Rarely, in severe sodium deficiency, infusion of hypertonic saline may be necessary. Central venous pressure should be observed carefully during such infusions, and the patient should be observed for evidence of left heart failure. Preferably, in this situation, the pulmonary capillary wedge pressure should also be monitored.

In the normal person the ingestion of large amounts of water lowers serum osmolality. A small serum reduction of 3 or 5% results in a maximum dilute urine (for example, less than 75 mOsm) in defense of serum concentration. In the syndrome of inappropriate secretion of antidiuretic hormone, the serum osmolality is reduced and the urine osmolality is greater than the osmolality appropriate for the concomitant tonicity of plasma or for the given solute and water intake. This syndrome can occur secondary to anesthesia and to the stress and trauma of surgery.

Clinically, in the syndrome of inappropriate secretion of antidiuretic hormone, the skin turgor and BP are normal, indicating that volume depletion is not evident. The picture is one of water intoxication. Early in the course of the syndrome, anorexia, nausea, vomiting, and irritability occur; later, there are muscular weakness, stupor, and convulsive episodes. The serum electrolytes, such as sodium ion, are low because of water retention. Blood urea nitrogen often is low. A BUN of less than 10 mg% (unusually low in an adult) in the presence of hyponatremia strongly suggests a diagnosis of inappropriate se-

Table 17–3. **Electrolyte Disturbances Indicated by Measurement of Osmolality***

Electrolyte Disturbance	Serum Osmolality	Urine Osmolality
Dehydration	Elevated	Elevated
Sodium depletion	Low	Low
Inappropriate secretion of antidiuretic hormone	Low	Inappropriately elevated

*From Gazes P. C.: *Postgrad. Med.* 49:184, 1971.

cretion of antidiuretic hormone syndrome rather than the true low-salt syndrome. The syndrome of inappropriate secretion of antidiuretic hormone with hyponatremia and renal salt loss is not related to renal or adrenal disease. Because total body sodium is normal in these patients, salt administration may be harmful; the disorder can be corrected by restricting fluid intake to between 500 and 700 ml/day.

Hypokalemia can produce arrhythmias, especially in the digitalized patient. Hyperkalemia can occur in the presence of renal failure.

Hypovolemia and Hypervolemia

An electrolyte disturbance and fluid loss can cause hypovolemia. Blood loss commonly produces hypovolemia and hypotension immediately after operation. However, it must be recognized that in blood loss the hematocrit initially may be near normal due to a shrunken plasma volume. Serial determinations of the hematocrit are more meaningful than a single determination. When blood transfusion is necessary, packed red cells are preferable to whole blood in the cardiac patient who can tolerate only a limited amount of I.V. fluid. However, in acute hemorrhagic shock, intravascular volume is critical, and type-specific whole blood, balanced salt solutions or plasma expanders may be more beneficial than red cell transfusions alone.

Aggressive therapy with blood and fluid transfusions can cause hypervolemia with heart failure, especially since water excretion is impaired by reduced renal blood flow and glomerular filtration immediately after major surgery.

Hypotension

Hypotension may be due to hypovolemia as mentioned above or myocardial failure caused by systolic dysfunction. To assess either volume deficit or pump failure, a challenge of 100 to 200 ml of fluid can be given. If the CVP is less than 12 cm H_2O, a trial of fluid replacement is given with dextran at a rate of 20 ml/minute. If the CVP exceeds 5 cm H_2O during this period, the fluid is discontinued because heart failure rather than hypovolemia is present. Ideally, as mentioned previously, a Swan-Ganz catheter should be inserted to measure the pulmonary artery diastolic and pulmonary capillary wedge pressures, which reflect left ventricular function and may be elevated in the presence of a normal CVP. If myocardial failure is present, the digitalization status should be reviewed and diuretics and vasodilators should be given if necessary. If other measures fail, cardiac output may be increased by I.V. administration of dopamine (Intropin) in doses of 2 to 5 µg/kg/minute and increasing accordingly. More recently, dobutamine (Dobutrex) has become popular, and is often more appropriate for heart failure and hypotension because it has an inotropic effect and peripheral arterial dilating effect. This latter effect reduces afterload. In addition, dobutamine reduces preload by reducing the pulmonary capillary wedge pressure.

Myocardial infarction, cardiac tamponade (following thoracic procedures), arrhythmias, or catecholamine depletion due to drugs also can cause hypotension. The postoperative signs and findings of myocardial infarction often are atypical. Pain may be absent or obscured because of sedatives and narcotics, and total enzyme determinations can be confusing because of skeletal muscle and liver trauma. The CPK and LDH isoenzymes, radionuclide, and echo studies have improved tremendously the accuracy of detecting an acute myocardial infarction in this setting. These studies and frequent ECGs should be made, especially in the presence of pain in the chest, shoulder, back, or arm; hypotension; congestive heart failure; arrhythmias; dyspnea; rales; gallops; or neck vein distention at the 45-degree position. In fact, daily tracings up to 2 to 4 days for comparison with the baseline preoperative tracing should be performed in patients who have hypertension, coronary artery disease, and a prior infarction. Most postoperative myocardial infarctions occur in the first 3 days following surgery.

Oliguria

Oliguria (urine volume less than 400 ml/24 hours) is usually one of three types: prerenal, renal (parenchymal), or postrenal (obstructive uropathy). Extracellualr fluid volume depletion, such as from hemorrhage, prolonged dehydration, or sodium depletion, often produces prerenal oliguria. In addition, in the cardiac patient congestive failure is an important factor. Because of such events, oliguria can occur postoperatively in the cardiac patient. Hypotension may cause prerenal or, if prolonged, renal parenchymal oliguria such as acute renal failure. The following suggest that the oliguria is prerenal rather than acute renal failure: ratio of urine to plasma osmolality of 1.2 or greater, ratio of urine to plasma urea of 10 or greater, ratio of urine to plasma creatinine of 15 or greater, spot urine sodium concentration of less than 10 to 15 mEq, or good response to diuretics or to correction of volume deficits. In the final analysis, one should use good clinical judgment and the patient's response to therapy to distinguish between oliguria due to prerenal and acute renal failure.

Respiratory Depression

The prolonged effects of anesthesia or the indiscriminate use of opiates can cause respiratory depression and suppression of the cough reflex. Ventilatory failure occurs most often after abdominal surgery within the first few days, especially in the aged, or if the patient is obese or has chronic pulmonary disease along with cardiac disease. Early signs of pulmonary failure should be suspected if the pulse and respirations are rapid and the patient appears restless and anxious. The x ray of the chest may not be of aid, but blood gas studies (O_2, CO_2 and pH of arterial blood) are diagnostic. Blood gases also should be used for following the patient's progress during therapy. Oxygen is most important in treating ventilatory failure. At times an endotracheal tube connected to a mechanical ventilator may be necessary. Hypercarbia is the primary indication for mechanical support. If artificial ventilation is required for several days, a tracheostomy may be required.

Pulmonary complications can be prevented by encouraging deep breathing and by frequent use of suction. Sterile precautions should be used when suctioning, and infections should be treated immediately.

Arrhythmias and Congestive Heart Failure

Excessive fluid administration is the most frequent cause of postoperative heart failure. The myocardial depressant effect of anesthetic agents and the postoperative increased metabolic demands also are contributing factors. The postoperative management of arrhythmias and congestive heart failure is the same as the preoperative and operative management, which was described in detail previously in this chapter. Often arrhythmias clear by correction of extra-cardiac factors such as an electrolyte imbalance or fever.

Fever

Fever may be due to lung infection (especially secondary to atelectasis), urinary tract infection, bacterial endocarditis, pulmonary emboli, or wound infection. Gram-negative sepsis can produce shock; thus, when infections are noted, every attempt should be made to isolate the microorganisms and to give appropriate antibiotic therapy. At times antibiotics must be administered empirically.

Thrombophlebitis and Pulmonary Embolism

Thrombophlebitis and pulmonary embolism may be prevented by frequently moving the patient, use of elastic stockings, and early ambulation. Prophylactic low-dose heparin (5000 units subcutaneously every 12 hours) postoperatively appears to diminish this risk in patients 40 years of age or older who are having major general, urologic, gynecologic, or orthopedic surgery[50] (see Chap. 9). Larger adjusted doses such as 10,000 units every 8 hours may be necessary prophylactically for hip replacement.

Because pulmonary embolism may not be classic (with chest pain, hemoptysis, and the usual x ray findings), it should be suspected when sudden dyspnea, tachycardia, hypotension, weakness, syncope, arrhythmias, or unexplained fever occur. One should not wait for the leg signs of thrombophlebitis to develop, since they often do not occur or may appear after an embolism. Ventilation perfusion scanning and selective pulmonary angiography are the most definitive procedures available for diagnosis. When pulmonary embolism has occurred or is suspected, or evidence of thrombophlebitis appears, heparin should be given for several days and then replaced by an oral anticoagulant such as warfarin. In certain cases, such as with massive pulmonary embolism and shock, thrombolytic agents (streptokinase, urokinase and more recently tissue plasminogen activators[51]) have proved valuable and will probably often replace the need for pulmonary embolectomy. Ligation or clipping of the inferior vena cava or insertion of an umbrella or filters is seldom necessary, unless anticoagulant therapy fails to halt emboli formation.

DENTAL AND ORAL SURGICAL PROBLEMS IN PATIENTS WITH CARDIAC DISEASE

It is important that the dentist or oral surgeon and physician discuss the problem. The physician should tell the patient to inform the dentist of his cardiac problem. Many cardiovascular drugs can cause adverse reactions; for example, an antihypertensive agent may potentiate the response to vasoconstricting drugs. Patients with congenital or rheumatic heart disease, as well as valvular prosthesis, who require extraction of teeth, periodontal procedures, or other oral surgery, should have antibiotic therapy for prevention of bacterial endocarditis (see Table 17–2).

Preliminary sedation with an anti-anxiety agent orally at least 45 minutes before the procedure can be used in tense individuals, especially those with coronary and hypertensive cardiac disease. Tranquilizers such as Valium may be preferable, especially if the patient has been using them with good relaxation. However, many now do not often advise oral premedications. Nitrous oxide and O_2 (up to 50 to 50%) is often used by general practitioners. Most oral surgeons use Valium I.V., with Demerol titrated according to the patient's apprehension. Local anesthesia is generally best; however, for some extensive procedures, especially in a tense person, a general anesthesia in the hospital may be indicated. In addition, in certain instances a number of separate procedures can be avoided by performing all of them at one time under general anesthesia. Vasoconstrictors allow better anesthesia and decrease toxicity by slowing the absorption of the local anesthetic. They also permit the use of a smaller volume of the anesthetic agent. A possible disadvantage associated with the use of vasoconstrictors is systemic reactions following the administration of drugs such as epinephrine. Reactions may include anxiety, tachycardia, palpitation, and BP elevation. In extreme situations, these adverse effects may proceed to the development of pulmonary edema and ventricular fibrillation. However, such reactions are seldom seen when the concentration of epinephrine is 1:100,000, which gives optimal vasoconstriction. One milliliter of this solution contains 0.01 mg of epinephrine. The dose of 4 to 6 ml of anesthetic solution containing 0.04 to 0.06 mg of epinephrine is much less than that used for cardiovascular emergencies, which range from 0.2 mg to 1.0 mg. Therefore, epinephrine is used in practically all cases, with caution being exercised primarily in elderly patients and in those with diabetes, hyperthyroidism, hypertension, and other cardiovascular diseases. Norepinephrine and phenylephrine are seldom used as vasoconstrictors and are less effective than epinephrine, and require two to three times the concentration. Lidocaine (Xylocaine), 2% with epinephrine 1:100,000, or mepivacaine hydrochloride (Carbocaine hydrochloride), 2% with levonordefrin (Neo-Cobefrin) 1:20,000, are often used today and are available in Carpules of 1.8 ml. Carbocaine is similar in pharmacologic activity to lidocaine but has a slightly longer duration of action, and thus reduces the need for a vasoconstrictor. Although no clinical evidence exists to verify it, Carbocaine appears to be more toxic. A 3% solution of Carbocaine is used when there is a definite contraindication to use of a vasoconstrictor.[52] Total dose of lidocaine or Carbocaine should not exceed 400 mg. Each 1.8-ml Carpule of these 2% solutions has only 36 mg of the drug. Toxic reactions to both agents include apprehension, excitement, convulsions, drowsiness, tremor, dizziness, blurred vision, and possible respiratory arrest. The ester agents (such as procaine) are vasodilators and produce early CNS stimulation. The nonesters (such as lidocaine and Carbocaine) are mild vasoconstrictors and tend to be CNS depressants in the same doses as the ester agents. Therefore, the early excitability of the nonesters may be transient or nonexistent, with the CNS depression being the first clinically evident reaction. Use of an aspiration syringe to avoid intravascular injection is advisable, thereby keeping the incidence of side effects and anesthetic failure at a minimum. Oxygen is the most important initial treatment for toxicity.[53]

Periodontal or oral surgical procedures in cardiac patients requiring general anesthesia should be done in the hospital. Intravenous narcotics and short-acting barbiturates should not be given to such patients in the office, except in small, titrated doses for premedication. Morphine can produce hypotension, bradycardia, and respiratory depression. The short-acting barbiturates can produce an abrupt fall in BP accompanied by apnea, and can depress myocardial contractility.

The dentist or oral surgeon should have sufficient basic medical knowledge to enable him to treat a cardiovascular emergency in his office until the services of a physician can be obtained. An accurate diagnosis of the cause of the emergency is not necessary for beginning treatment. A careful history should be taken concerning known cardiac disease and recent symptoms. Specific attention should be given to the drug history, including drug allergies. It is important to know whether the patient is taking an anticoagulant, for bleeding may occur. Dental procedures can be safely performed without undue bleeding if the prothrombin time is in the therapeutic range of 20 to 30% activity or two times control level measured in seconds in the patient receiving an oral anticoagulant.[54] Effective hemostasis should be achieved with sutures, gauze dressings, and pressure. Diuretics and other antihypertensive agents may predispose to orthostatic hypotension and faintness when the patient is suddenly tilted. They may also be potentiated by drugs given in the dental office.

The dentist or oral surgeon should be familiar with the technique of cardiopulmonary resuscitation. The following equipment should be available in their offices for cardiac emergencies: BP cuff and stethoscope, pharyngeal airway, O_2 with mask, nasal catheter, and Ambu bag or other method of positive-pressure O_2 delivery. Epinephrine (Adrenalin), narcotics, atropine, and nitroglycerin are important drugs that should be available. If the patient has an anginal attack, 0.32 mg (1/200 grains) of nitroglycerin should be given sublingually and repeated in 5 minutes, if necessary. The patient should be given oxygen if the pain persists or if he becomes dyspneic. If the pain persists longer than 15 minutes, his physician should be called, and Demerol, 50 to 75 mg I.M., should be given. Persistent dyspnea can be due to heart failure. In such instances, sitting up is better for the patient, and O_2 should be administered. In the event of extreme dyspnea, morphine, 8 mg, or Demerol, 50 to 75 mg, may be given I.M. Other drugs such as digitalis should be given only by the physician. Naturally, prosthetic dental appliances should be removed to give an open airway and also to reduce the sense of suffocation. Syncope may be due to a benign faint, arrhythmia, or a transient cerebral ischemic episode. The patient should immediately be placed in the recumbent position and have his legs elevated. The airway should be maintained and O_2 started. If breathing stops, mouth-to-mouth resuscitation or the Ambu bag should be used, and external cardiac massage begun if a major pulse cannot be palpated or if the heartbeat is not audible. It is of great importance that the dentist or oral surgeon maintain his poise and remain with the patient until the emergency is over or until assistance arrives. Periodic emergency drills by the dentist and his staff will greatly reduce confusion and indecision when an actual emergency occurs (Table 17–4).[55]

Surgical mortality in cardiac patients, as in noncardiac patients, is caused by hemorrhage, uncontrolled infections, inadequate surgery, pulmonary emboli, or other complications. However, the complications are more prevalent and more poorly tolerated in cardiac patients. Skinner and Pearce[2] gave three

Table 17–4.   Standard Operating Procedure for Cardiac Arrest*

Dentist	Nurse or First Assistant
State diagnosis and notify office staff of emergency	Check vital signs
Check pupils; secure airway	Maintain airway
If asystole or ventricular fibrillation, begin CPR	Begin 100% oxygen
Use defibrillator, if needed	Control resirations
Supervise sequence of actions	Assist as directed
Second Assistant	**Secretary**
Bring emergency cart	Call nearest physician
Insure patent vein	Call emergency medical service (EMS)
If ECG available, apply leads	Call hospital emergency room
Secure defibrillator	Notify patient's physician
Place saline pads on chest and place paddles if available	Inform family that emergency has occurred and that everything possible is being done
Get stretcher and portable oxygen	Assist as directed
Supervise record of medications and activities	
Assist as directed	

*Adapted from Emergencies in Dentistry, a manual reproduced by the College of Dental Medicine and Area Health Education Center (AHEC), Medical University of South Carolina, Charleston, S.C., 1978.

categories of information that are most sensitive for predicting mortality: (1) Severity of the surgical procedure. (2) Cardiac functional capacity—class I, 4% mortality; class II, 11% mortality; class III, 25% mortality; class IV, 67% mortality. In view of the abandonment of the functional classification for a new classification (New York Heart Association) of the patient's overall cardiac status, this category for predicting mortality can be changed as follows based on cardiac status: uncompromised, 4% mortality; slightly compromised, 11% mortality; moderately compromised, 25% mortality; severely compromised, 67% mortality. However, in view of recent developments, these percentages for each class have been reduced by almost 50%. (3) Mortality increased in sequence in rheumatic heart disease, hypertensive heart disease, arteriosclerotic heart disease, and pulmonary heart disease.

It has always been difficult to decide whether a patient with cardiac disease can tolerate anesthesia and surgery. In spite of available data, this decision is most often based on the physician's personal experience.

REFERENCES

1. Hunter P.R., Endrey-Walder P., Bauer G.E., et al.: Myocardial infarction following surgical operation. *Br. Med. J.* 4:725, 1968.
2. Skinner J.F., Pearce M.L.: Surgical risk in the cardiac patient. *J. Chronic Dis.* 17:57, 1964.
3. Danowski T.S., Bonessi J.V., Sabeh G., et al.: Probabilities of pituitary-adrenal responsiveness after steroid therapy. *Ann. Intern. Med.* 61:11, 1964.
4. Prys-Roberts C., Meloche R., Foex P.: Studies of anesthesia in relation to hypertension: I. Cardiovascular responses to treated and untreated patients. *Br. J. Anaesth.* 43:122, 1971.
5. Myers J.K., Horwitz L.D.: Hemodynamic and metabolic response after abrupt withdrawal of long-term propranolol. *Circulation* 58:196, 1978.
6. Nattel S., Rangno R.E., VanLoon G.: Mechanism of propranolol withdrawal phenomena. *Circulation* 59:1158, 1979.
7. Goldman L.: Noncardiac surgery in patients receiving propranolol: Case reports and a recommended approach. *Arch. Intern. Med.* 141:193, 1981.
8. Smulyan H., Weinberg S.E., Howanitz P.J.: Continuous propranolol infusion following abdominal surgery. *JAMA* 247:2539, 1982.

9. Jenkins L.L., Graves H.B.: Potential hazards of psychoactive drugs in association with anesthesia. *Can. Anaesth. Soc. J.* 12:121, 1965.
10. Veith R.C., Raskind M.A., Caldwell J.H., et al.: Cardiovascular effects of tricyclic antidepressants in depressed patients with chronic heart disease. *N. Engl. J. Med.* 306:954, 1982.
11. Edwards R.P., Miller R.D., Roizen M.F., et al.: Cardiac responses in imipramine and pancuronium during anesthesia with halothane or enflurane. *Anesthesiology* 50:421, 1979.
12. Palumbo, P.J.: Blood glucose control during surgery. *Anesthesiology* 55:94, 1981.
13. Galloway J.A., Bressler R.: Insulin treatment in diabetes. *Med. Clin. North Am.* 62:663, 1978.
14. Tinker J.H., Tarhan S.: Discontinuing anticoagulant therapy in surgical patients with cardiac valve prostheses. *JAMA* 239:738, 1978.
15. Goldman L., Caldera D.L., Nussbaum S.R., et al.: Multifactorial index of cardiac risk in noncardiac surgical procedures. *N. Engl. J. Med.* 297:845, 1977.
16. Detsky A.S., Abrams H.B., Forbath N., et al.: Cardiac assessment for patients undergoing noncardiac surgery. A multifactorial clinical risk index. *Arch. Intern. Med.* 146:2131, 1986.
17. Dripps R.D., Echenhoff J.E., Vandam L.D.: *Introduction to Anesthesia: The Principles of Safe Practice.* 6th ed., Philadelphia, W.B. Saunders Co., 1982, p. 17.
18. DelGuercio L.R.M., Cohn J.D.: Monitoring operative risk in the elderly. *JAMA* 243:1350, 1980.
19. Kuner J., Enescu V., Utsu F., et al.: Cardiac arrhythmias during anesthesia. *Dis. Chest* 52:580, 1967.
20. Fisch C., Oehler R.C., Miller J.R., et al.: Cardiac arrhythmias during oral surgery with halothane-nitrous-oxide-oxygen anesthesia. *JAMA* 208:1839, 1969.
21. Wells P.H., Kaplan J.A.: Optimal management of patients with ischemic heart disease for noncardiac surgery by complementary anesthesiologist and cardiologist interaction. *Am. Heart J.* 102:1029, 1981.
22. Logue R.B., Kaplan J.A.: The cardiac patient and noncardiac surgery. *Curr. Prob. Cardiol.* 7:2, 1982.
23. Dowdy E.G., Fabian L.W.: Ventricular arrhythmias induced by succinylcholine in digitalized patients. *Anesth. Analg.* 42:501, 1963.
24. List W.F.M.: Succinylcholine-induced cardiac arrhythmias. *Anesth. Analg.* 50:361, 1971.
25. Rogers M.C.: Anesthetic management of patients with heart disease. *Mod. Concepts Cardiovasc. Dis.* 52:29, 1983.
26. Knapp R.B., Topkins M.J., Artusio J.F., Jr.: The cerebrovascular accident and coronary occlusion in anesthesia. *JAMA* 183:332, 1962.
27. Arkins R., Smessaert A.A., Hicks R.G.: Mortality and morbidity in surgical patients with coronary artery disease. *JAMA* 190:485, 1964.
28. Tarhan S., Moffitt E.A., Taylor W.F., et al.: Myocardial infarction after general anesthesia. *JAMA* 220:1451, 1972.
29. Steen R.A., Tinker J.H., Tarhan S.: Myocardial reinfarction after anesthesia and surgery. *JAMA* 239:2566, 1978.
30. Rao T.L.K., Jacobs K.H., El-Etr A.A.: Reinfarction following anesthesia in patients with myocardial infarction. *Anesthesiology* 59:499, 1983.
31. Tinker J.H., Noback C.R., Vlietstra R.E., et al.: Management of patients with heart disease for noncardiac surgery. *JAMA* 246:1348, 1981.
32. Foster E.D., Davis K.B., Carpenter J.A., et al.: Risk of noncardiac operation in patients with defined coronary disease: The Coronary Artery Surgery Study (CASS) Registry experience. *Ann. Thoracic Surg.* 41:42, 1986.
33. Adler A.G., Leahy J.J., Cressman M.D.: Management of perioperative hypertension using sublingual nefidipine. Experience in elderly patients undergoing eye surgery. *Arch. Intern. Med.* 146:1927, 1986.
34. Goldman L., Caldera D.L.: Risks of general anesthesia and elective surgery in the hypertensive patient. *Anesthesiology* 50:285, 1979.
35. Weitz H.H., Goldman L.: Noncardiac surgery in the patient with heart disease. *Med. Clin. North Am.* 71:413, 1987.
36. Shulman S.T., Amren D.P., Bisno A.L., et al.: Prevention of bacterial endocarditis. A statement for health professionals by the Committee on Rheumatic Fever and Infective Endocarditis of the Council on Cardiovascular Disease in the Young. *Circulation* 70:1123A, 1984.
37. Kennedy H.L., Whitlock J.A., Sprague M.K., et al.: Long-term follow-up of asymptomatic healthy subjects with frequent and complex ventricular ectopy. *N. Engl. J. Med.* 312:193, 1985.
38. Perlroth M.G., Hultgren H.N.: The cardiac patient and general surgery. *JAMA* 232:1279, 1975.
39. Berg G.R., Kotler M.N.: The significance of bilateral bundle branch block in the preoperative patient: A retrospective electrocardiographic and clinical study in 30 patients. *Chest* 59:62, 1971.

40. Kunstadt D., Punja M., Cagin N.: Bifascicular block: A clinical and electrophysiologic study. *Am. Heart J.* 86:173, 1973.
41. Rooney S.M., Goldiner P., Muss E.: Relationship of right bundle-branch block and marked left axis deviation to complete heart block during general anesthesia. *Anesthesiology* 44:64, 1976.
42. Thomsen T.R., Dalton B.C., Lappas D.G.: Right bundle-branch block and complete heart block caused by the Swan-Ganz catheter. *Anesthesiology* 51:359, 1979.
43. Goldberg A.H., Maling H.M., Gaffney T.E.: The effect of digoxin pretreatment on heart contractile force during thiopental effusion in dogs. *Anesthesiology* 22:974, 1961.
44. Shimasato S., Etsten B.: Performance of digitalized heart during halothane anesthesia. *Anesthesiology* 24:41, 1963.
45. Mauney F.M., Jr., Ebert P.A., Sabiston D.C.: Postoperative myocardial infarction: A study predisposing factors, diagnosis and mortality in a high risk group of surgical patients. *Ann. Surg.* 172:497, 1970.
46. Carliner N.H., Fisher M.L., Plotnick G.D., et al.: The preoperative electrocardiogram as an indicator of risk in major noncardiac surgery. *Can. J. Cardiol.* 2:134, 1986.
47. Simon A.B.: Perioperative management of the pacemaker patient. *Anesthesiology* 46:127, 1977.
48. Batra Y.K., Bali I.M.: Effect of coagulating and cutting current on a demand pacemaker during transurethral resection of the prostate: A case report. *Can. Anaesth. Soc. J.* 25:65, 1978.
49. Shapiro W.A., Roizen M.F., Singleton M.A.: Intraoperative pacemaker complications. *Anesthesiology* 63:319, 1985.
50. Collins R.C., Scrimgeour A., Yusuf S., et al.: Reduction in fatal pulmonary embolism and venous thrombosis by perioperative administration of subcutaneous heparin. Overview of results of randomized trials in general, orthopedic and urologic surgery. *N. Engl. J. Med.* 318:1162, 1968.
51. Goldhaber S.Z., Meyerovitz M.F., Markis J.E., et al.: Thrombolytic therapy of acute pulmonary embolism. Current status and future potential. *J. Am. Coll. Cardiol.* 10:96B, 1987.
52. Hiatt W.: Local anesthesia: History; potential toxicity; clinical investigation of Mepivacaine. *Dent. Clin. North Am.* July 1961, p. 243.
53. Moore D.C., Bridenbough L.D.: Oxygen: The antidote for systemic toxic reactions from local anesthetic drugs. *JAMA* 174:842, 1960.
54. Waldrep A.C., McKelvey L.E.: Oral surgery for patients on anticoagulant therapy. *J. Oral Surg.* 26:374, 1968.
55. Emergencies in dentistry. Manual reproduced by the College of Dental Medicine and Area Health Education Center (AHEC), Medical University of South Carolina, Charleston, S.C., 1978.

Appendix: Usual Dosage of Drugs Used for Cardiovascular Disease

Drug	Preparations* Tablets	Capsules	Injectables	Dosage
Abbokinase (urokinase)			250,000 IU per vial	2,000 IU/lb priming dose I.V. over 10 min, then 2,000 IU/lb/hr continuous infusion for 12 hr
Activase (alteplase, recombinant)			20, 50 mg vial	60 mg I.V. over first hr (10 mg bolus) 20 mg I.V. over second hr 20 mg I.V. over third hr
Adrenalin (epinephrine)			10-ml 1:10,000 0.1 mg/ml disposable syringe or 1-ml ampule 1:1,000 1 mg/ml	5 ml-1:10,000 solution I.V., I.M., or intracardiac
Aldactone (spironolactone)	25, 50, 100 mg			50–100 mg orally daily in single or divided doses
Aldomet (methyldopa)	125, 250, 500 mg		250 mg in 5-ml ampule	250–750 mg orally t.i.d., 250–500 mg in 100 ml 5% dextrose in water I.V. infusion q 6 hr
Aminophylline (theophylline ethylenediamine)			500 mg in 20-ml ampule or 250 mg in 10-ml ampule	250–500 mg I.V. slowly or as I.V. infusion in 100 ml 5% dextrose in water, 250–500 mg q 12 hr by rectal suppositories
Apresoline (hydralazine HCl)	10, 25, 50, 100 mg		20 mg in 1-ml ampule	25–50 mg orally q.i.d., 20–40 mg q 4 hr I.M. or I.V.
Aquamephyton and mephyton (phytonadione)	5 mg		1 or 2.5-ml vial 10 mg/ml	5–10 mg orally, 5–25 mg I.M. or I.V. slowly not exceeding 1 mg/min
Aramine (metaraminol bitartrate)			10-ml vial or 1-ml ampule 10 mg/ml	100–200 mg in 500 ml 5% dextrose in water I.V. infusion

(Continued)

Appendix: **Usual Dosage of Drugs Used for Cardiovascular Disease**

Drug	Preparations*			Dosage
	Tablets	Capsules	Injectables	
Arfonad (trimethaphan camsylate)			10-ml ampule 50 mg/ml	500 mg in 500 ml 5% dextrose in water I.V. infusion
Aspirin	325 mg			325 mg orally once daily
Atromid-S (clofibrate)		500 mg		500 mg orally q.i.d.
Atropine sulfate			10-ml vial 1 mg/ml	0.6–1 mg I.V. or I.M. q 3–4 hr
Blocadren (timolol maleate)	10, 20 mg			10–20 mg orally b.i.d.
Bretylol (bretylium tosylate)			500 mg in 10-ml ampule	5–10 mg/kg I.V. (over a period greater than 8 min) or I.M., repeat in 1–2 hr, then 6–8 hr
Brevibloc (esmolol HCL)			10-ml ampule 250 mg/ml	50–200 µg/kg/min IV
Bumex (bumetanide)	0.5, 1, 2 mg		2-ml ampule or vial 0.25 mg/ml	0.5–5 mg orally once daily 0.5–1.0 mg I.V. or I.M.
Calan (verapamil HCl)	80, 120 mg SR 240 mg		2-ml ampule, 2.5 mg/ml	5–10 mg I.V. over 2 min, repeat in 30 min, 80–120 mg t.i.d. orally, SR 240 mg daily
Calcium chloride			10-ml ampule 100 mg/ml	5 ml I.V.
Capoten (captopril)	25, 50, 100 mg			25–150 mg orally daily
Cardene (nicardipine HCL)		20, 30 mg		20–40 mg t.i.d.
Cardioquin Tablets (quinidine polygalacturonate)	275 mg			275 mg orally b.i.d. or t.i.d.
Cardizem	30, 60, 90, 120 mg	SR 60, 90, 120 mg		30–90 mg orally q 6–8 hr SR 60–120 mg orally b.i.d.
Catapres (clonidine HCl)	0.1, 0.2, 0.3 mg			0.1–0.4 mg orally b.i.d., patch 0.1–0.3 mg

Drug	Tablet/Capsule	Injectable/Other Form	Dosage
Colace (dioctyl sodium sulfosuccinate)	50, 100 mg		100 mg orally b.i.d.
Colestid (colestipol HCl)			5–10 g (5-g packet or 500-g bottle) in milk, soups, or fruits, t.i.d.
Cordarone (amiodarone HCL)	200 mg		Loading dose 800–1600 mg orally daily 2 wk, then 200–600 mg daily
Corgard (nadolol)	20, 40, 80, 120, 160 mg		40–240 mg orally once daily
Coumadin (sodium warfarin)	2, 2.5, 5, 7.5, 10, 25 mg		10–15 mg daily for 2–3 days or 30–40 mg oral loading dose, then 5–10 mg daily depending on prothrombin time
Crystodigin (digitoxin)	0.05, 0.1, 0.15, 0.2 mg	1-ml ampule or 10-ml vial 0.2 mg/ml	0.7–1.4 mg oral or 1 mg I.V. or I.M. loading dose in 24 hr, maintenance 0.1–0.15 mg daily
Dalmane (flurazepam)	15, 30 mg		30 mg hs
Demerol (meperidine HCl)	50, 100 mg	30-ml vial, 50 mg/ml or Tubex 50, 75, 100 mg in 1 ml	50–100 mg I.V. or I.M. q 3–4 hr, 50–100 mg orally q 4 hr
Dextran 40 (Rheomacrodex)		10% in 5% dextrose in water or 0.9% sodium chloride	500-ml solution I.V. infusion
Diamox (acetazolamide)	125, 250 mg	500-mg vial dissolve in 5 ml sterile water	250 mg orally t.i.d. or rarely I.V.
Dibenzyline (phenoxybenzamine HCl)	10 mg		40–100 mg orally daily
Digibind (digoxin immune fab)		40 mg vial	Dosage varies according to digoxin amount—400 mg I.V. average dosage

(Continued)

Appendix: Usual Dosage of Drugs Used for Cardiovascular Disease

Drug	Preparations*			Dosage
	Tablets	Capsules	Injectables	
Digitalis leaf	100 mg			0.8–1.2 g loading oral dose in 24 hr, maintenance 0.1 g daily
Dilantin (sodium phenytoin)		30, 100 mg	2-ml ampule or syringe 50 mg/ml	100 mg orally q.i.d., 100 mg I.V.
Diulo (metolazone)	2.5, 5, 10 mg			2.5–10 mg orally once daily
Dobutrex (dobutamine HCl)			250 mg in 20 ml vial	2.5–10 µg/kg/min I.V. infusion
Dyrenium (triamterene)		50, 100 mg		50–100 mg orally b.i.d.
Ecotrin (enteric-coated aspirin)	325, 500 mg			325 mg orally once daily
Edecrin (ethacrynic acid and sodium ethacrynate)	25, 50 mg		50-mg vial dissolve in 50 ml 5% dextrose in water or in saline	50–150 mg orally daily, 25 mg I.V.
Enkaid (encainide HCL)		25, 35, 50 mg		25–75 mg orally q 6–8 h
Heparin sodium			1,000 to 20,000 units per ml in ampules, vials, or Tubex units	5,000–10,000 units I.V. q 4 hr or 5000 units initial dose and 20,000–40,000 by infusion per day, depending on Lee-White clotting or partial thromboplastin times
Hydrodiuril (hydrochlorothiazide)	25, 50, 100 mg			25–100 mg orally daily
Hygroton (chlorthalidone)	25, 50, 100 mg			25–100 mg orally daily
Hylorel (quanadrel sulfate)	10, 25 mg			10–50 mg orally bid
Hyperstat (diazoxide)			300 mg in 20-ml ampule	150–300 mg I.V. or 1–3 mg/kg at 5–15-min intervals as necessary

Drug	Tablet/Capsule	Injectable	Dosage
Hytrin (terazosin HCL)	1, 2, 5, 10 mg		1–5 mg orally once daily
Inderal (propranolol HCl)	10, 20, 40, 60, 80, 90 mg	capsules LA 60, 80, 120, 160 mg	1 mg in 1-ml ampule	10–60 mg orally q.i.d., 0.5–2 mg I.V., LA 60–160 mg orally once daily
Inocor (amrinone lactate)		20 ml ampule 5 mg/ml	0.75 mg/kg bolus I.V. 5–10 μg/kg/min maintenance I.V.
Intropin (dopamine HCl)		200 mg in 5-ml ampule	200 mg in 500 ml 5% dextrose in water I.V. infusion at rate of 2–50 μg/kg/min
Ismelin (guanethidine sulfate)	10, 25 mg		10–50 mg orally daily
Isoptin (verapamil HCl)	80, 120 mg SR 240 mg	2-ml ampule, 2.5 mg/ml	5–10 mg I.V., repeat in 30 min, 80–120 mg orally t.i.d., SR 240 mg daily
Isordil (isosorbide dinitrate)	2.5, 5, 10, 20, 30 mg		2.5–5 mg q 3–4 hr sublingually, 5–30 mg orally q.i.d.
Isuprel (isoproterenol HCl)	10, 15 mg glossets	0.2 mg in 1-ml ampule, 1 mg in 5-ml ampule	0.02–0.05 mg I.V. 1–2 mg in 500 ml 5% dextrose in water I.V. infusion, 5–15 mg sublingually q 4–6 hr
Kaochlor, Kayciel (potassium chloride)			20 mEq (15 ml or 1 tablespoonful) orally t.i.d.
Kaon Cl-10 (potassium chloride)	10 mEq		10–20 mEq orally b.i.d.
K-Dur (potassium cl)	15, 20 mEq extended release		20–40 mEq orally daily
K-Lor (potassium cl)			15–30 mEq packet orally 1–4 × daily
K-Lyte Cl/50 (potassium chloride)	50 mEq		50 mEq once daily dissolved in water

(Continued)

Appendix: Usual Dosage of Drugs Used for Cardiovascular Disease

Drug	Preparations*				Dosage
	Tablets	Capsules	Injectables		
K-Tab (potassium cl)	10 mEq extended release				20–80 mEq orally daily
Lanoxicaps (digoxin)		0.05, 0.1, 0.2 mg			0.6–1.0 mg orally loading 0.1–0.2 mg orally maintenance
Lanoxin (digoxin)	0.125, 0.25, 0.5 mg		2-ml ampule 0.25 mg/ml		0.75–1.5 mg oral or 0.75–1.0 mg I.V. or I.M. loading dose in 24 hr, maintenance 0.25–0.5 mg daily
Lasix (furosemide)	20, 40, 80 mg		2–10-ml ampule 10 mg/ml		20–240 mg orally daily, 20–40 mg I.V.
Levophed (levarterenol)			4 mg in 1 ampule		4 mg in 1 L 5% dextrose in water I.V. infusion
Librium (chlordiazepoxide HCl)		5, 10, 25 mg	100-mg ampule dissolve in 2 ml diluent		10–20 mg orally q.i.d., 25–100 mg I.M.
Loniten (minoxidil)	2.5, 10 mg				10–40 mg orally daily
Lopid (gemfibrozil)	600 mg	300 mg			600 mg orally b.i.d.
Lopressor (metoprolol tartrate)	50, 100 mg		5 mg in 5-ml ampule		50–100 mg orally b.i.d. 5 mg I.V. q 2 min × 3
Lozol (indapamide)	2.5 mg				2.5–5 mg orally once daily
Lorelco (probucol)	250, 500 mg				500 mg orally b.i.d.
Magonate (magnesium gluconate)	500 mg				500–1000 mg t.i.d.
Meticorten (prednisone)	5 mg				10–20 mg orally t.i.d. and subsequently reduce
Mevacor (lovastatin)	20 mg				20–80 mg orally once daily

Drug	Strength	How Supplied	Dosage
Mexitil (mexiletene HCL)	150, 200, 250 mg		150–300 mg orally q 6–8 hr
Midamor (amiloride HCl)	5 mg		5–10 mg daily
Minipress (prazosin HCl)	1, 2, 5 mg		1–5 mg orally t.i.d.
Minitran (nitroglycerin)			2.5, 5, 10, 15 mg/24 hr transdermal
Morphine sulfate		Tubex 2, 4, 8, 10, 15 mg in 1 ml	5–15 mg subcutaneously, I.M., or I.V. q 4 hr
Neo-Synephrine (phenylephrine HCl)		10 mg in 1-ml ampule	0.2–0.5 mg I.V. or 10 mg in 500 ml 5% dextrose in water I.V. infusion
Nico-span (nicotinic acid)	400 mg		400–800 mg orally t.i.d.
Nipride (sodium nitroprusside)		50 mg in 5-ml vial	0.5–10 μg/kg/min I.V. infusion
Nitro-Bid (nitroglycerin)	2.5, 6.5, 9 mg		2.5–9 mg b.i.d. or t.i.d. orally, 2% ointment 1–4 in. applied to skin q 8 hr
Nitro-Disc (nitroglycerin)			5–10 mg/24 hr transdermal
Nitro-Dur (nitroglycerin)			5, 10, 15, 20, 30 cm^2/24 hr (2.5–15 mg) transdermal
Nitroglycerin (glyceryl trinitrate)	0.15, 0.3, 0.4, 0.6 mg		0.15–0.6 mg sublingually
Nitrol unit dose (nitroglycerin, 2%)			1–2 in. applied to skin q 8 hr
Nitrolingual Spray (nitroglycerin lingual aerosol)			0.4 mg metered dose sprayed under tongue
Nitrostat (nitroglycerin)	0.15, 0.3, 0.4, 0.6 mg	8, 50, 100 mg in 10-ml ampule or vial	0.15–0.6 mg sublingually, 5—100 μg/min I.V. infusion
Normodyne (labetalol HCL)	100, 200, 300 mg		100–900 mg orally b.i.d.

(Continued)

Appendix: Usual Dosage of Drugs Used for Cardiovascular Disease

Drug	Preparations*			Dosage
	Tablets	Capsules	Injectables	
Norpace (disopyramide phosphate)		100, 150 mg CR 100,150 mg		100–150 mg orally q 6 hr, CR 100–300 mg b.i.d.
Persantine (dipyridamole)	25, 50, 75 mg			25–50 mg orally t.i.d.
Potassium chloride			Vials 20 and 40 mEq	40 mEq in 500 ml 5% dextrose I.V. infusion
Prinvil (lisinopril)	5, 10, 20 mg			20–40 mg orally once daily
Procan SR (procainamide HCl)	250, 500, 750, 1000 mg			250–1000 mg orally q.i.d.
Procardia (nifedipine)		10, 20 mg		10–40 mg orally t.i.d.
Pronestyl (procainamide HCl)		250, 375, 500 mg	10-ml vial 100 mg/ml, 2-ml vial 500 mg/ml	250–500 mg q 4–6 hr orally or I.M., 50 mg/min I.V. up to 1 g
Prostigmin (neostigmine methylsulfate)			1:2,000 solution 0.5 mg in 1-ml ampule	0.5–1 ml subcutaneously
Protamine sulfate			50 mg vial dissolve in 5 ml sterile water	50 mg I.V.
Questran (cholestyramine)				4 g (packets or in cans or as a fruit-flavored bar) orally t.i.d. in milk or fruit juice
Quinaglute Dura Tabs (quinidine gluconate)	324 mg			324 mg orally q 8–12 hr
Quinidex Extentabs (quinidine sulfate)	300 mg			300 mg orally q 8–12 hr
Quinidine gluconate			10-ml vial, 80 mg/ml	240 mg q 6 hr I.M.
Quinidine sulfate	100, 200, 300 mg	100, 200, 300 mg		200–400 mg orally q 6 hr
Regitine (phentolamine mesylate)	50 mg		5-mg vial dissolve in 1 ml sterile water	5 mg I.V., 50 mg orally q.i.d.

Drug	Tablet/Capsule	Injectable/Other Form	Dosage
Sectral (acebutolol HCL)	200, 400 mg		200–1200 mg orally once daily or divided b.i.d.
Serpasil (reserpine)	0.1, 0.25, 0.5, 1 mg	2-ml ampule or 10-ml vial 2.5 mg/ml	0.1–0.25 mg orally daily, 0.1 mg to 0.25 mg I.M. q 6–8 hr
Slow-K (potassium chloride)	8 mEq		24–80 mEq orally daily
Sodium Bicarbonate		50 mEq in 50-ml ampule	50 mEq I.V. every 10 min as needed
SOLU-Medrol (methyl prednisolone sodium succinate)		500 or 1,000-mg vial dissolve in diluent	30 mg/kg I.V. (for shock), may be repeated q 6 hr for 48 hr
Streptase (streptokinase)		50 ml infusion bottle or vial, 1.5 million IU	1.5 million IU over 60 min I.V.
Susadrin (nitroglycerin)	1, 2 mg		1–2 mg transmucosal t.i.d.
Tambocor (flecainide acetate)	100 mg		100–200 mg orally b.i.d.
Tenex (guanfacine HCL)	1 mg		1–3 mg orally once daily
Tenormin (atenolol)	50, 100 mg		50–100 mg orally once daily
Tensilon (edrophonium chloride)		10 mg in 1-ml ampule	5–10 mg I.V.
Tonocord (tocainide HCL)	400–600 mg		400–600 mg orally q 8–12 hr
Trandate (labetalol HCL)	100, 200, 300 mg		100–900 mg orally b.i.d.
Transderm-Nitro (nitroglycerin)			2.5–15 mg/24 hr transdermal
Trental (pentoxifylline)	400 mg		400 mg orally t.i.d.
Tridil (nitroglycerin)		50 mg in 10-ml ampule	50 mg in 500 ml 5% dextrose I.V. infusion at a rate of 5–160 µg/min
Valium (diazepam)	2, 5, 10 mg	2-ml ampule 5 mg/ml	5–10 mg orally q.i.d., 5 mg I.V. q 5 min up to 40 mg for cardioversion

(Continued)

Appendix: Usual Dosage of Drugs Used for Cardiovascular Disease

Drug	Preparations*			Dosage
	Tablets	Capsules	Injectables	
Vasotec (enalapril maleate)	2.5, 5, 10, 20 mg		2-ml vial 1.25 mg/ml	5–40 mg orally once daily or divided b.i.d.; 1.25 mg q 6 hr I.V.
Vasoxyl (methoxamine HCl)			20 mg in 1 ampule or 10-ml vial 10 mg/ml	3–5 mg I.V. or 10–15 mg I.M. as needed
Versed (midazolam HCl)			5-50 mg in 1-10 ml vials	3–5 mg I.M. for premedication
Visken (pindolol)	5, 10 mg			5–20 mg orally b.i.d.
Xylocaine (lidocaine HCl)			5-ml ampule 20 mg/ml or 25-, 50-ml vials 40 mg/ml	50 to 100 mg bolus I.V. 2–4 g in 1 L 5% dextrose in water I.V. infusion at a rate of 2–4 mg/min
Zaroxolyn (metolazone)	2.5, 5, 10 mg			2.5–10 mg orally daily
Zestril (lisinopril)	5, 10, 20 mg			5–40 mg orally daily

*Automated disposable syringes with usual doses for emergencies are available for many of the drugs.

INDEX

Note: Page numbers in *italics* refer to illustrations; page numbers followed by t refer to tables.

561

Liver, congestion of, 2
  enlargement of, in cardiac failure, 476
  evaluation of, 31
  tests of, in cardiac failure, 477
Löffler's disease, restrictive cardiomyopathy in,
    356–357
Loniten. *See* Minoxidil
Lonitenine. *See* Minoxidil
Lopid. *See* Gemfibrozil
Lopressor. *See* Metoprolol
Lorelco. *See* Probucol
Lovastatin (Mevacor), in lipoprotein control, 169
  usual dosage of, 556t
Lowenberg's sign, 314
Lown-Ganong-Levine syndrome, 432
Lozol. *See* Indapamide
Ludiomil. *See* Maprotiline
Lung capacity, total, in pulmonary disease, 306t
Lupus erythematosus, cardiac involvement in, 357
  in pericarditis, 380
Lutembacher's syndrome, 267. *See* Atrial septal de-
    fect

Magnesium gluconate (Magonate), usual dosage of,
    556t
Magnesium hydroxide, digitalis interaction with,
    515t
Magnetic resonance imaging, 12, 13
Magonate. *See* Magnesium gluconate
Mahaim fibers, in pre-excitation syndrome, 432
Malposition, 274. *See also* Transposition
Mammary souffle, 298
Maprotiline (Ludiomil), cardiac toxicity of, 361
  preoperative evaluation of, for noncardiac sur-
      gery, 525
Macroglossia, 24
Marey's reflex, 32
Marfan's syndrome, 24, 32
  aortic changes in, 323–324, *324, 325*
  diagnosis of, 323
  in pregnancy, 391
  mitral anulus in, 226
  mitral valve involvement in, 226
Means-Lerman scratch, in hyperthryoidism, 392
Medications, 2
Meperidine (Demerol), in acute myocardial infarc-
      tion, 114
  preoperative, 529
  usual dosage of, 553t
Mepivacaine hydrochloride (Carbocaine hydrochlo-
      ride), for dental surgery, 546
Mesocardia, 274
Metabolic equivalent (MET), activity expenditure
      of, 157, 158–159t
  definition of, 74
Metanephrines, urinary, in pheochromocytoma, 195
Metaraminol (Aramine), in cardiogenic shock, in
      acute myocardial infarction, 144
  usual dosage of, 551t
Methohexital (Brevital), for noncardiac surgery, 530
Methoxamine (Vasoxyl), usual dosage of, 560t
3-Methyl 0-desmethyl, 407
Methyl prednisolone sodium succinate (SOLU-
      Medrol), usual dosage of, 559t
Methyldopa (Aldomet), in hypertension, 200, 203t

  in hypertensive emergency, 205t
  usual dosage of, 551t
α-Methyltyrosine, in pheochromocytoma crisis, 195
Meticorten. *See* Prednisone
Metolazone (Diulo, Zaroxolyn), in cardiac failure,
      496, 498t
  in hypertension, 203t
  usual dosage of, 554t, 560t
Metoprolol (Lopressor), for hypertension, 203t
  in acute myocardial infarction, 115, 153
  in angina, 91, 91t
  in hypertension, 198, 201
  usual dosage of, 556t
Mevacor. *See* Lovastatin
Mexiletine (Mexitil), in arrhythmias, 405t, 406
  in ventricular arrhythmia prevention, in acute
      myocardial infarction, 140t
  usual dosage of, 557t
Mid-expiratory flow, maximum, in pulmonary dis-
      ease, 306t
Midamor. *See* Amiloride
Milrinone, in cardiac failure, 509
Minipress. *See* Prazosin
Minitraix. *See* Nitroglycerin
Minoxidil (Loniten), in cardiac failure, 503
  in hypertension, 202, 203t
  usual dosage of, 556t
Mitral anulus, calcified, 226
Mitral insufficiency, 215–229
  acute, 228–229
    murmur of, 229
    valve replacement in, 229
  calcified mitral anulus and, 226
  chronic, 227–228
  congenital, 227
  connective tissue diseases and, 226
  coronary artery disease and, 226
  end-systolic volume in, 227
  end-systolic wall stress/end-systolic volume ratio
      in, 227
  etiology of, 215
  heart catheterization studies in, 217–219, *220*
  in pregnant patient, 228
  left ventricular enlargement and, 227
  mitral valve prolapse and, 219–226, *222, 223,*
      224t
  parasternal pulsations in, 28
  rheumatic, 215–219, *217–220*
    cardiac characteristics of, *220*
  surgery for, 250t
  systolic murmur of, 30
  V wave in, 217, *220*
  valve replacement in, 227
Mitral regurgitation, end-systolic volume in, 227
  grade of, 218–219
  in pregnancy, 388
  in rheumatic mitral insufficiency, 215
  noncardiac surgery and, 534
Mitral stenosis, 229–235, *231–234*
  balloon mitral valvuloplasty in, 235
  cardiac output in, 234
  chest x ray in, 231
  digitalis and, 487
  echocardiogram in, 230, *231,* 231–232, *232*
  electrocardiogram in, 230–231